PRACTICE OF PÆDIATRIC ORTHOPÆDICS

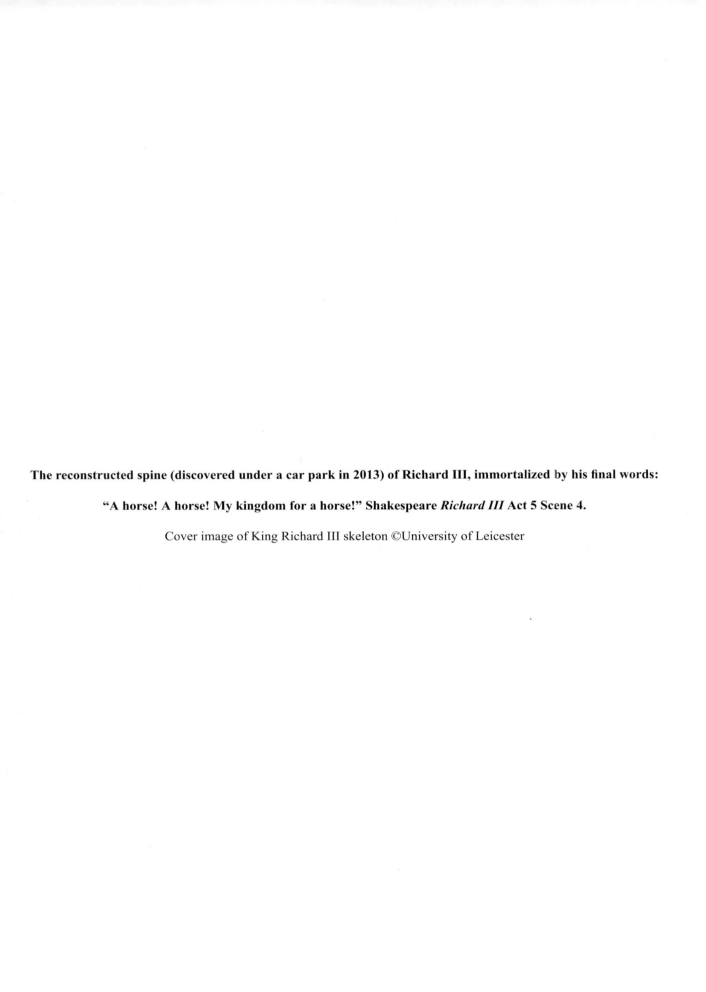

The reconstructed spine (discovered under a car park in 2013) of Richard III, immortalized by his final words:

"A horse! A horse! My kingdom for a horse!" Shakespeare *Richard III* Act 5 Scene 4.

PRACTICE OF PÆDIATRIC ORTHOPÆDICS

THIRD EDITION

Mohammad Diab, MD

Professor
Chief
Pædiatric Orthopædics
Department of Orthopædic
Surgery
University of California, San
Francisco
San Francisco, California

Lynn T. Staheli, MD

Emeritus Professor, Department
of Orthopædics
University of Washington School
of Medicine
Seattle, Washington
Emeritus Editor, Journal of
Pædiatric Orthopædics
Acquisitions Editor: Brian Brown

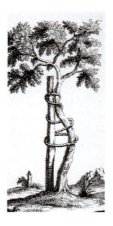

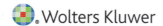

Philadelphia • Baltimore • New York • London
Buenos Aires • Hong Kong • Sydney • Tokyo

Product Development Editor: Dave Murphy
Marketing Manager: Daniel Dressler
Senior Production Project Manager: Alicia Jackson
Design Manager: Teresa Mallon
Manufacturing Coordinator: BethWelsh
Prepress Vendor: SPi Global

Third edition

9 8 7 6 5 4 3 2 1

Printed in China

Library of Congress Cataloging-in-Publication Data
Diab, Mohammad, author.
   Practice of pediatric orthopaedics / Mohammad Diab. — Third edition.
      p. ; cm.
   Preceded by Practice of pediatric orthopedics / Lynn T. Staheli. 2nd ed. c2006.
   Includes bibliographical references and index.
   ISBN 978-1-60831-505-5 (hardback)
   I. Staheli, Lynn T. Practice of pediatric orthopedics. Preceded by (work): II. Title.
   [DNLM: 1. Child. 2. Musculoskeletal Diseases—therapy. 3. Musculoskeletal System—physiopathology. 4. Orthopedic Procedures—methods. WS 270]
   RD732.3.C48
   616.70083--dc23
                                                                                    2015020388

LWW.com

RRS1509

DEDICATION

"To our families, for whose support we are profoundly grateful."

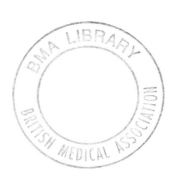

Preface

The mind is not a vessel to be filled, but a fire to be kindled.

Plutarch

This is a book founded upon principles and guided by practicality. It was conceived by Dr. Lynn Staheli with the goal of presenting the work of the pædiatric orthopædic surgeon in a simple but never simplistic, direct as opposed to sinuous, and most importantly readable form. We have adhered faithfully to Ockham's Principle of Parsimony, willing to sacrifice comprehensiveness at the altar of clarity for what is first and foremost a teaching tool and not a surgical manual or a research compendium. The language is directive because brevity begets clarity.

Figures are rudimentary in order that they may be accessible to the reader, who might imagine drawing them, and not to distract from the essential information. Peaks and valleys are emphasized: let the reader fill in what lies between. We acknowledge when consensus has not been reached and uncertainty leads to variability. Where there is consensus, facts are presented. Controversy is acknowledged in so far as it influences understanding and management. Where there is clinical equipoise, no recommendation is given to avoid prejudice.

We hope that the reader will find the book useful and that our patients and colleagues will accept it in gratitude for all they have taught us.

Mohammad Diab, MD
Lynn T. Staheli, MD

PREFACE TO SECOND EDITION

This second edition of the *Practice of Pædiatric Orthopædics* (PPO) was designed to build upon the strengths of the first edition. The basic objectives are the same: to provide a guide to learning the essentials of this specialty quickly and efficiently. As with the first edition, I designed, wrote, and illustrated PPO utilizing desktop publishing technology that made possible a full-color, extensively illustrated book that is affordable.

This edition was greatly enhanced by my coauthors. Each is an acknowledged expert in their fields and each contributed substantially to improving their chapters.

Royalties for this publication will be donated to Global-HELP Organization to make health care publications available without charge for use in developing countries.

The new features and instructions for readers are detailed below:

NEW FEATURES

- Coauthors contributed information and edited content.
- Text is updated and expanded.
- New illustrations have been added.
- Illustrations have been updated and improved.
- Topic discussion and procedures consolidated.
- Upper limb and hand chapters separated and expanded.
- Contents presented on end sheets to simplify access.
- Publication reformatted for production in Adobe InDesign.
- Anticipated readership expanded to include general orthopædists, residents, nurses, therapists, and students.

PREFACE TO FIRST EDITION

The *Practice of Pædiatric Orthopædics* (PPO) was designed to make learning children's orthopedics efficient and pleasant. This book provides core information, references, and e-mail access to experts. I designed, wrote, and illustrated PPO utilizing desktop publishing technology that made possible a full-color, extensively illustrated book that is affordable. To insure accuracy and clarity, each section was reviewed by at least two consultants. Consultants are acknowledged authorities.

The general features of PPO are listed below. Please read—*Instructions to Readers*. 2001

GENERAL FEATURES

- Designed for general orthopedists and residents.
- Provides core information on pædiatric orthopædics.
- 37 consultants edited content and may accept e-mail consultations.
- Current references are provided.
- Compact, efficient design, with over 400 pages and 2,500 illustrations.
- Practical, how to book details common problems.
- Management recommendations are whole child oriented.
- Mainstream approach to management—safe and proven.
- Management recommendations are current.
- Trauma and procedures are presented in greatest detail.
- Flowcharts are added to guide management.

Table of Contents

INTRODUCTION

Orthopædic derives from *L'Orthopedie* (1741) by Nicholas Andry de Bois-Regard (1658–1742). It is derived from Greek ορθος: "straight" and παις (root παιδ–): "child." Andry was a Professor of Theology before becoming a Professor of Physick in the Faculty of Medicine at the University of Paris. The remainder of the title explains his purpose: "*Or, the art of correcting and preventing deformities in children: by such means, as may easily be put in practice by parents themselves, and all such as are employed in educating children.*" The book emphasized simple remedies even a child's caretaker could administer, such as straightening by bracing [A]. Nowhere is surgery mentioned.

GROWTH

Growth distinguishes the child [B].

Joint

Joints may be fibrous, for example, syndesmosis and symphysis, or synovial, in which the skeletal elements are in contact but not in continuity: they are draped by hyaline cartilage of which the purpose is motion and not structure. Innervation of synovial joints is of two types.

- Myelinated group A fibers in the capsule detect joint position and motion.
- Unmyelinated group C fibers in blood vessels of the synovial membrane transmit pain. Joint injury or disease results in effusion, which stretches these fibers and hurts. The child accommodates by placing the joint in the position that maximizes volume and thereby reduces pressure, for example, flexion, lateral rotation, and abduction in an infected hip.

In children, a third type of articulation occurs, synchondrosis, during coalescence of ossification centers or bony segmentation: persistence may cause dysfunction, for example, tarsal coalition.

Joints develop first as a cleft in mesenchyme, which chondrifies and cavitates by the end of 3rd month. The process is regulated by the HOX family of genes. Joint development requires motion; hence, joint dysplasia in neuromuscular conditions characterized by akinesia or dyskinesia, such as arthrogryposis.

Bone

Timing of ossification influences care of the child. Imaging of hip dysplasia is facilitated by appearance of the proximal epiphysis of the femur, absent at birth. Patellar ossification after the 2nd year may delay diagnosis of its disorders. The multiple secondary ossification centers of the elbow appearing at different ages obfuscate the unfamiliar.

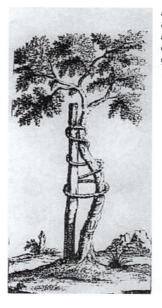

A Tree. The enduring symbol from an engraving on the frontispiece of *L'Orthopedie*. A straight stake is tied to a crooked sapling to partially correct it and guide its growth.

Stage	Definition	Comment
Early embryo	0–2 weeks	Before implantation
Embryo	2–8 weeks	Organogenesis Anomalies — problems of formation
Fetus	8 weeks to birth	Problems of growth
Infant	Birth to 2 years	Latin *in-* "not," *fari*: "to speak"
Child	2 years to puberty	Growth influences treatment Treatment influences growth
Adolescent	Transition to maturity	Childhood disease and treatment resemble adult

B Stages of growth.

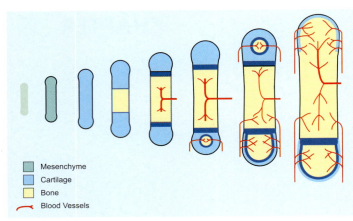

Mesenchyme	
Cartilage	
Bone	
Blood Vessels	

C   Endochondral ossification Mesenchyme turns into cartilage that turns into bone.

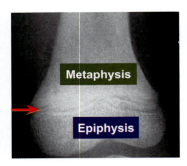

D   Physis Röntgenogramme shows physis (*red*) interposed between metaphysis and epiphysis.

Metaphysis

Epiphysis

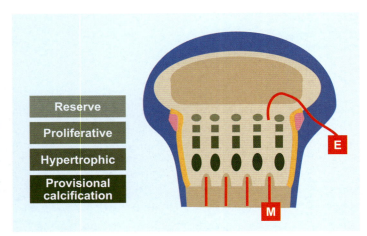

Reserve

Proliferative

Hypertrophic

Provisional calcification

E

M

E   Physis architecture E: epiphysial artery supplies the resting zone. Interruption of this may explain growth disturbance after fracture. M: metaphyseal blood supply loops back acutely at the impervious physis, leading to sludging that increases likelihood of bacterial concentration and infection. The physis is supported by the ring of La Croix (*orange*), which is continuous between the periosteum at the metaphysis and the epiphysis and which is constricted by the groove of Ranvier (*pink*).

Intramembranous ossification Mesenchymal stem cells give rise to osteoblasts that secrete osteoid that mineralizes directly without an intervening cartilage model. In achondroplasia, this process is spared.

- Relatively normal size of clavicles results in broad shoulders; of fibulæ, it results in ankle varus; of skull, it results in a large head.
- Disordered endochondral ossification is seen as a "champagne pelvis," resulting from constriction at the triradiate cartilage amidst flat bones produced by intramembranous ossification.
- Constriction of the midface with unfettered surrounding osseous growth disrupts breathing.
- Constriction of the foramen magnum compresses the brainstem.

Intramembranous ossification also is the mechanism responsible for periosteal appositional growth (bone width) and fracture healing.

Endochondral ossification During the 6th week of gestation, mesenchymal stem cells differentiate into chondrocytes to form a model of the future skeleton. During the next week, periosteum forms, and by the 8th week, vascularization is under way [C]. Vascularization ushers in ossification and the fetal period. Secondary ossification of the epiphyses begins after birth, with the exception of the distal femur, which is present at birth. In between the primary and secondary ossification centers is interposed the physis.

Physis

This also is known as growth plate and epiphysial plate [D]. On one side is the secondary ossification center that sits "upon" it (Greek επι-), called epiphysis. The epiphysis forms the articular end of a bone: when alone, it is referred to as "head," when paired, it is known as "condyle." On the other side of the physis is the metaphysis (Greek μετα-: "beside," next to). Where it separates an ossification center that grows "away" from the main bone under traction from an attached muscle, this is known as an apophysis (Greek απο-: "away").

The physis has four zones [E]. In the resting zone, SOX-9 is coexpressed with COL2A1, its regulatory target, resulting in a high concentration of type II collagen. Proliferation is under the influence of several regulatory factors such as insulin-like growth factors and fibroblastic growth factors. Due to stress concentration between cartilage and bone, physeal fracture occurs through the zone of provisional calcification, which may be distinguished from the hypertrophic zone. Injury to the reserve and proliferative zones, such as by a crushing mechanism (Salter-Harris V) or at an irregular physis with irregular shape (e.g., Poland hump at the distal tibia), will cause growth disturbance.

Longitudinal growth occurs by bone deposition at the metaphysis. After the 1st year of life, the physis becomes impervious to metaphyseal vessels, which are turned back in sharp loops: this results in slowing of flow that concentrates bacteria and increases the likelihood of infection. The physis is surrounded by a ring of perichondrium (La Croix): thinning of this at the commencement of puberty may destabilize the physis in slipped capital femoral epiphysis. The perichondrial ring is constricted by a groove (Ranvier), which supplies physeal chondrocytes and epiphysial osteoblasts.

Rate of Growth

The child is growing most rapidly at birth [F]. By 2 years, growth plateaus, increasing again at the pubertal growth acceleration. A child is half adult height by 2 years, and three-fourth by the end of the 1st decade. The head is disproportionately large at birth: accommodate for this when immobilizing a child with a suspect neck injury, so that the cervical spine may be neutralized and not flexed. The trunk grows earliest, while the lower limbs lag behind, achieving half of adult length by 4 years. The upper:lower body segment ration is 1 by maturity.

Growth may be influenced mechanically according to the Heuter-Volkmann law: compression of the physis retards growth, while distraction accelerates it. This may be harnessed for limb lengthening. Growth also is retarded physiologically by denervation, for example, hemiplegic cerebral palsy, and accelerated by hyperæmia, for example, congenital vascular malformation.

PRINCIPLES OF DISEASE

Definition and classification aid understanding.

Syndrome A group of anomalies that present in a predictable manner and due to a single cause.

Association A group of anomalies that occur together but are not related by a common cause.

Malformation This refers to an abnormality that arises during the period of organogenesis. There are five types [A].

Dysplasia This is used for abnormal structure due to an intrinsic tissue defect, for example, diastrophic dysplasia, or for abnormal shape due to an extrinsic cause, for example, of the hip

Disruption Abnormal event occurs late in gestation after normal growth and development established, for example, amniotic band syndrome.

Deformation Extrinsic factors produce disease superimposed upon a normal part, for example, idiopathic scoliosis.

Sequence A group of anomalies that arise downstream from a single initial event.

Field defect A group of anomalies that are geographically linked or restricted.

Diseases affecting the musculoskeletal system have been variably classified by the salient clinical feature, for example, Friedreich ataxia; geographically, for example, nail–patella syndrome; by röntgenographic appearance, for example, chondrodysplasia punctata; by pathogenesis, for example, osteogenesis imperfecta; by eponym, of which countless examples exist. We are evolving toward a fundamental and unifying approach based upon the molecular basis of disease [B].

Structural gene The product has a mechanical function. Osteogenesis imperfecta is caused by a mutation in type I collagen, which is the principal collagen supporting the extracellular matrix of bone.

Tumor regulatory gene The product stimulates cell growth and differentiation or prevents cell death, affecting the cell cycle. Neurofibromatosis type I is caused by a mutation in neurofibromin, which is a tumor suppressor inhibiting p21 ras oncoprotein.

Developmental gene The product is involved in cell development or patterning. Nail–patella syndrome is caused by a mutation in LMX1B, which plays a rôle in dorsoventral patterning of the vertebrate limb.

Nerve and muscle function gene Mutation in dystrophin causes muscular dystrophy.

Protein processing gene The product is an enzyme, of which mutation results in accumulation of precursors or abnormal products. The quintessential example is mucopolysaccharidoses, which are characterized by intracellular accumulation and urinary excretion of mucopolysaccharides due to deficiency in degradative lysosomal enzymes.

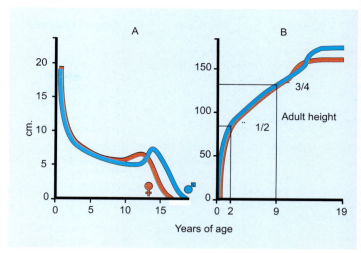

F Growth Rate A: absolute rate. B: variation of height with age.

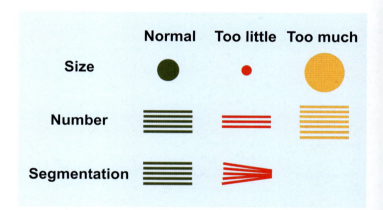

A Malformation types. This simplified method includes too little, too much, too few, too many, and failure of segmentation.

Gene	Examples	Clinical features
Structural	Marfan syndrome Osteogenesis imperfecta	Phenotypes change with time as structure wears out, superimposing degenerative changes on congenital abnormalities
Tumor regulatory	Multiple exostosis Neurofibromatosis	Overgrowth of cells and tissue type in which gene is expressed. Malignant potential
Developmental	Achondroplasia Cleidocranial dysplasia Nail–patella syndrome	Abnormal embryonic development results in malformation present at birth
Nerve or muscle	Charcot-Marie Tooth Duchenne syndrome Rett Spinal muscular atrophy Friedreich ataxia	Musculoskeletal system normal at birth, develops abnormalities secondary to neuromuscular imbalance Muscle and central nervous disorders more severe for example, shortened life-span, than peripheral nervous disorder
Protein processing	Gaucher syndrome Mucopolysaccharidosis Osteopetrosis	Enzyme replacement may alter natural history
Chromosomal defect	Down syndrome Turner syndrome	Multiple genes affected, resulting in multiple abnormalities in multiple systems

B Classification by type of gene mutation (Alman) An attempt to bring order to a disparate group of conditions.

Distinguishing features of pædiatric orthopædic surgery

The original

Horizontal

Growth

More nonoperative care

More casts

More diseases

More multidisciplinary

Less long-term follow-up

Better surgical outcomes in the uninvolved child

Parents

A Distinctive features of pædiatric orthopædic surgery.

Chromosomal defect This affects multiple genes on a whole, such as trisomy 21, or part of a chromosome.

Not all mutations can be classified. Some products can be included in more than one category. How a given mutation exerts its effect is understood in some and unclear in others.

CARE OF THE CHILD

Pædiatric orthopædic surgery is a horizontal discipline [A]. Its domain is the child as a whole, traveling across the broad landscape of the body and navigating disparate diseases within a defined age echelon. This contrasts with the direction of our discipline as a whole, where specialization has turned it vertical, where the surgeon is focused on a single system or part "from cradle to grave." Delicate is the balance between caring for the child as a whole, interconnected person and developing sufficient skill and experience to care most optimally for the affected part.

The approach to a child, and to the family, is unique in many ways.

- Sit down, at eye level with a small human being (child), and take some time to ease anxiety brought on to a child by an authority figure.
- Minimize exposure. Uncover only the part necessary to examine, and limit traffic, to reduce the sense of vulnerability in the child.
- Retain the parents, whose presence will reassure the child and whose input is essential when a child cannot or will not speak.
- Close the door so that the child feels safe.
- Focus on the child, even when the parent is giving the history. Talk to the child first and last.
- Ask children to come in sports clothes or a bathing suit. A gown is a foreign object.
- Listen to the child. While parents advocate and consent for their children, their concerns and perceptions may differ from their children's. Additionally, children often bring a simple clarity to complex decision making that eludes their parents.
- Take every and all opportunities to examine the child. Watch the child walk into the office (gait, affect, pain, stature, proportion). Assess how well a child who complains of pain moves about in the room, or surmounts the examining table. How does the child who is supine use or rest the limbs? Ask the child to walk on the heels and toes, perform a deep knee bend, and walk "like a duck," thereby testing strength against body weight and doing so without touching the child.
- Start by checking the normal side, or perform a screening examination, so that the child is assured you are not there to inflict more pain.
- Consider as an examining table using a parent's lap, which will comfort and calm a baby.
- Choose your words carefully. The language of a 12-year-old is simple and direct, not technical and not convoluted.
- Involve the child in decision making; sequestration engenders suspicion.
- Avoid unnecessary or excessive treatment, which will invade childhood and may expose the child to risk.
- Weigh hope and a desire for parental agency against "medicalization" (devices, therapies, consultants, new treatments) of a handicapped child.
- Enlist the parents. They are an ally who will care for the child at home, who will comply with instructions, and who will ensure scheduled follow-up. Their vigilance is normal and in the interest of the child.
- Pay attention to a parent's intuition. They know the child better than you do.
- Acknowledge and accept that often the most benign presentation will be the most time consuming. It takes time and patience to educate and convince parents of normal variants such as flexible flat foot and in-toeing, which is the most reason for consultation of a pædiatric orthopædic surgeon.
- Measure childhood in dog years. Every year in a child's life represents a big change, physiologically, emotionally, socially. How much does

treatment of a dislocated hip change between 6 months of age (soft tissue) and 18 months of age (bone)? A child's rapid evolution presents many children within the same childhood. How different is the same child at 10 years of age and 2 years later during puberty?

- Observation is a form of active management. It is not neglect, benign or otherwise. It admits that sometimes the entire picture may not be revealed at an initial encounter. It allows time for a family to come to grips with a diagnosis and elective treatment options when these are serious and to become comfortable with their child's surgeon. It gives natural history, which is very dynamic in a growing child, some more time to declare itself. Insisting on finding out an answer by evaluating further may not be benign, for example, an MRI may require an anæsthetic. Remember the English poet and statesman John Milton: "They also serve who only stand and wait" (*On His Blindness*, 1655).

UPPER LIMB

The upper limb positions the hand for bimanual activity within the field of vision. For many anomalies of the upper limb, normal function and appearance are unattainable. Management focuses on the preservation or enhancement of motion to meet activities of daily living, at a minimum access to the face and perineum. Goals for the dominant hand include pinch and fine motor function. Goals for the nondominant hand include grasp and release to stabilize objects for the dominant hand. The critical nature of sensibility and mobility in the hand influences surgical incisions and dissection.

DEVELOPMENT

Morphologic description of the embryo provides a gross understanding of development [A]. Lodged within this is an orderly, sequential expression of genes known as a developmental cascade, which is under the control of HOXD genes expressed in successive overlapping fields. The apical ectodermal ridge releases fibroblast growth factors that induce the zone of polarizing activity, located in the posterior mesenchyme of the bud, to secrete sonic hedgehog to establish anteroposterior (radioulnar) polarity in the developing limb. Dorsal ectodermal expression of the WNT7A, which induces mesodermal LMX1B, and suppression of WNT7A in the ventral ectoderm by EN1 determine the dorsoventral axis of the limb.

Anomalies may be classified according to abnormality of development [B]. Upper limb anomalies are features of several syndromes [C].

Week	Development
3	The upper limb bud originates as a core of mesenchyme draped by ectoderm from Wolff crest opposite the 5 lowest cervical vertebrae on the ventrolateral surface of the embryo. The leading edge is thickened into apical ectodermal ridge, which directs longitudinal limb growth. The limb bud at this stage is perfused by the marginal sinus.
4	The hand plate is visible.
5	Mesenchymal cells condense into blastemas, which form the cartilage models of the bones of the limb. Nerves enter from the spinal cord.
6	The ulnar artery branches from the central brachial artery to reach the hand.
7	The upper limb rotates 90 degrees around a longitudinal axis, "before" which are the thumb and radius (Latin pre-), to turn the apex of the elbow posterior and determine its dermatomal pattern. Endochondral ossification and joint cavitation begin. The mesenchyme differentiates into dorsal and ventral muscles, which represent the extensors and flexors.
8	The apical ectodermal ridge fragments as the digits begin to separate by apoptosis.

A Embryonic development of the upper limb Most anomalies of the upper limb form during the embryonic period.

Type	Example
Failure of formation	Limb deficiency
Failure of differentiation	Syndactyly, camptodactyly, trigger thumb, clinodactyly, delta phalanx
Duplication	Polydactyly
Overgrowth	Macrodactyly
Undergrowth	Thumb hypoplasia, Poland
Constriction	Amniotic band syndrome
Generalized skeletal abnormalities	Syndromes

B Classification of anomalies This may be used as an organizing framework. One-third of hand anomalies are bilateral. One-fourth of children with hand anomalies have a nonhand anomaly, most often in the lower limb. One-sixth of children have an affected relative.

Deficiency

Cornelia de Lange
Holt-Oram
Poland
Split hand/split foot
Thrombocytopenia-absent radius
VACTERL

Failure of Differentiation

Apert
Arthrogryposis
Oculodentodigital
Pfeiffer

Duplication

Orofacial digital syndrome
Ellis-van Creveld
Rubinstein-Taybi

Undergrowth

Brachydactyly A-E
Hand–Foot–Genital
Oto-palato-digital

C Syndromes characterized by upper limb anomalies *Cf.* Syndromes chapter.

EVALUATION

Observation

Hand function progresses in an orderly fashion [D]. The function of each upper limb is more independent than that of the lower limbs; thus, a short arm causes less functional difficulty than a short leg. Look for deformity, asymmetry, anomaly. What is the resting position? Watch how the child uses the upper limb—toys are helpful. Does the child have bimanual function? Does the child guard? Does the child express hand dominance? Determine functional limitations, such as bringing the hand to the mouth. What is the muscular tone? Are there contractures or spasticity? Ask about medical comorbidities that may be features of a generalized condition.

Physical Examination

A detailed motor and sensory assessment may not be possible in a young child. Ask the parents. Perform gross tests, such as distinguishing textures. Check passive and active motion. Look for signs of laxity, including elbow and metacarpophalangeal hyperextension, and thumb on volar forearm. Examine the entire child for other anomalies that may suggest a syndrome. Bring the child back for a second evaluation.

DEFICIENCY

Distinguish congenital from acquired deficiency [E]. Failure of formation may be transverse or longitudinal [F]. Symbrachydactyly is a transverse deficiency. Examples of longitudinal deficiency is radial clubhand, of central is split hand, and of postaxial is ulnar clubhand, and of intercalary is phocomelia.

Symbrachydactyly

Cause may be disruption of vascular ingrowth during limb development. Digits are "short" (Greek βραχυς) and webbed "together" (Greek συν-). Mildest is short, webbed but well-formed fingers. Cleft hand is characterized by absence of central digits [G]. Monodactyly refers to loss of fingers, marked by remnants or "nubbins," with preservation of the thumb. Digital remnants lack a nail remnant, distinguishing this from constriction deficit. Peromelia (Greek πηρος: "disabled, incapacitated") is most severe, with absence of all digits.

Treatment depends upon what remains. Metacarpal spaces may be created for basic pinch. A hand plate may be fitted to a mobile wrist. Free vascularized toe transfer has variable success.

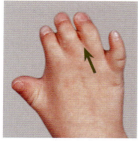
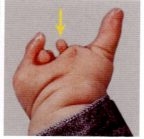
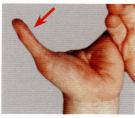

G Types of symbrachydactyly Digits may be short, webbed, and functional (*green*). Central deficiency, with digital remnants, characterizes cleft hand (*yellow*). The thumb is normal in monodactyly (*red*).

Preaxial Deficiency

There are six types.

- N. Hypoplasia or absence of thumb. Wrist and radius are normal.
- 0. Hypoplasia or absence of thumb. Carpal anomaly. Normal distal radius. Proximal radius may be normal, dislocated, or synostosed with the ulna.
- 1. As 0, except distal radius shortening >2 mm.
- 2. Hypoplasia or absence of thumb. Carpal anomaly. Distal and proximal radial hypoplasia.
- 3. As 2, except absence of distal epiphysis of radius.
- 4. Hypoplasia or absence of thumb. Carpal anomaly. Absent radius [H].

The radial nerve and artery follow bone deficiency. Tethering by the radial anlage may dislocate the ulna. Half of cases are bilateral, most of which are associated with a syndrome, for example, Holt-Oram, thrombocytopenia-absent radius, and VACTERL.

Soft tissue stretching may be achieved by serial splinting or casting. Pollicization of the index substitutes for nonfunctional thumb. Centralization or radialization of the ulna supports the hand when there is significant radial hypoplasia. This is contraindicated in elbow stiffness, which may prevent accessing the mouth by a straightened hand and wrist, which previously were more functional in the deviated and shortened position.

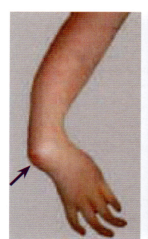
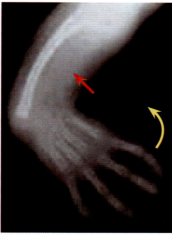

Age		Function
1	M	Clenches hand
2	O	Opens hand
3	N	Holds objects
6	T	Independent sitting Bimanual function
9	H	Early finger pinch
12	S	Prehension
1.5	Y	Piles blocks
2	E	Fine motor function, e.g., buttons clothing
3	A	Hand dominance
4	R	Throw a ball
5	S	Catch a ball

D Developmental milestones for the upper limb.

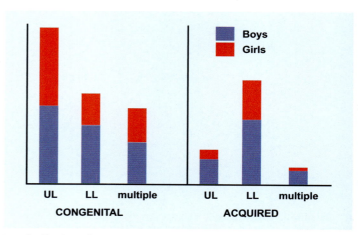

E Distribution of pædiatric amputees Upper limb–acquired deficiency is rarer than congenital. UL: upper limb; LL: lower limb.

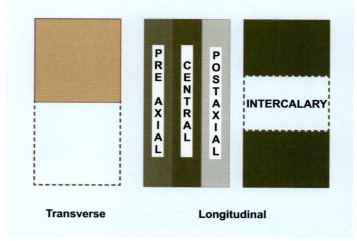

F Classification of failure of formation.

H Radial dysplasia Absence of radius (*red*) produces a radial clubhand (*yellow*) and a prominent end of ulna (*blue*).

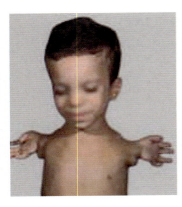

I Phocomelia Severe longitudinal humeral and ulnar deficiency makes the upper limbs resemble the flippers of a seal.

Postaxial Deficiency

Ulnar deficiency differs from radial deficiency in being 1/10 as common, in showing autosomal dominant inheritance, in rarely being associated with a syndrome, and in being typically unilateral. In addition, the consequences to the hand are milder, whereas the elbow is more severely affected. There are four types.

- I. Hypoplasia of the ulna, with preservation of proximal distal physes and minimal deformity.
- II. Absent distal ulna, with radial bowing. This is most common.
- III. Complete absence of ulna.
- IV. Absent ulna with humeroradial synostosis.

Thumb and carpal anomalies occur variably. Excise the ulnar anlage and perform a corrective radial osteotomy for ulnad deviation of the wrist. Fuse the proximal ulna to radius to create a single bone forearm: this stabilizes the head of the radius, thereby improving elbow function, and reduces bowing of the forearm.

Phocomelia

The appellation describes resemblance of the severely shortened limb to that of a "seal" (Greek φωκη). An epidemic in Europe developed after thalidomide became an over-the-counter drug in Germany (1957) for nausea in pregnancy. It is rare today and may be due to true intercalary deficiency or severe axial deficiency [I].

FAILURE OF DIFFERENTIATION

Syndactyly

The upper limb develops as a zeugopod (arm), then stylopod (forearm), and then autopod (hand). This is associated with sequential expression of HOXD9 and HOXD10 (zeugopod) followed by HOXD11 and HOXD12 (stylopod), which in turn give way to HOXD13 (autopod). Mutation in HOXD13 on 2q31.1 results in failure of programmed interdigital apoptosis and syndactyly.

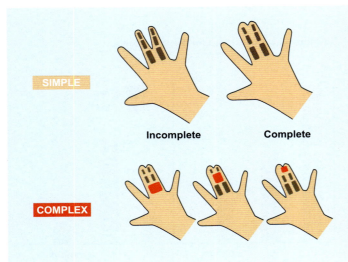

SIMPLE

Incomplete   Complete

COMPLEX

A Classification of syndactyly This is an anatomic classification. Simple involves only skin. This fusion may be incomplete, leaving variable parts of the digits free, or complete. Complex involves bone, which may be fused at different levels.

Syndactyly has been classified according to affected tissue and extent of joining [A]. When osseous abnormalities are more than side-to-side fusion, such as accessory bones, it is referred to as "complicated." Syndactyly is most common in the third web, by contrast with the second web in the foot. It may be associated with syndromes such as Apert.

There are several principles of surgical separation [B].

- Full-thickness, local, dorsal, or volar skin flaps to avoid contracture and "web creep."
- Zigzag incisions to avoid longitudinal contracture.
- Operate on only one side of a digit, to avoid vascular insufficiency.
- Correct underlying osseous deformity.
- Relaxed closure to avoid vascular constriction.

Symphalangism

This refers to failure of cavitation of the interphalangeal joints, usually of the ulnar digits. Three types have been distinguished:

- Affected digits is normal in length.
- Brachysymphalangism, in which the digit is "short" (Greek βραχυς).
- Symphalangism associated with syndromes.

Digits are gracile and lack cutaneous creases. There is loss of motion and narrowing of the joint on röntgenogramme, to which the cartilaginous bridge is invisible. Release, for example, by capsulectomy, has limited success. Arthrodesis is unnecessary. Children adapt to the stiffness.

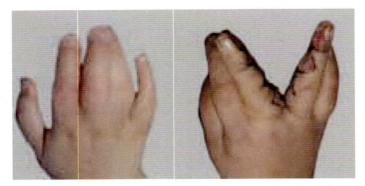

B Separation of syndactyly The completely joined middle and ring fingers were separated by zigzag incisions.

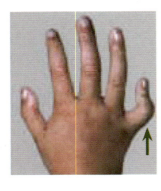

C Camptodactyly Flexion of the proximal interphalangeal joint of the smallest finger (*green*) is a sagittal plane deformity (Greek καμπτος: "bent, crooked").

Camptodactyly

This refers to contracture of the finger in the sagittal plane [C]. Smallest finger and proximal interphalangeal joint are most affected. In a subset of patients, the condition is genetic, linked to 3q11.2-q13.12. This also is known as streblomicrodactyly (Greek στρεβλος: "bent, crooked"). There are three types of camptodactyly.

- I. Congenital
- II. Progressive, presenting in the second decade
- III. Affecting multiple digits and associated with other conditions, in particular arthrogryposis

Intrinsic imbalance due to muscle anomaly, for example, errant lumbrical insertion or hypoplastic tight flexor digitorum superficialis, produces secondary soft tissue contracture and osseous deformity, such as condylar blunting.

Initial management is stretching and splinting. If this is unsuccessful, release anomalous muscle insertion or transfer flexor digitorum superficialis to the extensor retinaculum when the deformity is flexible. For rigid deformity, add wide capsular release and consider osteotomy.

Trigger Thumb

The flexor pollicis longus develops a nodular swelling (Notta) that restricts and ultimately obstructs excursion at the entrance of the tendon sheath. This is not congenital. Cause is unknown. One-fourth are bilateral.

The thumb may click and hurt with forcible interphalangeal extension, as the nodule squeezes abruptly past the first anular pulley, or it may be held in fixed flexion. The mobile nodule is palpable as the interphalangeal joint is manipulated. To compensate for lack of interphalangeal extension, the metacarpophalangeal joint may become hypermobile, extending abnormally to better position the pulp of the thumb during opening of the hand.

Observe trigger thumb during the 1st year of life, as most resolve spontaneously. Resolution is unlikely after the 2nd year, which is an indication for operative section of the first anular pulley. Demonstrate full interphalangeal extension to confirm acceptable release. The surgical site may be traversed by the radial digital nerve [D], which may be endangered by a percutaneous method. By 3 years of age, development of diffuse contracture at a flexed interphalangeal may limit surgical result. For patients with hyperextension of the metacarpophalangeal > 60 degrees, some advocate concomitant advancement of the volar plate.

Clinodactyly

In contrast with camptodactyly, the finger in clinodactyly (Greek κλινη: "that upon which one *reclines*, a couch," whence "*clinic*") is deformed in the coronal plane [E]. Most affected is the smallest finger. This deformity tends to be bilateral and associated with syndromes, for example, 80% of children with trisomy 21. It is classified.

- Simple, due to osseous deformity, or complex, which has associated soft tissue contracture.
- Uncomplicated, when the deformity is < 45 degrees, or complicated when > 45 degrees associated with rotation.

Because of the plane of deformity, this leads to dysfunction when severe. For significant digital overlap, perform an opening wedge osteotomy rather than closing, which may relax the extensor to produce a mallet finger.

Delta Phalanx

The name describes the shape of a triangular bone, like the Greek letter delta (Δ), which on its short side is flanked by a C-shaped bracket epiphysis (*cf.* Foot chapter). Most affected are the middle phalanx of the longest finger [F] and the thumb, where it may form a triphalangeal thumb. The bone produces a coronal plane deformity.

Excise an accessory delta phalanx in triphalangeal thumb early, before secondary deformity sets in. Physeolysis with fat interposition is an effective detethering in the child who has enough growth remaining to overcome a deformity that is not severe. For severe deformity in the older child, opening osteotomy with bone graft is indicated.

Kirner Deformity

Progressive volad and radiad curving of the distal phalanx of the smallest finger [G]. Cause of this growth disturbance is unknown. It tends to be bilateral and affects girls more than boys toward the end of the first decade. It is characteristic in appearance, which is the principal problem it poses because it causes no disability. Phalangeal osteotomy at the end of growth is indicated rarely.

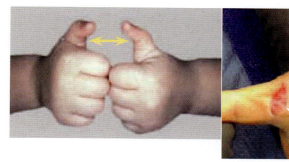

D Trigger thumb Both thumbs are stuck in interphalangeal flexion (*yellow*). A transverse incision in the metacarpophalangeal flexion crease becomes invisible after healing. The radial digital nerve may traverse the surgical site (*white*).

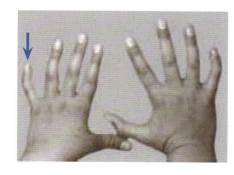

E Clinodactyly Coronal plane deformation of the smallest fingers (*blue*) is distinguished from camptodactyly, which occurs in the sagittal plane.

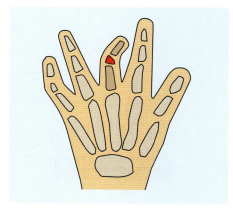

F Delta phalanx The triangular middle phalanx of the longest finger (*red*) is an osseous cause for digital deformity.

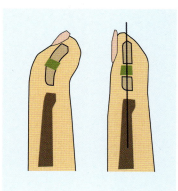

G Kirner deformity Correction by osteotomy.

	Preaxial	Central	Postaxial
Prevalence	Common	Rare	Common
Inheritance	Variable	Variable	Autosomal dominant
Ethnicity	Whites		Blacks 10 × Whites
Associated condition	Often	Syndactyly Foot anomaly	Rare
Surgical repair	Difficult	Complex	Simple

A Polydactyly Distinguishing features.

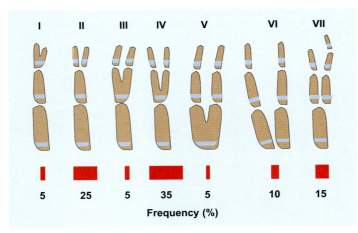

B Thumb polydactyly Classification according to osseous duplication. Type VII represents a triphalangeal thumb with or without duplication.

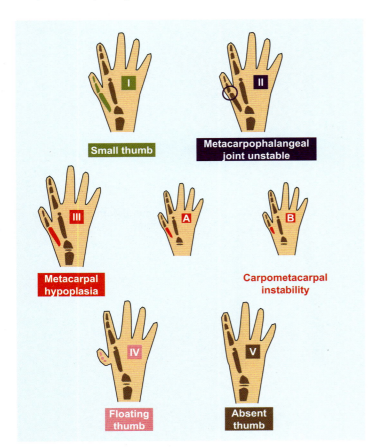

C Classification of thumb hypo-/aplasia.

DUPLICATION

Polydactyly

This is the most common anomaly of the upper limb. It may be preaxial, central, or postaxial [A]. It may be subtyped as A: full digital development, and B: rudimentary or pedunculated digit. Central lesions often are polysyndactylies.

Thumb polydactyly has been classified according to osseous involvement [B]. While most are sporadic, type VII may be syndromic. A subset of triphalangeal thumb is caused by an autosomal dominant heterozygous mutation in a sonic hedgehog regulatory element (ZRS) that resides in intron 5 of the LMBR1 gene on 7q36.3.

For postaxial polydactyly, type B may be suture ligated or excised. Counsel family that the former, which is performed simply in the neonatal nursery, may be followed by a residual bump that does not interfere with function. For type A, reconstruct collateral ligament and hypothenar muscle attachments as indicated.

Principles of thumb polydactyly reconstruction include the following:

- Timing is influenced by the development of pinch, toward the end of the 1st year.
- Reconstruct the collateral ligament connected to the excised thumb.
- Transfer thenar muscles, for example, in type IV, opponens and abductor insert on radial digit while adductor inserts on ulnar digit.
- Perform chondroplasty of a widened metacarpal of metatarsal.
- Recognize pollex abductus, and release the abnormal connexion between flexor pollicis longus and extensor pollicis longus. This is one cause of postoperative angulation, which is the most common complication of excision of thumb polydactyly.

OVERGROWTH

Macrodactyly

Overgrowth may be static, which remains proportionate as the child grows, or progressive, which is more common and characterized by growth acceleration. The longest finger is most affected. Half of cases involve more than one finger. There are four types.

- Associated with nerve territory–oriented lipofibromatosis. This is most common. Overgrowth is driven by a digital (single finger affected) or peripheral (more than one finger affected) nerve, which is enlarged, is tortuous, and has fibrofatty infiltration.
- Associated with neurofibromatosis. Overgrowth is neurotrophic.
- Associated with hyperostosis. There is no neural abnormality. The driver is primary bone overgrowth.
- Associated with hemihypertrophy.

Surgical management may be divided into three categories.

- Growth modulation. Timing of physeodesis is difficult. This addresses only length.
- Reduction. This may be of bone, by segmental excision, or of soft tissue, which risks neurovascular structures and stiffness.
- Amputation. This may be partial or of the ray. It may be performed in conjunction with digit or toe transfer.

Counsel the patient and family that multiple procedures may be necessary and that normal function is unrealistic.

UNDERGROWTH

Thumb Hypo-/a-plasia

This also may be considered within the spectrum of preaxial deficiency. It is classified according to severity [C].
- I. The thumb is small but otherwise muscles and joints are normal.
- II. Metacarpophalangeal joint is unstable. Thumb is adducted. Thenar muscles are underdeveloped.
- III. This is subtyped according to degree of metacarpophalangeal hypoplasia and presence of carpometacarpal instability (B and C).

Thenar muscles are absent. There is dysplasia of trapezium and scaphoid, as well as styloid process of radius.

- IV. The thumb, consisting of rudimentary phalanges, floats at the side of the hand, connected by its neurovascular pedicle. Thenar muscles are absent. There is dysplasia of trapezium and scaphoid, as well as styloid process of radius.
- V. Thumb is absent. This is most common.

Type I needs no treatment. Central to surgical decision making is the metacarpophalangeal joint. Reconstruction is possible when the joint is stable. An unstable joint is an indication for pollicization.

Poland Syndrome

This autosomal dominant disorder is characterized by unilateral chest hypoplasia, including unilateral hypoplasia or absence of pectoralis major muscle, most commonly the sternocostal head [D], as well as digital anomalies, including brachydactyly, oligodactyly, and syndactyly.

Other features include costal and vertebral anomalies, as well as absence of hypoplasia of shoulder muscles, including latissimus dorsi, serratus anterior muscle, and rotator cuff. It occurs on the right side in three-fourths of cases. Boys are affected thrice as often as girls. Most are sporadic, with a small subset demonstrating autosomal dominant inheritance.

The disorder may be regarded as part of the subclavian artery dysplasia complex, as evidenced by reports of dextrocardia in left-side cases (*cf.* Pseudarthrosis of the Clavicle).

A lower limb counterpart includes gluteal hypoplasia with brachysyndactyly of the toes.

Orthopædic management resides in the hand. Plastic reconstruction of the chest may be necessary, in particular for breast asymmetry and nipple absence.

CONSTRICTION

Amniotic Band Syndrome

This is sporadic and may be associated with other anomalies, for example, clubfoot. Amniotic bands encircle the member perpendicular to the longitudinal axis, presenting as an anular soft tissue constriction [E]. Anatomy is normal proximal. More than 80% occur distal to the wrist. There are four types.

- I. Simple constriction ring without distal anomaly. Consider release of constriction ring.
- II. Distal swelling and hypoplasia. Excise constriction ring with local flaps.
- III. Distal syndactyly. Separate syndactyly.
- IV. Amputation. Reconstruction should be individualized, including bone lengthening, web deepening, and free vascularized toe transfer.

GENERALIZED SYNDROMES

Arthrogryposis

Hypokinesia *in utero* results in muscle hypoplasia, joint stiffness, and deformity (*cf.* Syndromes chapter).

Evaluation The upper limb assumes a classic posture [A]. In the distal form of the disorder, the hand is principally affected, with relative sparing of the elbow and shoulder. There is minimal muscle action. Intelligence and sensation are normal. These factors significantly improve hand adaptation and surgical outcomes.

Management Physical therapy for stretching and occupational therapy for adaptive training. Consider realignment, by soft tissue release or osteotomy, to improve functional position and not motion, of which any gain may be lost in the absence of muscle action. Lengthen biceps or triceps, but this will add to weakness. Consider supracondylar humeral osteotomy. If there is sufficient passive elbow motion, unilateral pectoralis major transfer may facilitate one hand reaching the mouth, while the other remains in extension to reach the perineum for independent care and to use an assistive ambulatory device.

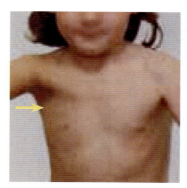

D Poland syndrome The sternocostal head of right pectoralis major is absent.

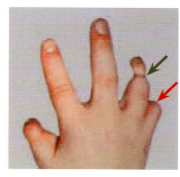

E Amniotic band syndrome There is distal hypoplasia (*green*) and amputation (*red*).

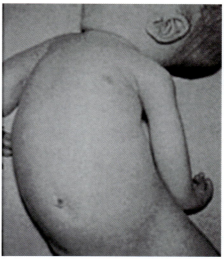

A Arthrogryposis The upper limb is held in a typical posture, including shoulder adduction and internal rotation, elbow extension, wrist flexion, and digital mild camptodactyly.

Level	Classification	Ability
0	No use	Not used
1	Passive help—poor	Uses limb to stabilize weight
2	Passive help—fair	Holds onto object placed in hand
3	Passive—good	Hold and stabilize object for use by other hand
4	Active help—poor	Weak grip
5	Active help—fair	Good grip
6	Active help—good	Manipulates object
7	Spontaneous use—limited	Performs bimanual function
8	Spontaneous use—complete	Use of hand independent of other hand

A House classification This is a functional assessment of hand use in cerebral palsy.

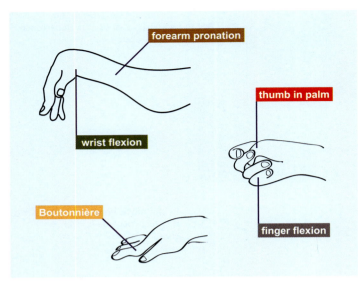

B   Common hand deformities in cerebral palsy Deformities may be combined and vary in severity.

Level	Spasticity	Ability
1	Minimal	Full active extension of the fingers with wrist 0- to 20 degree flexion
2	Moderate	Full active extension of the fingers only with wrist at >20 degree flexion
2A		Active wrist extension with fingers flexed
2B		No wrist extension due to extensor paralysis
3	Severe	No finger extension

C   Zancolli classification of spasticity This assesses active finger and wrist extension.

Cerebral Palsy

About half of children with cerebral palsy have a problem with hand function. Impairment correlates with disease severity; for example, most affected are those with tetraplegia. Disability results from limited voluntary control, including spasticity, sensory, and cognitive impairment, contractures, and deformity, to which contribute soft tissue and bone. The classic classification systems was developed by House and colleagues [A].

Evaluation   Ask the family and therapists, who know the patient more broadly and for longer. Determine cognitive status, which is essential to outcome, in particular as pertains to postoperative rehabilitation. The classic posture of the upper limb is shoulder internal rotation, elbow flexion, forearm pronation, wrist flexion, finger flexion or boutonnière deformity, and thumb-in-palm [B]. Since examination may be difficult, focus on stereognosis, that is, tactile discrimination of size, shape, and texture, which is the most common sensory deficit. Level of function may be assessed by several instruments [C].

Management   Passive range of motion, splinting (including night and day), and casting prevent and may correct contracture. Pharmacologic treatment may be central, for example, baclofen administered intrathecally or *per orem*, or peripheral, including botulinum toxin and phenol injection into muscle. The two approaches may be used synergistically, for example, botulinum toxin potentiates casting and splinting.

Operative treatment may be divided into muscle reconstruction or ablation. Reconstruction, including muscle lengthening and transfer, restores function to a cognitively spared child with flexible deformity. Ablation includes neurotomy, to permanently disable a spastic muscle without significant underlying contracture in a child with low functional demand, or fusion, which is an end treatment when soft tissue release and muscle balancing cannot control severe, rigid deformity.

For reconstruction, the child must be cooperative and compliant with evaluation and postoperative rehabilitation. As a result, intervention is delayed until after 5 years of age, when the child is old enough to comprehend and be motivated.

Elbow   Chronic flexion contracture may require plastic reconstruction for antecubital closure. Z-lengthen biceps brachii, fractionally lengthen brachialis, and release brachioradialis. Protect radial nerve and lateral antebrachial cutaneous nerve, although the latter may be cut if it resists elbow extension.

Forearm   No operative treatment is indicated for supination beyond neutral. For active supination, perform a pronator quadratus and flexor–pronator aponeurotic release. For no active supination but an active pronator teres, transfer the muscle through the interosseous membrane to the dorsolateral radius.

Wrist and fingers   Wrist flexion may be caused by weak wrist extensors, spastic wrist flexors, or spastic digital flexors. For active wrist extension but spastic wrist flexors, lengthen flexor carpi ulnaris, and radialis, and release palmaris longus. Transfer a deforming extensor carpi ulnaris to extensor carpi radialis brevis to enhance wrist extension. For finger flexor spasticity, fractionally lengthen these if the fingers may be extended with <45 degrees of wrist extension, or release the flexor pronator origin if wrist flexion > 45 degrees is necessary for digital extension. Rigid deformity is addressed by carpal fusion.

For flexible boutonnière deformity without dynamic metacarpophalangeal flexion deformity, perform a central slip tenotomy.

Thumb   Sequential release includes thenar muscles, first dorsal interosseous, flexor pollicis longus lengthening, and soft tissue stabilization or fusion of the metacarpophalangeal joint. Weak thumb abduction may be addressed by extensor pollicis longus or brachioradialis transfer.

WRIST

Kienböck Disease

Osteochondritis of the lunate, also known as lunatomalacia (Greek μαλακος: "soft"), is rare in children. Microtrauma conspires with force concentration at the distal corner of radius brought about by a negative ulnar variance to injure the bone. The condition may be associated with dermatomyositis and athetoid cerebral palsy, which is characterized by increased motion under high tone.

Evaluation Presentation includes insidious onset pain and tenderness over lunate, with wrist swelling and stiffness.

IMAGING Röntgenogrammes show sclerosis, collapse, and irregularity of contour of lunate and allow measurement of ulnar variance [A].

Management Most children may be treated symptomatically, with resolution without sequela over months to a few years. Radial shortening osteotomy to address negative ulnar variance and reduce stress on the lunate is indicated for persistent or unacceptable pain, or for carpal deformity.

Madelung Deformity

Growth disturbance of the volar–ulnar part of the distal radial physis leads to volar translation of the hand and wrist associated with dorsal prominence of the distal ulna. Prepubescent girls are primarily affected. More than half of cases are bilateral and of asymmetric severity. Madelung deformity may be primary or secondary; for example, it is a feature of Léri-Weill dyschondrosteosis and Turner syndrome (*cf.* Syndromes chapter).

Evaluation Ask about family history, as one-third of cases show an autosomal dominant pattern of inheritance, with variable expression and penetrance. Wrist pain, stiffness, and deformity are accompanied by the characteristic hand displacement.

IMAGING Obtain bilateral röntgenogrammes on the same image to allow comparison. Posteroanterior projection shows increased radial inclination (normal 20 to 25 degrees) and ulnar variance [B]. Lateral projection shows increased volar tilt of distal radius (normal 10 to 15 degrees) and relative subluxation of the distal ulna dorsal to the proximal carpal row. CT may provide a clearer understanding of the three-dimensional nature of the deformity.

Management Release of Vickers ligament, *via* a volar approach, reduces tension that is implicated in the genesis of pain. In addition, early release combined with bridge resection may remove a retardant force to growth, thereby altering the natural history of progressive deformation by allowing the volar–ulnar physis to grow again.

Osteotomy of the distal radius corrects orientation of the articular surface [C], when insufficient growth remains for release and physeolysis. Distraction osteogenesis with an external fixator may facilitate multiplanar correction and enables restoration of radial length.

For severe deformity that prevents restoration of a congruent wrist, radioscaphocapitate arthrodesis is indicated. Deformity of the distal radioulnar joint may be addressed by distal radioulnar fusion (Lauenstein): avoid resection of the distal ulna (Darach), which may be followed by gradual ulnar migration of the wrist.

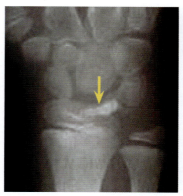

A Kienböck disease. This 9 year old gymnast with dermatomyositis developed wrist pain. There is sclerosis, collapse and irregular contour of lunate is obvious (*yellow*).

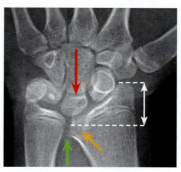

B Madelung deformity There is lucency and premature fusion (*orange*) at the locus of growth disturbance, triangular distortion of the distal epiphysis, and pyramidilization (*red*) of the wrist as it sink into the defect, with apex at the lunate. Distal radial height is increased (*white*) by retardation of ulnar growth (normal 12 to 15 mm). Interosseous space is widened, into which lunate may displaced. Vickers ligament attaches immediately distal to the osteophyte arising from the ulnar aspect of the distal metaphysis of radius (*green*).

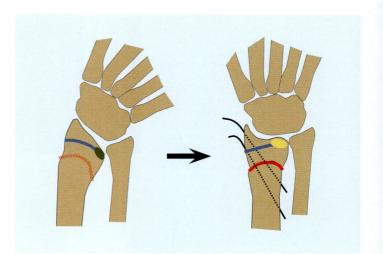

C Correction of Madelung deformity This correction is performed through a volar approach. Vickers ligament and physeal bridge (*green*) are excised with fat interposition (*yellow*). The dome shape of osteotomy (*red*) allows simultaneous correction of radial inclination as well as radial and dorsal translation, which improves articular support of lunate. Fixation is with divergent wires, due to the inherent stability of the wide surface area of the osteotomy.

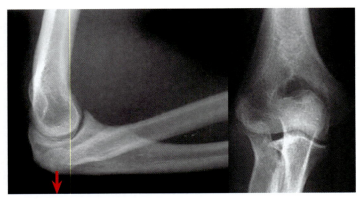

A **Atraumatic dislocation of radial head** The proximal radius is thin and deformed; capitulum is blunted. Posterior direction is most common.

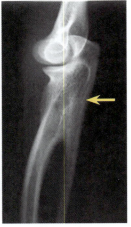

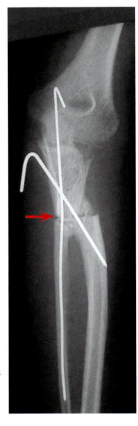

B **Congenital radioulnar synostosis** Proximal radius and ulna fail to differentiate (*yellow*). Perform a rotational osteotomy (*red*) through the synostosis. Incision is along subcutaneous border of ulna. Subperiosteal interval is safe, including away from posterior interosseous nerve. Nail the ulna antegrade with a wire, around which osteotomy is rotated to 45 degrees of pronation or supination and cross-fixed with a wire into the radius. Monitor after operation for compartment syndrome, which is a risk of acute forearm rotation. If signs develop, remove the cross wire and relax the forearm. Rerotate the forearm after bleeding, swelling, and risk subside.

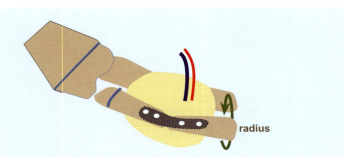

C **Mobilization of radioulnar synostosis** Through a subanconeus approach, synostosis is excised. Proximal radius is cut: it is shortened to reduce its dislocated head to capitulum, the distal fragment is supinated (*green*) to take its synostosis surface away from the ulna's, and fixed with a plate. Profunda humeri vessels of the fasciofat graft are anastomosed to radial recurrent vessels. The fasciofat graft, like a lateral arm flap, includes a skin bridge to monitor viability.

FOREARM

Congenital Dislocation of the Head of the Radius

This may be isolated or associated with other anomalies, such as nail–patella syndrome, hereditary multiple exostosis, and osteogenesis imperfecta (*cf.* Syndromes chapter). Most are bilateral.

Evaluation Limited forearm rotation and a palpable prominence over the displaced radial head bring the child to medical attention, typically around 5 years of age. Posterior dislocation is most common and limits extension of the elbow; anterior dislocation limits elbow flexion. The dislocated radial head becomes progressively more prominent with growth. Shortening of the radial side of the forearm makes the ulna more prominent at the wrist. Bilateral involvement and a family history distinguish this from traumatic dislocation, for example, as part of Monteggia fracture (*cf.* Trauma chapter).

IMAGING Röntgenogrammes show relative lengthening of ulna associated with a hypoplastic capitulum and proximal radius, of which the epiphysis is underdeveloped and deformed in childhood and which becomes tapered like "sucked candy" by maturity [A]. Differentiate traumatic dislocation, which is characterized by normal development of capitulum and proximal radius, including epiphysis, without shortening of radius.

Management Most presentations are so mild that education and symptom control *pro re nata* suffice. Reduction of atraumatic dislocation of the radial head is unsuccessful due to radiocapitular dysplasia: incongruence leads to persistent instability. Rarely, excision of the radial head is indicated, to alleviate pain and reduce prominence more than to improve motion. Delay this until maturity, to reduce heterotopic ossification that may require repeat excision. Cubitus valgus, ulnar neuritis, and weakness are theoretical concerns that have eluded demonstration.

Congenital Radioulnar Synostosis

This may be categorized as a failure of differentiation of proximal radius and ulna. Longitudinal segmentation of radius and ulna proceeds from distal to proximal. Radioulnar synostosis is detectable at neonatal examination. Alternatively, like congenital dislocation of the radial head presentation may be delayed due to absence of pain and adaptation of the child: radioulnar synostosis comes to light when forearm rotation becomes noticed by third parties, such as when drawing at school. Half are bilateral.

Distinguish traumatic synostosis. This follows and correlates with the energy of fracture, or it may be iatrogenic from surgical dissection. It may occur at any level of the forearm. It is more common in the setting of head injury.

Evaluation There is no forearm rotation. Hand position may be stuck in any degree of pronation or supination. Wrist may be hypermobile to compensate. Another compensatory mechanism is shoulder abduction for loss of pronation.

IMAGING Röntgenogrammes show fusion of proximal radius and ulna that extends beyond the bicipital tuberosity [B].

Management In a patient with unilateral synostosis, the unaffected forearm may compensate for loss of motion on the synostosed side.

OSTEOTOMY Surgical correction is indicated for a patient with bilateral synostosis who is unable to compensate for physical demand [B]. Perform a rotational osteotomy through the synostosis to achieve the goals of pronation of the dominant side to write and use a keyboard, and supination of the nondominant side to receive, for example when accepting change, and for support, for example when carrying objects.

EXCISION This promises restoration of motion. Interposition of synthetic material, for example silicone, or biologic material, for example autograft fat, or allograft or autograft fascia wrapped around the radius, has not been durable. Interposition of a vascularized fasciofat flap, obtained from lateral aspect of the same arm, has shown success in limited series [C]. The problem and solution resemble tarsal coalition (*cf.* Foot chapter).

SHOULDER

Sprengel Anomaly

During the 2nd to 3rd fetal months, the scapula migrates from adjacent to the fourth to sixth cervical vertebrae caudad. Failure of descent (not elevation) strands the scapula between the neck and shoulder. The scapula is small; its inferior angle is rotated medialward such that the glenoidal cavity is directed downward. One-third of cases are associated with an omovertebral bone (Greek ωμος: "shoulder"), which connects superomedial border of scapula with lower cervical vertebrae, and which is a homolog of the suprascapular bone in lower vertebrates, in particular Amphibia [A]. Boys are thrice as affected as girls. It is sporadic, with rare subsets of autosomal dominant inheritance.

Evaluation This is detectable at neonatal examination. The patient has a firm fullness in the neck. Shoulder abduction is limited: downward projection of the glenoidal cavity shifts the glenohumeral arc inferior, while hypoplasia and contracture of spinoscapular muscles reduces scapulothoracic motion. An omovertebral bone further restricts motion. Serratus anterior weakness results in winging, which worsens the appearance. Bilateral presentation is less disfiguring due to symmetric neck contour, but more disabling due to difficulty raising a hand above the horizon.

IMAGING Röntgenogrammes show relative elevation of a dysplastic scapula. A lateral or oblique view of the cervical spine screens for vertebral anomalies and may show the omovertebral bone, which is confirmed by CT. An MRI visualizes the spinal cord for neural lesion, and a fibrous connexion with the cervical spine.

Management Physiotherapy preserves and maximizes shoulder motion. Unacceptable appearance and limited shoulder motion are indications for operation. Optimal age is the first decade, when contractures are less unyielding and when nerves, including brachial plexus, are more tolerant of stretch. Muscle release is extraperiosteal to avoid osseous regrowth. Cutting the clavicle decompresses the brachial plexus when the scapula is mobilized significantly.

SCAPULOPLASTY (MᶜBURNEY, SANDS) This is indicated for mild deformity, in which neck fullness is more significant than displacement of the body and winging of the scapula and than shoulder abduction above the horizon. Release levator scapulæ and rhomboid minor, protecting transverse cervical artery and dorsal scapular nerve. Identify scapular attachment of omovertebral bone: release this and draw it distal to liberate it for extraperiosteal excision. Reflect supraspinatus to the greater scapular notch, protecting the transverse scapular artery and suprascapular neurovascular bundle. Reflect subscapularis off deep surface of the scapula. Excise the superior angle of scapula. Reattach supraspinatus to the spine of the scapula.

REPOSITIONING (GREEN, WOODWARD) This is indicated for more severe deformity. Division of the clavicle, with preservation of its periosteal sleeve, reduces the risk of brachial plexus compression with scapular distalization. This is performed supine, after which the patient is turned prone.

Release trapezius, protecting spinal accessory nerve. Release adhesions tethering scapula to the thorax. Release latissimus dorsi. Reposition scapula, including suture of superomedial corner to spinous processes of T11-T12 to rotate glenoid out of varus, thereby shifting the glenohumeral arc toward more abduction. The scapula may be held in place by a pocket fashioned in latissimus dorsi and by suture to adjacent ribs. Reattach muscles to new sites based upon the distalization [C].

OSTEOTOMY (KÖNIG) Because of a return of the scapula toward its original position with time as the soft tissue reconstruction gives way, osteotomy has been advocated to provide more secure healing [D]. The scapula is divided 1 cm lateral to vertebral border, leaving its muscular attachments undisturbed. The medial half is tensioned distalward to deliver an omovertebral bone, which is excised. Subscapularis and adhesions are freed from the lateral half, which is distalized and secured to the medial half by sutures or wire through offset drill holes. Excise the superomedial angle, leaving levator scapulæ free.

Anomaly
Omovertebral bone
Congenital scoliosis
Cervical spina bifida
Diastematomyelia
Costal fusion
Syndromes, e.g., Klippel-Feil, Poland

A Anomalies associated with Sprengel anomaly. These are seen in half of cases.

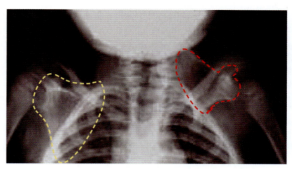

B Sprengel anomaly. The left scapula is dysplastic, rotated, and elevated.

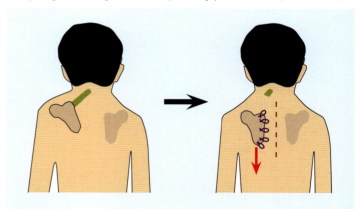

C Soft tissue repositioning. A midline linear incision is used (*brown*). Omovertebral bone (*green*) is resected. Muscular attachments are released extraperiosteally and reattached (*blue*) in the new scapular position (*red*).

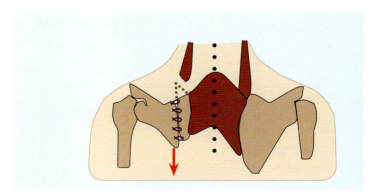

D Vertical osteotomy. Osseous union may be more reliable than soft tissue reconstruction. The lateral half of the scapula is distalized (*red*) and fixed in the new position to the medial half by suture or wire (*blue*). The superior angle of the medial fragment is excised (*green*), leaving levator scapulæ free.

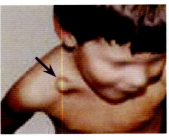 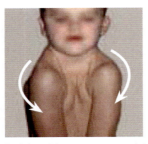

E Congenital pseudarthrosis of the clavicle. This presents as a painless prominence at the midclavicle (*blue*). Absent clavicles in cleidocranial dysplasia result in shoulder hypermobility (*white*).

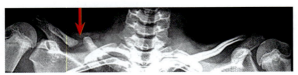

F Congenital pseudarthrosis of the clavicle. Medial and lateral ossification centers of right clavicle failed to coalesce (*red*). Medial end is displaced superior, where it is prominent under skin.

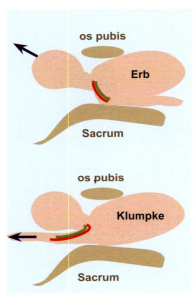

G Dystocia. When a child obstructed in the birth canal at the shoulders is pulled by the head, the upper brachial plexus may be stretched and injured (*red*). This disproportionately affects the proximal upper limb. Pulling the child by the arm, by contrast, will put tension on the lower brachial plexus (*red*). The focus of disability is the hand.

Risk Factor
Birth weight >5 kg
Maternal diabetes
Multiparity
Breech
Second stage of labor >60 minutes
Assisted delivery
Manual traction during delivery
In utero torticollis
Shoulder dystocia

H Risk factors for brachial plexus birth injury. Injury may occur during delivery, during descent into the canal or *in utero*. This explains injury in small babies and absent dystocia, and the fact that only 1/2 of cases have an identifiable risk factor.

Poor prognostic sign
Preganglionic injury
Total plexus involvement
2 weeks: no sign of early recovery
6 months: no recovery of elbow flexion, wrist and digital extension

I Poor prognostic signs. These aid counseling of family and decision making.

Congenital Pseudarthrosis of the Clavicle

The clavicle is the first bone to ossify and the last to fuse into one. Medial and lateral primary centers of ossification appear by the 6th fetal week. A third, secondary ossification center appears toward the end of the second decade at the sternal end and unites with the rest of the bone by the middle of the third decade.

Failure of coalescence of the two primary ossification centers of the clavicle leaves a central defect. Contributing to this failure may be pulsation of the subclavian artery, whence the concept of subclavian artery dysplasia syndrome. The lesion is predominantly right sided (95%). The right subclavian artery arises from the innominate artery, and its third portion is intimately apposed to the clavicle. By contrast, the left subclavian artery arises from the arch of aorta at a lower level and is more remote form the clavicle on its way to the upper limb. Left-sided lesions have been reported in association with dextrocardia.

Evaluation The pseudarthrosis produces a painless prominence over the clavicle [E], associated with narrowing of the shoulder. Fatigue and pain may develop in the older child as the demands of sports heighten. Distinguish cleidocranial dysplasia, in which bilateral failure of coalescence of the primary ossification centers or aplasia of the clavicle is associated with hypermobility of the shoulders, such that they may be brought together anteriorly in the midline, as well as other stigmata absent from congenital pseudarthrosis of the clavicle (*cf.* Syndromes chapter) [F].

IMAGING Röntgenogrammes show a midclavicular defect with anterior and superior angulation. Occasionally, osseous irregularity may raise the specter of infection or tumor.

Management The indication to treat is unacceptable appearance and pain with activity. Explain to the patient and family that a bump will be traded for a scar and a slightly narrower shoulder. Resect the sclerotic ends of each fragment, compress with a plate, and augment with autogenous iliac crest bone graft. Stay within and preserve the periosteal sleeve: this will improve union rate and reduce the risk of brachial plexus injury due to anatomic distortion.

Brachial Plexus Birth Injury

Traction during dystocia may stretch and thereby injure the brachial plexus [G]. Several risk factors have been identified [H]. Injury may affect part of the brachial plexus or the entire brachial plexus. Partial injury may affect the upper trunk (C5-C6; Erb), which is most common; the lower trunk (C8-T1; Klumpke); or it may be mixed.

There are three types of neural injury.

- Apraxia is characterized by temporary loss of function that is followed by spontaneous resolution without sequela.
- In axonotmesis, the axon and myelin sheath are disrupted but the nerve remains in continuity: there is Wallerian degeneration and recovery over several months.
- Neurotmesis refers to complete nerve discontinuity, which makes spontaneous recovery unlikely.

Natural history Eighty percent show spontaneous recovery during the first year. Return of partial antigravity upper trunk muscle strength in the first 2 months indicates complete recovery by 2 years. There are several signs indicative of a poor prognosis [I]. Recovery of elbow flexion and shoulder abduction are better than of shoulder external rotation.

Evaluation The upper limb hangs by the side of the body or has an abnormal posture. There is reduced or no spontaneous movement of the upper limb. Moro reflex is asymmetric. Deep tendon reflexes are absent.

Determine if the lesion is pre- or postganglionic, because this is prognostic. The dorsal root ganglion contains the sensory cell body. The motor cell body is in the spinal cord. Preganglionic lesions represent avulsions from the spinal cord, which will not spontaneously recover. Signs include Horner syndrome (miosis, ptosis, anhidrosis, enophthalmos), elevation of the hemidiaphragm (phrenic nerve), and winging of the scapula (long thoracic nerve).

Upper brachial plexus injury produces a "waiter tip" posture of the upper limb: shoulder adduction and internal rotation, elbow extension, forearm pronation, wrist and digital flexion reflect loss of antagonists, for example, supraspinatus, deltoid, biceps, supinator, long extensors. Lower trunk injury manifests as elbow flexion, wrist extension, and clawing of the hand.

Measure motion. Palpate the posterior shoulder for a dislocation. Check for scapular winging. There may be associated fracture of the clavicle or humerus, as a sign of dystocia. At 3 to 6 months, a child in the supine position who cannot remove a towel from the face ("towel test"), lacking sufficient flexion and abduction, is a microsurgical candidate.

Sensation and strength may be graded systematically [J, K].

IMAGING Röntgenogrammes are unrevealing. MRI visualizes neural elements, for example, presence of roots in the neural foramina or meningocœles (root avulsion), and allows study of the glenohumeral joint for dysplasia without or with dislocation [L].

TESTS Electromyography and nerve conduction studies early may be used to measure injury and track recovery, both of which may be achieved by physical examination.

Management During observation for recovery, passive range of motion exercises are essential to prevent contracture and secondary osseous deformity. Passive stretch also reduces muscle hypoplasia and atrophy. Isolate glenohumeral motion to stretch the shoulder joint capsule by stabilizing the scapula. Enlist a physical therapist. Botulinum toxin facilitates stretching.

Nerve surgery This is indicated after 3 months in total plexus injury or in the presence of Horner syndrome, and after 6 months in postganglionic injury if there is no clinical sign of recovery [M].

AVULSIONS Perform a nerve transfer [N].

RUPTURES Nerve transfer may offer better outcomes than use of an autogenous peripheral nerve graft, for example, sural, to bridge the defect.

NEUROMA This is the most common lesion. Excision and grafting with autogenous sural nerve has superior results to neurolysis. The rôle of collagen matrix tubes has not been defined.

Soft tissue surgery This assumes no significant osseous deformity, which soft tissue reconstruction cannot overcome [O].

RELEASE Consider contracture release after 1 year of age, in order to preserve motion for later muscle transfer and to prevent secondary osseous deformity. Slide subscapularis off its origin on scapula *via* a posterior vertebral border approach. Indications for open reduction, as well as glenoid osteotomy for early dysplasia and dislocation, are in flux.

MUSCLE TRANSFER After 2 years of age, combine internal rotation release, including pectoralis major and subscapularis (Sever) as well as joint capsule, with transfer of latissimus dorsi and teres major to the rotator cuff at the greater tubercle (L'Episcopo) in order to restore shoulder abduction. Identify and protect the axillary nerve, which is at risk during this procedure. An alternative transfer for is lower trapezius augmented by tendo Achilles allograft to infraspinatus. Durability of muscle transfer is a concern.

Bone surgery This is indicated in the older child (>5 years) in whom improved positioning of the hand is the goal when shoulder motion is limited by advanced glenohumeral dysplasia.

HUMERAL OSTEOTOMY Perform a humeral osteotomy proximal to deltoid eminence, *via* a direct anterior approach and fixed with a plate, to recover external rotation. Adjust this to maintain sufficient internal rotation for perineal access.

FOREARM ROTATIONAL DEFORMITY A child with upper recovery but persistent C8-T1 palsy will present with supination contracture of the forearm. If there is >60 degrees of passive pronation, reroute the biceps brachii around the neck of radius to covert the muscle from supinator to pronator.

If passive motion is limited due to extensive contracture, place medullary wires in radius and ulna, which are cut and rotated into 25 degrees of pronation, where they are held by a cast until union.

Type	Sensation
S0	No reaction to pain
S1	Reaction to pain, none to touch
S2	Reaction to heavy touch, none to light touch
S3	Normal

J Sensory grading system (Narakas).

Grade	1	2	3	4	5
Abduction	0	0–30 degrees	30–60 degrees	>60 degrees	Full
External Rotation	0	0 degrees	0–20 degrees	>20 degrees	Full
Hand to Neck	0	0 degrees	Difficult	Easy	Normal
Hand to Spine	0	0 degrees	to S-1	to T-12	Normal
Hand to Mouth	0	Trumpet	Partial trumpet	<40 degree abduction	Normal

K Grading of motor function (Mallet).

Type	Finding (MRI)
I	Normal
II	>5 degree glenoid retroversion
III	Posterior subluxation of humeral head
IV	Pseudoglenoid
V	Deformity of humeral head
VI	Dislocation
VI	Growth arrest of proximal humerus

L Glenohumeral dysplasia (Waters) This develops secondary to muscle imbalance and chronic contracture. Recognition of this approaches hip dysplasia.

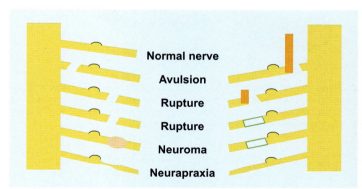

M Nerve surgery for obstetric brachial plexus injury Rupture may be treated by nerve transfer (*orange*) or grafting (*green*). The former has the advantage of a single microsurgical interface. Neurapraxia recovers without operation.

Nerve	Recipient	Function
Ulnar flexor carpi ulnaris motor branch	Musculocutaneous	Biceps brachii
Medial pectoral nerve	Musculocutaneous	Biceps brachii
Spinal accessory nerve	Suprascapular	Supraspinatus
Radial motor branch to long head of triceps	Axillary	Deltoid

N Nerve transfer for upper brachial plexus birth injury Spinal accessory nerve is transferred distal to innervation of trapezius.

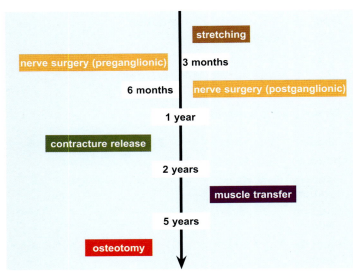

O   **Algorithm for treatment of brachial plexus birth injury.**

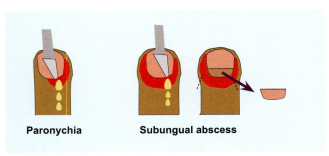

Paronychia   Subungual abscess

A   Nail infections Incising the nail wall for paronychia. If puss extends subjacent to the nail plate, remove part of this to complete drainage.

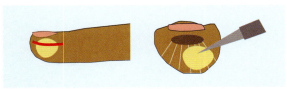

B   Felon Lateral incision dorsal to neurovascular bundle (*red*). Follow with a blunt instrument to evacuate the abscess. Do not cut the septa with scalpel. Do not advance scalpel deep in order not to contaminate flexor tendon sheath or interphalangeal joint. Leave gauze to wick pus.

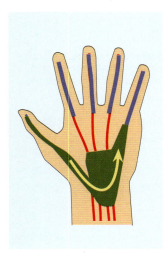

C   Flexor tenosynovitis Infection spreads rapidly along tendon sheaths (*blue*). Radial and ulnar bursæ (*green*) communicate to spread infection from the thumb to smallest finger (*yellow*).

HAND INFECTION

The most common pathogens are *Staphylococcus aureus* and *Streptococcus pyogenes*.

Cellulitis

Inspect the skin for breach. Rule out deep infection, for example, there should be painless motion of the digits and wrist. Draw the perimeter on the skin to aid follow-up. Treat with intravenous followed by oral antibiotics. Reduction of pain, recession of erythema, and return of cutaneous wrinkling indicated recovery.

Paronychia

This represents an infection lodges between nail plate and nail wall. Most are caused by *Staphylococcus aureus*; however, nail biting and thumb sucking introduce anærobes. Treatment begins with warm soaks in dilute soap solution, a cotton wisp between nail wall and plate, to allow it to lift away with growth, and oral antibiotics if necessary. Severe infection is incised and drained [A].

Felon

This represents a closed space infection of the digital pulp, which is divided into compartments by vertical septa that stabilize the pad. Abscess in a confined space may lead to a mini–compartment syndrome, which may lead to necrosis of the skin and pulp, and spread to bone, joint, and flexor tendon. The infection develops spontaneously in 1/2 of patients, with no history of penetrating or other injury. Treatment consists of incision and drainage [B].

Herpetic Whitlow

Type I or II herpes simplex is the most common viral infection of the hand, caused typically by direct inoculation from gingivostomatitis. Clear vesicles are surrounded by erythema with tenderness but no swelling or distortion of the finger tip. A Tzanck test shows multinucleated giant cells in a smear taken from an unroofed vesicle. Do not incise and drain: this may lead to bacterial superinfection, or to systemic viral spread, for example, herpetic encephalitis. Protect the area, and observe for resolution over 3 to 4 weeks.

Flexor Tenosynovitis

Deep infections are introduced by a penetrating injury, they may be contiguous, for example, from a felon, or rarely they may be hæmatogenous. The infection travels rapidly through the tendon sheath, making this a surgical emergency. There are four cardinal signs (Kanavel):

- Flexed posture of the digit.
- Fusiform swelling along the volar digit.
- Tenderness along flexor tendon.
- Pain on passive extension.

In 80% of people, the thumb and smallest finger tendon sheaths communicate *via* radial and ulnar bursæ [C], which may produce a horseshoe abscess. Second to fourth tendon sheaths are independent. In children, and for a presentation within the first 24 hours, intravenous antibiotics alone may suffice. Incise and drain an unresponsive infection.

Deep Space Infection

There are four deep spaces in the hand.

- Dorsal subaponeurotic
- Subfascial web
- Thenar
- Midpalmar

Dorsal subaponeurotic and subfascial web spaces communicate: tracking of infection between them may form a "collar-button" abscess. Because of dorsal location of the lymphatics of the hand, and because of the thickness and unyielding nature of palmar skin, deep palmar infection may manifest as dorsal erythema and swelling. This may be distinguished from cellulitis by pain with passive extension of inflamed flexor tendons. Ultrasonogramme also aids diagnosis and is easy on the child. Treatment is incision and drainage.

GENERAL

Ekblom AG, Laurell T, Arner M. Epidemiology of congenital upper limb anomalies in 562 children born in 1997 to 2007: a total population study from Stockholm, Sweden. *J. Hand Surg. Am.* 35(11):1742–1754, 2010.

Manske PR, Oberg KC. Classification and developmental biology of congenital anomalies of the hand and upper extremity. *J. Bone Joint Surg. Am.* 91(Suppl 4):3–18, 2009.

Swanson AB, Swanson GD, Tada K. A classification for congenital limb malformation. *J. Hand Surg. Am.* 8(5 Pt 2): 693–702, 1983.

DEFICIENCY

Bayne LG, Klug MS. Long term review of the surgical treatment of radial deficiencies. *J. Hand Surg. Am.* 12(2):169–179, 1987.

Bayne LG. Congenital hand deformities: ulnar club hand (ulnar deficiency). In: Green DG, ed. *Operative Hand Surgery.* New York: Churchill Livingstone; 1982.

Eaton CJ, Lister GD. Toe transfer for congenital hand defects. *Microsurgery* 12(3):186–195, 1991.

Goldfarb CA, Manske PR, Busa R, Mills J, Carter P, Ezaki M. Upper-extremity phocomelia reexamined: a longitudinal dysplasia. *J. Bone Joint Surg Am.* 87(12):2639–2648, 2005.

James MA, McCarroll HR Jr, Manske PR. The spectrum of radial longitudinal deficiency: a modified classification. *J. Hand Surg. Am.* 24(6):1145–1155, 1999.

Miura T, Nakamura R, Horii E. The position of symbrachydactyly in the classification of congenital hand anomalies. *J. Hand Surg. Br.* 19(3):350–354, 1994.

O'Rahilly R. Morphological patterns in limb deficiencies and duplications. *Am. J. Anat.* 89(2):135–193, 1951.

FAILURE OF DIFFERENTIATION

Baek GH, Kim JH, Chung MS, Kang SB, Lee YH, Gong HS. The natural history of pediatric trigger thumb. *J. Bone Joint Surg. Am.* 90(5):980–985, 2008.

Hefner RA. Inheritance of crooked little fingers. *J. Hered.* 20(8):395–398, 1929.

Kemp T, Ravn J. Über erbliche hand-und fussdeformitaeten in einem 140-koepfigen geschlecht, nebst einigen bemerkungen ueber poly-und syndaktylie beim menschen. *Acta Psychiat. Neurol. Scand.* 7:275–296, 1932.

Kjaer KW, Hansen L, Eiberg H, Utkus A, Skovgaard LT, Leicht P, Opitz JM, Tommerup NA. 72-year-old Danish puzzle resolved—comparative analysis of phenotypes in families with different-sized HOXD13 polyalanine expansions. *Am. J. Med. Genet.* 138(4):328–339, 2005.

Kirner J. Doppelseitige verkrummungen des kleinfingerendgliedes als selbstandiges krankheitsbild. *Fortschritte auf dem Gehiete der Rönigenstrahien.* 36:804–806, 1927.

Larner AJ. Camptodactyly: a 10-year series. *Eur. J. Dermatol.* 21(5):771–775, 2011.

DUPLICATION

Frazier TM. A note on race-specific congenital malformation rates. *Am. J. Obstet. Gynecol.* 80:184–185, 1960.

Furniss D, Lettice LA, Taylor IB, Critchley PS, Giele H, Hill RE, Wilkie AOM. A variant in the sonic hedgehog regulatory sequence (ZRS) is associated with triphalangeal thumb and deregulates expression in the developing limb. *Hum. Mol. Genet.* 17(16):2417–2423, 2008.

Tupper JW. Pollex abductus due to congenital malposition of the flexor pollicis longus. *J. Bone Joint Surg. Am.* 51(7):1285–1290, 1969.

Wassel HD. The results of surgery for polydactyly of the thumb. A review. *Clin. Orthop.* 64:175–193, 1969.

OVERGROWTH

Cerrato F, Eberlin KR, Waters P, Upton J, Taghinia A, Labow BI. Presentation and treatment of macrodactyly in children. *J. Hand Surg. Am.* 38(11):2112–2123, 2013.

Tsuge K, Ikuta Y. Macrodactyly and fibro-fatty proliferation of the median nerve. *Hiroshima J. Med. Sci.* 22(1):83–101, 1973.

UNDERGROWTH

Blauth W. The hypoplastic thumb. *Arch. Orthop. Unfallchir.* 62(3):225–246, 1967.

Buck-Gramcko D. *Congenital Malformations of the Hand and Forearm.* London, UK: Churchill Livingstone; 1998.

Poland A. Deficiency of the pectoral muscle. *Guys Hosp. Rep.* 6:191, 1841.

CONSTRICTION

Patterson TJ. Congenital ring-constrictions. *Br. J. Plast. Surg.* 14:1–31, 1961.

GENERALIZED SKELETAL ABNORMALITIES

Gschwind C, Tonkin M. Surgery for cerebral palsy: Part 1. Classification and operative procedures for pronation deformity. *J. Hand Surg. Br.* 17(4):391–395, 1992.

House JH, Gwathmey FW, Fidler MO. A dynamic approach to the thumb-in palm deformity in cerebral palsy. *J. Bone Joint Surg. Am.* 63(2):216–225, 1981.

Tonkin M, Freitas A, Koman A, Leclercq C, Van Heest A. The surgical management of thumb deformity in cerebral palsy. *J. Hand Surg. Br.* 33(1):77–80, 2008.

Tonkin M, Gschwind C. Surgery for cerebral palsy: Part 2. Flexion deformity of the wrist and fingers. *J. Hand Surg. Br.* 17(4):396–400, 1992.

Zancolli EA, Zancolli ER Jr. Surgical management of the hemiplegic spastic hand in cerebral palsy. *Surg. Clin. North Am.* 61(2):395–406, 1981.

WRIST

Carter PR, Ezaki M. Madelung's deformity. Surgical correction through the anterior approach. *Hand Clin.* 16(4):713–721, 2000.

Dannenberg M, Anton JI, Spiegel MB. Madelung's deformity. *Am. J. Roentgen. Radium. Ther. Nucl. Med.* 42(5):671–676, 1939.

Laffosse JM, Abid A, Accadbled F, Knör G, Sales de Gauzy J, Cahuzac JP. Surgical correction of Madelung's deformity by combined corrective radioulnar osteotomy: 14 cases with four-year minimum follow-up. *Int. Orthop.* 33(6):1655–1661, 2009.

Vickers D, Nielsen G. Madelung deformity: surgical prophylaxis (physiolysis) during the late growth period by resection of the dyschondrosteosis lesion. *J. Hand Surg. Br.* 17(4):401–407, 1992.

ELBOW

Almquist EE, Gordon CH, Blue AI. Congenital dislocation of the head of the radius. *J. Bone Joint Surg. Am.* 51(6):1118–1127, 1969.

Blodgett WE. Congenital luxation of the head of the radius. Report of two cases. Analysis of fifty-one cases. *Am. J. Orthop. Surg.* 3:253–270, 1905.

Green WT, Mital MA. Congenital radio-ulnar synostosis: surgical treatment. *J. Bone Joint Surg. Am.* 61(5):738–743, 1979.

Kanaya F, Ibaraki K. Mobilization of a congenital proximal radioulnar synostosis with use of a free vascularized fascio-fat graft. *J. Bone Joint Surg. Am.* 80(8):1186–1192, 1998.

SHOULDER

Cavendish ME. Congenital elevation of the scapula. *J. Bone Joint Surg.* 54(3)-B:395–408, 1972.

Eulenberg M. Casuistische mittelheilungen aus dem gembeite der orthopadie. *Arch. Klin. Chir.* 4:301–311, 1863.

Fawcett J. The development and ossification of the human clavicle. *J. Anat. Physiol.* 47:225–234, 1913.

Gilbert A, Tassin JL. Surgical repair of the brachial plexus in obstetric paralysis. *Chirurgie* 110:70–75, 1984.

Green WT. The surgical correction of congenital elevation of the scapula (Sprengel's deformity). *J. Bone Joint Surg. Am.* 39-A:1439–1448, 1957.

Haerle M, Gilbert A. Management of complete obstetric brachial plexus lesions. *J. Pediatr. Orthop.* 24(2):194–200, 2004.

Hale HB, Bae DS, Waters PM. Current concepts in the management of brachial plexus birth palsy. *J. Hand Surg. Am.* 35(2):322–331.

König F. Eine neue operation des angeborenen schulterblatthochstandes. *Beitr. Klin. Chir.* 94:530–537, 1914.

L'Episcopo JB. Tendon transplantation in obstetrical paralysis. *Am. J. Surg.* 25:122–125, 1934.

Lloyd-Roberts GC, Apley AG, Owen R. Reflections upon the aetiology of congenital pseudarthrosis of the clavicle. With a note on cranio-cleido dysostosis. *J. Bone Joint Surg. Br.* 57(1):24–29, 1975.

Mallet J. Obstetrical paralysis of the brachial plexus. *Rev. Chir. Orthop. Reparatrice Appar. Mot.* 58(Suppl 1):166–168, 1972.

Matsuoka T, Ahlberg PE, Kessaris N, Iannarelli P, Dennehy U, Richardson WD, McMahon AP, Koentges G. Neural crest origins of the neck and shoulder. *Nature* 436(7049):347–355, 2005.

McBurney CH, Sands A. Congenital deformity due to malposition of the scapula. *N Y Med. J.* 47:582–583, 1888.

McMurtry I, Bennet GC, Bradish C. Osteotomy for congenital elevation of the scapula (Sprengel's deformity). *J. Bone Joint Surg. Br.* 87(7):986–989, 2005.

Narakas AO. Brachial plexus surgery. *Orthop. Clin. North Am.* 12(2):303–323, 1981.

Sever JW. Obstetric paralysis: report of eleven hundred cases. *JAMA* 85:1862–1865, 1925.

Sprengel RD. Die angeborene verschiebung des schulterblattes nach oben. *Arch. Klin. Chir.* 42:545–549, 1891.

Woodward JW. Congenital elevation of the scapula: correction by release and transplantation of muscle origins. *J. Bone Joint Surg. Am.* 43(2):219–228, 1961.

INFECTION

Doyle JR. Anatomy of the finger flexor tendon sheath and pulley system. *J. Hand Surg. Am.* 13(4):473–484, 1988.

Kanavel AB. *Infections of the Hand. A Guide to the Surgical Treatment of Acute and Chronic Suppurative Processes in the Fingers, Hand, and Forearm.* Philadelphia, PA/New York: Lea & Febiger; 1912.

SPINE

Converse to adults, deformity commands the largest proportion of spine care in children. Back pain, while not infrequent, in most children will have no identifiable cause.

EMBRYOLOGY AND DEVELOPMENT

At the end of the 2nd week, the embryo is trilaminar, composed of endoderm (which gives rise to the gut) adjacent to the yolk sac, ectoderm adjacent to the amnion, and mesoderm in between.

Ectoderm gives rise to the nervous system. The notochord appears during the 3rd week, at the beginning of *gastrulation*. The notochord (of which the vestige is the nucleus pulposus) induces the formation of the neural plate. The neural plate begins to fold into the neural tube in the 4th week from its center rostrad and caudad, a process known as *neurulation*. During neurulation, there is *disjunction* of the superficial ectoderm, which goes on to form the skin.

Paired blocks of mesoderm, known as somites, give rise to the musculoskeletal system [A]. The part of a somite that forms bone is known

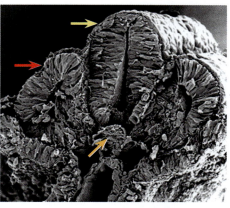

A Scanning electron micrograph of an embryo Somite, *red*. Neural tube, *yellow*. Notochord, *orange*. [http://php.med.unsw.edu.au]

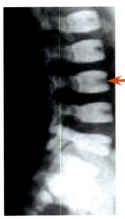

B   Vertebral intersegmental development The vertebral bodies form as intersegmental structures. As blood vessels grow between somites, their final position is midvertebral. The site of blood vessel entry and somite fusion may appear radiographically as an anterior notch in the vertebral body of the child (*red*).

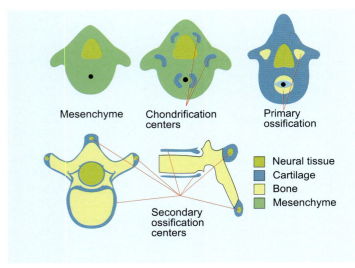

C   Vertebral development Chondrification leads to ossification, which is complete by maturity. From Moore (1988).

as a sclerotome and that which forms muscle is a myotome. During the 4th week, the sclerotome grows around the notochord to become the vertebral body and anulus fibrosus and around the neural tube to form the vertebral arches.

The rostral half of one sclerotome fuses with the caudal half of the adjacent one to form each vertebra. This intersegmentation means that original vascular ingrowth between somites ends in midvertebral segmental blood vessels. Anterior notching of vertebrae in the immature spine marks the site of somite fusion [B].

During the 7th to 8th weeks, paired *chondrification* centers appear around the notochord, which will fuse during the process of *ossification* to form the centrum of the vertebral body; around the neural tube, where they fuse to form the neural arch; and at each transverse and spinous processes, where their rôle is apophyseal [C]. Fusion of the neurocentral junction occurs by 5 years of age, at which time the final capacity of the vertebral canal is determined.

Differential growth of the spinal cord and vertebral column leads to *ascension* of the conus medullaris to its adult level at L1 by the first few months of age. This is accompanied by formation of the cauda equina, as lumbosacral nerves travel to reach their respective intervertebral foramina. The spinal cord is anchored to the coccyx by the filum terminale.

In the coronal plane, the spine is straight throughout growth. In the sagittal plane, the spine evolves from a single curve at birth to a triple curve.

A knowledge of embryology and its nomenclature aids an understanding of disease.

- Dysrrhaphism refers to a "bad" "groove," a general term for midline, that is, spine anomaly
- Schisis refers to "splitting, cleavage, or *schism*" of the spine. Two types are distinguished, myeloschisis: "splitting of the medulla, or spinal cord," and rhachischisis: "splitting of the osseous spine."
- Spina bifida is the general term for "splitting of the spine." This may be aperta: "open," in which nerve has escaped the confines of bone, or occulta: "closed," characterized by retention of nerve within an open osseous canal (a benign, often radiographic finding most frequently located at the lumbosacral junction that affects up to ¼ of the normal population).
- Spina bifida aperta includes myelomeningocœle, which results from incomplete neurulation.
- Premature disjunction leads to migration of mesoderm into the neural tube, where the mesodermal cells are induced to form fat and ultimately a lipomyelomeningocœle.
- Failure of disjunction accounts for cutaneous signs of dysrrhaphism, such as hairy patch or sinus.
- Failure of ascension may result in tethered cord.
- Adhesion between endoderm and ectoderm results in split cord malformation, such as diastematomyelia or neurenteric cyst.
- Hyperkyphosis may be observed for the first 2 years for the normal development of sagittal contour during growth.
- Fusion of the spine before 5 years of age, that is, before ossification of the neurocentral junction, risks iatrogenic stenosis of the vertebral canal.
- Development of the vertebrae is associated most closely with that of the neuraxis, genitourinary system, and heart. As a result, an insult to one system may insult them all, and evaluation of one should include evaluation of the others.

EVALUATION

History and Physical Examination

Sit down, and take some time to gain the confidence of the child (and family): the spine is a site of awkwardness and vulnerability. Examine the whole patient. Is this an isolated problem of the spine, or part of a generalized disorder? Look at other systems, such as the skin, where *café au lait* spots suggest neurofibromatosis or a midline stigma points to dysrrhaphism.

History Directly and independently include the child, who may express a different complaint from parent or referring physician. For example, the child may be more concerned about the appearance of spine deformity than the pædiatrician, who may be focused on long-term consequences. Ask the family, which may reveal a genetic disorder. Because of the gravity of diagnosis, many other disciplines have become involved in spine care; be considerate as you navigate this world with patient and family.

Physical examination Develop a standard approach, including the following:

- Age. This is the most important patient characteristic in any disease.
- Other measure(s) of maturity [A].

Progression of spine deformity is proportional to growth.

- Gender. Certain conditions are more frequent or have a different natural history according to gender.
- Gait. This may be influenced by pain or neural function.
- Pain. This traditionally has been underestimated in children and in certain conditions (e.g., scoliosis).
- Palpation. In particular tenderness, and step-off (e.g., spondylolisthesis).
- Lower limb length discrepancy. This may produce an apparent or secondary spine deformity.
- Plane of deformity. Evaluate spine in three dimensions: coronal, transverse, and sagittal.
- Trunk asymmetry. Include the shoulder, scapula, ribs, breast, flank, iliac crest.
- Spine balance. Plumb line dropped from inion to natal cleft [B].
- Spine motion, including Adams forward bend test.
- Neural examination. Spine deformity may be primary or secondary to a neural lesion.
- Skin. Look for cutaneous signs of decompensation in the setting of deformity [B] and for a midline sign of dysrrhaphism.

Imaging

Röntgenogramme is the fundamental screening modality for spine deformity and for back pain. The latter also may be screened with scintigramme, which may detect a radiographically occult lesion [C].

Scintigramme allows a dynamic or physiologic assessment of bone: the phosphorus attached to technetium (^{99m}Tc) medronic acid is taken up by bone undergoing turnover, as in an active spondylolysis that has potential to heal or in inflammation induced by infection.

Single photon emission computed tomography (SPECT) allows localization of scintigraphic uptake in a vertebra, for example, the pars interarticularis in spondylolysis.

Computed tomography (CT) gives the best detail of vertebral architecture [D]. It confirms spondylolysis. In neurofibromatosis, it reveals osseous erosion. In tumors, it defines margins. In complex deformity, it allows understanding of the three-dimensional shape of the spine and aids planning of operative treatment.

Magnetic resonance imaging (MRI) shows the soft tissue, in particular neural, intervertebral disc, muscle, ligament. Indications for MRI include abnormality on physical examination, such as weakness or upper motor neuron sign, as well as symptoms or signs of atypia such as thoracic hyperkyphosis, early age of presentation.

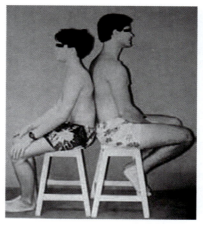

A   Maturity Maturation is variable. Girls mature earlier and more predictably than boys. The ethnic spectrum is broad. These two boys are 16 years old.

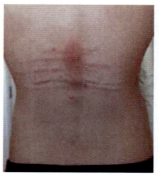

B   Skin decompensation The skin shows stretch marks and callus over an inflexible kyphosis. This is an objective sign that the deformity is significantly impacting (and will impact) the patient's function, such as sitting against the back of a chair.

Imaging method	Indication
Röntgenogramme	Osseous deformity
Oblique röntgenogramme	Lumbosacral spondylolysis
Ferguson view röntgenogramme	Spondylolysis Lumbosacral fusion
Scintigramme	Back pain—initial screening Osseous activity—spondylolysis, infection, tumor
SPECT (single photon emission CT)	Spondylolysis
CT (computed tomography)	Osseous deformity—operative planning Osseous architecture—fracture, spondylolysis, tumor
MRI (magnetic resonance imaging)	Soft tissue detail—neural lesion, disc, tumor, infection Osseous activity—spondylolysis, infection, tumor

C   Imaging methods and their indications These are not a substitute for history and physical examination. Obtain judiciously: incidental findings may lead to unnecessary intervention.

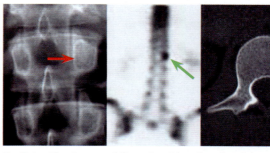

D   Osteoid osteoma of the spine Distortion of pedicle on röntgenogramme (*red*) was associated with focal increased uptake on scintigramme (*green*). CT scan showed a geographic, sclerotic lesion in the pedicle (*yellow*), guiding excision.

BACK PAIN

Prevalence

Drawing upon engineering and aviation, in medicine, back pain resembles a "black box." Up to 1/3 of children complain of back pain; the incidence increases in adults to >2/3 in adults.

Causes

In more than three-quarters of these, no cause can be identified; such children are said to have "overuse" or "growing" or idiopathic pain, in the same way they may complain of other sites in the skeleton [A]. The most common identifiable cause is spondylolysis, followed by deformity such as hyperlordosis. Less than 10% of children will present with a significant arthropathy, infection, neural lesion, or tumor, which should assure the physician to take a measured approach to evaluation and management.

CANDIF

One CANDIF (ferentiate) "good," or benign or idiopathic, from "bad" back pain, which should raise concern for an identifiable cause.

- Constant. Come and go pain typically is mechanical, from overuse.
- Associated symptoms or signs. This includes abnormality detected on physical examination, such as neural deficit or deformity.
- Nocturnal. Pain that arouses a child from sleep is more concerning than pain that interferes with falling asleep, which is typical of overuse pain.
- Duration. Follow-up a patient with pain <3 months. The physician may be at odds with the patient, who may regard duration >3 months to be evidence that something is amiss, since the pain has not resolved spontaneously. Educate the patient that a significant morbid process accounting for pain would manifest in other ways after several months or years.
- Intensity. Take note of pain that is worsening inexorably, as opposed to pain that may wax and wane within a stable range.
- Focal. Focal pain is more likely to have a structural cause. Pain that is diffuse, or that radiates in a nonanatomic distribution, is more typical of overuse.

Evaluation

History and physical examination are the foundation. Image judiciously: results may be misleading, they may raise anxiety unnecessarily, they may lead to unhelpful "treatment", and they add cost.

- Röntgenogramme. This is the first-line modality, particularly useful for spondylolysis and deformity. It also shows loss of height in discitis.
- Scintigraphy (including SPECT). For spondylolysis and occult process. This may be a screening tool for "serious" disease.
- MRI. For tumor, infection, or neural lesion (in particular in association with radiculopathy).
- CT. In the evaluation of back pain, this often serves a confirmatory rôle, such as to define spondylolysis or to characterize extent of osseous involvement by tumor.

Laboratory analysis is useful for infection, inflammatory arthritis, and blood tumors. C-reactive protein is the best measure of acute infection. Inflammatory arthritis may affect other joints (in particular knee and hand) and shows elevation of erythrocyte sedimentation rate. Complete blood count with differential screen for leukæmia.

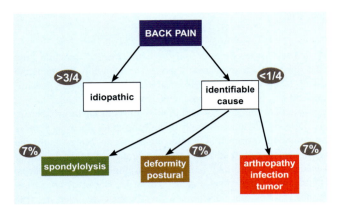

A Back pain A simplified ætiologic algorithm.

Management

Idiopathic back pain is best managed according to general principles.

- Establish the diagnosis by exclusion.
- Educate and reassure the patient and family. Education may include a physiotherapist on modalities for back health.
- Activity modification. Avoid what makes it worse, such as a back pack that is >15% body weight.
- Light aerobic exercise, including participating in P.E.
- Weight reduction and control.
- Stretching. This may begin under the guidance of a physiotherapist but should continue as part of a more "holistic" approach, such as yoga.

Encourage "lifestyle" techniques that may be adopted by a child into adulthood, rather than medical interventions with which the child may not be compliant or which will be regarded as temporary. This is of particular importance because the majority of adolescents who complain of back pain and have a family history of such will experience back pain as adults.

Juvenile Idiopathic Arthritis

The majority of patients will be HLA-B27 positive (ANA and RF negative). Up to a third of patients with seronegative spondyloarthropathy will have a family history. Other characteristic signs include the following:

- Schober test for spine stiffness. Forward bend is associated with <4 cm of lumbar spine excursion due to syndesmophytes.
- Enthesitis, for example, at tendo-Achillis
- Cutaneous stigmata, for example, psoriasis
- Visceral involvement, for example, uveitis, enteritis

Management of back pain in this setting is secondary to management of the primary disease, by a rheumatologist.

Developmental Lordosis

Strain on facet joints in the hyperlordotic lumbar spine is a cause of back pain around the turn of the decade [B]. It is flexible, transient, and resolves spontaneously. Treatment consists of education and assurance, with postural training by antilordotic exercises.

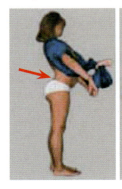
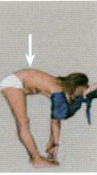

B Physiologic lordosis of puberty This results from hyperflexibility of the lumbar spine as the trunk settles upon the pelvis.

DISCITIS

Discitis represents infection of the metaphyseal region of a vertebra. By contrast with tumor, to which the intervertebral disc may be impervious, infection will traverse and erode the disc. The term places emphasis on the loss of disc height on röntgenogrammes [A].

Clinical Features

Presentation may be obscure and result in delayed diagnosis. It is one of the causes for refusal to walk in an infant. The preadolescent may complain primarily of abdominal pain; only in the second decade does the complaint reliably localize to the spine. Constitutional symptoms and signs, stiffness of the spine, and elevated inflammatory markers suggest the diagnosis. Paraspinous muscle splinting may be assessed in the prone position with the hips extended and the knees flexed: moving the pelvis from side to side causes a synchronous movement of the lumbar spine (Goldthwaite sign). Severe or untreated disease may be complicated by extension to paravertebral soft tissues, such as psoa abscess.

Imaging Röntgenogrammes take more than a week to show reduced disc height [A]. Scintigramme shows increased uptake of adjacent vertebrae at onset of disease [A] and will hasten diagnosis. MRI is indicated only if uncertainty persists, as it may introduce confusion with more morbid process such as tumor and lead to unnecessary intervention such as aspiration or biopsy.

Management

If the child does not present with systemic illness, immobilization alone in brace or pantaloon cast may be sufficient [B], while the spine, well vascularized, in a healthy child recovers spontaneously. Antibiotics may be added to shorten disease duration and avoid complications; they are indicated unequivocally in systemic illness. Regimen follows general principles for musculoskeletal infection.

- Initially target gram-positive organisms.
- Venous antibiotics for systemic illness and until the disease is controlled.
- Conversion to oral antibiotics after clinical and laboratory response.
- Continuation of treatment until normalization of ESR.
- Change of antibiotics, further imaging, aspiration, or biopsy for atypical course or lack of response.

Prognosis

Disc recovery is inversely proportional to age at presentation [C]. Despite outcomes that include residual disc narrowing, sagittal plane deformity, and spontaneous fusion, function is not significantly impacted during childhood.

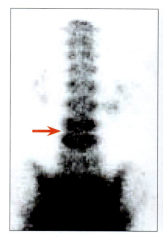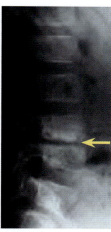

A   L3-L4 discitis Scintigramme at presentation shows increased uptake (*red*). After 2 weeks, lateral röntgenogrammes shows narrowing of the disc (*yellow*).

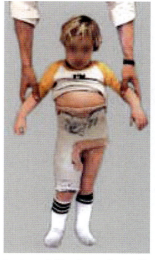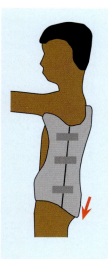

B   Immobilization reduces discomfort Most complete immobilization includes the back and one limb to immobilize the lumbosacral spine (**left**). A "long" (*red*) TLSO is better tolerated.

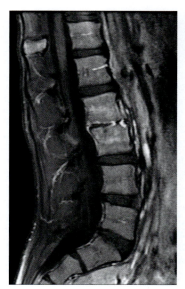

C   Outcome of discitis Persistent loss of disc height and mild focal kyphosis 2 years after successful treatment.

Category	Comment
Idiopathic	Cause unknown Most common type Subdivided by age: infantile, juvenile, adolescent
Congenital	Vertebral anomaly
Neuromuscular	Upper neural lesions—cerebral palsy Lower neural lesions—spina bifida
	Myopathies—muscular dystrophy
Syndromic	Skeletal dysplasias Marfan syndrome Neurofibromatosis (of von Recklinghausen)
Secondary	Pain Lower limb length discrepancy

A   Classification of scoliosis.

Abnormality	Comment
Genetic	Up to 75% concordance in monozygotic twins 10% in first–degree relatives Chromosome mapping to multiple loci
Hormonal	Growth leads to progression ↓ Melatonin ↑ Calmodulin
Neural	Dorsal column: abnormal proprioception Oculovestibular system: abnormal nystagmus to caloric testing cerebral cortex: abnormal evoked potentials ↑ Chiari malformations
	Myopathies—muscular dystrophy
Structural	Growth disturbance of anterior column leads to loss of sagittal contour until buckling lateralward and rotation
Serologic	Abnormality of platelets

B   Causes of idiopathic scoliosis Scoliosis is multifactorial, and most cases are new spontaneous.

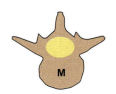

C   Growth of the vertebral canal Volume doubles from birth (0) to 5 years of age, at which point volume is 95% of maturity (M).

Characteristic	Comment
Specific and sensitive	Nonspecific: normal variation in population Too sensitive: referral of untreated curves
Applied to at risk population	Applied to all children
Cost:benefit ratio	~33% increased cost of management ~0.2% indication for bracing
Early intervention alters natural history	Treatment effect of bracing difficult to quantify Manipulative and alternative modalities debatable

D   Screening of scoliosis Essential characteristics of an effective screening test. Screening for scoliosis is recommended twice for girls and once for boys in the first half of the second decade.

SCOLIOSIS

Scoliosis is ancient. It is named and discussed extensively in the Hippocratic Corpus, including the scamnum for correction. It permeates Western literature and art: Shakespeare recounts how the Duke of Gloucester lamented his back, "Where sits deformity to mock my body." While it is defined as angulation in the coronal plane >10 degrees, scoliosis is a three-dimensional deformity including rotation in the transverse plane and alteration of sagittal alignment. It may be divided into causative categories [A].

IDIOPATHIC SCOLIOSIS

Idiopathic refers to "disease" (Greek παθος) that arises on its "own" (Greek ιδιος), that is, cause unknown. Despite the name, several causes have been speculated [B]. Idiopathic scoliosis is the most common deformity of the back. It affects approximately 1% of children, approximately 90% of whom never require active treatment. Progression is proportional to growth, necessitating follow-up through maturity. It is defined as ≥5 degrees, and averages 1 degree *per mensem* during growth and 1 degree *per annum* after maturity for curves >50 degrees.

Evaluation

Essential to evaluation is exclusion of other cause, determination of growth potential, characterization of curve (including magnitude and flexibility), estimating risk of progression, and by extension likelihood of treatment.

History

- Age. This is one measure of growth, which correlates with progression of deformity. Children in the first decade have a higher incidence of neuraxis lesion. Fusion arrests growth. Significant growth of the spinal canal concludes by 5 years of age [C], before which focal operation for vertebral anomaly should be postponed if possible in order to avoid stenosis. Clinically significant growth of the thoracic spine concludes as the child transitions into the second decade, by which point the 50% threshold of thoracic volume has been traversed and before which fusion will have a deleterious effect on pulmonary function.
- Gender. Scoliosis affects both genders equally, but progression in girls is approximately five times than in boys.
- Other measures of growth. Growth amplifies deformity. Girls grow fastest in the 7 months before menarche and stop significant growth 2 years postmenarche. Menarche is variable, including according to activity and ethnicity. It occurs after peak growth velocity, that is, after the curve acceleration phase, the time of greatest risk of progression. It applies to only half of children. Boys grow later and less predictably, in particular a greater variability in cessation of growth.
- Complaints. Pain traditionally has been underestimated in children, and in scoliosis in particular, where it affects 2/3 (twice the background rate). This may be related to fatigue of muscles attempting to rectify the spine. On the other hand, abnormal pain or other complaint (e.g., neural change) may be a sign that the scoliosis is not idiopathic.
- Family. Such a history may suggest greater risk of progression. A susceptibility to develop scoliosis has been linked to the gene GPR126 on chromosome 6, which is highly expressed in cartilage and is associated with height and trunk growth.
- Ethnicity. Caucasians are most affected.
- Screening [D]. This developed from the observation that the thoracic spine and its deformity may be seen on röntgenogramme of the chest obtained during tuberculosis screening. It no longer is practised in the United Kingdom or Canada, and in only half the United States. Greater than 99% of referrals consist of normal variants, scoliosis <10 degrees ("schooliosis") or <25 degrees (no treatment).

Physical examination Develop a standard approach, including the following:

- Gait. This may indicate pain (antalgic), a generalized disease or associated findings (e.g., ataxia).
- Maturity. Tanner scale of secondary sex characteristics has not been bettered by any other system [A]. It is the simplest, fastest, and cheapest method. It may be performed in office (not off-site) and is least morbid (e.g., no radiation from röntgenogrammes). Progression is greatest in the first two stages. Stage 3 coincides with menarche. Stage 4 marks end of significant spine growth. Plane of deformity. Examine coronal (from back and front), transverse (forward bend), and sagittal (from side) planes.
- Palpation. For tenderness, step-off, crepitus, and including the paraspinous soft tissues.
- Trunk asymmetry, including the shoulder, scapula, rib, breast, flank, iliac crest. Asymmetry may be a secondary sign of spine deformity, or it may be a normal variant (5 to 15 mm). Correlate trunk asymmetry with other signs, including direct palpation of the spinous processes. Coronal curvature in the chest elevates the shoulder and below the chest will indent the flank [B]. Rotation will push the scapula, breast, and ribs out, which may be accentuated by sagittal plane deformity such as loss of thoracic kyphosis. Rotation is proportional to risk of deformity progression. Angle of trunk rotation may be measured on forward bending with a scoliometer [C].
- Trunk shift [B]. Project the surface of thorax vertically relative to the iliac crests. This carries an increased risk of deformity progression.
- Spine balance [B]. Even in the setting of trunk shift, a child with idiopathic scoliosis will bring the head back toward midline to balance it on the pelvis. Imbalance may be a subtle indicator of neural abnormality.
- Spine motion, including Adams forward bend test. This is performed ideally from the front (not the back) so that the entire coronal contour may be evaluated by varying the degree of bend without changing the examiner's position, as well as from the side. Asymmetry or limitation may be a sign of pain, neural lesion, or associated abnormality such as hamstring tightness.
- Neural examination, including central signs such as altered gait, lower limb hyperreflexia, clonus, and abnormal abdominal reflex [D]. The latter is a superficial reflex for the thoracic spinal cord. Presence or absence is normal; asymmetry suggests a spinal cord lesion. It is explained evolutionarily as a mechanism to thicken the abdominal wall to protect subjacent viscera.
- Other deformity. For example, in cavus, the arch may point to the primary problem (proximalward to the spinal cord).
- Skin. Note the apothegm that "the skin tells the story." Look for cutaneous signs of decompensation in the setting of deformity, such as stretch marks (rapidity of change in back shape) and callus (in response to unrelieved pressure due to lack of flexibility). Look for a midline stigma of underlying neural lesion, such as hairy patch or sinus. The former may be regarded as an early functional outcome sign, which may influence intervention. The latter is an indication for magnetic resonance imaging.
- Laxity. Signs of hyperlaxity may be present, including elbow extension <0 degrees, placement of the thumb on volar forearm, extension of metacarpophalangeal joints >90 degrees, extension of the knee <0 degrees, flexion of the ankle >30 degrees, and the ability to place palms flat on floor during forward bending with knees straight. As an example, an increased incidence of private variants in fibrillin-1 gene, causing nonsynonymous amino acid substitutions, has been found in a subset (4%) of children with adolescent idiopathic scoliosis who present with more severe and more progressive curves, as well as hyperlaxity without other sign of Marfan syndrome (cf. Syndromes chapter).

Stage	Girl	Boy
1	Prepubertal	
2	Breast bud	Sparse + downy hair scrotal skin texture + pigment
3	Breast elevation subjacent contour	Dense + coarse hair
4	Areolar mound	Triangulation of hair
5	Adult	Hair extends to thighs

A   Tanner scale consists of five stages Distinctive and practical features. P: progression of spine deformity.

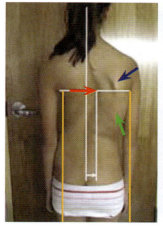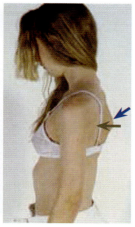

B   Trunk asymmetry Apex dextrad curvature (*red*) produces a right posterior thoracic prominence (*green*) and scapular protraction (*blue*). The trunk shifts dextrad (*orange*) relative to the pelvis. Despite trunk shift, balance is maintained, as evidenced by a plumb line (*white*) dropped from inion to natal cleft. Sagittal alignment is changed as the thoracic spine rotates out of kyphosis (*brown*).

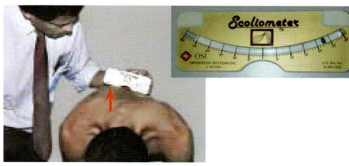

C   Trunk inclination The scoliometer is grooved in its center to accommodate spinous processes as the examiner runs it continually along the entire spine. Observe inclination of a silver ball along a curvilinear slot marked in degrees.

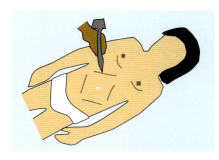

D   Abdominal reflex Stroke each quadrant of the relaxed abdomen. Reflex contraction of abdominal muscles draws umbilicus toward the stimulation.

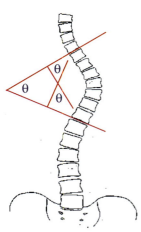

E Angles of Cobb and trunk rotation (ATR) Measure the maximum angle from end vertebra to end vertebra (θ). Draw a line tangent to end plates. Because lines may meet beyond field of view, draw orthogonal lines to obtain the angle. Missed rate begins to rise significantly after 7 degrees of ATR, equivalent to 20-degree Cobb angle.

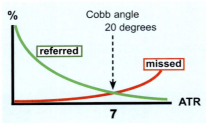

Sign	Comment
Risser	Divide iliac apophysis into quarters 1–4; fusion of apophysis is 5. Most progression occurs before appearance of iliac apophysis.
Triradiate cartilage	Closed marks cessation of spine growth. Open allows no differentiation of maturation stage.
Distal phalangeal epiphyses	Capping of distal phalanges by epiphyses marks beginning of curve acceleration phase. Fusion marks end of significant progression. Fusion coincides with menarche, triradiate closure, absent Risser.
Tanner-Whitehouse RUS	Complex method based upon multiple sites in radius, ulna, and small bones of the hand. Selection of distal phalangeal epiphyses is a simplification.

F Radiographic signs of maturity This is in constant flux. Risser noted that the iliac apophyses could be seen serendipitously at the bottom of spine röntgenogrammes. Evaluation of the distal phalangeal epiphyses is the current favorite method.

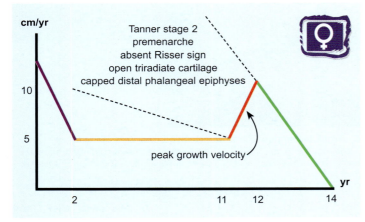

G Growth curve for a girl Note the features associated with peak growth velocity, during which the spine goes through the curve acceleration phase.

H Vertebral rotation This may be graded according to location of spinous process and of pedicles as viewed in coronal plane. Beyond d, or grade ++++, spinous process projects beyond vertebral body. In grade +++ and ++++, concave pedicle has disappeared.

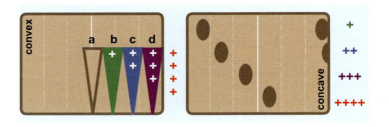

Imaging Röntgenogrammes are the foundation. Measure curve magnitude in degrees after the method of Cobb [E]. Note that measurement error is approximately 5 degrees, which has not been improved by digital imaging. In order to reduce referrals for which orthopædic management is not indicated, a minimum of 7 degrees on scoliometer has been identified to correspond with a Cobb angle of 20 degrees.

Obtain full-length röntgenogrammes to determine spine balance. Sagittal balance is represented by a vertical line between midpoint of C7 and superoposterior corner of S1. In the coronal plane, this vertical line should pass through S1 spinous process. Imbalance is measured in centimeters: ≤2 cm is within normal range.

Posteroanterior projection reduces breast exposure to radiation, which, after reflection of its majority off the skin, declines with travel through tissue, reaching the breasts last. Shield the breasts when it does not impact analysis of the deformity. Include the clavicles to assess shoulder height, which influences operative technique and outcomes. Include the iliac apophyses and triradiate cartilages to aid determination of maturity [F]. Add röntgenogramme of the hand for evaluation of the distal phalangeal epiphyses. Note that calculation of maturity is nuanced and multifactorial [G]. The iliac crests also allow assessment of limb length discrepancy.

Röntgenogrammes identify stable and neutral vertebrae. The former is bisected by the central sacral line. The latter show no rotation, defined as symmetric pedicles and midline spinous process [H]. Rotation is a risk factor for progression and must be considered in addition to curve magnitude. The apical vertebra is least stable and most rotated. Limit fusion to vertebrae that at least are crossed by the central sacral line. Pedicle screws have promoted fusion before reaching the neutral vertebra, because of direct vertebral rotation.

Determine flexibility on röntgenogrammes. Prone posteroanterior view simulates the operating room. Bending views will show opposite inclination at flexible discs, which may be spared fusion. Bending views also show whether the planned lowest instrumented vertebra can become <15 degrees oblique (greater associated with progression) and enters the stable zone.

Computed tomography is useful for complex osseous architecture. In idiopathic scoliosis, this applies to severe deformity rather than vertebral anomaly, which is not a feature. CT provides detail in the postoperative spine, for example, for pseudarthrosis. CT with myelogramme evaluates the instrumented spine for vertebral canal encroachment, for example, by implants in the setting of neural compromise. For other neurologic evaluation, myelography has been replaced by magnetic resonance imaging. Pedicle dimensions may be measured on CT to aid operative planning.

Magnetic resonance imaging is indicated when an abnormality of the neuraxis is suspected in the so-called "idiopathic" setting. Principal risk factors are as follows:

- abnormal physical examination
- age <10 years
- kyphosis >40 degrees for thoracic curves

There is debate about association between neural lesion and other signs of atypia, such as apex left thoracic curve, rapid progression (moderate estimate >3 degrees *per mensem*), male gender, dystrophic curve (short and sharp, Harrington factor >5 degrees/segment), or otherwise unusual appearance curve (e.g., long and sweeping akin to a neuromuscular presentation).

Classification

Morphologic Curves are divided into six types [I]. Main refers to a structural thoracic curve in the setting of an upper structural thoracic curve. Major refers to a structural curve when thoracic and lumbar regions are affected independently, and the largest of two or three structural curves. Nonstructural refers to a compensatory curve that may be spared fusion.

- Main thoracic. Structural thoracic curve.
- Double thoracic. Two structural thoracic curves.
- Double major. Structural thoracic + lumbar curves.
- Triple major. Two thoracic + thoracolumbar/lumbar structural curves.
- Thoracolumbar or lumbar curve.
- Thoracolumbar or lumbar + thoracic structural curves.

Thoracic curves are modified based upon kyphosis:

- − hypo-, defined as <10 degrees
- N, normal
- + hyper-, defined as >40 degrees

Lumbar curves are modified based upon whether central sacral line:

- A bisects the apical pedicles.
- B touches apical vertebral pedicles.
- C is medial to the apical vertebra.

Classification applies order based upon pattern recognition, but variability argues against dogma. An alternative is the descriptive approach.

- Curve magnitude. This is defined in the coronal plane. Sagittal plane is most predictive of functional outcome. Appearance is most influenced by rotation in the transverse plane.
- Type of curve. This is a geographic assessment based upon location of apical vertebra: thoracic, which may be single or double (termed main and upper); lumbar; combined thoracic and lumbar; and thoracolumbar (T12-L1 apex).
- Flexibility of curve. This is based upon intervertebral disc inclination. Discs that are inflexible are part of a structural curve. Flexible discs are part of what may be a compensatory curve that rectifies or does not progress upon treatment of the structural curve and as such may be spared direct treatment. Curves flexible to <25 degrees also may be excluded.
- Relation to midline. A curve that crosses the midline is structural. A curve that is returning to the midline from a structural curve, for example, the lumbar spine returning to the pelvis, represents compensation by the flexible spine.
- Sagittal contour. Thoracic curves may be associated with hypokyphosis, lordosis, or hyperkyphosis. This is more difficult to correct than coronal curvature. Increased power of instrumentation exposes anterior overgrowth and loss of thoracic kyphosis with increasing coronal correction. Sagittal contour is essential to determination of end instrumented vertebrae. Sagittal balance correlates more directly with functional outcome than coronal balance. Hyperkyphosis of the thoracic spine may be the most sensitive predictor of associated neural lesion.
- Coronal and sagittal balance. Imbalance is associated with poor functional outcome, most in the sagittal plane.
- Rotation in the transverse plane. This is predictive of progression, in addition to curve magnitude. It may serve as an alert that a flexible curve may not be compensatory.
- Atypia. This may be an indication for MRI of the neuraxis.

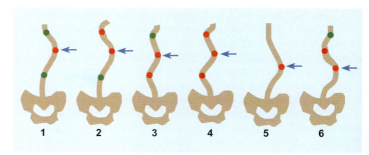

I Classification of scoliosis—morphologic Fusion is indicated for structural curve, represented by *red. Green* signifies a compensatory curve that may be spared. Main and major curves are structural and largest (*blue*).

Type	Comment
Infantile <3 years	• <5% • Boys 2 times girls • Most thoracic curves apex left • Extrinsic cause suggested by associated "packaging" signs including torticollis, plagiocephaly, hip dysplasia • Resolving or progressive—calculate Rib–Vertebral Angle Difference and Phase
Juvenile 3–10 years	• High rate of associated neural lesion ≤1/3 • High rate of progression ≤2/3
Adolescent >10 years	• >80% of all cases

J Classification of scoliosis—clinical Three types are distinguished according to age.

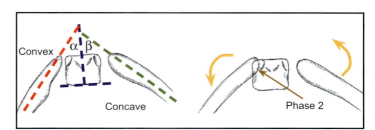

K Rib–vertebral angle difference (RVAD) and phase Determine angle subtended by the axis of the rib (*red, green*) and vertical axis of the body of the apical vertebra (*blue*). RVAD = α − β. The difference results from hinging of the ribs as the spine curves away from the convex set toward the convex set. Greater than 80% of curves with RVAD <20 degrees will not progress. RVAD >20 degrees is associated with >80% progression.

On the right, the curve is in phase 2, which is defined as overlap of the convex rib head with apical vertebra (*brown*) and in which progression is certain. Such a curve is termed "progressive" type. Phase 2 is a manifestation of rotation displacing the apical vertebra anterior to the apical rib so far that the overlap becomes radiographically visible even in the incompletely ossified skeleton. Phase 1, exemplified by the figure on the left, is defined as no overlap: such curves do not progress and are known as "resolving."

Clinical Idiopathic scoliosis may be classified according to age [J].

INFANTILE This is rare and distinct from juvenile, which may be considered a graver form of adolescent. It may be divided into two types: resolving and progressive. The former is unique in potential for spontaneous correction, which along with associated packaging signs suggest a unique cause, at least for this subgroup. Progression may be predicted by the rib–vertebra angle difference and phase [K].

JUVENILE This is distinguished by a high rate of associated neural lesion (up to 1/3) and the highest rate of progression (up to 2/3). The former is an indication for MRI of the neuraxis. The latter adds urgency: more patients will require treatment, earlier and more aggressively.

Natural History

Understanding of natural history is founded in the classic studies from the University of Iowa [A]. While they are revered due to their 50-year follow-up, which is unrivaled in orthopædic surgery, there is not absolute clarity.

Progression The principal determinants of progression are growth and curve magnitude. Risk of progression to surgery is what patients and parents most want to know. Progression has been the most consistent outcome measure in the literature of idiopathic scoliosis. Deformity has the potential to progress during growth. All juvenile idiopathic scoliosis >20 degrees progresses [B]. If the threshold of 30 degrees is crossed in the first decade, scoliosis will progress beyond 50 degrees (to fusion) despite nonoperative treatment (bracing).

Pulmonary function This is the principal concern of thoracic scoliosis. Curve magnitude, location, and rotation conspire to produce pulmonary disease, of which essential features are spinal encroachment upon thoracic viscera, reduced thoracic dimensions, and disruption of mechanics of ribs and respiratory muscles (intercostal and diaphragm). Alveolar and pulmonary vascular hyperplasia cedes to hypertrophy toward the end of the first decade, as growth moves from increasing numbers to increasing size of preexisting structure.

Diminution in pulmonary function testing, in particular total lung capacity and forced vital capacity as measures of restrictive lung disease, may be observed at 60 degrees of scoliosis. Clinically apparent pulmonary dysfunction, such as dyspnœa on exertion and sleep hypopnœa or apnœa, occurs at 90 degrees. Spine fusion with instrumented correction of deformity in idiopathic scoliosis may arrest pulmonary decline or even improve function by up to 10%. By contrast, costal osteotomy or thoracotomy, for example, for anterior approach, may reduce pulmonary function by a similar amount, although the effect may be temporary.

Back pain This is the principal concern of lumbar scoliosis. Back pain affects 2/3 of children with scoliosis. It is related to fatigue of muscles resisting progressive deformity and imbalance. Spine fusion reduces pain but not for every patient and not always completely. Long-term pain is related to degenerative changes at facet joints and intervertebral discs that are malaligned (abnormal force vector) or spared fusion (force concentration). Untreated severe scoliosis is associated with increased pain quantitatively; for example, in the Iowa experience, it occurred "frequently or daily" 50% more than controls. There is a qualitative increase in back pain as well, such as less physically demanding employment and more frequent disability claims. Controversy and lack of further granularity remain, in large part due to the difficulty of measuring an effect when back pain is so prevalent in the general population.

- Thoracic curves progress more than lumbar or thoracolumbar curves.
- Curves > 50 degrees tend to progress, but ~ 1/3 do not.
- Progression of curves averages ~ 30 degrees
- Curves > 90 degrees do not progress.
- Thoracic deformity > 90 degrees significantly impairs pulmonary function.
- Lumbar deformity increases back pain.

A   Natural history of scoliosis The Iowa experience.

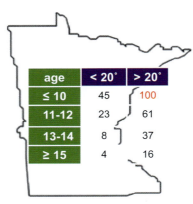

age	< 20°	> 20°
≤ 10	45	100
11-12	23	61
13-14	8	37
≥ 15	4	16

B   Progression is influenced by growth and curve magnitude The Minnesota experience drew attention to the at-risk group of juvenile scoliosis with significant curvature. This has been refined to progression in <10 years of age >30 degrees to severe deformity and fusion.

Appearance The Iowa studies noted that untreated patients with scoliosis were more self-conscious of appearance. For surgically treated patients, the Spinal Appearance Questionnaire and the Scoliosis Research Society Appearance domain show large effect size, demonstrating that they are sensitive enough to measure treatment effects. By contrast, Scoliosis Research Society Activity, Pain and Mental domains show small effect sizes and standardized response means, demonstrating an immeasurable effect on these functional outcomes by operation. Appearance matters, both to patients and because it is the factor most effectively treated.

Management

The pillars of management are education, observation, bracing, and surgery. Education is all encompassing. For example, educate parents that "doing nothing" by observation is a legitimate form of treatment, as most curves do not progress significantly and as such do not cause long-term disability. Patient characteristics that drive management are curve magnitude and age.

Observation 10 to 30 degrees Obtain röntgenogrammes every 6 months through maturity.

Bracing 30 to 50 degrees Institute at 25 degrees for the high-risk child, in particular in the first decade. This is the standard of care for the growing skeleton. The principle that underpins bracing is application of contralateral forces through the ribs or flank against the limbs of the spine on either side of the apex. The multiplicity of braces and regimens exemplifies the axiom that permeates surgery: "Where there is variability there is uncertainty." The Boston brace as well as full-time wear (as opposed to night time) have the broadest experience [A]. While a curve may be corrected in a brace, success of bracing is defined as arrest of progression. Factors associated with brace failure include thoracic lordosis, high thoracic apex, obesity and poor compliance, as well as curve >30 degrees in the first decade.

- Custom brace fabrication to the patient and röntgenogramme.
- Wean to full-time wear, defined as >20 hours *per diem*.
- Doff brace day before serial follow-up röntgenogrammes.
- Don brace until maturity.

Such treatment at such a critical developmental period carries a psychosocial cost that, while difficult to measure (unlike, e.g., angle of scoliosis), is real and may endure after cessation of active care.

Casting 30 to 50 degrees This is indicated for infantile idiopathic scoliosis. Serial casts are applied every 2 to 4 months from 2 to 4 years of age under general anæsthesia. Reduction of spine deformity is based upon derotation as opposed to direct force. Distinctive features of the cast include minimal padding, stable purchase on the pelvis as the foundation, and windows to allow for dynamic correction. Success is defined as continual curve correction to resolution (cure), arrest of progression that is maintained by casting followed by bracing, or delay of operation. Assessment of efficacy is impacted by limited experience given rarity of condition, uncertainty about natural history, as well as significant intra- and interobserver error in RVAD and phase determination.

Operation 30 to 50 degrees fusionless Patients in the first decade with a curve >30 degrees, and premenarcheal girls with curves >40 degrees, have a high likelihood of progression to fusion despite bracing. In the former group, fusion in the first decade limits growth of the spine and thereby reduces thoracic volume enough to negatively impact clinical pulmonary function. The latter group is approaching the magnitude for fusion with significant growth remaining, including the curve acceleration phase before menarche. For these groups, operation is an alternative. The goal of fusionless surgery is to tether the convexity of a curve, which is growing more rapidly. This may arrest progression (as an internal brace) or allow for correction with concave growth, at which point the tether may removed. The latter distinguishes this modality from bracing.

Growth modulation by physeal tethering is well established, in particular at the distal femur and proximal tibia for *genu valgum et varum*. Application of the technique in the spine differs in that implants are placed between bones across a motion segment, which theoretically increases the risk of failure. There are two types of fusionless operations, performed by telescope or open on the anterior spine, which may restore kyphosis in the thoracic region but has the potential to reduce lordosis in the lumbar region. As with *genu valgum et varum*, implant removal is indicated if there is anatomic correction.

VERTEBRAL BODY STAPLING [B] This is indicated for juvenile idiopathic scoliosis 30 to 39 degrees. Vertebral end plates and intervertebral discs are spanned by a two- or four-pronged NiTiNOL staple, which is inserted ice-cold and with straight tines that return to the original curved shape as the memory metal warms to body temperature. The innovation of curved NiTiNOL has eliminated the complication of staple back out. The procedure has the advantage of sparing the intercostal vessels, which may be mobilized away during insertion of, and rest between, staples.

SCREW AND CORD [C] The ideal candidate is a child with a curve 40 to 60 degrees and having more than 2 years of growth remaining. The latter may be estimated as premenarche in a girl and no facial hair in a boy, or according to the arithmetic method as under 12 years for a girl and under 14 years for a boy. Other measures of significant growth potential include open triradiate cartilage and no Risser sign.

Hydroxyapatite coating of vertebral body screws is designed to reduce pullout. Screw insertion requires intercostal vessels ligation. Washers support screw fixation. A flexible polyester cord fixed to the screws is tensioned to effect a partial reduction and resist convexity growth.

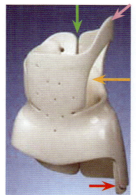

A Boston brace Thoracolumbosacral orthotic (TLSO) is custom fabricated based upon patient shape and röntgenogramme from hard plastic lined by dense foam with pads placed according to morphology of curve. It opens in the back (*green*), is indented to fit the waist above the iliac crests, and includes opening (*orange*) and greater trochanteric extension (*red*) to allow three-point bend. Note that the highest extension is axillary (*pink*) reducing effectiveness for curves with apex above T6.

Wean to full-time wear, defined as >20 hours per diem. Doff brace day before serial follow-up röntgenogrammes. Don brace until maturity.

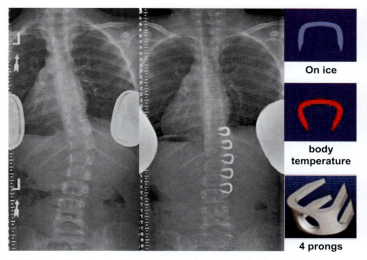

On ice

body temperature

4 prongs

B Vertebral body stapling Correction in 7-year-old girl with 32-degree thoracolumbar curve. NiTiNOL (NIckel–TItanium Naval Ordnance Laboratory), a memory metal, has eliminated implant back out.

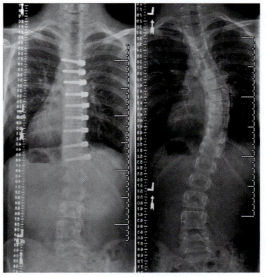

C Screw and cord Correction by tethering the convex side of the spine, which is growing more rapidly. While overall correction is complete, segmental correction varies because segmental growth – normal and asymmetric – is variable.

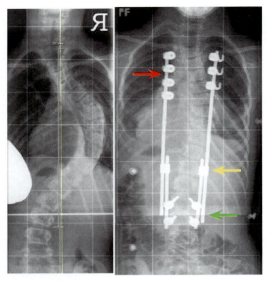

D   Growing rods A 7-year-old girl with 75-degree thoracic curve. Two rods and pedicle screws at a lower end fusion (*green*) improve stability. Modification of upper anchors to the ribs (*red*) increases number of anchors at flexible sites and reduces spine dissection, potentially reducing implant failure and fibrosis. Use of standard implants lengthened at side–side connectors (*yellow*) simplifies index procedure and procedure at maturity.

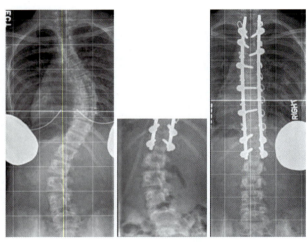

E   Selective fusion The lumbar curve was spared because it was flexible <25 degrees. Early residual curvature spontaneously corrected by 1 year. Transverse process wires at the top instrumented vertebra avoid interference with superjacent facet joints and midline dissection. Screws at the ends reduce construct pullout. Apical screws aid reduction of deformity. There are two anchors at every level, including transverse process wires that are safe and cheap.

Operation >50-degree fusionless Indication for fusionless operation is juvenile scoliosis having curve magnitude too great for vertebral body stapling or screw and cable.

GROWING RODS [D] This is the original fusionless operation. The goal is deformity correction and its maintenance while allowing growth of the spine. It is mechanically disadvantaged: end fixation with intervening motion fails approximately 15% of the time. Advances to enhance stability include the following:

- Two contoured rods with or without cross-links, compared with one straight rod
- End fusion of two vertebrae, compared with anchoring to a single vertebra at each end
- Pedicle screws, compared with laminar hooks

Unlike vertebral body stapling or screw and cable, which rely on spontaneous growth of the concave spine, growing rods lengthen the spine by active distraction. It is biologically disadvantaged: after implantation and initial distraction (which achieves the most elongation), the rods are distracted every 4 months through the same incision. Repeated opening of a scarred wound results in an infection rate up to 10%. Multiple procedures, prolonged instrumentation, and infection lead to fibrosis, possible heterotopic ossification, and stiffening of the spine. At maturity, or as close as is reasonable based upon patient tolerance of multiple procedures and complications, definitive fusion is performed.

Operation >50-degree fusion Indication for fusion is risk of progression regardless of growth, as the spine decompensates into advancing deformity. The goals of operation are safety, fusion, and correction.

- Safety. "To do no harm" is the primary ethical imperative. Pertinent factors are discussed under *Complications*.
- Fusion. This is augmented by osseous graft and decortication.
  — Autogenous graft from iliac crest adds time and pain (although the latter may not be clinically significant compared with overall pain of operation) and may add a separate incision. Autogenous graft also may be obtained by harvest of spinous processes, and from ribs, as part of thoracoplasty. Allogenous graft is as effective as autogenous, saves time but adds cost (although the latter may not be significant relative to overall cost of operation, including implants) and does not require second incision. Bone graft substitutes and adjuvants are not indicated in primary operation.
  — Decortication simulates fracture to stimulate adjacent vertebrae to heal to one another. This may be performed with burr or gouge. The latter lifts strips of bone from transverse processes and laminæ that may bridge vertebrae without the heat of a motorized tool.
  — Facet joint excision aids fusion and correction.
  — Selective fusion maximizes remaining motion of the spine and reduces risk. As in the assessment of maturity, selection of fusion levels cannot rely on any single factor nor can it be formulaic; rather, it is a synthesis of several concepts [E, F].

Principle	Comment
Structural curve	*Fuse.*
Compensatory curve	Bending röntgenogrammes show opposite bending of intervertebral discs and curve <25 degrees. *Spare.*
Stable vertebra	Each end vertebra must be crossed by center sacral line.
Neutral vertebra	Pedicle screw instrumentation may shift this by vertebral derotation to limit fusion.
Sagittal contour	End vertebrae must be out of kyphosis.
Rotation	May represent a structural component independent of coronal magnitude or flexibility
Shoulder height	Extend fusion proximalward in order to pull down a shoulder elevated opposite apex of thoracic curve.
Thoracolumbar junction	T12 lowest instrumented vertebra associated with increased risk of junctional kyphosis–stop at L1
Obliquity	Obliquity of lowest instrumented vertebra >15 degrees may be associated with progression and poor long term outcome.

F   Selection of fusion levels

- Correction. This is achieved by instrumentation, osteotomy, and vertebral resection.
  — Akin to cement technique in arthroplasty, posterior instrumentation has developed in generations [G]. Harrington introduced a rod with lamina hooks at end ratchets for reduction of scoliosis by distraction. Luque used lamina wires for segmental fixation and translation. Wires also may be applied to spinous and transverse processes. Cotrel and Dubousset reduced the spine by rod rotation applied through lamina and pedicle hooks and added cross-links between two rods to enhance construct stability. Pedicle screws are most stable, which reduces anchor failure at ends of fusion to; in addition, they enable correction of the third dimension of deformity by vertebral derotation, both at the apex to improve appearance and at the ends to shift the neutral vertebra in order to minimize fusion and maximize preservation of motion.
  — While pedicle screws are the most stable anchor, correction is more related to ante-operative flexibility and number of anchors. Optimal correction for ante-operative flexibility is ≥ 1.5 anchors/ level.
  — In scoliosis correction, Ponte modification of Smith-Petersen osteotomy enhances restoration of lumbar lordosis. Pedicle subtraction osteotomy includes the pedicle as it extends across the three columns of the spine to correct focal kyphosis in revision operation. Vertebral resection is reserved for severe and stiff deformity and for congenital disease.
  — It remains debated whether rib osteotomy, for example, thoracoplasty to reduce posterior prominence and improve appearance, and rib resection, for example, in concavity to aid curve correction, improve functional outcome, particularly in light of potential deleterious impact on pulmonary function.

Posterior approach to the spine is the oldest, most familiar and most versatile. Posterior osteotomies have equalized levels of fusion with anterior approach. Posterior osteotomies have reduced the need for anterior operation to loosen a stiff curve. Posterior circumferential dissection makes vertebral resection possible without, and even easier than, adding an anterior approach. Anterior approach has a rôle.

- It may enable better correction and even overcorrection to limit fusion levels, as it allows pushing against the deformity in contrast with pulling from behind [H]. Pushing more readily translates a lowest instrumented vertebra that is not crossed by the center sacral line and reduces obliquity of the subjacent spared vertebra. The isolated major thoracolumbar or lumbar curve is ideal for anterior operation [I].
- Absence of posterior elements for sufficient surface area for fusion, or previous posterior pseudarthrosis.
- In the immature spine, continued anterior growth about a posterior fusion axis may produce the "crankshaft phenomenon." Pedicle screws, which lock the anterior column to posterior instrumentation, have made this obsolete. In addition, fusionless modalities have reduced indications for fusion in the first decade.
- The increased primary morbidity of the anterior approach must be balanced by its significantly lower rate of infection compared with the posterior approach.

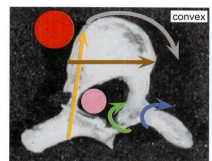

G   Vertebral anchors Vertebral body is rotated (*gray*) toward convexity. Concave pedicle is narrower and shorter. Pedicle screw (*orange*) navigates between spinal cord (*pink*) and great vessel (*red*). Laminar hook or wire (*green*) enters canal. Transverse process hook or wire (*blue*) avoids canal. Vertebral body screw (*brown*) serves as an anterior anchor.

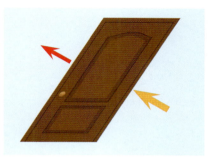

H   Spine as door Leaning door is more easily rectified by pushing (*orange*), akin to anterior correction of the spine, than pulling (*red*), as is the mechanism in posterior correction.

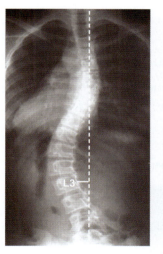
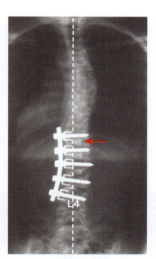

I   Anterior operation Overcorrection spares L4 and brings it horizontal (*red*). One or two rods may be used, with vertebral body screws and staples. Intervertebral cages, in this case allogenous fibula (*green*), support sagittal contour to maintain lordosis.

Complication	Rate
Hæmorrhage requiring transfusion	<10%
Infection	1%
Neural injury	<1%
Superior mesenteric artery syndrome	<<1%
Pancreatitis	<10%
Pseudarthrosis	2%
Reoperation	10%

A Complication rate Primary spine fusion with instrumentation for adolescent idiopathic scoliosis is safe.

Modality	Comment
Somatosensory-evoked potential	Spinal cord—dorsal column and medial lemniscus pathway. Continuous. **Alarm**: ↓50% amplitude, ↑10% latency
Motor-evoked potential	Spinal cord—corticospinal tract. Triggered. Most sensitive to injury. Most sensitive to blood pressure, inhalation anaesthetic, body temperature, younger age. **Alarm**: ↓80% from 1 muscle site
Electromyography	Nerve root. • Spontaneous. **Alarm**: high frequency high amplitude trains • Triggered by direct implant stimulation. **Alarm** : ≤6 mA suggests osseous breach
Wake up test	Non-specific assessment of motor function. *Post facto.* Requires patient comprehension and risks excessive movement.

B Neural monitoring during spine surgery There are four modalities.

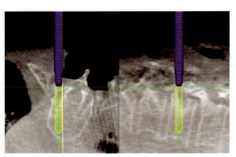

C Operative CT Navigation aids instrumentation. Drill sleeve is *blue*, length is measured by *green* ruler, and location of selected width pedicle screw is projected as *yellow*.

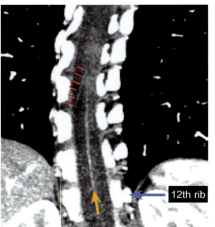

D CT angiogramme Segmental medullary artery of Adamkiewicz (*red*) arises from the 10th intercostal segmental vessels and travels proximalward to the spinal artery (*orange*). This patient underwent anterior convex instrumentation that skipped the 10th vertebra.

12th rib

Complications

Complications are rare but potentially spectacular [A].

Hæmorrhage This may be limited by:

- Positioning with the abdomen free to reduce external pressure on the vertebral venous plexuses (e.g., Relton-Hall frame).
- Hypotensive anæsthesia. This must be balanced with normal blood pressure or hypertension to protect spinal cord perfusion, in particular during correction and fluid shifts over time.
- Surgical technique, including subperiosteal dissection, diathermy, wound packing.
- Antithrombolytic agents *per venam*, as well as gelatin, thrombin, and other agents *in situ*.
- Autogenous blood recovery system.

Infection The skin is the single greatest barrier to infection, and spinal deformity wounds are large. Infection rate is approximately 1%, compared with up to 15% for neuromuscular scoliosis. Infection may be limited by:

- Sterile technique, including Chlorhexidine and bleach for skin.
- Antibiotics. Administer within 30 minutes of incision and every 4 hours thereafter, to account for hæmorrhage. Postoperative administration may be single dose and should not exceed 24 hours. Mixture of antibiotics in allogenous osseous graft or lavage may be effective.
- Efficacy of other practices, such as limiting personnel, use of a sterile adhesive drape, changing of clothing and instruments, occluding suction when not in use, is difficult to demonstrate.
- Treatment includes incision and drainage, irrigation, and débridement of wound and spine. Remove loose osseous graft. Replace loose anchors. Insert drains, which are removed when the wound is sealed. Retain implants until robust fusion, at which point implant removal allows cure.

Neural injury This is the gravest concern for the patient and family.

- Minor injury includes positional neurapraxia. Most frequent is compression of the lateral femoral cutaneous nerve at the anterior iliac crest, but motor neurapraxias may occur, such as femoral nerve compression at the brim of the pelvis.
- Major injury may be central, at the spinal cord level, or peripheral, at the nerve root level. Neural monitoring includes somatosensory and motor-evoked potentials and electromyography [B]. Wake-up test may supplement these modalities. Keep implants out of the canal. Operative imaging, with image intensifier, röntgenogrammes, or CT, aids instrumentation [C]. Consider CT angiography in preparation for anterior instrumentation in order to look for dominant perfusion of the spinal cord from the side of operation [D]. Temporarily and atraumatically clamp intercostal vessels before ligation to ensure no change in neural signals.
- The risk of major neural injury is under 1%. Most children will demonstrate at least partial recovery. Ischæmic injury, such as after intercostal vessel ligation, shows least recovery.
- Treatment is complex and multifactorial. Observe positional neurapraxias, which recover spontaneously. In the event of neural signal changes, consider reversal of operative steps, for example, replace implant or relieve correction. Raise blood pressure, blood count, and body temperature. Modify anæsthetic agents. Administration of steroids *per venam* is controversial. CT myelogramme will outline vertebral canal in case of encroachment. Lumbar catheter will decompress vertebral canal in the event of spinal cord swelling.

Superior mesenteric artery syndrome This also is known as "cast syndrome," from its occurrence after the application of extension casts for spinal fracture. This is caused by compression of the third part of the duodenum between superior mesenteric artery and aorta (angle <25 degrees) when the trunk is stretched after the spine is corrected. It typically occurs in tall and thin girls (less mesenteric fat), who present with nausea and vomiting, epigastric pain, and abdominal distension. Evaluation includes a dynamic contrast radiography. Treatment consists of left decubitus or prone positioning, intravenous fluids, abdominal rest and decompression, and in persistent cases total parenteral nutrition. Extremely rarely, division of the ligament of Treitz to release the duodenum, or duodenojejunostomy to bypass the point of obstruction, may be necessary.

Pancreatitis This is underdiagnosed after spinal fusion, because pain, nausea, loss of appetite are nonspecific. Theories include pancreatic hypoperfusion, altered anatomy, or complement activation, for example, by an autogenous blood recovery system. The presentation may resemble that of superior mesenteric artery syndrome, from which it is distinguished by elevated serum lipase (more sensitive and specific) and amylase. Treatment includes abdominal rest, intravenous fluids and, if persistent, hyperalimentation.

Progression of deformity In the instrumented curve, this may be due to pseudarthrosis or the crankshaft phenomenon. In the latter, posterior fusion acts like an axis about which the spine may turn with continued anterior growth to produce progressive deformity. The phenomenon does not occur after peak growth velocity and curve acceleration phase. Operations on children before these time points should include anterior fusion to avoid crankshaft. In the spared spine, curve progression may be seen in younger patients in whom fusion was performed in the early stages of development of structural curvature. Alternatively, this may occur after zealous correction that exceeds the degree to which the spared spine can compensate. This prioritizes spine balance over curve correction.

Pseudarthrosis The rate of pseudarthrosis after spinal deformity surgery is up to 2% in children, compared with up to 10 times in adults [E]. Principal causes are surgical technique and infection. Most present within the first 3 years, including persistent pain, progression of deformity, and implant failure. CT gives detail of pseudarthrosis and implant failure. Management consists of exploration of the entire spine, as multiple pseudarthroses may be present, possible opposite approach for a fresh bed for grafting, and revision instrumentation as necessary.

Venous thromboembolism, a serious complication of adult spine surgery, occurs so rarely in children that it does not warrant prophylaxis. Overall rate of secondary operation during childhood is approximately 10%.

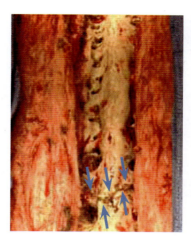

E Pseudarthrosis This was discovered at implant removal for chronic infection.

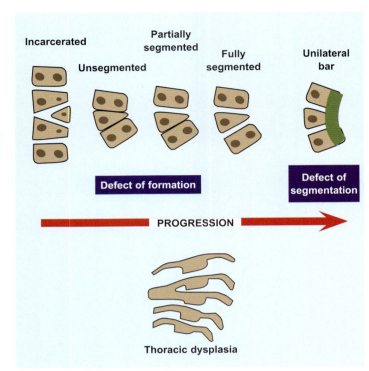

A **Simplified classification of congenital scoliosis** Heterogeneity and multiplicity undermine utility, leading to continual efforts to subclassify.

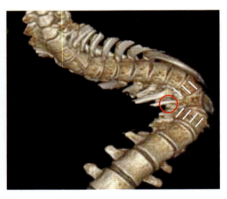

B **CT of congenital scoliosis** Unilateral bar (*red*) opposite hemivertebra (*white*) is associated with greatest progression.

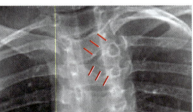
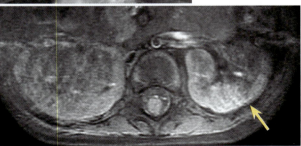

C **Incarcerated hemivertebra** Outlined by red. No progression over 3 years. MRI spine also showed solitary kidney (*yellow*).

CONGENITAL SCOLIOSIS

This is defined as scoliosis produced by vertebral anomaly. It is classified based upon presence of tether around which growth may accelerate deformity and growth potential at vertebral physes [A].

Evaluation

Because development of the vertebrae is associated most closely with that of the neuraxis, genitourinary system, and heart, evaluation must encompass all these systems, including appropriate subspecialist referral. Vertebral anomaly may be seen in association with other anomalies, such as exemplified by VACTERL (Vertebra, Anal atresia, Cardiac anomaly, Tracheo-Esophageal fistula, Renal anomaly, Limb anomaly). In addition, congenital scoliosis may represent one part of a greater regional disorder that results in thoracic dysplasia, including chest wall and viscera.

Imaging Röntgenogrammes provide the initial assessment of type and magnitude and subsequent assessments of progression. CT defines osseous anatomy and is essential during operative preparation [B]. MRI evaluates the neuraxis for associated lesion, which is seen in approximately 1/3 of patients [C]. Abdominal ultrasonogramme screens the renal system. Echocardiogramme screens the heart.

Management

Observation Progression depends upon growth, in particular during infancy and puberty, and type of anomaly. Follow progression with serial röntgenogrammes. Three-fourths of curves will progress significantly, and up to 1/2 will require operative treatment. Postpone operative treatment, if necessary, until after 5 years of age, if possible: consider observation of the supine rather than the upright spine, following flexibility and ensuring that compensatory curves have not become stiff. Bracing is ineffective.

Operation After 5 years of age, balance the goal of further longitudinal growth with focal operation on an isolated lesion before secondary structural deformation of the spine occurs. The former approach will consist of a limited fusion while the latter may require extension over a broad segment of the spine.

POSTERIOR FUSION This is safest. The ideal indication is a second decade child and a curve that is sufficiently flexible and mild–moderate that a fusion will not be too long to balance the spine.

ANTERIOR AND POSTERIOR FUSION This is indicated for a child in the first decade. It may be performed to obtain greater correction and thereby limit levels of fusion, and in order to prevent crankshaft, although the latter is less of a concern in congenital scoliosis due to circumferential growth disturbance compared with idiopathic scoliosis.

VERTEBRAL RESECTION This may be performed by simultaneous anterior and posterior approach performed with the young patient in the decubitus position when the anomaly is discrete or staged anterior followed by posterior in the older patient with severe deformity. Alternatively, this may be performed by a posterior approach [D].

- Insert anchors before resection.
- Identify and excise anomalous posterior elements.
- Disarticulate and excise corresponding rib heads.
- Excise corresponding transverse processes.
- Ligate thoracic nerve roots as necessary.
- Develop interval between spine and pleura or peritoneum, placing circumferential retractors.
- Identify cranial and caudal intervertebral discs. Discs serve as limits of resection, which begins by discectomy.
- Insert temporary rod to stabilize spine.
- Resect bone. This may be *in toto* in a young patient with a discrete anomaly, or sequentially starting with pedicles and removing posterior cortex of vertebral body last to protect spinal cord.
- Complete instrumentation, including anterior support as indicated.
- Reduction must be controlled and must not lengthen the spine.

THORACIC INSUFFICIENCY SYNDROME

The chest is deformed *in toto*: it can support neither pulmonary function nor pulmonary growth. Thoracic dysplasia with pulmonary insufficiency drive management in the first decade of life, which is aimed at restoring and maintaining thoracic volume in order to support lung development and function. Congenital scoliosis (incorporated in the term "spondylothoracic dysplasia") may be one component and is treated secondarily.

Evaluation

Röntgenogrammes measure thoracic dimensions as well as spine curvature. CT allows calculation of chest and lung volume. Spirometry may be limited by patient participation given age and disease burden.

Management

Thoraco(s)tomy and expansion The thorax is opened according to location of deformity, including costal and spine anomalies [A]. Cranial hook and cap are attached to the ribs, circumferential and forgiving to tolerate motion during respiration. Caudal implants may be attached to the ribs, lumbar spine by means of lamina hooks, or pelvis by looping over and into iliac crest.

While the procedure has the potential to rescue affected children from pulmonary collapse, it carries the significant costs of multiple procedures, implant failure, infection, and fibrosis of the chest wall with time.

Secondary Scoliosis

Scoliosis represents the effect on the spine of a primary problem [A] and as such is not structural. This type is distinguished by:

- Complete resolution ("cure") by complete treatment of the underlying disorder
- Absence of vertebral rotation

Lower limb length discrepancy Tilting of the pelvis results in obliquity of takeoff of the lumbar spine, which curves back toward the midline in order to balance the head on the pelvis. Curvature of the spine will not become structural because not enough time in a day is spent erect with both feet on the ground to tilt the pelvis.

EVALUATION Place a block under the respective foot to bring the pelvis horizontal. Alternatively, examine the spine sitting or in the prone position. The deformity will thereby be eliminated. Side bending shows that the spine can be curved opposite to the presenting deformity. Röntgenogrammes with a block under the foot equal to the discrepancy will show a straight spine.

MANAGEMENT This follows general principles for lower limb length discrepancy. Do not let concern for scoliosis lead to unnecessarily treatment, for example, shoe lift.

Pain Scoliosis may be the presenting sign for several inflammatory disorders. Curvature of the spine splints against pain. In contrast to scoliosis secondary to lower limb length discrepancy, the deformity may not be influenced by position (if pain is not) and may not be flexible (opposite bending may exacerbate pain).

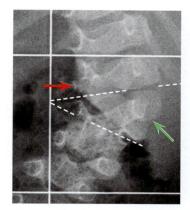
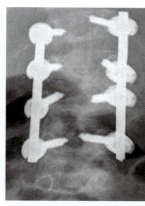

D Posterior vertebral resection for congenital scoliosis MRI confirmed incompletely ossified unilateral bar (*red*) and hemivertebra (*green*). After removal of posterior elements, anterior hemivertebra was resected *in toto* by following planes through intervertebral discs (*white*).

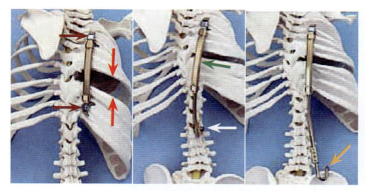

A Vertical Expandable Prosthetic Titanium Rib (VEPTR) Thoracotomy permits expansion of the chest by a growing implant (*green*) that anchors to the ribs (*brown*), lumbar lamina (*white*), or iliac crest (*orange*). [www.pmda.go.jp].

Primary cause		Comment
Lower limb length discrepancy		Compensatory to lumbosacral obliquity produced by pelvic tilt
Pain	Infection	Discitis
Pain	Deformity	Spondylolisthesis
Pain	Tumor	Osseous, e.g., osteoid osteoma Neural

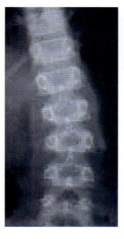

A Secondary scoliosis The deformity is not structural and resolves with resolution of the primary disorder. It is distinguished by limitation to a coronal plane deformity with absence of transverse plane deformity. Imaging shows no vertebral rotation.

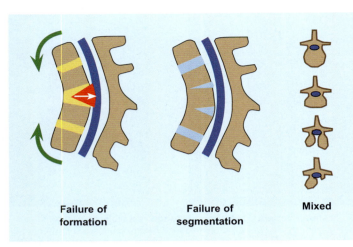

A Classification of congenital kyphosis Increasing flexion of the spine can propel a hemivertebra into the vertebral canal, where the spinal cord is draped over and restricted by the gibbus. Variability of anomalies is captured under the mixed type.

Failure of formation | Failure of segmentation | Mixed

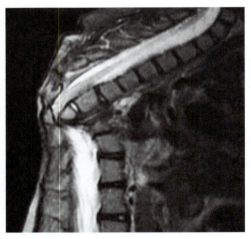

B Congenital kyphosis This presents the highest neural risk of spine deformity in children.

CONGENITAL KYPHOSIS

Like congenital scoliosis, it is defined as kyphosis produced by vertebral anomaly. It is classified as failure of formation, failure of segmentation, and mixed, including rotatory type [A]. It may be distinguished from congenital scoliosis in being rarer and graver, because the plane of deformity deflects the vertebral column directly toward the spinal cord while simultaneously restricting its motion.

Evaluation

Like congenital scoliosis, evaluation must encompass neuraxis, genito-urinary system, and heart. Failure of formation and mixed types are more progressive, and present a greater neural risk, than failure of segmentation. While the tether in failure of segmentation creates deformity, the lack of tether in failure of formation allows sagittal displacement of the hemivertebra toward the neuraxis. Mixed lesions may include rotatory subluxation or dislocation, which also compromises the vertebral canal. Most patients with congenital kyphosis are asymptomatic in the first decade. Adolescents may complain of back pain due to subjacent lumbar hyperlordosis, which is compensatory to maintain sagittal balance. Progressive deformity, or trauma in the setting of severe deformity, may present with neural deficit. Neurologic examination is essential. Evaluate flexibility by draping the small child over the knee or by asking the older child to push up with the hands in the prone position. Associated scoliosis tends to be mild and is treated secondarily.

Imaging Röntgenogrammes provide the initial assessment of type and magnitude, and subsequent assessments of progression. Hyperextension röntgenogrammes evaluate flexibility. CT defines osseous anatomy and is essential during operative preparation. MRI evaluates the vertebral canal for encroachment and neuraxis for injury [B]. Urodynamic testing is helpful in the setting of neural changes.

Management

Observation Progression depends upon growth and type of anomaly. Follow progression with serial röntgenogrammes. Bracing is ineffective.

Operation The young deformed spine is technically challenging to instrument. Incomplete ossification makes excision difficult: gristle is tougher than bone.

POSTERIOR FUSION This is safest. It is indicated in the child <5 years of age with curve <50 degrees. The tether produced by fusion may lead to spontaneous improvement of deformity with anterior growth, although this is unpredictable as it is inherently abnormal. A hooked construct does not lock the anterior column, thereby not interfering with its potential for growth. Hooks by definition are placed in the vertebral canal, where there is less space available for cord than in scoliosis.

VERTEBRAL RESECTION This is indicated for severe deformity and in the event of neural deficit, in which decompression is necessary. Posterior approach with circumferential dissection is more direct than the addition of an anterior approach, which is farthest from the site of deformity, and safer, as the great vessels and viscera fall forward away from the deformity.

KYPHOSIS OF SCHEUERMANN

Normal thoracic kyphosis is 20 to 50 degrees. Increasing lumbar lordosis compensates for thoracic hyperkyphosis, as in Scheuermann ("Shoyer-man") disease [A]. Hip flexion contracture will drive the spine into lordosis. Sagittal balance is more directly related to functional outcome than coronal balance.

Clinical Features

Pathogenesis This is an osteochondrosis, a growth disturbance producing vertebral wedging, shortening of the anterior column, and kyphosis. Because this is an undergrowth phenomenon, the spine does not buckle to produce concomitant rotation. Scheuermann implicated manual labor in pathogenesis ("apprentice kyphosis"), although the rôle of abnormal load is unclear. There is an undefined heritable component.

Evaluation Onset is in the second decade. Boys are affected more. The disease occasionally occurs in the lumbar spine. Pain is characteristic: this occurs at the apex of deformity and/or at an associated lumbar spondylolysis. Patients are significantly disturbed by the appearance. Scheuermann kyphosis "peaks" with forward bending [B], in contrast with postural round back, which is less severe, more flexible, less acute, and not painful. The skin at the apex of deformity may be roughened due to prominence and lack of flexibility of the spine: this is a sign of decompensation and serves as a functional extraskeletal indication for treatment. There may be associated scoliosis: this tends to be small, not significantly progressive, and as such does not drive management. Compensatory hyperlordosis of the lumbar spine to maintain sagittal balance increases the risk of spondylolysis.

Imaging Röntgenogrammes:

- Allow measurement of kyphosis, after the method of Cobb. This includes lateral fulcrum hyperextension to assess flexibility.
- Show end plate irregularity associated with anterior wedging of vertebrae. The end stage is Schmorl nodes [C]: these represent vertical herniation of intervertebral disc through end plate into vertebral body, where bone may be necrotic.
- Show associated spondylolysis and scoliosis.
- Must be full length standing to enable assessment of spine balance, which is of particular importance in operative cases.

MRI provides detail but may not influence management.

Management

Natural history is not well understood, making treatment recommendations variable. Nonoperative treatment includes the following:

- Symptom control, including activity modification and nonnarcotic analgesics.
- Stretching exercises, focused on the spine (hyperextension), proximal muscles, and posture ("tuck" chin "don't poke" nose).
- Thoracolumbosacral orthotic (TLSO), although evidence for effectiveness, and compliance, are poor.

Operative treatment is indicated for progressive and severe deformity. There is no consensus, influences including pain, patient's perception of appearance, and degree (>75 degrees is a moderate guideline). Issues of relevance to spine fusion with instrumentation include the following:

- Anterior approach for stiff curves. The rate has been reduced by greater understanding and acceptance of posterior osteotomies, in particular Ponte modification of Smith-Petersen [D].
- Multiple (this is diffuse deformity) posterior osteotomies to allow shortening of posterior column by compression instrumentation. This overcomes severity and stiffness of curves, reduces risk of lengthening of the anterior column and associated neural risk, and decreases cantilever force thereby reducing implant failure (which is more frequent than in scoliosis operation).
- Fusion from lordosis to lordosis and stable to stable vertebra. Stopping fusion at a kyphotic level, or posterior to sagittal balance line, risks implant failure and adjacent segment kyphosis.

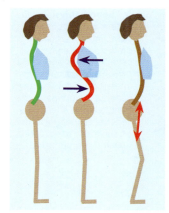

Normal
Scheuermann kyphosis
Neuromuscular disorders

A Spine alignment Spine and pelvis alignment is interconnected. The spine compensates to maintain balance. Note chest dimensions: Scheuermann kyphosis increase thoracic volume unless severe, by contrast with lordosing conditions of the thoracic spine, which reduce pulmonary space.

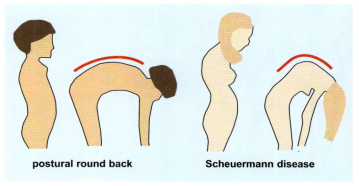

postural round back   Scheuermann disease

B Postural round back from Scheuermann kyphosis Scheuermann kyphosis is exacerbated to a focal angulation with spine flexion.

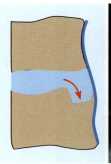 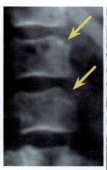 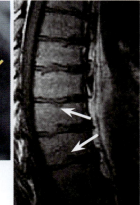

C Schmorl nodes These may be a feature of this osteochondrosis. They may be associated with an increased likelihood of pain.

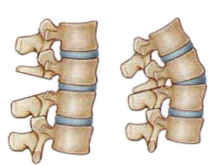

D Posterior osteotomy for Scheuermann kyphosis Resection of adjacent articular processes, ligamentum subflavum with or without spinous processes allows segmental correction (1 degree/mm bone up to 10 degrees/level) of nonfocal kyphosis by shortening posterior column without lengthening anterior column.
[www.srs.org]

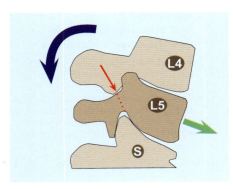

A Spondylolysis With hyperextension of the spine, inferior articular process of superjacent vertebra strikes and (eventually) fractures pars interarticularis of affected vertebra. If both parts are fractured, the affected vertebra can slip forward on subjacent spine, taking with it the entire trunk.

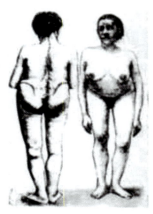

B Spondylolisthesis Neugebauer's original sketch (1895):
• lumbar hyperlordosis
• vertical sacrum
• lumbosacral kyphosis
• lumbosacral step off
• cordiform buttocks
• hip flexion
• knee flexion
• secondary painful scoliosis

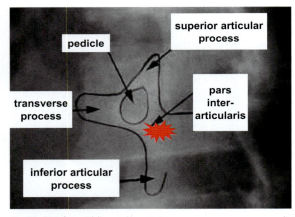

C Scotty dog Oblique view röntgenogramme exposes pars interarticularis.

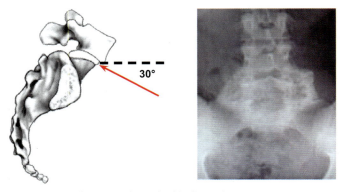

D Ferguson view X-ray beam (*red*) is directed tangent to L5-S1 intervertebral disc for a true orthogonal view of the lumbosacral junction, thereby highlighting fusion mass on röntgenogrammes.

SPONDYLOLYSIS AND SPONDYLOLISTHESIS

Greek σπονδυλη: "*spondyle*," is Latin *vertebra*. Greek λυσις: "*lysis*," is equivalent to Latin *fractura*. Greek ολισθεσις, anglicized as "*olisthy*," means "slipping." Greek πτωσις: "*ptosis*," means "falling down," used of both the eyelid and a vertebra.

Pathogenesis

Spondylolysis refers to a fracture of the pars interarticularis caused by the inferior articular process of the superjacent vertebra during hyperextension of the lumbar spine [A]. In 2/3 of patients, this represents a stress or fatigue type of fracture; however, up to 1/3 of athletes recall a sudden event. Unilateral spondylolysis is stable and more likely to heal with nonoperative treatment. Bilateral spondylolysis disengages the neural arch from the body, which may allow the body with superjacent vertebral column to "slip" relative to the ipsilevel neural arch and remaining subjacent vertebral column. Hyperlordosis and horizontalization of sacrum increase traction and likelihood of olisthy. The traumatic mechanism is reinforced by the fact that spondylolysis occurs with increased frequency in children who participate in certain sports that involve hyperextension with axial loading of the lumbar spine, such as gymnastics, and the fact that it has not been described in the nonambulatory. A genetic predisposition is suggested by familial and racial features (e.g., Eskimos an order of magnitude more than Whites) and by increased incidence in certain diseases (e.g., Marfan syndrome).

Evaluation

History and physical examination Spondylolysis occurs in approximately 5% of the population. Boys are two to three times more affected than do girls. In >80%, L5 is affected. The majority are asymptomatic. However, it is the most common identifiable cause of back pain, which results from micromotion and the inflammatory response of attempted healing. Pain is exacerbated by hyperextension of the lumbar spine, which when performed in single limb stance helps localize a unilateral lysis as the child cannot accommodate for pain by shifting away. Causes of pain in spondylolisthesis include tension on the broken bone, neural compression (foraminal or central), and shear on the intervertebral disc. Spondylolisthesis is two to three times more frequent in girls, which is consistent with the principle that natural history is worse in the gender in which a disease is rarer. Its *forme pleine* is well illustrated in the original sketch of Neugebauer [B]. Phalen and Dickson (1961) described hamstring tightness limiting swing phase to produce a short-stride, shuffling, toe–toe, crouched gait. Children are at highest risk of olisthy during growth acceleration of puberty, although clinically significant progression is <10%.

Imaging Oblique röntgenogrammes bring the pars interarticularis orthogonal to the x-ray beam, thereby exposing spondylolysis. In the Scotty dog representation [C], the transverse process is the nose, the ear is the superior articular process, the eye is the pedicle, the forelimb is the inferior articular process, and the neck is the pars interarticularis. Spondylolysis is said to appear as a collar or a broken neck. Bilateral spondylolysis may be seen on lateral projection röntgenogramme.

Ferguson view, taken with beam directed tangent to L5-S1 intervertebral disc, is a true orthogonal view of the lumbosacral junction and is essential to evaluation of L5-S1 fusion [D]. Standard anteroposterior projection may produce an upside down "Napoleon hat" superimposition of L5 as it has slipped in front of S1.

For spondylolisthesis, several measurements aid assessment [E–G].

• Grade (severity). Myerding divided the top of S1 into quarters. Taillard distinguished olisthy <50% as stable from olisthy >50%, which is unstable. Such reductiveness is functional and akin to, for example, dividing physeal fractures after Salter and Harris into without (I + II) and with (III + IV) articular extension. When the affected vertebra slips off the subjacent one (>100%), this is known as spondyloptosis.

- Sacral inclination. Angle subtended by a tangent to posterior S1 relative to the vertical. The greater the sacral inclination, the more vertical is the axis of body weight, which increases shear on L5 pars interarticularis and L5-S1 intervertebral disc, thereby increasing risk of olisthy.
- Sacral slope. Angle subtended by the horizontal and a line tangent to the top of S1. Increasing sacral slope is associated with increasing shear force. As L5 disengages from S1—in the extreme in spondyloptosis—sacral slope and inclination reduce as the pelvis retroverts.
- Olisthy angle. Angle subtended by a tangent to L5 and a perpendicular to the posterior S1 tangent. This is a measure of lumbosacral lordosis (positive value) or kyphosis (abnormal, stated as a negative value). The latter is an indication of instability, as L5 has begun its fall off S1, and is associated with >50% olisthy.
- Pelvic incidence [G]. Angle subtended by a perpendicular to the top of S1 and a line drawn from the center of S1 to the center of rotation of the hips. If femoral heads are not superimposed, take the midpoint between their centers. Assuming pelvis rotation centered at the hips, pelvic incidence is constant and as such is a patient characteristic. The normal range is 45 to 60 degrees. Increasing pelvic incidence means increasing lordosis and increasing shear force leading to tensile failure. Decreasing pelvic incidence means decreasing lordosis and compressive failure ("nut-cracker" mechanism). Ideal balance is achieved when pelvic incidence equals lumbar lordosis, akin to a thoracic inlet angle equal to cervical lordosis at the upper end of the spine.
- Pelvic tilt [G]. Angle subtended by the vertical and a line drawn from the hip center(s) to the center of the top of S1. By contrast with pelvic incidence, reduction in pelvic tilt brings the lumbosacral junction more vertical, thereby increasing shear force on pars interarticularis and intervertebral disc. Unlike pelvic incidence, pelvic tilt can be altered, for example, with physiotherapy targeted at retroversion of the pelvis to reduce lumbar lordosis to relieve back pain.
- Flexion and extension lateral views aid in determination of flexibility of the olisthy.
- Full length lateral röntgenogramme assesses spine sagittal balance. This is essential to operative planning. For a balanced spine, spondylolisthesis needs no reduction. By contrast, pull L5 back and restore lumbosacral lordosis if that is what is necessary to correct sagittal imbalance. If sagittal balance is not restored, a flexible pædiatric spine may compensate by increasing lumbar lordosis; however, a degenerating, stiffening lumbar spine as the child transitions to adult will expose sagittal imbalance, which now is locked by a fusion at the lumbosacral junction.

Scintigraphy provides a measure of osseous metabolism; as such, it may detect an active spondylolysis that has potential to heal, which may influence decision to brace [H]. Single photon emission computed tomography (SPECT) allows localization of scintigraphic uptake in a vertebra, that is, to the pars interarticularis [I]. Positive scintigramme defines an "acute" spondylolysis.

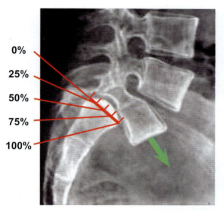

E Spondylolisthesis—grading after Myerding Types I-IV according to % olisthy.

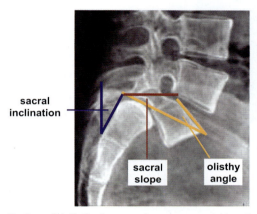

F Spondylolisthesis—angular assessment Note that secondary osseous deformity in chronic conditions introduces imprecision to measurements based upon tangents.

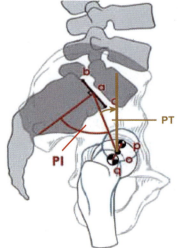

G Pelvic incidence (PI) and pelvic tilt (PT) The assessment of spondylolisthesis has expanded to include the hips. [https://neurosurgerycns.wordpress.com]

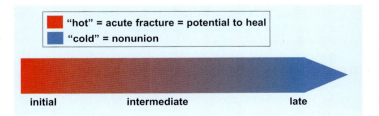

H Scintigraphic activity of spondylolysis Increased uptake (*red*) and/or early detection is an indication for bracing to allow healing of lesion without operative intervention.

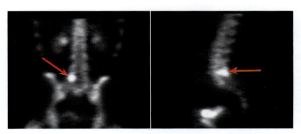

I Single photon emission computed tomography SPECT shows that increased uptake occurs focally in the posterior elements on the right side of L5, at the pars interarticularis.

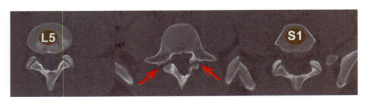

J   CT of Spondylolysis Bilateral atrophic L5 spondylolysis, which appears as an "extra facet joint sign" between L5-L4 and L5-S1 facet joints.

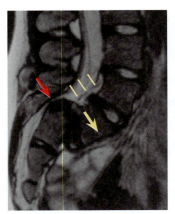

K   MRI of spondylolisthesis Note course of L5 nerve root (*yellow*), visible in its descent as part of the cauda equina and in cross section resembling a "target" as it exits the neural foramen. Note severe central canal stenosis (*red*), which influences decompression in risk of neural or dural injury and in indication for sacral ostectomy.

Factor	Comment
L5 lesion	Increased lordosis leads to increased shear force at fracture
Bilateral lesion	Increased motion and instability at fracture
Chronic	Fracture nonunion

L   Factors associated with nonhealing of spondylolysis

Factor	Comment
Olisthy > 50%	Unstable
Lumbosacral kyphosis	Unstable
Growth acceleration of puberty	Growth amplifies deformity Follow patients through maturity
Gender	Female
Increased sacral inclination Increased sacral slope Decreased pelvic tilt	Radiographic assessment essential

M   Factors associated with progression of spondylolisthesis

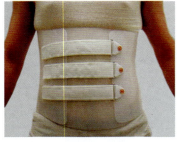

N   Brace for spondylolysis This differs from a deformity brace in being antilordotic, fabricated to 15 degrees, and simple, having no pads or openings.

Computed axial tomography provides the best osseous detail in spondylolysis [J]. It has a rôle when the clinical presentation is consistent with spondylolysis but scintigramme, as the initial screening test, is negative. It also can definitively follow healing of spondylolysis.

Because of availability, broad scope, and lack of radiation, MRI often is used as a screening test for back pain in children. Its greatest utility lies in the discovery of a "prelysis" state, as evidenced by increased T2 signal in the pars interarticularis without fracture. Such patients are braced to heal the lesion as prophylaxis against spondylolysis. Like positive scintigramme, high signal change defines an acute spondylolysis. MRI is most utilized in operative preparation [K].

Management

General principles

- Successful treatment is defined as resolution of symptoms, even in the setting of persistent spondylolysis or pseudarthrosis after spondylolisthesis fusion.
- Healing of spondylolysis is least likely for L5, bilateral, chronic spondylolysis [L].
- Nonoperative management suffices for the majority (>80%) of patients with stable lesions.
- Several factors are associated with olisthy and its progression [M].
- Decompression is indicated for neural symptoms and signs. These may be central, such as bladder dysfunction assessed by cystometrogramme, or foraminal, such as radiculopathy. They tend to be features of unstable olisthesis.
- Instrumentation aids fusion and enables controlled reduction. It is essential for unstable lesions, and after decompression, which is destabilizing.
- Circumferential fusion with instrumentation of unstable olisthesis reduces pseudarthrosis and saves a level.
- Reduction includes both translation and angulation. The former is more likely to result in stretch neuropathy. Goals of reduction are restoration of sagittal balance and moving from instability to stability. Complete reduction is not necessary, and increases neural risk. Reduction also reduces pseudarthrosis by restoring stability as well as providing compressive force and greater surface area for osseous graft. Operative casting and traction for reduction may be regarded as historical, although proponents of the latter point to reduced neural risk due to its gradual nature. Reduction must be preceded by decompression to reduce neural risk.
- Sagittal balance is the most sensitive measure of quality of life. Röntgenogrammes must include full length standing views. Operation must restore global alignment in addition to addressing focal oilsthesis.

Spondylolysis

Management depends upon two features: activity of lesion and symptoms.

- Symptomatic care.

This is in dictated for:
— Chronic lesion
— Acceptable symptoms and signs

This consists of:
— Activity modification, for example, stop offending sport
— Exercises, including pelvic tilt and others antilordotic to the lumbar spine, hamstring, and iliopsoa stretching
— Nonsteroidal anti-inflammatory agents
Brace [N].

This is indicated for:
— Hyperintensity on scintigramme or MRI, suggesting potential to heal. This represents immobilization of an acute fracture.
— Unacceptable pain.

The protocol consists of two consecutive phases:
— Full time for 3 months with no sports
— Full time for 3 months with sports

- Operative treatment.

This is indicated for unacceptable pain despite symptomatic care or bracing. It consists of the following:

— usion *in situ* [N]. This is advocated for L5 lesion. Motion at L5-S1 is least in the lumbar spine. L5-S1 is most affected by degenerative disc disease. Repair of L5 is technically difficult because transverse processes are small (if used as site for cranial anchor) and because this is the most lordotic part of the lumbar spine, making access difficult. A midline posterior approach or a paramedian approach may be utilized [O]. The latter consists of bilateral incisions in deep fascia followed by splitting of erector spinæ for a direct approach to partes interarticulares, facet joints, and transverse processes. It is said to be easier than retraction of the robust column of muscle at the lumbosacral junction against the iliac crests. In addition, disruption of midline soft tissues may be destabilizing. Excise L5-S1 facet joint. Place osseous graft obtained from ilium through same cutaneous incision from sacral alæ to L5 transverse processes with or without interlaminar grafting. Instrumentation may aid fusion and substitutes for postoperative immobilization. These must be balanced against increased risk, time, and cost. Absent instrumentation, supplement with postoperative brace, including the hip to immobilize the lumbosacral junction.

— Repair. No motion is sacrificed. Midline posterior approach, for any level. Anchor cranial (pedicle or transverse process) and caudal (lamina or spinous process) to the spondylolysis, or place a screw through the spondylolysis [P]. Débride spondylolysis. Lay graft obtained from the ilium through same cutaneous incision across spondylolysis. A wire may be looped around transverse process as a cranial anchor; this has evolved to a screw in the pedicle, which preserves the transverse process for complete decortication and fusion. The screw may be connected with a rod to a laminar hook as a caudal anchor or to a spinous process wire or cable as the caudal anchor. The latter caudal anchor achieves compression across the spondylolysis while trading rigidity for lower profile to permit a wider surface area for fusion.

Spondylolisthesis <50% This is stable. As such, treatment follows spondylolysis.

- An exception is bracing based upon osseous activity, because there is no expectation of healing.
- Repair is controversial, with the balance of operative treatment weighted toward fusion.
- Instrumentation is controversial. Stability argues against. Stability means lordosis is preserved, obviating the need for reduction. Instrumentation may aid fusion across a wide gap under tension.

Spondylolisthesis >50% The following characteristics dictate management.

- Instability. Operative treatment is indicated primarily.
- Instability. Instrumentation and reduction are stabilizing.
- Severity of olisthy leads to kyphosis and increases likelihood of sagittal imbalance. Instrumentation with reduction correct angular deformity and restore balance.
- Severity of olisthy is associated with significant central and foraminal neural compression, which requires decompression and in turn instrumentation. Excision of the posterior superior corner of S1 allows for adequate decompression without the need for excessive reduction.

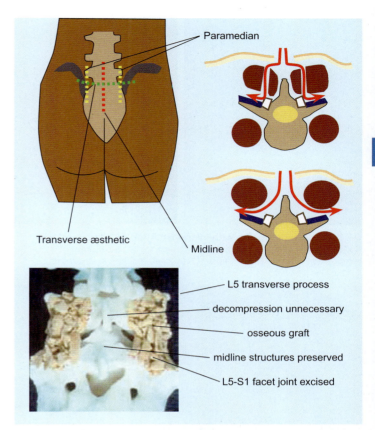

O Surgical approach for spondylolysis fusion Midline is the standard. It is extensile and provides full exposure for fusion for decompression and for instrumentation. Paramedian give direct access for fusion *in situ* but is not extensile and does not allow decompression.

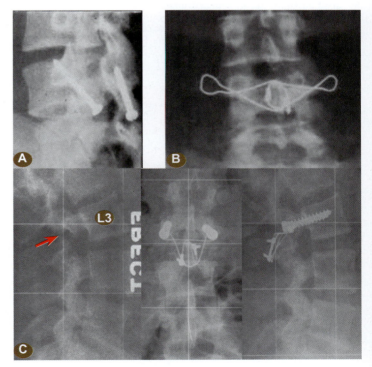

P Repair of spondylolysis.
A—Buck placed a screw through and across the pars interarticularis.
B—Scott compressed the fracture by a wire passed around transverse and spinous processes.
C—Débridement, compression, and grafting of L3 spondylolysis (*red*) resulted in successful repair (*orange*).

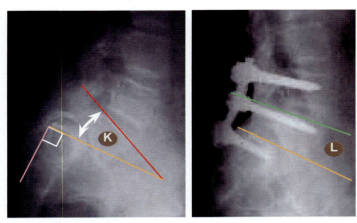

Q L4-S1 posterior fusion with instrumentation L4 provides fixation stability to aid reduction and increased surface area to aid fusion in compression. Lumbosacral kyphosis (k) has been reduced to lordosis (L).

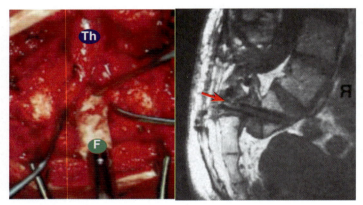

R L4-S1 posterior fusion with instrumentation Fibula allograft (F) as anterior instrumentation via posterior approach to enhance construct stability. After decompression, cannulated drill prepares central channel into which fibula is tamped between neural elements (Th).

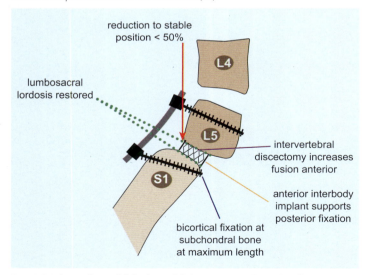

S L5-S1 circumferential fusion with instrumentation This allows saving of a motion segment.

For L5-S1 spondylolisthesis >50%, there are two principal approaches.

- Posterior fusion with instrumentation. This extends from L4 to S1 [Q]. L4 is indicated for construct stability, which aids fusion and reduction, as well as reducing implant failure. Distal fixation may be enhanced by anchoring into the ilium and by anchoring through S1 into the body of L5 [R]. Extension to L4 increases surface area for fusion, in particular after decompression removes posterior elements of L5, and allows compression upon graft rather than tension to L5.
- Circumferential fusion with instrumentation. This saves a motion segment by limiting to L5-S1. Stability is enhanced by circumferential instrumentation, including anterior interbody support [S]. Fusion is enhanced by providing interbody surface area under anterior compression.

Summary of management [T]

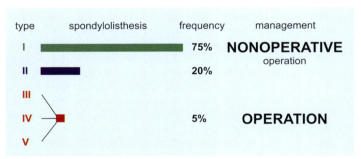

T Spondylolisthesis Most cases are stable, and nonoperative management is effective in most cases.

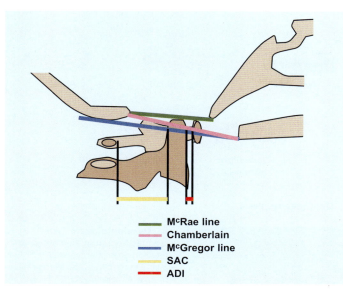

A   Relational lines of the upper cervical spine They describe relationship of the spine to the skull and the spine to the spinal cord.

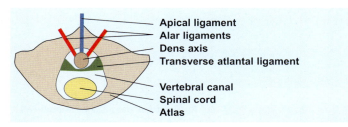

B   Ligaments of the dens They allow the atlas to rotate about the dens for neck motion but restrict dens translation to protect the spinal cord.

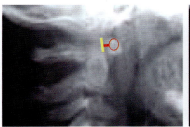
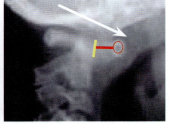

C   Atlantoaxial instability Neutral and flexion lateral views of the cervical spine show an increase of the interval between posterior surface of the anterior arch of atlas (*red ring*) and the anterior dens axis (*yellow line*) due to rupture or laxity of the transverse atlantal ligament.

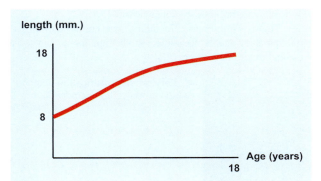

D   Growth of dens axis The dens axis ossifies mostly over the first decade but continues over the second decade.

CERVICAL SPINE

Essential to understanding the cervical spine are anatomic and radiographic relationships [A].

- McRae, Chamberlain, and McGregor lines describe the entrance to the skull. Chamberlain and McGregor lines relate to the hard palate, which may be difficult to see. In addition, they allow for the dens to be above in the normal state ($\leq$1.5 mm and $\leq$4.5 mm, respectively). McRae line is most reliable: it is drawn from opisthion to basion and defines the foramen magnum, above which the dens never reaches in the normal state. Basilar impression is defined as tip of dens above McRae line. Chiari malformation is defined as >5 mm downward displacement of cerebellar tonsils; $\leq$5 mm is considered benign tonsillar ectopia.

- SAC. Space available for cord. Posterior dens to anterior surface of posterior arch. Normal is $\geq$13 mm.

- ADI. Atlantodental interval, measured from posterior surface of anterior arch of atlas to anterior dens. The dens is waisted where it is retained by the transverse atlantal ligament against the anterior arch of atlas to within 5 mm. [B]. Flexion is a stress view [C]. Atlantoaxial instability is defined as ADI >5 mm. This may be due to anomaly of the dens axis (*q.v.*) or to ligamentous laxity, as typified by Down syndrome (*q.v.*).

- The alar ligaments connect dens to occipital condyles and check side–side movement of the skull when it turns. The apical ligament connects the tip of dens with the anterior margin of foramen magnum; it is a vestigial intervertebral structure containing elements of notochord.

- Dens axis development. The tip of dens may not reach the arch of atlas until the end of the first decade and continues to grow through the second decade. Early imaging may mistake normal development for hypoplasia [D].

- Pseudosubluxation. Ligamentous laxity allows <5 mm of anterior translation of C2-C3 and less frequently C3-C4 in the first decade [E].

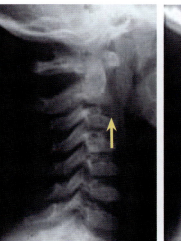
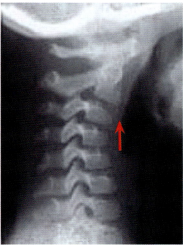

E   Pseudosubluxation Anterior translation of C2 on C3, and less frequently C3 on C4, <5 mm is normal in a child, due to ligamentous laxity.

Anomaly of the Dens Axis

Aplasia is rare [A].

Hypoplasia is associated with skeletal dysplasia, in particular the type II collagenopathies and the mucopolysaccharidoses [B].

Os odontoideum refers to separation of a well-developed rounded bone from the body of axis [B]. It represents a nonunion of fracture of the dens. The mechanism is hypothesized to include disruption of a tenuous blood supply to the base of the dens together with traction applied to the fragment by the alar ligaments. Indications for treatment include pain, evidence of instability, and neural change. Direct osteosynthesis with a dens screw if the fragment is sufficiently large stabilizes the fracture; posterior atlantoaxial fusion sacrifices motion but is technically easier.

Klippel-Feil Syndrome

This is a generalized disorder defined by Klippel and Feil (1912) based upon anomaly of the cervical spine.

Type	Features
1	Autosomal dominant mutation in growth differentiation factor 6 gene on chromosome 8q22.1. GDF6 is a member of the transforming growth factor β superfamily, regulating neural induction and patterning of ectoderm by interaction with bone morphogenetic proteins.
2	Autosomal recessive mutation in the mesenchyme homeobox 1 gene on chromosome 17q21. MEOX1 plays a rôle in mesoderm induction and regional specification, including somitogenesis as well as myogenic and sclerotomal differentiation.
3	Autosomal dominant mutation in GDF3 gene on 12p13.1. Distinguished by skeletal and ocular manifestations, including microphthalmia, iritis, and retinal coloboma.

Pathogenesis Klippel-Feil, Sprengel anomaly and Chiari malformation have been linked as defects in postotic neural crest cells, which give rise to the osseous and muscular connexions between head and shoulder girdle.

Evaluation

- Failure of segmentation of the cervical spine is the essential feature, which results in
- Short webbed neck with low hairline
- Reduced cervical motion, with or without torticollis

While the triad focuses on the neck [C], associated findings in up to 1/3 of patients include the following:

- Genitourinary anomalies. Screen with renal ultrasonogramme.
- Cardiac anomalies. Refer to cardiologist.
- Sensorineural and conductive deafness. Audiology testing.
- Synkinesia (involuntary or "mirror" movement associated with voluntary movement of a remote part of the body).
- Foramen magnum dysplasia associated to Chiari malformation.
- Other skeletal abnormalities, including extracervical spine deformity, facial asymmetry, Sprengel anomaly, carpal and tarsal coalition.

Röntgenogrammes establish failure of segmentation [D]. CT defines anomalous architecture. MRI characterizes the occipitocervical junction and associated neural lesions.

Management Educate the family to modify activity, that is, avoid contact sports. Surgical treatment is targeted at:

- Deformity. Due to location, rigidity, and potential for adjacent decompensation, intervention is indicated for any progression.
- Brainstem compression, as evidenced by neural dysfunction, in particular Chiari malformation and basilar impression.
- Painful adjacent segment hypermobility/instability. This rarely occurs during childhood.

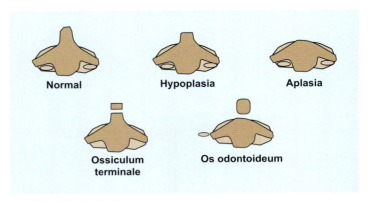

A Odontoid dysplasia

Normal   Hypoplasia   Aplasia

Ossiculum terminale   Os odontoideum

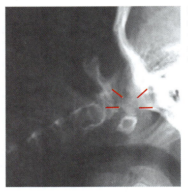

B Os odontoideum Dens separate (*red*) from the body of axis retained against anterior arch of atlas. Discontinuity allows migration of atlas anteriorward.

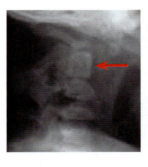

D Radiographic features of Klippel-Feil syndrome Failure of segmentation of upper cervical spine (*red*).

Cervical Intervertebral Disc Calcification

Cervical disc calcification is a rare, idiopathic condition characterized by neck pain and stiffness, with or without torticollis and fever. Röntgenogrammes show calcification. Pain resolves spontaneously by 1 month on average but may persist for several months. Calcification resolves over several years with no significant sequelæ.

Evaluation Röntgenogrammes are characteristic [A].

Management This is symptomatic, including rest, collar, and nonsteroidal anti-inflammatory agents. Recognize the benign course and resist aggressive evaluation or intervention.

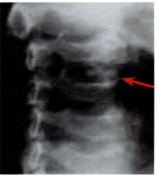

A Cervical disc calcification Although cause is unknown, the disorder has a more benign clinical course than imaging might suggest.

TORTICOLLIS

Torticollis describes a "twisted neck." It has multiple lay names—*wry-neck, cock-robin deformity*—because it long has been recognized, including as a symbol of beauty in Western art after the bust of Alexander the Great. It may be divided into several types [A].

Type	Comment		
Muscular torticollis	contracture of SCM		neck stiffness
Osseous	normal SCM		neck stiffness
Traumatic	pain	new onset	neck stiffness
Inflammatory	pain	new onset	neck stiffness
Tumor	pain	new onset	neck stiffness
Gastrointestinal	pain	systemic signs	normal motion
Ocular	normal SCM		normal motion
Neural	normal SCM		normal motion
Other	"idiopathic"		

A   Types of torticollis SCM: sternocleidomastoid muscle.

Osseous

Pathogenesis Vertebral anomaly mechanically tilts the head.

Evaluation Röntgenogrammes of the spine early in life are difficult to interpret and will not provide sufficient detail to characterize an osseous anomaly, such as hemivertebra. CT or MRI is necessary, which will require anæsthesia. As a result, this diagnosis should be one of exclusion that is pursued if deformity is severe or progressive, if it is otherwise complicated, for example, in the setting of a syndrome, or if it will affect management.

Management This follows principles for congenital deformity correction.

Ocular

Pathogenesis This is produced by paralysis of extraocular muscle, most often obliquus oculi superior innervated (trochlear nerve), of which the primary action is intorsion (or internal rotation) to maintain horizontal vision during looking up and down. The child turns the head to keep the field of vision horizontal in compensation for the palsy.

Evaluation Diagnosis typically is made after the first year of age, after sufficient head and postural control have become established. The neck is normal, including normal motion and sternocleidomastoid muscles. On physical examination, covering the uninvolved eye will rectify a hypertropia in the affected eye; by contrast, covering the affected eye will correct a hypotropia in the normal eye.

Management Refer to an ophthalmologist.

Neural

Pathogenesis Abnormal sensory input, in particular visual in a posterior fossa lesion, or asymmetric neural signals to cervical paraspinous muscles.

Evaluation Physical examination reveals associated primary neural or secondary other system abnormalities. The difficulty of performing an accurate neurologic examination in an infant delays diagnosis. Neck motion and sternocleidomastoid muscles are normal. MRI of the head and cervical spine is the imaging modality of choice.

Management Refer to a neurologist.

Tumor

Pathogenesis Vertebral deformation mechanically, or inflammatory pain secondarily, tilts the head.

Evaluation Eosinophilic granuloma collapses bone into vertebra plana. This may be asymmetric, producing torticollis. Osteoid osteoma or osteoblastoma may cause a child to splint because of pain. As with osseous anomaly, röntgenogrammes of the spine may not provide sufficient detail to characterize the morbid process: CT and MRI are necessary.

Management This follows principles for benign tumors [B].

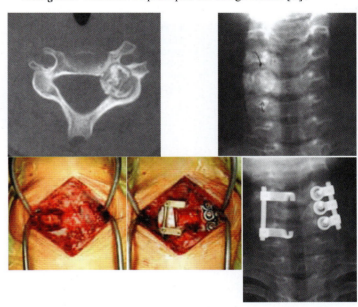

B   Tumor causing torticollis Cervical osteoblastoma. Preoperative imaging shows destruction of the lateral mass, abutting the canal for the vertebral artery. This was excised *en bloc*. Spine was fused and instrumented for stability.

Gastrointestinal

This is known as Sandifer syndrome, a gastrointestinal disorder with neurologic features of which torticollis is one.

Pathogenesis Abnormal posturing occurs with gastrœsophageal reflux (e.g., hiatal hernia), against which a child splints into torticollis.

Evaluation The condition must be considered in the setting of:

- No sternocleidomastoid contracture
- Normal cervical motion
- Extracervical dystonia
- Irritability
- Other signs of gastrointestinal dysfunction such as failure to thrive

Diagnosis may be established by pH study for œsophagitis, motility study for reflux, and endoscopy with biopsy as necessary.

Management Refer to a gastroenterologist.

Other

This category includes paroxysmal type.

Pathogenesis Vestibular system dysfunction has been implicated but not proven.

Evaluation The characteristic profile is as follows:

- Head and neck examination is normal.
- Girls are more often affected.
- It occurs in the first 3 years of life.
- The course is episodic.
- The torticollis may be bilateral.

Management Educate parents and assure them that this is a benign process that resolves spontaneously without sequelæ.

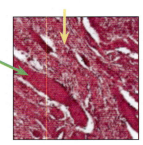

A Pathogenesis Fibrosis (*yellow*) of muscle (*green*) has led to the concept of *in utero* compartment syndrome.

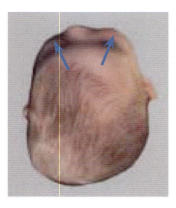

B Plagiocephaly Plagiocephaly and other "packaging" problems are associated with muscular torticollis. Arrows show malar blunting, also seen on CT performed to evaluate for osseous cause.

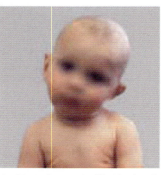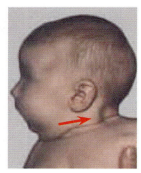

C Muscular torticollis The head tilts toward and rotates away from the contracted sternocleidomastoid muscle (*arrow*)

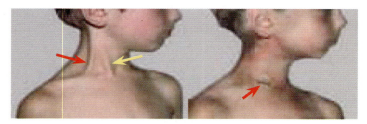

D Surgical approach Bipolar release through discreet incisions.

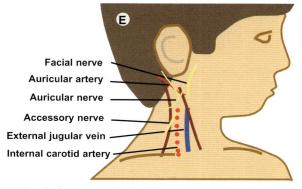

Facial nerve
Auricular artery
Auricular nerve
Accessory nerve
External jugular vein
Internal carotid artery

E Surgical anatomy This includes major and minor blood vessels, as well as motor and sensory nerves.

Muscular Torticollis

This is distinguished as

- Congenital
- Painless
- Associated with other deformities of the head, in particular plagiocephaly

It is the most common form seen by a surgeon.

Pathogenesis Compartment syndrome has been implicated, due to swelling and fibrosis of the sternocleidomastoid [A]. Evidence of a problem of "packaging" includes high prevalence in breech babies of primiparous mothers and associated signs of intrauterine crowding such as plagiocephaly [B], hip dysplasia, and metatarsus adductus.

Evaluation Contracture of sternocleidomastoid tilts the head toward and rotates the head away, in the process limiting neck motion [C]. The muscle is prominent and firm. Screen hips with ultrasonogramme or röntgenogrammes after 3 months of age. Packaging problems resolve spontaneously, as does muscular torticollis in >90% in the first year of life.

Management The benignity of natural history should temper treatment. Physiotherapy and other manipulative techniques (e.g., place cot against the wall to force the child to rotate against contracted sternocleidomastoid to look into room) in the first year are unproven. Surgical release should be delayed to allow natural history to play out. Operation consists of sternocleidomastoid section, which may be percutaneous or open, located at either or both poles, and involving excision of a small segment or Z-lengthening.

Surgical considerations There is no consensus, and approach is influenced by the following:

- Recurrence. Some believe that this may be reduced by delaying intervention. Others regard delay to be associated with poor outcome due to secondary contracture and deformity that may become permanent and that are not addressed by operation on the sternocleidomastoid, such as facial asymmetry from chronic traction. Recurrence is the reason given for bipolar (sternal, clavicular, as well as mastoid ends) section. Others counter by exsection of 1 cm of the distal poles, and include all surrounding fascia and other adhesions, which also conspire to contract the neck. Removing the entire muscle is excessive.
- Cosmetic concerns. "Percutaneous," endoscopic or open approaches are equivalent, as incisions are small and may be made transverse to the muscle along von Lager lines [D]. Concern that distal polar section or exsection may leave an ugly divot in the neck has led to Z-lengthening of the sternal head of the muscle; however, this technique adds complexity and may increase the risk of recurrence.

Anatomic considerations

- Auricular artery and nerve are at risk with release of the proximal pole [E].
- Facial nerve limits the anterior extent of a proximal incision
- The spinal accessory nerve pierces the muscle in its middle, away from any incision.
- At the heads of the sternocleidomastoid, the external jugular courses in the superficial interval. The deep interval lodges the internal carotid artery: complete release of the distal poles should leave only pulsating fat in the surgical bed, demonstrating release of surrounding fascia and adhesions, which are thought to account for recurrence after, and therefore dissatisfaction with, this unipolar approach. This may be unfamiliar territory, intimidating the orthopædic surgeon from dissecting deep.
- Raise flaps in this region of mobile skin and release all regional adhesions that may not be part of the muscle *per se* but have developed secondarily.
- Do not repair the deep fascia: augment closure of only superficial fascia and skin with glue.

Controversy continues in aftercare. Place the patient in a soft collar. Allow the wound 1 week to heal, then mobilize the neck under supervision of a physiotherapist until the patient has comfortable and full motion.

Atlantoaxial Rotatory Displacement

This is distinguished as:

- Acquired. It may follow inflammation of soft tissue of the neck, or trauma.
- Painful.
- Involvement of the contralateral sternocleidomastoid muscle, which contracts to rectify the neck and is elongated.

This is typed [A]:

- I. Rotation without displacement.
- II. Rotation with ≤5-mm displacement.
- III. Rotation with >5-mm displacement.
- IV. Rotation with posterior displacement. This may include fracture of dens axis.

Pathogenesis Venous drainage of the pharynx toward the periodontoidal vertebral plexus, where there are no lymph nodes to divert flow, leads to inflammatory hyperæmia that produces ligamentous laxity and spasm of paraspinous muscles. Nontraumatic torticollis first was described by Bell (1830); it is named after Grisel (1930), who implicated venous drainage and described enucleation of the atlas to correct the deformity. Traumatic extreme motion of the neck may shift and squeeze meniscus-like synovial membrane between atlas and axis, resulting in pain inhibition and a mechanical block to reduction.

Evaluation There is a history of infection or trauma; the latter may be activity related (e.g., wrestling) or may occur after head and neck surgery. The contralateral sternocleidomastoid muscle is contracted, painful, and elongated. Neck twisting may distort röntgenogrammes: the most useful view is a lateral of the skull (with which atlas is reduced), which may show increased atlantoaxial interval. CT will show displacement, and dynamic CT will show fixed or incomplete rotation of atlas relative to axis [B].

Management Infectious AARD resolves with treatment of the infection. Support the neck in a collar. This may be the most common form of torticollis, as it often is managed by the pædiatrician without involvement of the orthopædic surgeon. Traumatic AARD may persist. Correction or stabilization of deformity is indicated to eliminate risk of neural injury [C].

- 0 to 1 week. Soft collar and symptom control, such as rest and anti-inflammatory medication. The majority resolves clinically; imaging is not necessary given the benign and typical course.
- 1 to 4 weeks. Reduction. Start with traction in hospital, aided by relaxants. While halo is more invasive, it allows rotational as well as longitudinal force, and halter risks chin ulcer. Confirm reduction with CT. After reduction, halo–vest is worn for 3 months to reduce resubluxation.
- >1 month. Chronic AARD is unlikely to resolve. There is a gray zone of time during which some advocate manipulative reduction under anæsthesia. The head is held by halo and rotated gently, slowly, and fully with neural monitoring.
- >3 months. Persistent AARD despite closed methods is treated by atlantoaxial fusion. Sublaminar wiring of an H-graft at atlas with axis spinous process wiring (Gallie) or atlantoaxial sublaminar wiring (Brooks) introduces implants into a canal of which the volume may be reduced by the subluxation. Transarticular screws from axis into atlas (Magerl) avoid this, are more stable, and may be reductive [D].

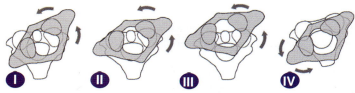

A Types of atlantoaxial rotatory displacement Scintigramme at presentation shows increased uptake (*red*). After 2 weeks, lateral röntgenogrammes shows narrowing of the disc (*yellow*).

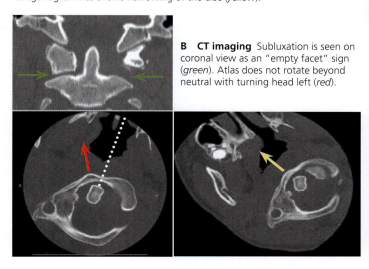

B CT imaging Subluxation is seen on coronal view as an "empty facet" sign (*green*). Atlas does not rotate beyond neutral with turning head left (*red*).

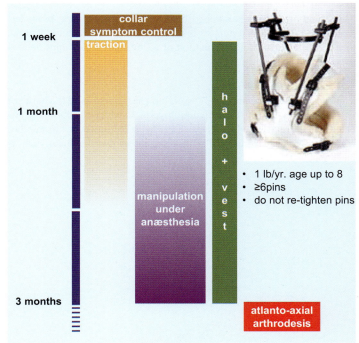

C Treatment protocol for atlantoaxial rotatory displacement

- 1 lb/yr. age up to 8
- ≥6 pins
- do not re-tighten pins

atlanto-axial arthrodesis

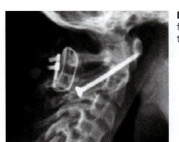

D Atlantoaxial arthrodesis Brooks fusion combined with Magerl transarticular screws.

ASSOCIATED NEURAL DISORDERS

Neural disorders may be associated with spine and other musculoskeletal deformity, such as cavus or unilateral calf asymmetry, vertebral anomaly, pain, and mixed upper and lower neuropathy.

Evaluation After physical examination, MRI is the imaging modality of choice. CT (with myelography) characterizes osseous architecture, including vertebral canal and for severe deformity, in preparation for operation.

Management Neurosurgical. Occipitocervical decompression of Chiari malformation. Section of thickened and contracted filum terminale to release tethered cord. Fenestration and drainage of syrinx. Resection of septum and release of adhesions for diastematomyelia.

Chiari Malformation

Brainstem compression associated with hindbrain and other neural anomalies [A]. Type I is defined as displacement of cerebellar tonsils >3 mm below foramen magnum. Type II is associated with myelomeningocœle.

Syrinx

This is defined as a morbid cavity in the spinal cord distinct from dilatation of the central canal, which is termed hydromyelia. They may occur in conjunction with Chiari malformation and will resolve with foramen magnum decompression. Treatment depends upon symptoms and size. The asymptomatic patient with a small syrinx is followed with serial MRI. Large syringes may require fenestration and subarachnoid, peritoneal, or pleural shunting [B].

Tethered Cord

The conus medullaris is retained below L2 by a contracted filum terminale [C]. The filum terminale is thickened such that it can indent the theca, and fatty, including formation of a fibrolipoma that appears as a mass on MRI.

Diastematomyelia

The term refers to a "through" "split" of the "spinal cord." There are two hemicords, in contrast with diplomyelia, in which the cord is duplicated. Girls are affected thrice as often. Most lesions occur in the thoracic cord and are connected with a stigma of dysrrhaphism such as hairy patch [D].

Chiari type	Features
I	Cerebellar tonsils below foramen magnum
II	Multiple hindbrain anomalies
III	Occipitocervical encephalocœle
IV	Absence of cerebellum

A Chiari malformation Types and features.

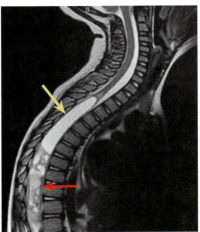

B Syrinx and tumor Six-year-old boy presented with scoliosis associated with hyperkyphosis. MRI shows tumor (*red*) and syrinx (*yellow*).

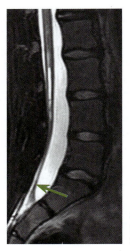

C Tethered cord Conus medullaris, with syrinx, is tethered to the level of L4 by a thickened filum terminale (*green*).

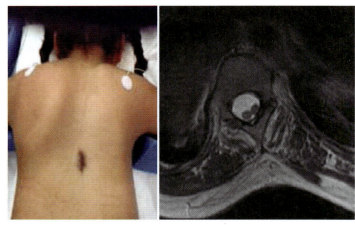

D Diastematomyelia Hairy patch associated with thoracic lesion.

TUMOR

Primary tumors may be divided into benign or malignant and may affect the hard tissue—bone—or soft tissue—neural elements [A]. Less than 10% of primary bone tumors occur in the spine, of which half occur in childhood. Vertebral tumors may affect the body or the neural arch [B]. The latter may produce radiculopathy, thereby mimicking disc herniation. Tumors of the spine may produce deformity, in particular scoliosis, which may be distinguished by:

- Focal pain
- Marked reduction in motion
- Rapid progression
- Absence of rotation

Cervical lesions may present with torticollis (*q.v.*).
Surgical treatment may be:

- Intralesional excision, such as curettage and bone grafting. While appropriate for benign tumors, this may be complicated by recurrence in aggressive lesions such as osteoblastoma.
- *En bloc* resection. This reduces recurrence but may risk surrounding neurovascular structures (e.g., vertebral artery in the cervical spine, the dura mater requiring patch grafting) and may produce instability (in particular kyphosis) necessitating fusion.

Consider contemporaneous spine fusion with instrumentation for *en bloc* resection, complete laminectomy, facetectomy. Follow partial excision for postsurgical deformity, in particular kyphosis in the thoracic spine.

Benign Osseous Tumors

Osteoid osteoma and osteoblastoma Osteoid osteoma is defined as <2 cm and is less aggressive than osteoblastoma, which most often is located in the spine. Pain is worst at night. The tumor releases prostaglandins, which explains its inflammatory nature and pain; prostaglandin inhibitors (e.g., ibuprofen) are both diagnostic and therapeutic, although not in all children. Delay in diagnosis can be longer than a year, in part because more than half are invisible on röntgenogrammes. SPECT shows intense uptake. CT will show the pathognomonic target lesion, consisting of a sclerotic margin surrounding a separate sclerotic nidus (hence the old term "sclerosing nonsuppurative osteomyelitis"). This modality localizes the lesion for radioablation or laser coagulation [C] and defines architecture for surgical resection.

Aneurysmal bone cyst Röntgenogrammes show an expansile heterogeneous geographic lesion [D]. Preoperative embolization reduces operative blood loss.

Eosinophilic granuloma Ten percent of lesions occur in the spine. Replacement of vertebral body by tumor results in collapse into vertebrae plana [E]; recognition of this deformity will aid in differentiation from more aggressive tumors, such as Ewing sarcoma. Indication for surgical intervention is neural deficit resulting from large or multiple lesions. The natural history of the majority of lesions, which are solitary and associated with normal neural function, is spontaneous regression with reconstitution of vertebral height. Management is supportive, including bracing. Residual osseous deformity usually is acceptable.

Osteochondroma This has a predilection for the cervical spine. Ten percent of patients with hereditary multiple exostosis have spine involvement. Symptoms are due to mass effect, including pain and neural deficit, which may be successfully treated with resection.

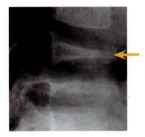

E Eosinophilic granuloma Vertebra plana, with preservation of the intervertebral disc.

Osseous Tumors	Neural Tumors
Benign	**Benign**
Eosinophilic granuloma	Neurofibroma
Osteoid osteoma	Lipoma
Aneurysmal bone cyst	Spinal cysts
Osteoblastoma	**Malignant**
Neurofibromatosis	Astrocytoma
Osteochondroma	Ependymoma
Malignant	Mixed glioma
Ewing sarcoma	Ganglioglioma
Lymphoma of bone	
Leukæmia	

A Vertebral (bone) and spinal cord tumors

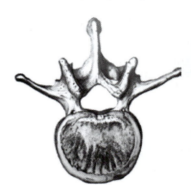

Posterior elements
Osteoid osteoma
Osteoblastoma
Aneurysmal bone cysts
Osteochondroma

Anterior elements
Eosinophilic granuloma
Giant cell tumor
Hæmagioma

B Geographic distribution of benign osseous tumors Tumors may affect the thoracolumbar spine (*green*) or the cervical spine (*beige*). Other tumors that affect the spine do not occur in children (*gray*).

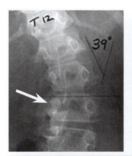
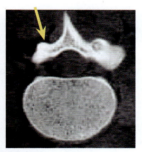

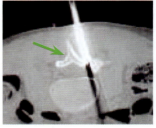

C Osteoid osteoma The lesion produces nonspecific sclerosis of the pedicle on röntgenogramme (*white*) but is well defined on CT (*yellow*) and is treated with radioablation (*green*).

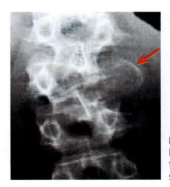

D Aneurysmal bone cyst Expansile lesion with sclerotic margin located at the concave apex of a painful secondary scoliosis.

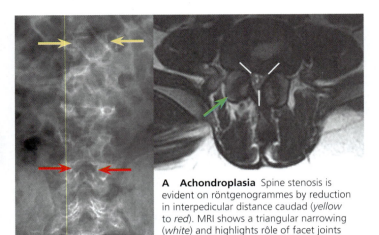

A Achondroplasia Spine stenosis is evident on röntgenogrammes by reduction in interpedicular distance caudad (*yellow* to *red*). MRI shows a triangular narrowing (*white*) and highlights rôle of facet joints (*green*) and the need for their excision to adequately decompress the vertebral canal.

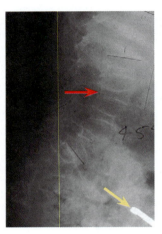

B Osteogenesis imperfecta Codfish vertebrae (*red arrow*) are characteristic. Note the femoral Rush rod (*yellow*).

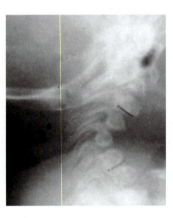

C Diastrophic dysplasia Cervical kyphosis is characteristic and grave. Neural risk is an indication for early surgical intervention.

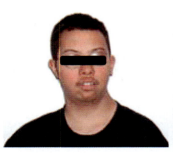
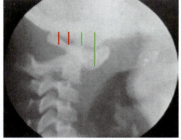

D Down syndrome Torticollis is a sign of atlantoaxial instability, as patient splints to stabilize cervical spine. Operative image shows space available for cord is reduced (*red*) as atlantodental interval increases (*green*).

Spine in Other Disease

The spine is affected characteristically in the skeletal dysplasias and in several syndromes. General principles of spine deformity include the following:

- Increased incidence
- Increased magnitude
- Increased progression, earlier onset, more and more rapid
- Increased neural risk, from disease and operative treatment
- Increased technical demand, including more frequent anterior fusion in addition to posterior fusion and more complications.

Achondroplasia

Lumbar spine Stenosis is the most common spine problem in achondroplasia. It results from hypoplasia of the neural arch and may be seen on röntgenogrammes as a reduction in interpedicular distance caudad in contrast with normal increase [A]. Reduction in vertebral canal volume and intervertebral foramen diameter is exacerbated by lumbar hyperlordosis, which in turn is worsened by thoracolumbar kyphosis or hip flexion contracture. Children typically present in the second decade: there is a spectrum of pain, claudication, radiculopathy, and neural deficit, including abnormal urodynamics. Flexion of the lumbar spine, such as interrupting play to squat, provides relief by increasing space available for nerves. Treatment consists of decompression and fusion with instrumentation to the pelvis. There is not enough space for laminectomy without disruption of facet joints to suffice.

Foramen magnum By contrast with the flat bones of the skull, which form by intramembranous ossification, this part of the skull forms by endochondral ossification, which is abnormal in achondroplasia. Foramen magnum stenosis may be treated based upon absolute diameter compared with published normative CT data for achondroplasia. Functional treatment is based upon demonstration of an abnormal sleep apnea study. Foramen magnum decompression with ventricular drainage improves sleep study metrics.

Kyphosis This most commonly affects the thoracolumbar junction. The natural history includes spontaneous improvement during infancy for flexible deformity. Kyphosis (no consensus on magnitude, certainly >50 degrees) persistent beyond 5 years of age is treated with single-stage circumferential fusion performed *via* a posterior approach and including circumferential instrumentation.

Osteogenesis Imperfecta

Severity and incidence of spine deformity is proportional to severity of disease. Biconcave vertebral bodies are characteristic and known as "codfish vertebra" [B].

Basilar impression This is a feature of type III. It is defined as tip of dens above McRae line on lateral röntgenogramme. The base of the skull settles from the level of the atlanto-occipital joints to the level of atlantoaxial joints on open mouth view. Because this occurs gradually, most patients are asymptomatic. Symptoms and signs relate to brainstem and upper cervical cord compression. Fundamental to treatment is surgical decompression.

Scoliosis Cause relates to loss of extracellular matrix integrity, including osseous fragility and ligamentous laxity. There is a relative lack of rotation and associated hyperkyphosis [B]. Early operative intervention for progressive curves <50 degrees is motivated by poor purchase of anchors and primary distortion of spine architecture.

Fragilitas ossium In its most subtle form, osteogenesis imperfecta may be silent during childhood and manifest as premature osteoporosis in the adult, including vertebral compression fracture.

Diastrophic Dysplasia

The name was proposed to highlight "twisting" of feet and spine, including scoliosis, lumbar hyperlordosis, and kyphosis. Risk of neural injury from cervical kyphosis necessitates early surgical intervention [C]. Anterior fusion with strut grafts addresses kyphotic tension on posterior fusion and frequent deficiency of posterior elements.

Atlantoaxial Instability

Altlantoaxial instability (AAI) is a feature of Down syndrome, several skeletal dysplasias (pseudoachondroplasia, type II collagenopathies), and the mucopolysaccharidoses. Pathogenesis includes connective tissue laxity and odontoid dysplasia.

Down syndrome In 1983, Special Olympics recommended radiographic screening before participation. This position was endorsed in 1984 by the American Academy of Pediatrics. Because patients with Down syndrome can move spontaneously between radiographic stability and instability without clinical manifestation and because all reports of neural injury from AAI demonstrated at least several weeks of prodrome, in 1995, the recommendation for screening was retired. In addition, surgical treatment has a high complication rate, making clear indications essential. Educate caregivers about symptoms and signs of AAI, including deformity (in particular torticollis), stiffness, myelopathy [D]. Follow patients clinically. Absent clinical manifestation, screening is not recommended lest it yield a radiographic false positive. The moderate position consists of clinical observation for ADI 5 to 10 mm and atlantoaxial posterior spine fusion with instrumentation for ADI >10 mm.

Type II collagenopathies and mucopolysaccharidoses While these two groups contain distinct diseases, which may include other spine deformity such as scoliosis and kyphosis [E], odontoid dysplasia resulting in AAI is the most significant spine abnormality, both in its high incidence (up to 1/2 of patients) and treacherous consequences. Abnormality of type II collagen produces spondyloepiphysial dysplasia and Kniest syndrome; lysosomal enzyme deficiency forms the basis of Morquio and Hurler syndromes. Upper cervical cord compression may be mistaken for typical delay in motor milestones resulting from generalized skeletal dysplasia, including lower limb deformity. Abnormal ossification makes röntgenogrammes difficult to interpret. Dynamic MRI shows the dens and vertebral canal, including constriction and any signal change in the spinal cord. Because the dens is dysplastic, follow reduction of atlas on axis during tightening of implants with image intensification to guard against posterior displacement of atlas.

Marfan Syndrome

Scoliosis This is a major diagnostic criterion. Approximately 1/2 of patients will develop scoliosis >30 degrees. Bracing is ineffective. Treat according to general surgical principles.

Dural ectasia This is one of the major diagnostic criteria. It is significant clinically in genesis of back pain. Its surgical significance rests in the fact that it results in osseous erosion, which undermines anchors and may account for high historic rates of pseudarthrosis due to instability of constructs. MRI is essential to evaluate this [F].

Spondylolisthesis This is part of the differential diagnosis of back pain. Olisthy is attributed to connective tissue laxity. Treat according to general principles.

Neurofibromatosis

The spine is affected in type 1 (of von Recklinghausen).

Scoliosis Scoliosis affects approximately 1/3 of patients. It may resemble idiopathic scoliosis, or it may be dystrophic [G], of which characteristics include the following:

- Short sharp curvature.
- Severe rotation.
- Osseous erosion by neurofibromata, which distorts anatomy, is destabilizing to the extreme of dislocation and impairs fixation.
- Rapid progression, which dictates early surgical intervention.

Kyphosis This is associated with dystrophic scoliosis. It also may occur in the cervical spine, where potential for severe angulation and instability dictates aggressive surgical management.

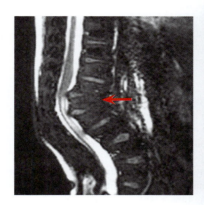
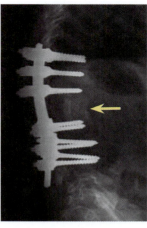

E   Hurler syndrome Six-year-old girl with progressive thoracolumbar kyphosis (*red*) was treated by posterior approach vertebral column resection, anterior strut grafting (*yellow*), and posterior instrumentation.

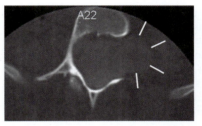

F   Marfan syndrome Dural ectasia eroding pedicles, thereby compromising fixation.

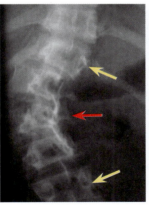

G   Neurofibromatosis Note the severe rotation (*red*) two segments away from relatively neutral vertebrae (*yellow*) in this dystrophic scoliosis.

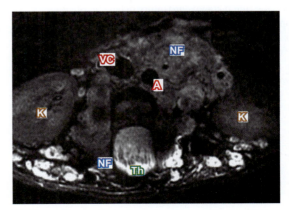

H   Neurofibromatosis Paraspinous neurofibroma (NF) has eroded posterior elements such that they cannot accept implants for fixation, and allowing theca (Th) to balloon. K: kidney, A: aorta, VC: vena cava.

Pseudarthrosis, a fundamental feature of neurofibromatosis, necessitates circumferential fusion for spine deformity, in particular the dystrophic type. CT defines osseous architecture, while MRI defines neurofibromata and neural architecture [H]. The latter is essential to reducing risk during spine manipulation from traction upon intraspinal lesions.

Caudal Dysgenesis

This also is known as caudal regression syndrome and sacral agenesis. It represents a heterogeneous constellation of anomalies affecting the caudal spine and spinal cord, pelvic and abdominal viscera, and the lower limbs. It may be divided into without or with abnormal sacrum, the latter into without or with instability [I].

Evaluation One-fifth of mothers of affected children have insulin-dependent diabetes mellitus. Presentation includes multiple contractures of the lower limbs, dislocation of the hips, clubfoot, scoliosis, and kyphosis. Musculoskeletal deformities vary in severity with level of agenesis and resulting neural loss. Motor loss is disproportionate to sensory loss, which can remain protective despite significant severity. Cognition is spared. Appearance of severe contractures of the lower limbs has been likened to Buddha posture. There are associated anomalies of the hindgut and the urogenital system. Currarino syndrome represents an autosomal dominant form of the disease, caused by a mutation in the HLXB9 homeobox gene on chromosome 7q36.

Management Neural status guides management. While the presentation can be dramatic, the most prudent approach is restraint. Painless instability is better than painful stiffness. Deformities recur despite operative correction because contractures are tenacious. Aggressive surgical treatment is indicated for the ambulatory. For the others, limited operative procedures to aid posture and care, combined with orthotic support and mobility aids are tailored to the child.

Sacral Dimple

This represents an indentation, or "pit," that may be observed during the neonatal physical examination at or within 1 inch of the natal cleft, which may be distorted. It affects 3% of children.

Evaluation The benign anomaly must be differentiated from a midline sign of dysrrhaphism, such as hair, sinus, cutaneous tag, altered pigmentation, drainage.

Management Diagnostic dilemma may be resolved in the neonate by ultrasonogramme to evaluate the subjacent neural elements [J], in particular level of the conus medullaris and thickening of filum terminale tethering the spinal cord. After 4 months of age, ossification of the posterior elements of the spine obscures ultrasonogramme, necessitating MRI. Because the latter requires general anæsthesia in this age, be prudent in obtaining this.

Spinal Cord Injury

Spine deformity is the rule if spinal cord injury occurs before puberty. All children develop scoliosis, while 2/3 will develop kyphosis and 1/5 will develop lumbar hyperlordosis. The spine deformity tends to be progressive and most will require spine fusion with instrumentation including the pelvis. Less than 1/5 of children who sustain spinal cord injury after puberty will develop a paralytic deformity.

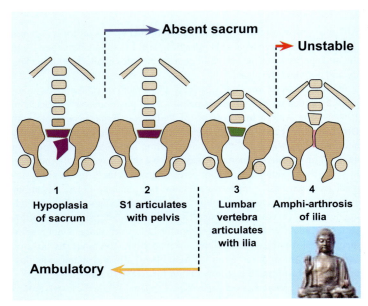

I Sacral agenesis The sacrum may be hypoplastic or absent (*blue*). The spine–pelvis relationship may be stable or unstable (*red*).

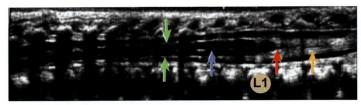

J Ultrasonogramme of neonatal spine for sacral dimple Spinal cord (*green*) and central canal (*blue*) are normal, as is level of conus medullaris (*red*) between L1 and L2. Cauda equina (*orange*) shows no thickened filum terminale.

BACK PAIN

Feldman DS, Straight JJ, Badra MI, Mohaideen A, Madan SS. Evaluation of an algorithmic approach to pediatric back pain. *J. Pediatr. Orthop.* 26(3):353–357, 2006.

Landman Z, Oswald T, Sanders J, Diab M, Spinal Deformity Study Group. Prevalence and predictors of pain in surgical treatment of adolescent idiopathic scoliosis. *Spine* 36(10):825–829, 2011.

IDIOPATHIC SCOLIOSIS—ADOLESCENT

Cotrel Y, Dubousset J, Guillaumat M. New universal instrumentation in spinal surgery. *Clin. Orthop.* 227:10–23, 1988.

Diab M, Landman Z, Lubicky J, Dormans J, Erickson M, Richards BS; Members of the Spinal Deformity Study Group. Use and outcome of MRI in the surgical treatment of adolescent idiopathic scoliosis. *Spine* 36(8):667–671, 2011.

Dolan LA, Weinstein SL. Surgical rates after observation and bracing for adolescent idiopathic scoliosis: an evidence-based review. *Spine* 32(19 Suppl):S91–S100, 2007.

Hamill CL, Lenke LG, Bridwell KH, Chapman MP, Blanke K, Baldus C. The use of pedicle screw fixation to improve correction in the lumbar spine of patients with idiopathic scoliosis. Is it warranted? *Spine* 21(10):1241–1249, 1996.

Harrington PR. Treatment of scoliosis: correction and internal fixation by spine instrumentation. *J. Bone Joint Surg.* 44(4):591–634, 1962.

Luque ER. Segmental spinal instrumentation for correction of scoliosis. *Clin. Orthop.* 163:192–198, 1982.

Negrini S, Minozzi S, Bettany-Saltikov J, Zaina F, Chockalingam N, Grivas TB, Kotwicki T, Maruyama T, Romano M, Vasiliadis ES. Braces for idiopathic scoliosis in adolescents. *Spine* 35(13):1285–1293, 2010.

Sanders JO. Maturity indicators in spinal deformity. *J. Bone Joint Surg.* 89(Suppl 1)-A:14–20, 2007.

Weinstein SL, Dolan LA, Spratt KF, Peterson KK, Spoonamore MJ, Ponseti IV. Health and function of patients with untreated idiopathic scoliosis. A 50-Year natural history study. *JAMA* 289(5):559–567, 2003.

Weinstein SL, Dolan LA, Wright JG, Dobbs MB. Effects of bracing in adolescents with idiopathic scoliosis. *N. Engl. J. Med.* 369:1512–1521, 2013.

IDIOPATHIC SCOLIOSIS—INFANTILE AND JUVENILE

Akbarnia BA, Breakwell LM, Marks DS, McCarthy RE, Thompson AG, Canale SK, Kostial PN, Tambe A, Asher MA. Dual growing rod technique followed for three to eleven years until final fusion: the effect of frequency of lengthening. *Spine* 33(9):984–990, 2008.

Crawford CH, Lenke LG. Growth modulation by means of anterior tethering resulting inprogressive correction of juvenile idiopathic scoliosis: a case report. *J. Bone Joint Surg.* 92(1):202–209, 2010.

Gupta P, Lenke LG, Bridwell KH. Incidence of neural axis abnormalities in infantile and juvenile patients with spinal deformity. Is a magnetic resonance image screening necessary? *Spine* 23(2):206–210, 1998.

James JIP. Idiopathic scoliosis; the prognosis, diagnosis, and operative indications related to curve patterns and the age at onset. *J. Bone Joint Surg.* 36(1)-B:36–49, 1954.

Klemme WR, Denis F, Winter RB, Lonstein JW, Koop SE. Spinal instrumentation without fusion for progressive scoliosis in young children. *J. Pediatr. Orthop.* 17(6):734–742, 1997.

Theologis AA, Cahill P, Auriemma M, Betz R, Diab M. Vertebral body stapling in children younger than 10 years with idiopathic scoliosis with curve magnitude of 30° to 39°. *Spine* 38(25):1583–1588, 2013.

Wynne-Davies R. Infantile idiopathic scoliosis. Causative factors, particularly in the first six months of life. *J. Bone Joint Surg.* 57(2)-B:138–141, 1975.

CONGENITAL SCOLIOSIS

Basu PS, Elsebaie H, Noordeen MH. Congenital spinal deformity: a comprehensive assessment at presentation. *Spine* 27(20):2255–2259, 2002.

Hedden D. Management themes in congenital scoliosis. *J. Bone Joint Surg.* 89(Suppl 1)-A:72–78, 2007.

Hedequist DJ, Emans J. Congenital scoliosis: a review and update. *J. Pediatr. Orthop.* 27(1):106–116, 2007.

Kawakami N, Tsuji T, Imagama S, Lenke LG, Puno RM, Kuklo TR, Spinal Deformity Study Group. Classification of congenital scoliosis and kyphosis: a new approach to the three-dimensional classification for progressive vertebral anomalies requiring operative treatment. *Spine* 34(17):1756–1765, 2009.

Lenke LG, Newton PO, Sucato DJ, Shufflebarger HL, Emans JB, Sponseller PD, Shah SA, Sides BA, Blanke KM. Complications after 147 consecutive vertebral column resections for severe pediatric spinal deformity: a multicenter analysis. *Spine* 38(2):119–132, 2013.

Marks DS, Qaimkhani SA. The natural history of congenital scoliosis and kyphosis. *Spine* 34(17):1751–1755, 2009.

McMaster MJ. Spinal growth and congenital deformity of the spine. *Spine* 31(20):2284–2287, 2006.

Mehta MH. The rib-vertebra angle in the early diagnosis between resolving and progressive infantile scoliosis. *J. Bone Joint Surg.* 54(2)-B:230–243, 1972.

Mehta MH. Growth as a corrective force in the early treatment of progressive infantile scoliosis. *J. Bone Joint Surg.* 87(9)-B:1237–1247, 2005.

Ruf M, Jensen R, Letko L, Harms J. Hemivertebra resection and osteotomies in congenital spine deformity. *Spine* 34(17):1791–1799, 2009.

Yazici M, Emans J. Fusionless instrumentation systems for congenital scoliosis: expandable spinal rods and vertical expandable prosthetic titanium rib in the management of congenital spine deformities in the growing child. *Spine* 34(17):1800–1807, 2009.

KYPHOSIS—CONGENITAL

McMaster MJ, Singh H. Natural history of congenital kyphosis and kyphoscoliosis. A study of one hundred and twelve patients. *J. Bone Joint Surg.* 81(10)-A:1367–1383, 1999.

Kawakami N, Tsuji T, Imagama S, Lenke LG, Puno RM, Kuklo TR, Spinal Deformity Study Group. Classification of congenital scoliosis and kyphosis: a new approach to the three-dimensional classification for progressive vertebral anomalies requiring operative treatment. *Spine* 34(17):1756–1765, 2009.

Noordeen MH, Garrido E, Tucker SK, Elsebaie HB. The surgical treatment of congenital kyphosis. *Spine* 34(17):1808–1814, 2009.

KYPHOSIS—OF SCHEUERMANN

Coe JD, Smith JS, Berven S, Arlet V, Donaldson W, Hanson D, Mudiyam R, Perra J, Owen J, Marks MC, Shaffrey CI. Complications of spinal fusion for Scheuermann kyphosis: a report of the Scoliosis Research Society Morbidity and Mortality Committee. *Spine* 35(1):99–103, 2009.

Lowe TG, Line BG. Evidence based medicine: analysis of Scheuermann kyphosis. *Spine* 32(19 Suppl):S115–S119, 2007.

Montgomery SP, Erwin WE. Scheuermann's kyphosis: long-term results of Milwaukee brace treatment. *Spine* 6(1):5–8, 1981.

Murray PM, Weinstein SL, Spratt KF. The natural history and long-term follow-up of Scheuermann kyphosis. *J. Bone Joint Surg.* 75(2)-A:236–248, 1993.

Riddle EC, Bowen JR, Shah SA, Moran EF, Lawall H Jr. The DuPont kyphosis brace for the treatment of adolescent Scheuermann kyphosis. *J. South. Orthop. Assoc.* 12(3):135–140, 2003.

Sachs B, Bradford D, Winter R, Lonstein J, Moe J, Willson S. Scheuermann kyphosis: follow-up of Milwaukee-brace treatment. *J. Bone Joint Surg.* 69(1)-A:50–57, 1987.

SPONDYLOLYSIS AND SPONDYLOLISTHESIS

Agabegi SS, Fischgrund JS. Contemporary management of isthmic spondylolisthesis: pediatric and adult. *Spine J.* 10(6):530–543, 2010.

Beutler WJ, Fredrickson BE, Murtland A, Sweeney CA, Grant WD, Baker D. The natural history of spondylolysis and spondylolisthesis: 45-year follow-up evaluation. *Spine* 28(10):1027–1035, 2003.

Bradford DS, Iza J. Repair of the defect in spondylolysis or minimal degrees of spondylolisthesis by segmental wire fixation and bone grafting. *Spine* 10(7):673–679, 1985.

Buck JE. Direct repair of the defect in spondylolisthesis. Preliminary report. *J. Bone Joint Surg.* 52(3)-B:432–437, 1970.

Hu SS, Tribus CB, Diab M, Ghanayem AJ. Spondylolisthesis and spondylolysis. *J. Bone Joint Surg.* 90(3)-A:656–671 2008.

Klein G, Mehlman CT, McCarty M. Nonoperative treatment of spondylolysis and grade I spondylolisthesis in children and young adults: a meta-analysis of observational studies. *J. Pediatr. Orthop.* 29(2):146–156, 2009.

Meyerding HW. Low backache and sciatic pain associated with spondylolisthesis and protruded intervertebral disc: incidence, significance, and treatment. *J. Bone Joint Surg.* 23(2):461–470, 1941.

Steiner ME, Micheli LJ. Treatment of symptomatic spondylolysis and spondylolisthesis with the modified Boston brace. *Spine* 10:937–943, 1985.

Taillard WF. Etiology of spondylolisthesis. *Clin. Orthop.* 117:30–39, 1976.

DISCITIS

Wenger DR, Bobechko WP, Gilday DL. The spectrum of intervertebral disk-space infection in children. *J. Bone Joint Surg.* 60A:100, 1978.

TUMORS

Beer SJ, Menezes AH. Primary tumors of the spine in children. Natural history, management, and long-term follow-up. *Spine* 22(6):649–658, 1997.

OTHER

Kim HW, Weinstein SL. Spine update. The management of scoliosis in neurofibromatosis. *Spine* 22(23):2770–2776, 1997.

Klippel M, Feil A. Un cas d'absence des vertebres cervicales avec cage thoracique remontant jusqua à la base du crane (cage thoracique cervicale). *Nouv. Icon. Salpetière* 25:223, 1912.

Lipton GE, Guille JT, Kumar SJ. Surgical treatment of scoliosis in Marfan syndrome: guidelines for a successful outcome. *J. Pediatr. Orthop.* 22(3):302–307, 2002.

Papaioannou T, Stokes I, Kenwright J. Scoliosis associated with limb-length inequality. *J. Bone Joint Surg.* 64(1)-A:59–62, 1982.

Vercauteren M, Van Beneden M, Verplaetse R, Croene P, Uyttendaele D, Verdonk R. Trunk asymmetries in a Belgian school population. *Spine* 7(6):555–562, 1982.

HIP

GENERAL

More than one-third of hip problems in adults have their origin during growth.

Development

The distal femur is the only epiphysis consistently present at birth. The proximal epiphysis of the femur appears by the 2nd month in girls (2 to 6 months) and the 4th month in boys (4 to 8 months). The apophysis of trochanter major appears by the 3rd year, while that of trochanter minor appears by the 9th year. The proximal femur develops from a cartilage model in continuity from head to trochanter major until separation at the neck by the 13th year [A]. The acetabulum grows in depth and width from the triradiate cartilage and by apposition from the edge [B]. A secondary ossification center at the edge of the acetabulum appears in the early second decade, known as os acetabuli. The trochanter major enlarges by physeal growth up to 8 years of age, after which growth is appositional.

Understanding growth of the hip elucidates disease and injury.

- Röntgenogramme for hip dysplasia becomes more reliable after appearance of the proximal epiphysis of the femur.
- Disease of the proximal femur epiphysis, such as Legg-Calvé-Perthes disease, affects the height and shape of the head, as well as the length of the neck.
- Injury to the cartilage between the head and trochanter major, as in antegrade nailing or curettage of lesion, results in growth disturbance of the neck of the femur [B].
- Fracture or injury of triradiate cartilage may result in premature closure and acetabular dysplasia.

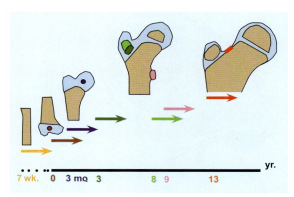

A Ossification of the femur Diaphysis (*orange*), distal epiphysis (*brown*), proximal epiphysis (*blue*), trochanter major (*green*), trochanter minor (*pink*), separation of proximal femur cartilage model (*red*).

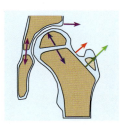
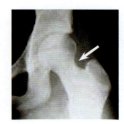

B Growth of the hip Acetabulum and trochanter major growth is physeal and appositional. Proximal femoral growth is physeal, while the neck grows by apposition of bone. Interference with the latter results in growth disturbance, as the thin neck seen on röntgenogramme after curettage of cervical cyst (*white*).

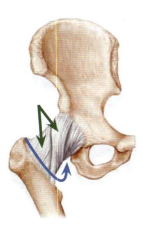

C Orientation of the hip joint The fibers of the hip joint capsule are rotated medialward. The anterior capsule is stouter and includes the Y-shaped iliofemoral ligament of Bigelow (*green*). Relaxation of the capsular fibers is maximized by lateral rotation and flexion, which is the position of comfort in painful conditions.

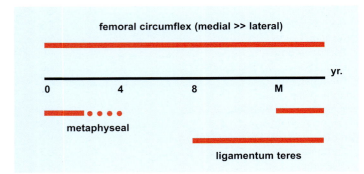

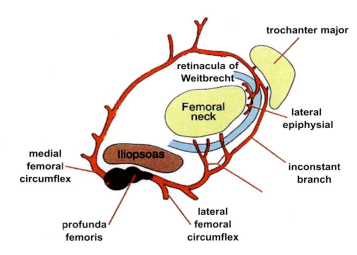

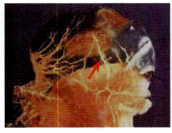

D Vascularity of the head of the femur Blood supply varies according to age. M: maturity. Transphyseal vessels (*red*) and lateral retinacular artery (*yellow*). There is variability, as evidenced by inconstant branch.

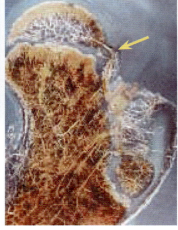

- Antegrade nailing for femur fracture is safe through trochanter major after 8 years of age. A case of a 10-year-old boy was included in Küntscher's original report on the technique.
- Os acetabuli is separated from the remainder of the acetabulum by horizontal or mildly oblique physeal cartilage; by contrast, a vertical orientation is seen with femoroacetabular impingement.

Evolutionarily, the forelimbs rotate laterally and the hindlimbs rotate medially. This results in medial twisting of the hip joint capsular fibers [C]. The universal response of a joint to injury or disease is effusion. The first and most consistently lost motion of a diseased hip is medial rotation: lateral rotation of the hip orients the capsular fibers parallel, thereby increasing volume of the hip joint to reduce pressure and stretch on pain fibers in the capsule.

Vascularity

In addition to growth disturbance, the immature proximal femur is susceptible to vascular injury. The head of the femur is perfused from three sources during childhood [D].

- In the neonatal period, metaphyseal vessels may traverse the physis to supply the head of the femur; after 4 years of age, the physis becomes impervious.
- Between 4 and 8 years of age, the head of the femur is dependent upon a single source: the circumflex vessels "travel around" the neck of the femur and are divided into medial and lateral based upon their direction of origin from the profunda femoris artery. The medial circumflex provides >80% of the blood supply to the head of the femur and enters the hip joint posterior to travel in the retinacula of Weitbrecht as the lateral epiphysial vessels. The lateral circumflex travels anterior and supplies the trochanter major in addition to the head of the femur.
- After 7 years of age, the artery of ligamentum teres reaches the epiphysis from the obturator artery.

After physeal closure, the metaphyseal blood supply returns.

Pathoanatomy

Select principles are essential to understanding hip deformity.

Cartilage Compression is good; shear is bad. Correct bone alignment to move oblique (shear) weight-bearing joint surface to horizontal (compression).

Acetabulum [E,F] The anterior wall overlaps the posterior wall approximately 50%. Margins of both walls meet at the lateral limit. In retroversion of the acetabulum, there is increasing overlap of the anterior wall until its margin overshadows that of the posterior wall to produce a crossover sign. The *sourcil* (named in French after its resemblance to an "eyebrow") represents the principal weight-bearing surface: osteotomy of the pelvis aims to place this horizontal. Pressure = Force/Area. The acetabulum should cover enough of the head of the femur to avoid abnormal stress concentration, in particular at the edge. The "teardrop" represents medial wall of acetabulum: widening suggests insufficient medial force from a subluxated head of femur, and displacement beyond the ilioischial line (of Köhler) is defined as *coxa profunda*: "deep hip."

Proximal femur [E,F] The top of the trochanter major is at the level of the center of the head of the femur. If the top is above this level, there is varus deformity; if the top is below this level, there is valgus deformity. The articulotrochanteric distance is measured from the top of the articular surface of the head of the femur to the top of trochanter major: it is increased in valgus, reduced in varus, and negative in severe varus. This assessment of varus and valgus is independent of rotation, which may distort measurement of neck–shaft angle. Tip of trochanter major is 2 radii lateral (offset) to the center of the head of the femur. "Protrusion" of the head of the femur beyond the ilioischial line is defined as *protrusio acetabuli*.

Femoral anteversion and neck–shaft angle vary *in utero*, are maximum at 2 years of age, and then decline until maturity [G]. The head is offset from the neck in coronal and sagittal planes [H]. The head–neck

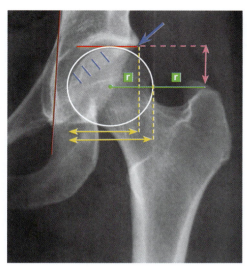

E Anatomic relationships in two dimensions.

Red: *sourcil*

Blue: anterior wall

Blue arrow: meeting of walls

White: head circumference

Green: radius

Yellow: coverage 0.8

Pink: articulotrochanteric distance (mm)

Brown: ilioischial line

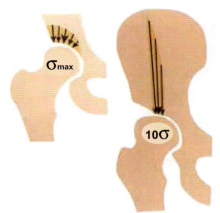

F Stress concentration
Reduction of coverage results in an order of magnitude increase in stress (σ) at *sourcil*. Subluxation, as measured by medial joint width (*green*), reduces coverage and congruity. The bone has reacted to stress concentration at *sourcil* (*red*).

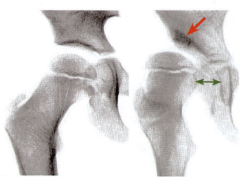

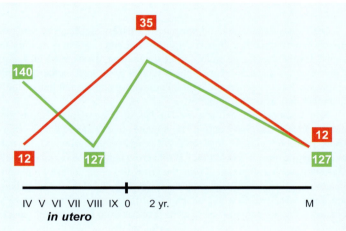

G Angulation of the proximal femur Mean values of neck–shaft angle (*green*) and neck anteversion (*red*) in degrees. Fœtal age in Roman numerals. M: maturity.

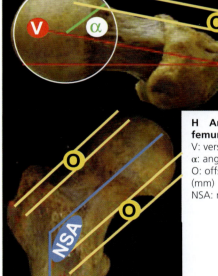

H Architecture of the proximal femur.
V: version of the neck (degrees)
α: angle of head–neck junction
O: offset of the head and neck (mm)
NSA: neck–shaft angle

junction subtends an angle (designated α) with the longitudinal axis of the neck in both planes. Lateral offset is reduced and α angle is increased in femoroacetabular impingement and slipped capital femoral epiphysis. The latter also is characterized by reduction in coronal plane offset, simulating varus deformity in the anteroposterior projection.

The head of the femur is spherical, which allows motion in all dimensions. More important than sphericity is congruity: while the latter may concede limitation in motion, matching articular surfaces prevent stress concentration. Incongruity despite cosphericity occurs in subluxation, leading to edge loading.

Distinguishing Features

The hip is a bone-dependent joint, in contrast with the knee (ligament dependent) and the shoulder (muscle dependent). It is enarthrodial, consisting of a "ball in socket" that allows motion in all directions, like the shoulder and in contrast with the knee, which is ginglymoid ("hinge-like"), and the symphysis pubica or sacroiliac joints, which as syndesmoses absorb motion more than they allow it. The hip, like the shoulder, may be distinguished by its axial location, which under cover of multiple layers of thick muscle makes it obscure to direct observation and palpation. It also may be distinguished by the precariousness of its blood supply, raising the specter of osteonecrosis in several of its disorders and management. Outside of trauma, the hip in a

I Congruity *versus* sphericity Incongruity (*red*) leads to stress concentration, which may result from subluxation in hip dysplasia (*brown*) or rotational osteotomy (*blue*).

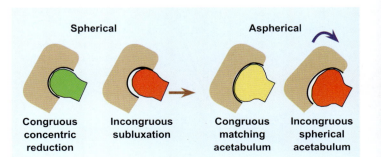

Spherical — Congruous concentric reduction — Incongruous subluxation — Aspherical — Congruous matching acetabulum — Incongruous spherical acetabulum

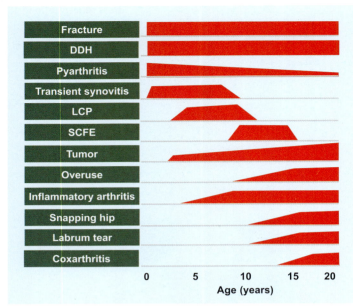

A Conditions affecting the hip by age DDH: developmental dysplasia of the hip. LCP: Legg-Calvé-Perthes. SCFE: slipped capital femoral epiphysis.

child demands more attention of the surgeon than any other joint. Like the glenoid cavity of the shoulder, the acetabulum is rimmed by a labrum. Like the cruciate ligaments of the knee, the hip joint is traversed by the ligamentum teres (also known as ligamentum capitis femoris), connecting the fovea centralis of the head of the femur with the fossa of the acetabulum.

EVALUATION

History

Is there a family history? Developmental dysplasia of the hip can be familial. Has there been an alteration of gait? The waddle of a dislocated hip may seem attractive in a young girl. Does the hip make noise or catch? Crepitus may be a sign of labrum tear.

Age Age is a universal discriminator of disease [A].

Onset In the acute presentation, it is imperative to rule out fracture, which occurs after an antecedent event, pyarthritis, and slipped capital femoral epiphysis, which carries urgency due to the fragile vascularity of the hip. Other conditions, such as Legg-Calvé-Perthes disease, tend to have a more insidious onset and chronic course.

Physical Examination

Observation Does the child appear ill? Distress and fear are signs of infection or trauma. Are there constitutional or other system symptoms or signs? Hyperactivity and small for age have been associated with Legg-Calvé-Perthes disease. Overweight is typical of slipped capital femoral epiphysis. Rash is associated with inflammatory and autoimmune conditions that may affect the joints.

Pain Is there pain, and where? The law of Hilton (John Hilton, surgeon at Guy's Hospital London, 1860) states that "a nerve which innervates a muscle that acts on a joint will innervate that joint and the skin overlying the muscle's insertion." While groin pain may have an intrapelvic origin, such as inguinal hernia, the groin also is the locus of hip pain. In addition, femoral and obturator nerves supply muscles inserting about the anteromedial knee, where hip pain manifests in isolation in up to 15% of cases. Buttock pain may be from the back or from hip abductor muscle fatigue. The latter also may manifest as lateral pain, which in turn may be produced by contracture of the iliotibial tract.

Pain that awakens from sleep is concerning, in particular for osteoid osteoma. Tenderness may be seen in apophysitis or apophyseal injury. Be careful of a "groin pull" in the peripubescent or associated with lateral rotation of the lower limb.

Gait Is there a limp, and if so what type? Reduced stance phase is seen in painful conditions such as trauma. Pain without an alteration in gait is less concerning. Abductor lurch (of Trendelenburg) results from weakness of pericoxal muscles [B]. Out-toeing gait is pathognomonic of slipped capital femoral epiphysis in a peripubescent child.

Palpation The hip joint is deep, and as such, points of tenderness are less revealing than more exposed joints such as the knee. Apophyses are accessible, including at iliac spines, tuberosity of ischium, and trochanter major in traumatic separation or irritation (overuse). Crepitus may be elicited from the hip joint, for example, labrum, or from pericoxal tissues, for example, a snapping psoa muscle in the groin or an iliotibial tract grating or "jumping" (*coxa saltans*) across trochanter major.

Motion

PSEUDOPARALYSIS Severity of disease or early age of onset may cause the child to quit the limb, out of pain and fear.

HIP ROTATION Medial rotation is the first and most characteristic motion lost in hip disease; this is followed by flexed posture or contracture. The prone position has three principal advantages [C]. It stresses a hip held in flexion. Comparison may be made as both hips may be moved simultaneously. The knee may be decoupled from the hip: the former may be moved without obligate motion of the latter, as occurs supine. Supine position allows assessment of rotation in the flexed position, which may be altered as the neck of the femur impacts acetabulum, as in slipped capital femoral epiphysis deformity.

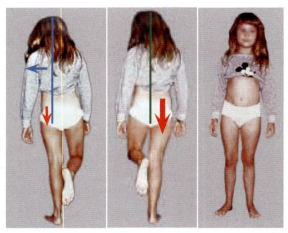

B Trendelenburg In developmental dysplasia of the hip, the abductor muscles are shortened and thereby weakened. In single limb stance, the patient reduces the lever arm of body mass by leaning toward the affected side (*blue*) to aid the contracting weakened hip abductors (*red*) to maintain the pelvis horizontal and avoid tilting and falling in the opposite direction. On the unaffected side, the head remains centered over the pelvis because the hip abductors are strong enough to maintain a horizontal pelvis with an unaltered lever arm. In two-limb stance, the affected limb is shortened. Gait may be observed as the child approaches the examination room. Trendelenburg elicited his sign during physical examination of a child with a dislocated hip (1895).

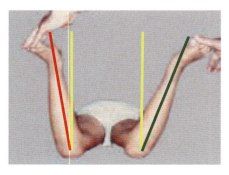

C Hip rotation prone Comparison may be made simultaneously of motion at both hips. Prone also exposes flexion contracture and allows isolation of movement of the knee from movement of the hip.

FLEXION In addition to losing medial rotation, the painful or diseased hip is held in flexion. This is exposed automatically when evaluating motion in the prone position. In the supine position, a contracture may be detected by the Thomas or the prone extension test [D]. Pain with flexion beyond 90 degrees, exacerbated by adduction and medial rotation, suggests impingement. By contrast, the same pain with the same manœuvre but with normal or increased motion is seen in hip dysplasia, due to damage of a deficient anterior wall of acetabulum.

EXTENSION Perform supine with pelvis at edge of table. The patient flexes contralateral hip while the examiner extends the hip and limb beyond table. Anterior deficiency of acetabulum, as in hip dysplasia, produces apprehension. Painful extension also may be seen in psoa abscess.

ABDUCTION–ADDUCTION Assess with fingers on anterior superior iliac spines as reference points, so that tilting of the pelvis does not mask contracture. Varus deformity of the hip, or growth disturbance of the head and neck of the femur, will lead to abutment of trochanter major against the ilium, thereby limiting abduction. Reduced adduction due to iliotibial tract contracture is assessed by Ober test: patient lateral; the examiner hand stabilizes the pelvis to keep it vertical; contralateral hip held by the patient in flexed position; and examined hip flexed, then abducted, and then extended while the examiner holds foot only. Contracture prevents the examined limb from adducting: the knee will remain suspended in abduction beyond midline.

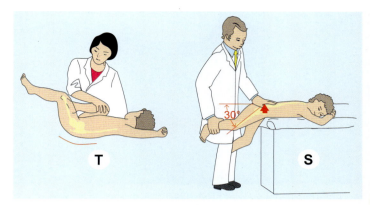

D Hip flexion contracture assessment In the Thomas test (T), maximal flexion of the contralateral hip eliminates lordosis of the lumbar spine, which can be a compensatory position for hip flexion contracture. In the prone extension test (S), gradually extend the hip until the hand on the pelvis begins to rise.

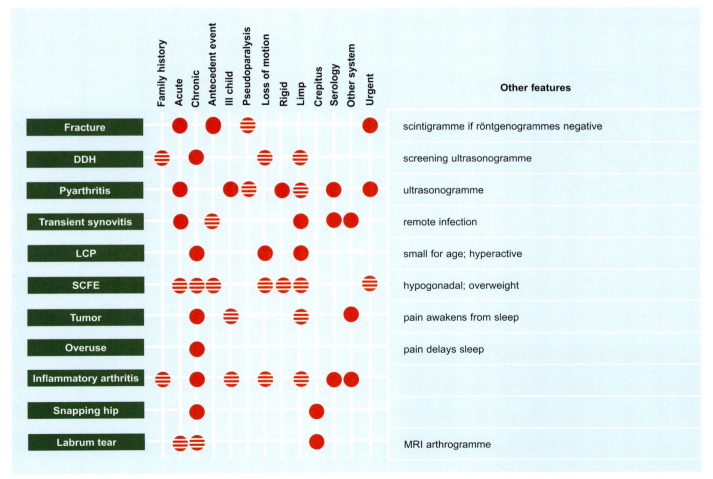

	Family history	Acute	Chronic	Antecedent event	Ill child	Pseudoparalysis	Loss of motion	Rigid	Limp	Crepitus	Serology	Other system	Urgent	Other features
Fracture		●		●		◒							●	scintigramme if röntgenogrammes negative
DDH	◒		●				◒	◒						screening ultrasonogramme
Pyarthritis		●		●	◒		●	●			●		●	ultrasonogramme
Transient synovitis		●		◒				●		●	●			remote infection
LCP			●				●		●					small for age; hyperactive
SCFE		◒	◒	◒			◒	◒	◒				◒	hypogonadal; overweight
Tumor		●		◒			◒		●					pain awakens from sleep
Overuse			●											pain delays sleep
Inflammatory arthritis	◒		●		◒		●		◒	●	●			
Snapping hip			●						●					
Labrum tear		◒ ◒							●					MRI arthrogramme

E   Diagnosis of hip disease Characteristic (solid) and possible features (striped). DDH: developmental dysplasia of the hip. LCP: Legg-Calvé-Perthes. SCFE: slipped capital femoral epiphysis.

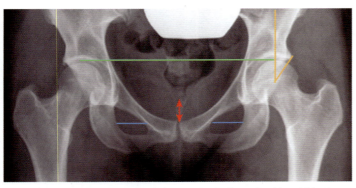

A   Anteroposterior view of pelvis Rotation is determined by width of obturated foramina (*blue*). Inclination is determined by coccygosymphyseal distance (*red*). Limb lengths are similar (*green*). Note angle between head center–edge of acetabulum (*orange*).

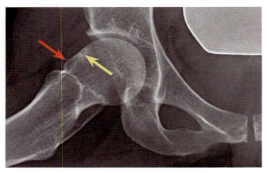

B   Lateral of proximal femur Note bump (*red*) on the neck with adjacent cyst (*yellow*), due to femoroacetabular impingement.

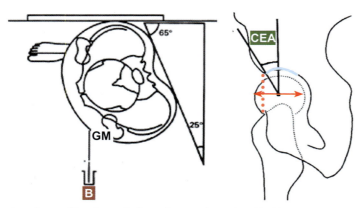

C   False profile of acetabulum The *sourcil* is outlined by blue. B: X-ray beam (*brown*). CEA: center–edge angle, subtended by a line drawn from the center of the head to anterior articular margin of acetabulum with a vertical line. Coverage (d:D) is measured as a ratio determined by a vertical line from the anterior articular margin of acetabulum (d) to the diameter of the head (D).

Imaging

Röntgenogrammes These are the foundation of imaging for the hip.

- In the anteroposterior projection of the pelvis, symmetry of the transverse diameters of the obturated foramina ensures neutral [A]. In the standing position, tip of coccyx to symphysis pubica distance 1 to 3 cm ensures correct pelvic tilt. The top of the femoral heads may be used to determine limb lengths, assuming a standing position with knees straight. Medial rotation of the lower limbs neutralizes anteversion of the femora for true coronal relationship with acetabula. The angle between a vertical through the center of the head of the femur and a line drawn from the center to the edge of the articular margin of acetabulum is a measure of coverage. The normal range is 25 degrees to 45 degrees: less represents insufficient coverage, as in developmental dysplasia of the hip, while more represents overcoverage, as in pincer impingement or *protrusio acetabuli*.

- Lateral projection of the proximal femora may be obtained by supine abduction with external rotation ("frog-leg"), placing the feet together with the knees flexed to 90 degrees [B]. In the painful or unstable hip, an easier and safer view is taken supine with the contralateral hip flexed 90 degrees and the x-ray beam directed "cross-table" at 45 degrees to the symptomatic limb. Soft tissue may obscure details. In the operating room, a lateral projection of the proximal femur may be obtained by flexing the hip to 45 degrees while preserving neutral rotation, and rotating the image intensifier 45 degrees away (modified Dunn).

- Supine abduction with medial rotation of the femora (von Rosen) assesses center of rotation of the head of the femur compared with acetabulum and simulates redirectional osteotomy of the acetabulum.

- The *faux profil* ("false profile") provides a true lateral of the acetabulum, based upon its version [C]. The patient stands with affected hip against the film, pelvis rotated 65 degrees toward affected side, and affected foot parallel to film. The angle between a vertical through the center of the head of the femur and a line drawn from the center to the edge of the articular margin of acetabulum is a measure of anterior coverage. Less than 20 degrees is abnormal.

- Version of acetabulum [D]. Normal version presents a symmetric opening of the cup to the front of the hip, seen on anteroposterior projection as an anterior wall that covers half of the posterior wall, which it meets at the lateral margin of acetabulum. In retroversion of the acetabulum, the anterior wall advances on the posterior wall, progressively crossing it from lateral to medial. Retroversion rotates the ischial spine anteriorward and medialward into profile. Note that projection of the walls of the acetabulum is influenced by pelvic tilt, which must be correct to correctly assess version of acetabulum and crossover.

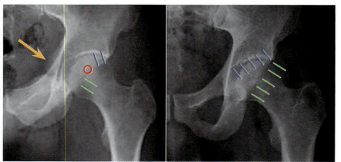

D   Version of acetabulum The acetabulum on the left is retroverted: the anterior wall (*blue*) crosses (*red*) the posterior wall (*green*), and the ischial spine is visible (*orange*). On the right, where version is normal, anterior and posterior walls do not cross, meeting at the lateral margin of acetabulum, and the ischial spine is hidden behind the acetabulum.

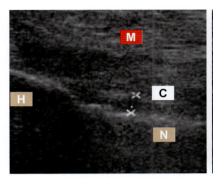
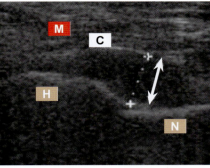

E Ultrasonography for hip effusion The joint capsule is elevated (*white*) off the femur by fluid. H: head of the femur. N: neck of the femur. C: capsule. M: muscle.

Ultrasonography This is the standard for screening and evaluation of hip dysplasia from neonatal period to 4 to 6 months. Ultrasonography is useful for evaluating the hip for effusion [E]. It is quantitative and qualitative, demonstrating volume of fluid and type (e.g., clear vs. turbid). It is harmless, is practical, and may be performed with the child awake, by contrast with MRI, which provides more detail at the expense of complexity and sedation. Other applications include assessment of severity of slipped capital femoral epiphysis, of head size and containment in Legg-Calvé-Perthes disease, and of neck continuity in coxa vara. This imaging technique is underutilized, despite the fact that it has the distinct advantage of being practicable by an orthopædic surgeon in office.

Scintigraphy This is a physiologic imaging modality, providing a measure of bone turnover and perfusion. After excluding pyarthritis by an ultrasonogramme showing no effusion of the hip, a scintigramme evaluates the lower limb for osteomyelitis as a cause of limp. Inflammatory conditions may be localized, such as osteoid osteoma of the proximal femur. Hypoperfusion may be detected, such as of a slipped capital femoral epiphysis with an acute or unstable or severe presentation, or of the proximal epiphysis of the femur during the initial ischæmic stage of Legg-Calvé-Perthes disease [F]. Hyperperfusion of the proximal physis of the femur may be an alert to a preslip state.

Arthrography Arthrogramme confirms articular penetration, as in arthrocentesis in infection or for diagnostic injection when a locus of pain is obscure. The technique aids operative evaluation of dislocation and reduction in developmental dysplasia of the hip. It provides further static definition of the deformed head of the femur in Legg-Calvé-Perthes disease [G] and permits dynamic assessment of hip motion. Arthrography enhances magnetic resonance imaging.

Magnetic resonance imaging This modality provides greatest detail, in particular of intra-articular structures such as labrum in developmental dysplasia of the hip [H], epiphysis with altered perfusion, physis in slipped capital femoral epiphysis, a mobile body after trauma, or effusion as a first or only sign of disease. Rapid sequence protocol assesses location of the head of the femur after reduction of a dislocated hip, without X-radiation. Balance this with less availability, less agency for the surgeon, increased cost, and the fact that in the first decade sedation may be necessary to avoid motion artifact. Gadolinium may be injected for arthrography or *per venam* to measure proteoglycan content of cartilage.

Computerized tomography CT gives the most accurate depiction of osseous architecture, in particular as part of preparation for osteotomy of the pelvis or femur in the setting of complex deformity. It is less distorted than MRI by metal, as in postoperative evaluation of implant placement or healing of osteotomy [I]. Rapid sequence protocol assesses location of the head of the femur after reduction of a dislocated hip, but with radiation exposure in contrast with MRI.

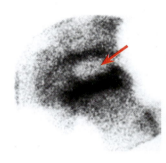

F Scintigraphy of the hip Focal lateral and anterior reduced uptake in the epiphysis (*red*) indicates ischæmic stage at presentation of Legg-Calvé-Perthes disease.

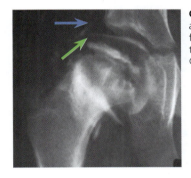

G Arthrography of the hip The articular surface is outlined showing flattening of the epiphysis (*green*) by the lateral acetabulum (*blue*) in Legg-Calvé-Perthes disease.

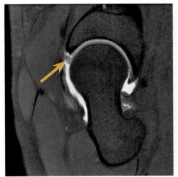

H MRI arthrography of the hip Gadolinium (*white*) fills the gap between acetabulum and anterior labrum, which is cystic and detached (*orange*) due to chronic stress concentration on a deficient anterior wall.

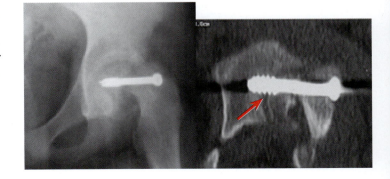

I CT to evaluate implant placement In this severe slipped capital femoral epiphysis, uncertainty about location of screw was resolved by CT, showing transarticular fixation (*red*).

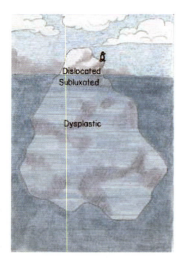

A   Spectrum of hip dysplasia Dislocated hips are usually diagnosed during infancy, but hip dysplasia may not become evident until adult life, when it presents as degenerative coxarthritis.

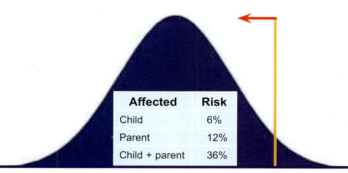

Affected	Risk
Child	6%
Parent	12%
Child + parent	36%

B   Inheritance of DDH Liability curve for affecteds. Polygenic inheritance follows a normal distribution: threshold (*orange*) above which a disease will be expressed (incidence) is lowered in first-degree relatives (*red*).

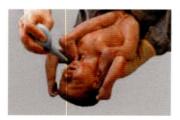

C   Breech This extrinsic cause of DDH represents a problem of packaging.

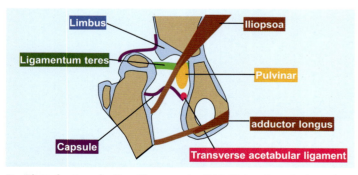

D   Obstacles to reduction These may be divided into extra-articular and articular.

Abduction	% normal
45 degrees	0%
60 degrees	<10
75 degrees	45%
90 degrees	45%

E   Hip abduction Normal infants will rarely have <60 degrees of hip abduction.

DEVELOPMENTAL DYSPLASIA OF THE HIP

Dysplasia refers to "bad" (Greek δυς) "formation" (Greek πλασσω) of the hip. The term developmental encompasses cases that are congenital, present "at birth," and those developing after birth, in which the neonatal evaluation is normal.

Incidence

Hip laxity affects up to 1% of neonates, whereas clinically detectable DDH affects 0.1% of the Caucasian population. The true incidence remains unclear [A]. Physical examination and even screening ultrasonography will have a certain miss rate for several reasons, including operator error, single evaluation of a developing condition in a developing skeleton, and the use of indirect measures as proxies for final outcomes. As a result, DDH may underlie up to one-third of adult coxarthritis.

Cause

The causes of DDH may be divided into intrinsic or extrinsic. The former represents polygenic inheritance ('problems of production'), in which a characteristic is controlled quantitatively by more than one gene (the quintessential example is height) [B]. The latter refers to 'problems of packaging', of which the most significant factor is breech, with oligohydramnios and primigravida uterus being relative factors [C]. Girls and the left hip are affected more. Incidence in Caucasians is 1%: it is five times more in Lappland and five times less in Africans.

Pathoanatomy

The acetabulum is shallow and maldirected. The proximal femur shows antetorsion and coxa valga. When either or both are sufficiently severe, the head of the femur will dislocate. Extra-articular obstacles to reduction include iliopsoa, which constricts capsule such that it will display an hourglass configuration with arthrography, and adductor longus [D]. Articular obstacles include labrum, which may be inverted and hypertrophied as the limbus, ligamentum teres, a thickened and tortuous ribbon, pulvinar, which expands (nature abhors a vacuum), and medial inferior capsule.

Evaluation

Physical examination This first is performed as part of neonatal screening, during subsequent routine evaluations, and as part of an orthopædic consultation. Take what the child will give: relax if there is resistance, and resume with no force when the child relaxes. Test for instability in the entire range of hip motion.

Hɪᴘ ᴄʟɪᴄᴋ This is normal. It refers to a fine short-duration feeling or sound that is a manifestation of laxity stressing the limits of motion. Differentiate from a "clunk," which represents the deep perception of a shift as the head of the femur dislocates and relocates. The sensation of the hip being displaced over the acetabular margin.

Cᴜᴛᴀɴᴇᴏᴜꜱ ᴄʀᴇᴀꜱᴇꜱ Asymmetry may be seen in long-standing dislocation in older children, where significant contracture has had time to develop. Asymmetric and extra creases affect approximately 50% of normal infants.

Hɪᴘ ᴀʙᴅᴜᴄᴛɪᴏɴ Abduction of the hip <60 degrees is concerning for DDH [E].

Bᴀʀʟᴏᴡ ꜱɪɢɴ Dislocation of a reduced hip [F]. With adduction of the hip, the head of the femur moves out over the rim of acetabulum. There is no need for posteriorward force: gravity will suffice.

Oʀᴛᴏʟᴀɴɪ ꜱɪɢɴ Reduction of a dislocated hip [G]. With abduction and anterior translation applied to the trochanter major, the head of the femur moves into the acetabulum. Prolonged dislocation may result in sufficient contracture to resist this manœuvre, producing an "Ortolani negative" hip. The only sign may be limited abduction. The symmetry of bilateral presentation may obscure detection.

Lᴏᴡᴇʀ ʟɪᴍʙ ʟᴇɴɢᴛʜ ᴅɪꜱᴄʀᴇᴘᴀɴᴄʏ The head of the femur, taking with it the rest of the limb, rests behind a dislocated hip, producing a lower limb length discrepancy [H].

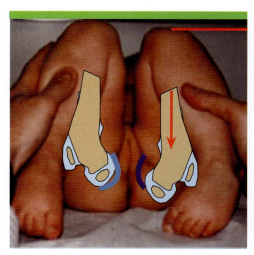

H Galeazzi or Allis sign Posterior displacement of the head and rest of the femur produces a limb length discrepancy that is exposed as differential knee heights.

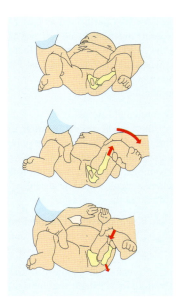 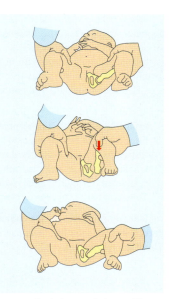

F Barlow sign A reduced hip is dislocated by adduction, posteriorward under force of gravity.

G Ortolani sign A dislocated hip is reduced by abduction with anterior translation applied to trochanter major, perceived as a "clunk."

LUMBAR LORDOSIS Dislocation in which the hips are displaced significantly craniad, and posteriorward is accompanied by anterior pelvic tilt and flexion contracture of the hips. The child compensates by hyperlordosis of the lumbar spine to maintain sagittal balance [I].

GAIT The dysplastic acetabulum, without or with subluxation, is silent in the first decade. Hip dislocation produces a Trendelenburg gait due to craniad displacement of trochanter major with shortening and thereby weakening of hip abductor muscles.

PACKAGING SIGNS As part of the extrinsic causation of DDH, other parts of the musculoskeletal system may manifest deformation, including plagiocephaly, torticollis, and metatarsus adductus. The natural history of these is benign, with spontaneous resolution without active treatment. A corollary is DDH as a packaging sign in association with congenital dislocation of the knee.

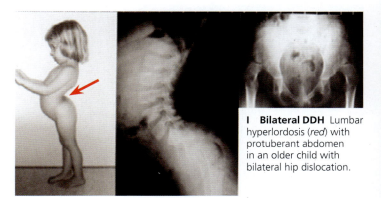

I Bilateral DDH Lumbar hyperlordosis (*red*) with protuberant abdomen in an older child with bilateral hip dislocation.

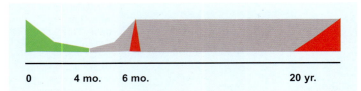

A Imaging of DDH Green: ultrasonography. Grey: röntgenography. Red: MRI.

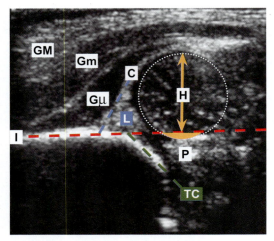

B Ultrasonography of the hip Developmental dysplasia of the hip with dislocation may be assessed by a portable ultrasonographic machine in the examining room. H: head of the femur, unossified. P: pulvinar and other fibrofatty tissue in fossa of acetabulum. TC: triradiate cartilage, hypoechoic. L: labrum. C: capsule. I: ilium, G: gluteus muscle, M: maximus, m: medius, m: minimus. Ilium line is the reference (red). Measure d:D ratio for coverage of the head of the femur (orange). Measure α (green) and β (blue) angles to assess depth of acetabulum and displacement of the head of the femur, respectively.

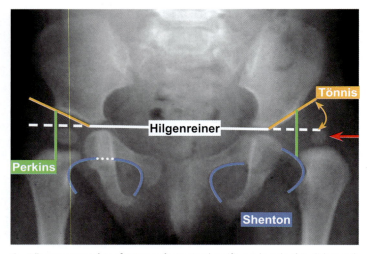

C Röntgenography of DDH Left proximal ossific nucleus (red) is dislocated into lower lateral quadrant.

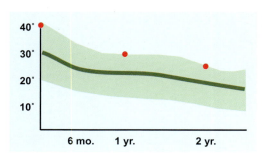

D Acetabular index by age This is measured in degrees. Light green bounds two standard deviations from the mean (dark green).

Imaging This varies according to age [A]. It is performed as part of neonatal screening, during subsequent routine evaluations, and as part of an orthopædic consultation. Take what the child will give: relax if there is resistance, and resume with no force when the child relaxes. Test for instability in the entire range of hip motion.

ULTRASONOGRAPHY Indications include the following:

- Screening tool. This is a practice in continental Europe.
- Infant at risk. This is the practice in the United States, in order to limit the false-positive rate. The definition of at risk varies: it may be restricted to breech girl, or it may include family history.
- Unclear physical examination, for example, if a fixed dislocation is suspected (Ortolani negative hip), where a clunk would be absent.
- To evaluate the success of brace treatment of the dysplastic hip.

Ultrasonography is not indicated when the physical examination detects a dysplastic hip, because imaging will not change management. There are two forms.

- Static [B]. This defines architecture. α (for "acetabulum") angle measures depth of acetabulum. This is mirrored by the β (next letter in the alphabet) angle, which measures deflection of the labrum by the head of the femur. d:D ratio measures coverage of the head of the femur by acetabulum.
- Dynamic. This evaluates stability and is an aid to the physical examination.

Normal α angle is >60 degrees. Most hips in range 43 degrees to 60 degrees "heal up" (Graf) without treatment. Normal d:D ratio is >0.5. Ratio <0.2 suggests failure of Pavlik harness. The static method describes architecture of the hip. The dynamic method may be considered the imaging extension of the physical examination: this, along with the fact that it is most operator dependent and is best assessed live (missed unless the surgeon is operator), makes it less useful.

RÖNTGENOGRAPHY This is the standard after 3 months of age, when the proximal femoral ossific nucleus is visible [C].

- Hilgenreiner line is the horizontal reference for the pelvis.
- Perkins line is a vertical mark of the lateral edge of acetabulum. In dislocation, the proximal femoral ossific nucleus lies lateral to this, with migration above Hilgenreiner line with increasing severity. If the nucleus has not ossified, medial corner of proximal metaphysis is medial to Perkins line in the normal hip.
- Shenton line is drawn along proximal metaphysis of the femur and margin of obturated foramen. Projected discontinuity between these two lines can highlight subluxation when dislocation is not apparent (e.g., when nucleus has not ossified).
- Acetabular index (of Tönnis) measures inclination of *sourcil*, a theme that arches over DDH regardless of age.

Normative data for acetabular index aid assessment of the dysplastic acetabulum without subluxation or dislocation [D]. The following are guidelines for abnormal (precision is evasive because measurement error is up to 10 degrees, due to observer, patient position, and projection):

- Index above 40 degrees in the first year of life.
- Index above 30 degrees in the second year of life.
- Index above 24 degrees by 24 months of age.

COMPUTERIZED AXIAL TOMOGRAPHY This is reserved for complex deformity, and when metal is present that would distort MRI. Be judicious in requesting this modality, due to radiation exposure early in life that is cumulative.

MAGNETIC RESONANCE IMAGING This has a bimodal application. It evaluates location of the head of the femur after closed or open reduction and immobilization of the infant hip, utilizing motion insensitive sequences that show sufficient detail despite sacrifice in resolution, avoiding need for anæsthesia. MRI has illuminated hip dysplasia in the teenager and young adult.

- Labrum. This is invisible to röntgenography or CT. Arthrography with gadolinium may highlight degenerative changes, such as tear or cyst.
- Impingement. This may be represented more accurately than by röntgenography, such as measurement of the α angle between the axis of the neck and a line drawn from center of the head to its junction with the neck in cam deformity of the proximal femur.
- Cartilage. Delayed gadolinium enhancement MRI of cartilage [E] is a measure of the biochemical composition of cartilage and as such of its health and mechanical properties. This contrasts with other structural or morphologic imaging modalities. An exogenous agent that may be nephrotoxic, the need for an exercise protocol to aid delivery to cartilage, and delay have stimulated development of other modalities. In sodium scanning, MRI may be used to measure relaxation times of the cation, which mirrors glycosaminoglycan concentration. Chemical exchange saturation transfer, T1r, T2 mapping, and diffusion-weighted MRI measure signal arising from protons as a biomarker, in particular hydroxyl and amide protons of glycosaminglycans. Ultrasonography shows healthy cartilage as homogeneously hypoechogenic with a well-defined chondrosynovial boundary, characteristics that are lost in degenerative arthritis.

Natural History

Untreated DDH may have the following outcomes [F, G].

- Acetabular dysplasia without subluxation. This presents in adulthood: cartilage degeneration results from stress concentration, according to the formula Pressure = Force/Area.
- Acetabular dysplasia with subluxation. This presents in childhood. Lack of concentric reduction significantly reduces surface area of contact, concentrating contact pressure. This is exacerbated by micromotion that shears cartilage.
- Acetabular dysplasia with dislocation. This in turn may be divided into without or with pseudoacetabulum. The former leads to functional disability produced by shortening and weakening of hip abductors, including Trendelenburg gait, fatigue pain, and restricted hip motion. The latter is associated with disabling pain due to osseous erosion between the head of the femur and ilium.

In one-third of patients treated for DDH (from bracing to operation), initial success will be followed by residual disease requiring secondary treatment. This is the rationale for long-term follow-up, through maturity. Treatment is mechanical and not more fundamental for a disease that has multiple causes, including genetic. Treatment aims to bring a dysplastic hip into the normative range and relies on it *sua sponte* to continue to grow appropriately once acetabulum and femur are correctly aligned. Such follow-up is akin to evaluation of height and weight at well checks by the pædiatrician: a child in the 50th percentile may fall off the charts with growth.

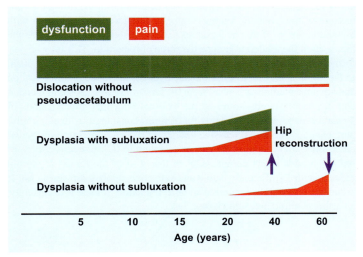

G   Dysfunction and pain from DDH.

E   Delayed gadolinium enhancement MRI of cartilage (dGEMRIC) Gadolinium concentrates in degenerated cartilage (*white arrow*). The extracellular matrix is depleted of glycosaminoglycans, of which negatively charged carboxyl and sulfate groups otherwise would repel the anionic contrast agent.

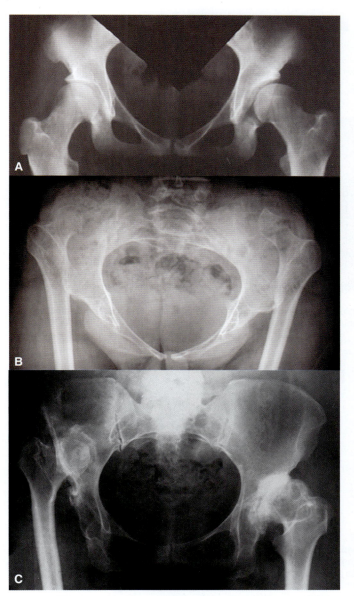

F   Natural history of untreated DDH A. Asymptomatic young adult treated for bilateral DDH from infancy with residual dysplasia without subluxation. B. Middle-aged adult with waddling gait and no pain, with bilateral high dislocations. Note pelvic inlet view due to hip flexion contractures, with associated lumbar hyperlordosis. C. Poor outcome of DDH, with bilateral severe hip pain. Left hip subluxation with end-stage degeneration, and right hip dislocation with pseudoacetabulum.

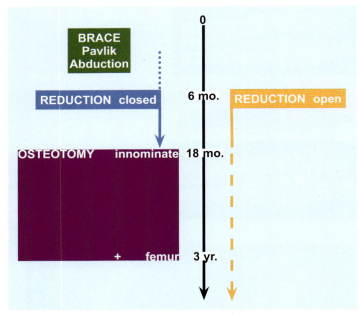

A Treatment of DDH according to age.

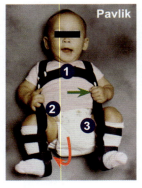

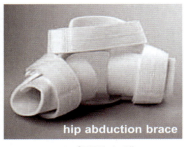

B Brace treatment of DDH 1: Allow comfortable passage of a finger under chest strap. 2: Adjust anterior strap (*green*) to flex hip to 90 degrees. 3: Keep posterior strap (*red*) loose enough that hip abducts to 45 degrees while allowing the knees to come together easily.

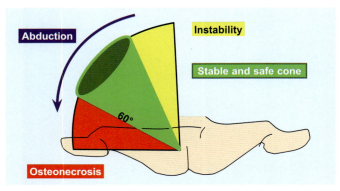

C Position of hip in closed reduction "Cone" emphasizes the three dimensions of stability, which must be achieved safely without excessive abduction in order to avoid osteonecrosis, or insufficient abduction such that the hip redislocates. Abduction >60 degrees brings the neck of the femur into contact with rim of acetabulum, where the medial circumflex artery can be occluded (*arrow*).

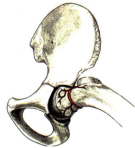

Management

Management is based upon age [A].

Birth to 6 Months

Pavlik harness This follows the principle of dynamic reduction: the child may move the limbs, which return to the favorable position for reduction and for stimulation of triradiate cartilage by the head of the femur when the child is still (including sleep). It is "simple, nondisturbing, and cheap" (Pavlik), hence its broad acceptance [B]. The straps, which are adjusted to maintain moderate force and to account for growth, are applied so that the hips are flexed to 90 degrees and abducted to 45 degrees while remaining readily adductable to neutral [B].

For the hip that rests located (Barlow or subluxatable), the harness is worn full time for 6 to 12 weeks. Treatment concludes once ultrasonographic or röntgenographic metrics have normalized, or if they have not done so by 12 weeks, at which point an alternative treatment is indicated.

For the Ortolani hip, the harness is applied and adjusted as necessary to convert to a Barlow hip over 3 weeks. Persistence of an Ortolani hip is a failure and an indication for alternative treatment. Restriction of the hip in a dislocated position may lead to deformation of the head of the femur and rim of acetabulum, worsening deformity. It also increases development of contracture of the hip. Both outcomes undermine subsequent treatment: the hip is more unstable, and contracture reduces likelihood of success with closed management.

There are other pitfalls of Pavlik harness. Do not overtighten the stirrups (e.g., to improve reduction of a very unstable hip): the posterior straps will abduct too much and risk the blood supply and osteonecrosis of the hip, while the anterior ones will hyperflex the hips and can cause a compressive femoral neurapraxia. While to the surgeon this is "simple" treatment, it may be confusing to parents: if you allow parents to remove the harness (e.g., to wash the child), spend time educating and follow-up with them to make sure they have reapplied the harness correctly.

The success rate of Pavlik harness is 80% to 90%. The Ortolani hip, bilateral disease, and increasing age reduce effectiveness. It is not indicated for teratic (e.g., arthrogryposis) or neuromuscular hip dysplasia.

Rigid immobilization This is indicated when Pavlik harness fails. For the persistent Ortolani hip, apply a hip abduction brace and follow Pavlik harness principles. For persistent abnormal imaging after 12 weeks of Pavlik harness treatment, apply a hip abduction brace full time until normalization of metrics. For a fixed dislocation (Ortolani negative hip), move to closed or open reduction.

6 to 18 Months

Closed reduction This is performed with general anæsthesia, in order to allow for arthrography and tenotomy of adductor longus. If there is contracture of the adductor longus origin, as determined by palpation with hip abduction, or if this necessitates excessive abduction to stabilize the hip, section the tendon to reduce the force of reduction. This may be performed through a stab incision after digital percutaneous isolation distal to the inguinal crease. Insert the blade over the lateral edge of the tendon and advance medialward away from the femoral vessels. A small incision and dissection avoids injury to the external pudendal artery (ramus of femoral artery), which accounts for at times considerable bleeding after percutaneous section. Excessive abduction risks compression of medial circumflex artery against the rim of acetabulum [C]. Excessive force of reduction adds direct compression of the head of the femur. If the hip reduces with a sufficiently stable and safe cone, apply a hip spica cast. If reduction is insecure, convert to an open reduction. If there is uncertainty, an arthrogramme may add clarity.

ARTHROGRAPHY Insert needle with trocar medial distal to inguinal crease raising the hand 30 degrees above the horizon directed at a point between anterior superior iliac spine and ipsilateral shoulder [A]. Alternatively, eliminate rotation of the hip and approach it laterally over trochanter major. Contact the neck of the femur (not the head and not the joint), relax force of insertion, and inject. Start with saline to confirm entry (so as not to obscure the joint by contrast reagent infiltrating the juxta-articular soft tissues), then just enough dilute contrast reagent to outline articular surfaces. Image intensifier assists. If there are significant obstacles to reduction, as evidenced by medial pooling of contrast due to lateral displacement of the head of the femur, open the hip. An inverted limbus may be a harbinger of persistent acetabular dysplasia despite successful reduction.

Open reduction The indication for this is articular obstacles to safe and stable closed reduction [B]. The hip may be approached anterior (Smith-Petersen) or medial [C]. The former is performed through an oblique incision in the "bikini line" (Salter). The latter, performed through a transverse incision centered on adductor longus origin one finger breadth distal to inguinal crease, may be divided according to relationship to the medial muscles of the hip (the adductor longus is sectioned). Ludloff described the "bloodless" approach between pectineus and adductor brevis. A more posterior medial approach travels between adductor brevis and adductor magnus. A more anterior medial approach follows the interval between pectineus and femoral vessels.

The anterior approach is familiar and utilitarian, including for osteotomy at an older age. Release of medial and posterior obstacles to reduction is blind to the medial femoral circumflex vessels, from which this approach is remote. A capsulorrhaphy is possible, which reduces redundancy of the dislocated hip capsule and adds a soft tissue restraint to redislocation. The medial is a more geographically direct approach to the obstacles to reduction. The medial femoral circumflex vessels are directly in its path, which lowers the risk of injury as these may be knowingly isolated and protected.

The anterior approach includes fractional lengthening of the iliopsoa at the brim of pelvis; the muscle is released from the trochanter minor in the medial approach. Do not make radial cuts, excise, or otherwise injure the limbus: just evert it out of the way. If you cannot see the entire acetabulum (horseshoe-shaped articular cartilage and fossa), take more time, and use a head lamp if necessary: all obstacles must be released completely, for a gentle and unequivocal reduction.

Immobilization in spica cast This follows closed or open reduction. The Latin term *spica* describes the manner in which strips of cast material are rolled in a crossing and layered pattern resembling an "ear of corn." The child is placed in the "human position" (which Salter contrasted with the frog-leg), to contrast with the original technique of Lorenz, in which the hip was forcibly and maximally abducted to ensure and maintain a reduction in the older child [D]. After the child is aroused and has been mobilized in the cast, an MRI is obtained to ensure maintenance of reduction [E]. The cast is applied for 3 months, with a change under anæsthesia at 6 weeks to accommodate growth and to permit physical examination of the hip as well as arthrography if necessary. After casting, a brace is worn until normalization of röntgenographic metrics or 18 months of age.

Traction There is no consensus. It is indicated for DDH with dislocation that is irreducible or requires considerable force to do so. Advocates point to gradual stretching of stiff pericoxal soft tissues such that closed reduction may be possible with less force and to a reduced rate of open reduction. The counterargument is based upon modern surgical techniques that significantly reduce risk and obviate the need for this closed method of treatment. Apply traction for 3 to 6 weeks, at home in 45 degrees of flexion and 30 degrees of abduction, with regular evaluation of the level of dislocation in order to estimate when the hip may dock without excessive force [E]. The debate surrounding traction for DDH resembles that surrounding halo traction for severe spine deformity.

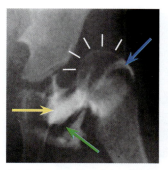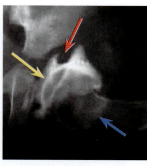

A Arthrography of the dislocated hip In the dislocated position (*white*), there is a medial contrast pool, which is eliminated with reduction (*yellow*). The ligamentum teres connects the head of the femur with fossa of acetabulum and displaces contrast (*green*). Contrast outlines zona orbicularis (*blue*) and limbus (*red*), which remains inverted despite reduction.

Extra-articular	Articular
Adductor longus	Capsule
Iliopsoa	Inverted limbus
	Ligamentum teres
	Pulvinar
	Transverse acetabular ligament

B Obstacles to reduction These may be grouped in two. Section tendons to lengthen iliopsoa (at the brim of pelvis by anterior approach or off trochanter minor by medial approach) and adductor longus. Excise pulvinar and ligamentum teres, which is a guide to the fossa of acetabulum and transverse acetabular ligament. The latter is sectioned along with the medial inferior capsule to expand the space for reduction of the head of the femur. Reflect an inverted limbus out of the way.

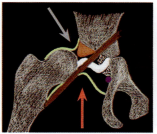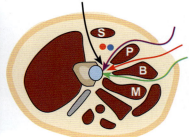

C Approach to the hip for open reduction The medial approach (*red*) is more direct than the anterior approach (*gray*). The anterior approach (*black*) is lateral to femoral vessels. There are three medial approaches (*purple, red, green*). P: pectineus. B: adductor brevis. M: adductor magnus. S: sartorius.

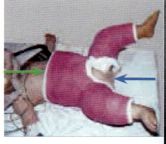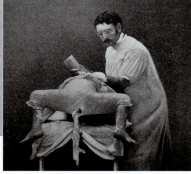

D Spica cast after closed or open reduction In the human position (*right*), hips are flexed to 90 degrees and abducted to 45 degrees, in contrast with the frog-leg position of Lorenz (*left*). The perineum is exposed (*blue*): reinforce the cast so that you do not restrict access with a dowel. Leave room for abdominal distension (*green*).

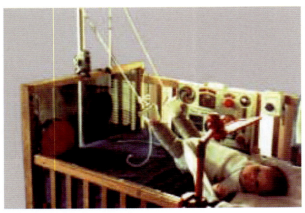

E **Traction** At home, reduces cost and stress for child and family.

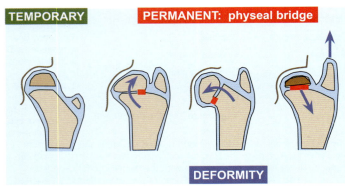

TEMPORARY   PERMANENT: physeal bridge

DEFORMITY

F **Osteonecrosis after closed or open reduction of the hip** The principal discriminator is formation and location of a physeal bridge.

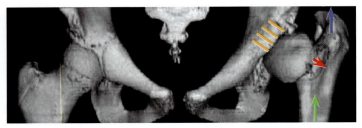

G **CT of hip** Three-dimensional reconstruction aids analysis of complex deformity, in this case consequent to osteonecrosis after open reduction of the left hip in infancy. The neck is very short (*red*), the anterior acetabulum is deficient (*orange*), the trochanter major is relatively overgrown (*blue*), and the limb is shortened (*green*).

Complications

OSTEONECROSIS This is the most grave complications. Early signs include the following:

- Failure of the ossific nucleus to appear after reduction
- Widening of the neck of the femur
- Fragmentation of the ossific nucleus

Osteonecrosis may be classified by time, as well as presence and location of physeal bridge [F]. The mildest form is characterized by no physeal bridge, limited to temporary irregularity of ossification that resolves spontaneously with no sequela. A lateral physeal bridge may not be apparent for several years, tilting the epiphysis into valgus. Less commonly, a medial physeal bridge shortens the neck into varus. Total epiphysis and physis involvement is least common but most severe, resulting in significant coxa brevis, relative overgrowth of trochanter major, and shortening of the limb [G].

In closed reduction, osteonecrosis was seen historically in up to 30% of cases, related to excessive force and abduction for reduction. Current practice has reduced this to <5%. After open reduction, the rate of permanent growth disturbance has been reported as high as 40%: this correlates with increasing age at operation beyond 1 year. Residual proximal femoral deformity results in dysfunction, for example, abductor weakness, and risks premature coxarthritis. Treatment includes the following:

- Intertrochanteric osteotomy to realign coxa vara
- Lengthening osteotomy for coxa brevis to restore offset
- Distal–lateral transfer of trochanter major to lengthen hip abductors
- Timed physeodesis of contralateral limb for length equalization
- Acetabular osteotomy if the head of the femur is uncovered

Other complications pale by comparison, including redislocation, bleeding from a percutaneous tenotomy site, hip stiffness after emerging from cast, and skin breakdown. Follow-up reduction with imaging to make sure that the hip remains located; a better molded cast with modification of the hip position (e.g., restoring flexion lost during original casting by a tiring assistant) as necessary usually suffice for redislocation. Bleeding from a percutaneous site will stop with reinforcement of dressing. Hip stiffness resolves in the normal child, as will skin breakdown. Counseling families of these possibilities will mitigate their negative effect.

18 months to 3 years

This marks a transition in surgical management from soft tissue reconstruction to osteotomy, based upon the concept that deformity will worsen and remodeling may be insufficient without realignment.

Open reduction This is indicated for the dislocated dysplastic hip and is performed through an anterior approach, because of concurrent innominate osteotomy. Cut the tendon of adductor longus separately. Expose the lateral surface of the ilium to reveal any pseudoacetabulum and identify the margin of the true acetabulum. Test the force of reduction. If this is excessive, plan to add a shortening osteotomy of the femur. If reduction is relaxed, as is typical in this age group, an innominate osteotomy will suffice. The rationale for innominate osteotomy follows the proverbial Sutton law (although the words were placed in Willie Sutton's mouth by a Mitch Ohnstad reporting on his trial): the acetabulum is where the deformity is.

Osteotomy The indication is a dislocated hip or persistent acetabular dysplasia without dislocation, as determined by an abnormal acetabular index [A]. There are two principal types in this age group [B].

Single innominate osteotomy (Salter) This is the original of the modern era. It redirects an acetabulum that fits the head of the femur (not too large, not too flat) but does not cover it sufficiently. Divide the apophysis of the ilium sharply and repair precisely to minimize later deformation. Because this is a distalizing osteotomy, perform a fractional lengthening of the iliopsoa at the brim of the pelvis to avoid increased pressure on the head of the femur. Expose medial and lateral tables of the ilium, as well as greater sciatic notch, through which a Gigli saw (made by the Florentine surgeon to cut the pelvis in dystocia) may be passed subperiosteally to avoid injury to sciatic nerve and superior gluteal artery. Cut the ilium by drawing the Gigli saw lateralward, emerging proximal to the anterior inferior iliac spine. Harvest the anterior ilium proximally as an autogenous tricortical structural graft, or use an allograft. Open the osteotomy so that it hinges along the arcuate and pectineal lines and symphysis pubica, akin to a door. Correction may be augmented by translating the distal fragment lateralward, which is possible due to laxity in this age group. Insert the graft, and fix it and the osteotomy with antegrade steel wires that are left long for later removal.

The length of the hinge restricts the extent and direction of correction. Lateral coverage is accompanied by obligate anterior coverage, which may lead to acetabular retroversion and femoral impingement. The instability produced by complete osteotomy of ilium requires fixation and a second operation for removal. In addition, the cut hemipelvis requires an opposite hemipelvis that is stable against which to hinge, thereby necessitating staged bilateral procedures.

ACETABULOPLASTY (PEMBERTON) This reshapes an acetabulum that is too large, indicating translation in addition to rotation of the head of the femur, and too shallow. It reduces the radius of curvature of the acetabulum as it deepens it. The approach is the same as for a single innominate osteotomy. Perform a curved osteotomy of medial and lateral tables of ilium beginning above the anterior inferior iliac spine and ending close but not into the triradiate cartilage, where the osteotomy hinges. Open the osteotomy and place a tricortical graft of appropriate height to correct the acetabular deformity. Compression of the graft by the incomplete osteotomy produces a stable interference fit.

The posterior column of the pelvis is not disrupted: this inherent stability obviates the need for implants and permits simultaneous bilateral procedures. The angle of osteotomy, as well as the extent of medial corticotomy, may be varied to decouple anterior from lateral coverage, allowing modulation of the former without restricting the latter. It is contraindicated when the head of the femur is large, such as hypertrophy from previous operation or Legg-Calvé-Perthes disease: in this setting, the osteotomy may drive the head out of the acetabulum, increasing subluxation and reducing coverage.

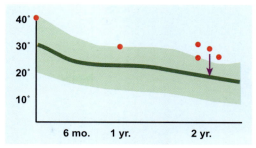

A Innominate osteotomy The procedure is indicated for persistent acetabular dysplasia, as measured by acetabular index (degrees), which is reduced into the normal range (*purple*).

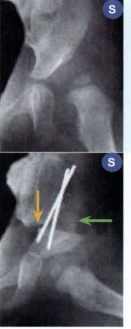

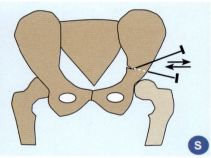

B Innominate osteotomy The Salter osteotomy (S) is linear and complete. The osteotomy may be opened and translated (*orange*) laterally. Because it is complete, the pelvis is destabilized, mandating internal fixation. The Pemberton osteotomy (P) is curved (*dots*) and incomplete. It hinges at the triradiate cartilage: because only the upper half of the acetabulum is displaced, a shallow acetabulum is reshaped to a smaller radius of curvature. Because the posterior column of the pelvis is preserved (*red*), no fixation is necessary. Both osteotomies are filled with a tricortical osseous graft (*green*).

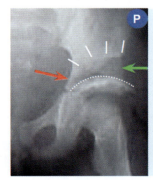

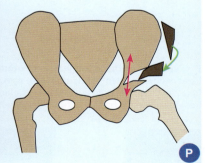

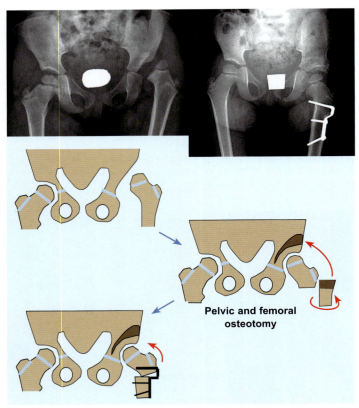

A   Femoral osteotomy, open reduction, and innominate osteotomy The overlap of fragments necessary to reduce the head of the femur is cut and grafted to the pelvic osteotomy. The femur is derotated and tipped into varus to complete correction and fixed with an offset blade plate.

Pelvic and femoral osteotomy

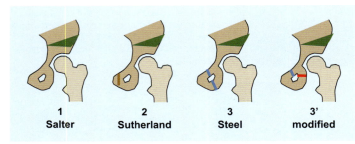

1	2	3	3'
Salter	**Sutherland**	**Steel**	**modified**

B   Evolution of the innominate osteotomy Salter was first. Parasymphyseal osteotomy (Sutherland) does not sufficiently improve mobility to justify dissection in an unfamiliar area. The triple (Steel) has been modified (*red*) to escape the hamstrings and thereby improve fragment mobility.

POSTOPERATIVE CARE Support the osteotomy with a spica cast or hip abduction brace for 6 to 12 weeks. Cast is standard, but brace is better tolerated by child and patient. Obtain röntgenogrammes 1 week after operation to ensure no displacement of osteotomy or graft. Six weeks are sufficient for osseous stability, but 12 weeks may be necessary for soft tissue remodeling in a very unstable hip.

Three to Six Years

There is no consensus on femoral osteotomy before this age, either to reduce the force of reduction and lessen the extent of soft tissue release, thereby reducing risk of osteonecrosis, or to better direct the proximal femur in order to stimulate remodeling of the acetabulum and thereby avoid innominate osteotomy. Three years of age is a guideline to long-standing DDH, beyond which dislocation may be associated with such severe pericoxal contracture that it cannot be released or overcome to permit safe and stable reduction. Shortening is necessary to sufficiently relax the soft tissue envelope [A]. Varus and derotation become more important with increasing age.

Cut the proximal femur. Perform an open reduction. Locate the head of the femur. Apply moderate tension to the distal femoral fragment and resect the overlap. Fix the femur with simple or blade plate. Perform an innominate osteotomy: use the resected femur as graft.

Six Years to Maturity

Treatment of a patient presenting with DDH with dislocation at this age is controversial. For unilateral disease, treat surgically for presentation in the first decade. For bilateral disease, do not operate. The rationale for the former is that asymmetry *per se* adds morbidity. Deformity (bone), contracture (soft tissue), and arthritis (cartilage) that accompany this late a presentation call for the prudent approach of acceptance and accommodation to the disease rather than treatment with outcomes that will be worse than the disease, including redislocation, pain, and stiffness.

Reconstructive osteotomy Treatment of persistent dysplasia without dislocation and without significant arthritis includes osteotomy of innominate bone and femur. Osteotomy of the femur may be indicated for correction of deformity resulting from growth disturbance after prior treatment. It also adds another locus for correction of severe deformity. Innominate osteotomy is more extensive because an older child will be stiffer and have a potentially more dysplastic acetabulum requiring further displacement to sufficiently cover the head of the femur. Add cuts to mobilize the acetabulum: hence the evolution of the single iliac osteotomy to the double then the triple [B].

TRIPLE INNOMINATE OSTEOTOMY The three cuts are of ilium, of os pubis, and of ischium. This has been modified to bring the cuts closer, based upon the principle that correction is most effective at the site of deformity, namely, the acetabulum, and in order to escape tethering by pericoxal soft tissue [C]. An open triradiate cartilage precludes periacetabular osteotomy. Cutting the ischium through the infra-acetabular

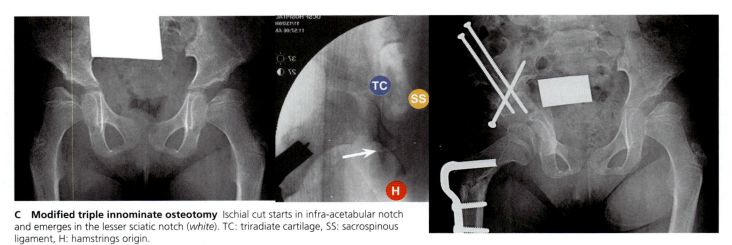

C   Modified triple innominate osteotomy Ischial cut starts in infra-acetabular notch and emerges in the lesser sciatic notch (*white*). TC: triradiate cartilage, SS: sacrospinous ligament, H: hamstrings origin.

Notch proximal to the tuberosity liberates the fragment from the hamstrings. The sacrospinous ligament remains a constraint to acetabular positioning. The iliac cut is the same as for the single osteotomy, as is the approach. Medial dissection is extraperichondrial to avoid injury to the triradiate cartilage. The os pubis is cut by a Gigli saw passed through obturated foramen round the superior ramus, subperiosteally to avoid the obturator neurovascular bundle. The ischium is cut by an angled osteotome passed distal and posterior between the neck of the femur lateral and tendon of iliopsoa medial to the infra-acetabular notch and driven horizontally into the lesser sciatic notch. The image intensifier aids location, direction, and extent of osteotomy. Complete disengagement of acetabular from the pelvis underlies the potency of this osteotomy. Conversely, pelvic disruption necessitates internal fixation, and wide displacement risks delayed or nonunion, in particular in the older child.

Salvage osteotomy This is indicated for persistent dysplasia without dislocation but with significant arthritis. It may serve as a bridge between reconstruction and ablation. In salvage osteotomy, a raw osseous surface is created to cover the head of femur, with joint capsule interposed. The hyaline cartilage surface is expanded to include a fibrous layer (to expect cartilage metaplasia is optimistic). Both types of salvage osteotomy start at the junction of lateral ilium and labrum, which is pried down to mark the level for the added osseous surface at, and not above (where it will result in a step off), the articular surface [D].

CHIARI OSTEOTOMY A complete iliac cut is angled inferior lateral to superiormedial in the coronal plane to complete the *sourcil* and retain the head of the femur. It is curved in the sagittal plane to follow the contour of the acetabulum. The femur is abducted as the distal fragment is displaced medialward to deepen the hip joint by means of the distal surface of the proximal fragment. Fix the osteotomy with screws.

STAHELI OSTEOTOMY This also is known as slotted acetabular augmentation and is a type of shelf procedure. Identify reflected head of rectus femoris, cut at the conjoined tendon, dissect off capsule, and preserve lateral attachment. Pry the labrum down and create a 1-cm deep slot parallel to its margin as wide as possible to maximize the weight-bearing surface. Harvest corticocancellous strips from the lateral table of the ilium. Cut strips to allow them to be contoured and of a length that will produce the desired center–edge angle based upon ante-operative röntgenographic planning, accounting for the depth of the slot. Place strips and secure them by sewing reflected head over them back to the conjoined tendon of rectus. Fill the space above the shelf with remaining osseous graft, which will be retained by the hip abductor muscles.

The Staheli procedure is least traumatic and has the advantage of augmenting the acetabulum; as a result, it may be considered for conditions in which the head of the femur is enlarged, including Legg-Calvé-Perthes disease. Because it is performed through an anterior approach, posterior coverage is limited and total coverage is incomplete, despite the appearance in an anteroposterior röntgenogramme.

Hip ablation Ablative procedures, hip arthrodesis and hip replacement, should be delayed as long as possible. They are a surrender to unacceptable dysfunction (principally pain) and terminal joint disease.

HIP ARTHRODESIS This is underutilized, increasingly unfamiliar to surgeons and unacceptable to patients, despite good outcomes, including ability to work and to bear children, a low rate of conversion to arthroplasty, and a willingness to have the same treatment again [E]. It relieves pain. It is durable: survivorship of hip arthrodesis is >20 years. It does not impose activity restriction. It may be converted reliably to a replacement, the principal determinant of success being function of abductor muscles. On the other hand, it eliminates motion. This alters function, both for daily living, such as donning socks, and for recreation. It alters gait, including visibly, characterized by short stance and prolonged swing, anterior pelvic tilt, and lumbar hyperlordosis. It transfers stress to low back and ipsilateral knee, which may become painful. The descent of arthroplasty, which provides pain relief without sacrificing motion, into younger age groups must be balanced by reduced longevity and multiple revisions [E].

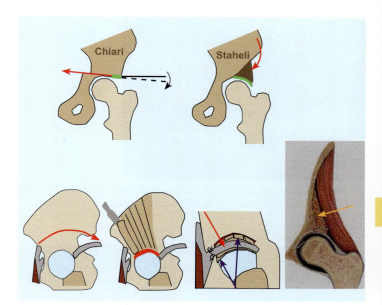

D   Salvage innominate osteotomy Chiari cut the ilium obliquely to match the sourcil and displaced the acetabulum medialward. Staheli used the reflected head of rectus (*red*) to secure corticocancellous strips slotted at the edge of acetabulum (*blue*) and completed by additional harvested bone (*orange*).

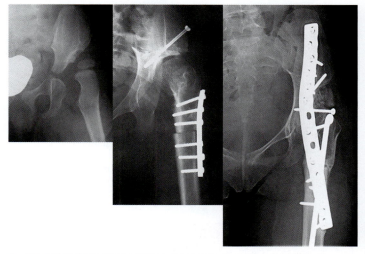

E   Hip arthrodesis The patient underwent six operations for DDH with dislocation from infancy to late teens, including a Chiari procedure to deepen a pseudoacetabulum, but pain persisted and was intolerable. The arthrodesis was performed through an anterior approach, where a plate may be applied as a tension band and the abductors are preserved for future reconstruction, and with the patient supine to ensure proper positioning of the limb: 20-degree to 30-degree flexion, 5-degree adduction, and 10-degree lateral rotation, and <2-cm limb length discrepancy. A femoral exsection (used as autogenous graft) was performed to return the head to the native acetabulum without stretching the sciatic nerve in anticipation of future reconstruction.

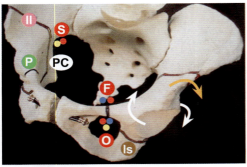

A   Periacetabular osteotomy There are four principal cuts. P: pubic, Is: ischial, PC: posterior column, Il: iliac. The major neurovascular bundles to the lower limb pass by the surgical field. S: sciatic, superior gluteal artery, F: femoral, O: obturator.

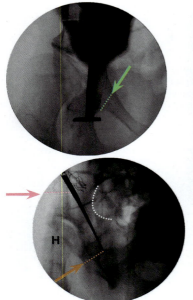

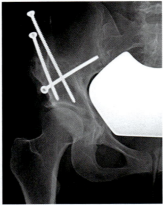

B   Technique of periacetabular osteotomies Ischial cut is reverse and incomplete, by an angled osteotome (*brown*). Pubic cut is complete by a Gigli saw (*green*). Iliac cut is complete (*pink*) to a point midway between greater sciatic notch (*white*) and acetabulum, whence posterior column cut (*black*) may be connected with ischial cut. H: head of femur.

Complication	Rate
Neural–major	1%
Vascular	<1%
Intra-articular osteotomy	1%
Loss of fixation	1%
Over-/undercoverage	≤10%
Nonunion	2%
Heterotopic ossification	≤10%
Neural - LFC	50%

C   Complications of periacetabular osteotomy The operation is safe, as complications have declined with experience.

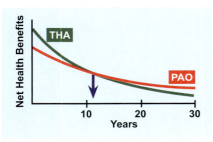

D   Net health benefits after periacetabular osteotomy In mild coxarthritis (CA), these become superior to total hip arthroplasty (THA) after approximately 10 years. Benefits are delayed with moderate coxarthritis (*blue*) and may not be realized in severe coxarthritis.

Maturity

The triradiate cartilage is closed; as a result, the posterior column may be preserved in redirectional innominate osteotomy.

Periacetabular osteotomy This is performed through an anterior approach with a 10-cm oblique incision [A]. Develop the superficial interval through sheath of tensor fasciæ latæ to avoid lateral femoral cutaneous nerve (akin to approaching the anterior aspect of distal radius through the sheath of flexor carpi radialis to avoid radial artery). Reflect iliopsoa off rectus femoris, which is preserved to avoid weakness, to expose anterior inferior iliac spine. Reflect iliocapsularis from underneath the rectus femoris, as well as the glutei minimus et medius, to expose the hip joint capsule. Follow iliopsoa tendon to trochanter minor. Dissect along medial table of the ilium into greater sciatic notch, staying subperiosteal to avoid sciatic nerve and superior gluteal artery, and leaving the lateral table and abductors undisturbed. Develop the interval between iliopsoa tendon and medial neck of femur posteriorward past obturator externus to the infra-acetabular notch. Reflect iliopsoa, which protects the femoral vessels, medialward beyond iliopectineal eminence, where the root of the os pubis may be exposed circumferentially subperiosteally in order to avoid the obturator neurovascular bundle.

Perform an anterior, medial, and lateral arthrotomy around the rectus femoris without detaching it, which has been associated with long term weakness. Inspect the labrum and repair or débride as indicated: the rate of labrum tear is low in the first two decades, increasing 10% *per* decade thereafter. Disease of the head and neck of the femur also may be addressed, such as cheilectomy.

Pass a Gigli saw through the obturated foramen and cut the os pubis from inside outward (antegrade cut may increase risk of obturator neurovascular injury). Insert an angled osteotome between iliopsoa tendon and medial neck of the femur to the infra-acetabular notch and cut the ischium posteriorward incompletely [B]. Cut the ilium beginning distal to the anterior superior iliac spine and ending lateral to the arcuate line at a point that bisects the posterior column. Cut the medial table of the posterior column midway between greater sciatic notch and acetabulum, ending at the incomplete ischial cut. Cut the lateral wall of the posterior column with an angled osteotome starting at the medial cut table. The posterior column remains in continuity, accounting for the inherent stability of the osteotomy.

Position the fragment, ensuring lateral and anterior coverage to place the *sourcil* horizontal without retroverting the acetabulum and producing impingement. The intraosseous nature of the osteotomy is key to its stability: fix with three to four screws. It also means that the osteotomy is free of soft tissue restraints that deny freedom to innominate osteotomies for the immature pelvis, where fragment positioning couples anterior and lateral coverage, thereby retroverting the acetabulum.

Complications of this osteotomy decline with experience [C]. Sciatic nerve injury is most grave; obturator and femoral nerve injuries are rarer. Femoral vascular injury may relate to exposure and manipulation of the vessels *via* an ilioinguinal approach. Intra-articular osteotomy may be avoided by image intensification. That impingement has such a high rate emphasizes the precision required for correct fragment positioning. Isolated pubic nonunion typically is asymptomatic, whereas ischial nonunion may require osteosynthesis. Heterotopic ossification is multifactorial, including genetic tendency, an inherent characteristic of the hip, and surgical trauma. Lateral femoral cutaneous is a compression neurapraxia from retraction and resolves completely in many, and enough in others not to matter to most patients long term.

Outcomes are related to amount of preexisting coxarthritis [D]. It is a hip preserving, not disease reversing, procedure. This differs from the expectation of remodeling after osteotomy in the immature pelvis. Patients with mild or moderate coxarthritis demonstrate improvement in general, hip-specific and sports functional outcome instruments. Severe coxarthritis is not benefited by periacetabular osteotomy, even as a temporizing procedure in a young patient, and is an indication for hip ablation.

LEGG-CALVÉ-PERTHES DISEASE

Despite the fact that shelves groan under the weight of its literature (Rang), Legg-Calvé-Perthes disease (LCP) remains obscure and a source of controversy. It is named after an American, who focused on the painless limp (1910), a Frenchman, who called it *coxa plana* after the residual deformity (1910), and a German, whose assistant took the first röntgenogramme (1898, published 1910). It also is known as Waldenström disease, after the Swedish surgeon who attributed it to tuberculosis (1909). It first was documented in Köhler's atlas, published 10 years after Röntgen discovered x-rays in 1895.

Pathoanatomy

The condition is consistent with avascular necrosis of the head of the femur, radiographically and pathologically [A]. Age of presentation supports this. Other factors implicated in causation include genetic predisposition, vascular anomaly (focal condition of the hip), and endocrine abnormality (a generalized disorder). Animal models of LCP demonstrate a repair response after revascularization that is characterized by osteoclastic bone resorption followed by a fibrovascularization without coupled bone formation, which may make the head of the femur fragile and put it at risk for deformity.

Ischæmia is transient, lasting weeks, and stimulates an inflammatory response, including pain, synovitis, and effusion. The dead bone eventually loses its structural integrity, whereupon it collapses, leaving behind a subchondral space known as a crescent sign in the midst of a radiodense epiphysis. Physeal injury may lead to bridge formation, which exacerbates growth disturbance. Resumption of blood flow permits resorption of dead bone of the epiphysis, which swells and appears fragmented on röntgenogramme. During this phase, the head of the femur is soft and susceptible to deformation, becoming flattened and widened, and in the most severe cases indented by the edge of acetabulum. After resorption of the dead bone, creeping substitution by new bone reconstitutes the head of the femur, which remodels with varying residual deformity that is dependent upon age of the child and extent of head involvement.

Both familial and isolated cases of LCP have been reported. A missense mutation in the gene encoding α-1 chain of type II collagen on chromosome 12q13 has been identified in affected members of a Japanese family segregating LCP.

Evaluation

The classic presentation is a small, hyperactive Caucasian boy who is constitutionally and socially disadvantaged (Wynn-Davies). Girls are affected one-fifth the time, but more severely. Peak age is 4 to 8 years, when the head of the femur is dependent on the medial femoral circumflex artery as sole blood supply. Ten percent are bilateral but asynchronous. Synchronous bilateral disease is the rarer dysplasia epiphysialis capitis femoris (Meyer), which has an earlier onset, is less deforming, and is characterized by a more rapid and complete resolution. Consider a generalized survey, including skeletal, in synchronous disease, to rule out a skeletal dysplasia such as spondyloepiphysial or multiple epiphysial dysplasia. Other conditions that feature irregularity of the proximal epiphysis of femur, such as metabolic and endocrine disorders, may be distinguish by nonskeletal symptoms and signs.

Physical examination There is a history of limp which is not "painless" so much as it is disproportionate to presentation: pain at onset may be severe, after which it evolves to mild and episodic. In long-standing disease with residual deformity, limp may be due to abductor weakness, manifesting as a Trendelenburg gait. The child is small for age. The hip is stiff. Medial rotation is lost first, most and universally, with coexistent adduction and flexion contractures.

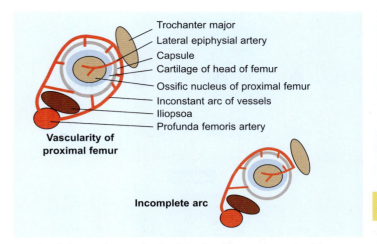

A Circulation to the proximal epiphysis of femur Anomaly of the redundant arcade of the proximal femur may make the head of the femur vulnerable to vascular insufficiency.

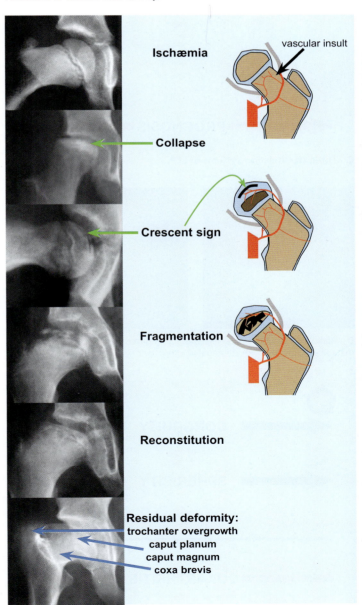

B Clinical stages of disease These form a predictable sequence.

Imaging Röntgenogrammes are fundamental and usually all that are needed for evaluation and management.

CLINICAL STAGE [B] While ischæmia is said to be radiographically silent, the inflammation that accompanies this stage may thicken the neck of the femur, which is the earliest radiographic sign. Ischæmia is followed by collapse, in which the epiphysis appears radiodense. Collapse may leave behind a crescent sign, which represents a subchondral fracture. Reperfusion ushers in bone resorption during the fragmentation stage, which lasts for months. During this stage, the epiphysis is soft and fragile: it is most susceptible to deformation and most responsive to treatment. After resorption, reconstitution of the epiphysis can commence, taking 1 to 2 years. Thereafter, the proximal femur remodels to a residual deformity during the remainder of growth.

RADIOGRAPHIC GRADE [C] There are three methods. They are descriptive, prognostic, and guide treatment. The original was devised by Caterall, whose divisions mirror perfusion of the head of the femur. Most vulnerable is the anterolateral region, furthest from the medial femoral circumflex artery, while last affected is the posteromedial region, closest to the artery. This method may be divided into anterior involvement in the first two grades and posterior involvement in the second two grades. It is prognostic in that outcome correlates negatively with extent of disease: poorest is seen with total head involvement. Salter and Thompson focused on the crescent sign, which delimits the extent of osteonecrosis. They simplify: in A, the crescent sign affects <50% of the head, while in B, it affects >50%. The specificity of this classification is its limitation: the crescent sign is present for a short time and is not always visible and not always in its entire extent. However, it is the earliest predictive sign. It is prognostic in the same way as the Caterall system. Herring emphasized the lateral pillar, which is a measure of the durability of the head against the edge loading of acetabulum during the time when it is softest and most vulnerable to fragmentation and which is a guide to treatment. The fovea bounds the central pillar by two lines drawn perpendicular to the physis.

RISK SIGNS [D] These negatively impact prognosis.

- Gage described a transradiant "V" formed by ossification of an extruded lateral epiphysis. This is a sign of indentation of the head of the femur, which carries risk of hinge abduction.
- Caterall described lucency of the lateral epiphysis, representing collapse of the lateral pillar.
- Rarefaction and cystic change in the subjacent metaphysis, which is affected by a widening zone of ischæmic injury.

Ultrasonogramme detects joint effusion as a manifestation of the inflammatory response to ischæmia. Scintigramme confirms ischæmia as reduced uptake in the epiphysis. MRI shows serpiginous or cavitary loss of signal in the epiphysis due to osteonecrosis. These modalities may aid earlier diagnosis but do not influence management.

Arthrography is an operative aid. It provides an image of the true contour and deformation of the unossified cartilage model, which may be assessed dynamically to determine center of rotation of the head of the femur relative to acetabulum.

Natural History

There is no treatment effect in children younger than 6 years, in whom outcomes are better [A]. By contrast, outcomes are grave for onset of disease in the second decade. Between these two age groups, outcome is dependent upon treatment. The younger head is more resilient to injury and has more potential to recover and longer to remodel. The most important prognostic factor is residual deformity and fit between the head of the femur and acetabulum. The former is divided into spherical, reduced sphericity, and flat. The latter is divided into congruent or incongruent. Physeal bridge adds growth disturbance to exacerbate deformity.

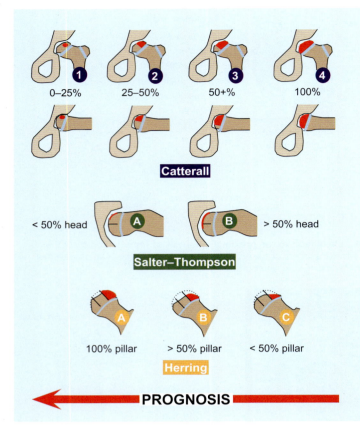

Catterall

< 50% head **A**   **B** > 50% head

Salter–Thompson

100% pillar   > 50% pillar   < 50% pillar

Herring

← **PROGNOSIS**

C   Three classification systems of LCP.

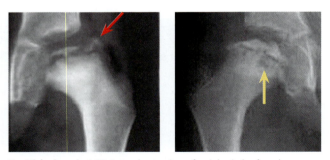

D   Risk signs in LCP Lateral extrusion of epiphysis (*red*) and metaphyseal cyst (*yellow*) are negative prognostic signs.

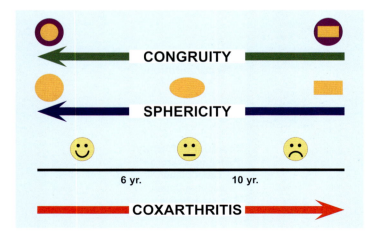

CONGRUITY

SPHERICITY

6 yr.   10 yr.

COXARTHRITIS →

A   Natural history of LCP Most important to outcome are age and residual deformity. Orange: head of the femur, which may be spherical, ovoid, or flat. Purple: acetabulum.

Management

Treatment is founded upon the principle of containment [A]. Containing the head of the femur within the confines of the acetabulum keeps the edge of the latter, where stress concentrates, away from the fragile bone and cartilage of the former, which otherwise may subluxate and become deformed. Redirect the femur so that the normally hard acetabulum may mold the soft head.

Nonoperative treatment Abduction and medial rotation of the thigh centers the head of the femur in the acetabulum. This may be achieved with cast or brace, without or with traction, without or with weight bearing. Such treatment must be maintained for fragmentation and for a variable amount of reconstitution, when the head is most susceptible to deformation. The temporal requirement makes this unrealistic when operative treatment may achieve this.

There is no consensus on activity restriction. Balance the logic of limiting force on a fragile head of the femur against the benefits of recreation, exercise, and maintaining as normal a childhood as possible.

Operative treatment The integrity of the lateral pillar informs operative treatment. If the lateral pillar demonstrates no collapse (A), then the epiphysis is sufficiently durable that it needs no help. If little of the lateral pillar remains (C) under the onslaught of the edge of acetabulum, then the head has been damaged beyond the benefits of containment. Treatment is beneficial in the second half of the first decade: before this, outcomes are not influenced by active treatment, while after this, outcomes are poor despite operative intervention. The decision to intervene is made during fragmentation. An essential challenge is timing: earlier is better, to minimize collapse and before swelling makes the head of the femur too big for the acetabulum to contain. This is may be the principal benefit of the crescent sign (if apparent): a type B is the first sign that intervention is indicated. Such a narrow window of time, and the narrowing range of age to treat, are seeds for nihilism among some surgeons.

The head of the femur may be redirected into the acetabulum by varus and derotation osteotomy of the femur (simulating the effect underlying the concept of cast or brace). Alternatively, the acetabulum may be redirected to take the edge away from the head of the femur [B]. Osteotomy of the femur has the theoretically advantages of reducing intra-articular pressure and intraosseous pressure. It accepts exacerbating the eventual deformity of the proximal femur as a price to protect the head and requires a secondary realignment procedure. Osteotomy of acetabulum treats the side of the hip joint that is not diseased, introducing a compensating deformity, which has implications long term if the acetabulum is retroverted or the *sourcil* is sloped downward, thereby creating femoroacetabular impingement. Add physeodesis of the trochanter major to slow its growth. An adduction contracture may be addressed by a concomitant adductor tenotomy.

Toward or at maturity, residual deformity may require operation, directed at reduced coverage due to an enlarged head, and relative overgrowth of the trochanter major due to growth disturbance of the proximal physis of the femur [C]. Stress concentration at the articular surface of the head presents as groin pain. Fatigue of shortened hip abductor muscles presents as peritrochanteric or buttock pain. Redirect the acetabulum by a periacetabular osteotomy, after ensuring that the head does not hinge with abduction. Offset may be increased by:

Distal and lateral transfer of the trochanter major. This is simplest and safest. Use a direct lateral approach. Release soft tissue such that only the hip abductors remain attached to the trochanter. Cut the trochanter in line with the superior margin of the neck toward the trochanteric fossa. Finish with an osteotome in order not to injure the medial femoral circumflex artery. Bluntly reflect remaining adherent soft tissue restraints. Resect the lateral corner of the distal fragment to aid displacement of the trochanter. Distalize and lateralize the trochanter until its top is at the level of the

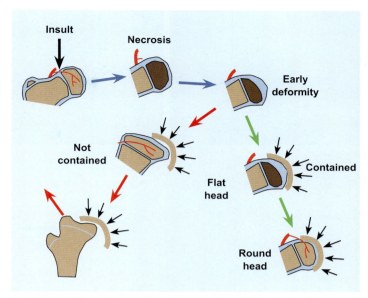

A Concept of containment in LCP Containing the head of the femur in acetabulum reduces deformity.

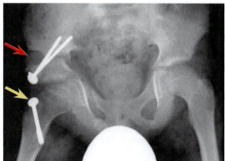

B Containment osteotomy for active LCP Triple innominate osteotomy (*red*) brings edge of acetabulum beyond articular surface of the head of the femur. Trochanter major physeodesis was performed with a screw (*yellow*).

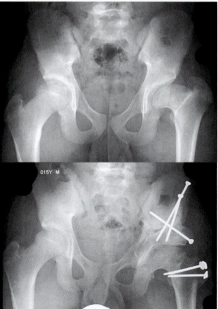

C Osteotomies for residual deformity in LCP Periacetabular osteotomy is combined with trochanter major transfer to cover the head of the femur and restore correct anatomic alignment of the proximal femur.

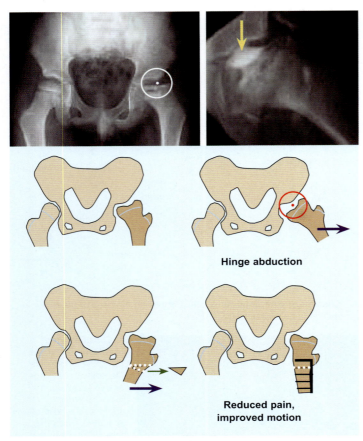

Hinge abduction

Reduced pain, improved motion

D Hinge abduction in LCP Center of rotation at point of contact between indentation of the head of the femur and edge of acetabulum (*white, red*) opens the medial joint, where arthrography shows contrast pool (*yellow*). Valgus osteotomy of the proximal femur is diagrammed.

center of the head of the femur. Fix with screws and washers, and support in a brace.

- Valgus osteotomy of the proximal femur. Use a direct lateral approach. Perform a transverse intertrochanteric osteotomy. Based upon ante-operative templating or intraoperative adduction of the lower limb, displace the distal fragment until the top of trochanter major is at the level of the center of the head of the femur. Fix with a plate.
- Lengthening osteotomy of the neck of the femur. Use a direct lateral approach. Cut the trochanter major. Cut the intertrochanteric region in line with the axis of the neck. Distalize the distal fragment and fix with a plate. Fix the trochanter in a position that places its top at the level of the center of the head of the femur. Graft the gap thereby left in the neck with part of the trochanter.

In addition to addressing the hip joint, assess and treat significant lower limb length discrepancy. If there is sufficient growth remaining, a timed physeodesis of the longer lower limb is simplest; otherwise, consider a femoral shortening osteotomy with internal fixation of the longer femur. The discrepancy is not great enough to warrant lengthening of the affected femur.

In milder deformity, innominate osteotomy may be avoided by performing an osteochondroplasty of the head of the femur by means of a surgical hip dislocation. The trochanter major may be transferred in association with this approach.

A requisite for redirection osteotomy is reduction of the head of the femur in acetabulum. This may be determined by röntgenogrammes of the hip in abduction without or with arthrography. If the head hinges, then either do not treat surgically or perform a valgus osteotomy of the proximal femur to bring up a rounder part of the head into contact and take indentation away from the edge of the acetabulum, thereby reducing pain and improving motion [D]. Add extension to the osteotomy as necessary to compensate for flexion contracture.

Medical treatment Bisphosphonates have a PO3-C-PO3 backbone, with a long side-chain that determines mode of action and a short side-chain that determines pharmacokinetics. As synthetic analogs of pyrophosphate, they bind with high affinity to hydroxyapatite. Non-nitrogenous bisphonates are absorbed by osteoclasts, which are induced to undergo apoptosis. Nitrogenous bisphonates kill osteoclasts by inhibiting protein prenylation.

In LCP, bisphosphonates delay osteoclastic resorption of necrotic bone during the fragmentation stage, which may permit more time for revascularization and new bone formation to occur before structural failure. While bisphosphonates are administered systemically, osteonecrosis may limit access of these agents due to absent perfusion. In an animal model, direct injection into the head of femur enhances efficacy.

Bisphosphonates are anticatabolic, which may limit fragmentation, but not anabolic, such as bone morphogenetic protein-2, which would aid reconstitution. Agents that block the inflammatory response elicited by ischæmia represent a third avenue for development of the medical treatment of this disorder.

Drug delivery may be systemic, which requires revascularization to reach the region of osteonecrosis and therefore presents a narrow therapeutic window. Alternatively, they may be injected directly into the affected bone, which allows earlier access before fragmentation of the femoral head begins.

SLIPPED CAPITAL FEMORAL EPIPHYSIS

This is the most common hip disorder of adolescence.

Pathoanatomy

In slipped capital femoral (upper) epiphysis (SCFE, SUFE), the proximal metaphysis of the femur displaces posteriorward and to a lesser degree lateralward relative to the capital epiphysis at the level and in the plane of the intervening physis. This produces a major apex anterior and a minor lateral rotation deformity that leaves the epiphysis in a relatively posterior position [A]. The sagittal plane deformity is accompanied by apparent varus in the coronal plane: corrective osteotomies should address primarily the former, which is the major plane of malalignment, rather than the latter. While the name of the disorder is misleading mechanically, it places emphasis on the source of morbidity. SCFE may be distinguished from transphyseal fracture [B], with the exception of the acute unstable subtype, where distinctions blur. Anatomic factors that conspire in pathogenesis include obesity with increased weight and widened gait as well as retroversion of the neck of the femur, which tilt the proximal physis of the femur vertical and amplify shear force. Physeal anticipation of puberty includes thinning of the perichondrium, which weakens the physis. Endocrinopathy, including hypogonadism, hypothyroidism, and renal osteodystrophy, or metabolic disorder, including radiation or chemical therapy, may weaken the physis.

Evaluation

The typical presentation is a 13-year-old boy who is obese and hypogonadal. Skeletal age is delayed 1 to 2 years. Boys are affected twice as often as are girls, whose mean presentation is 11 years. One-quarter of cases are bilateral: half are synchronous, while nonsynchronous cases present within 18 months. Always evaluate the other hip, and educate patients so that they come to medical attention if symptoms or signs develop. Pacific islanders are affected twice as often as Blacks, who are affected twice as often as Whites, who are affected twice as often as Asians. Atypical presentation is defined as a child outside of the 10 to 16 years' age range who is <50th percentile in weight. Evaluate the atypical patient for a generalized disorder of which SCFE is one feature, such as endocrinopathy.

History Ten percent are acute, which is defined as symptoms up to 3 weeks. Symptoms >3 weeks is chronic. Less than 25% (of the 10%) are true acute presentations; the other >95% are defined as acute or chronic presentations. The 2% to 3% of the total number of presentations that are purely acute carry the greatest morbidity [C]. These may be regarded as transphyseal fractures and treated as such.

Physical examination

WEIGHT BEARING Up to 10% have an unstable presentation, defined as inability to bear weight on the affected limb: such patients are at risk for osteonecrosis. Stable SCFE is characterized by ability to bear weight, producing an out-toeing gait due to loss of medial rotation. Severe deformity may weaken hip abductor muscles resulting in a Trendelenburg gait.

PAIN Pain in chronic stable SCFE may be misdiagnosed as a groin pull. Fifteen percent of patients present with knee pain.

MOTION Patients with unstable SCFE are intolerant of hip motion, including on physical examination and during imaging, and are at risk for osteonecrosis. Medial rotation is lost: this is most apparent in the supine position. With increasing deformity, the anterior apex abuts the edge of acetabulum such that obligate lateral rotation accompanies increasing hip flexion.

Imaging

RÖNTGENOGRAMMES AP pelvis and lateral of the affected proximal femur are the foundation. The AP pelvis allows survey of both hips. A cross-table lateral is indicated if the hip cannot be placed in the frog lateral position due to pain or if there is concern about displacement of an unstable SCFE with manipulation of the hip.

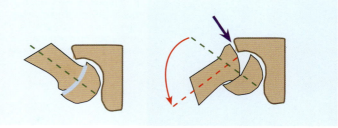

A   Deformity in SCFE The essential deformity is an extension type in the sagittal plane. The apex anterior deformity limits flexion as the prominent metaphysis abuts the edge of acetabulum (*blue*). Red arrow shows the loss between normal (*green*) and abnormal (*red*) flexion.

	SCFE	Transphyseal fracture
History	Antecedent symptoms in > 90%	Negative
Profile	Obese Hypogonadal	Nonspecific
Energy	Low	High

B   SCFE versus fracture   Most SCFE may be distinguished from fracture.

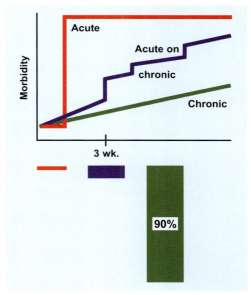

C   Temporal classification of SCFE The majority are chronic (*green*). Most acutes have a chronic history (*blue*). Acuity carries greatest morbidity.

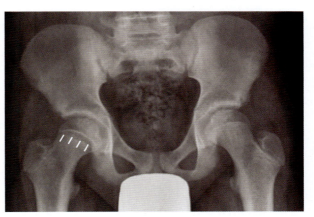

D   Preslip Widening of physis and rarefaction of subjacent metaphysis (*white*) are signs.

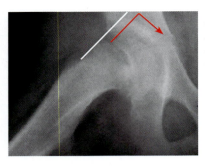

E   Epiphysis–neck relationship
The epiphysis (red) slips away from, and is not crossed by, a line (white) drawn along the anterior and lateral margin of the neck.

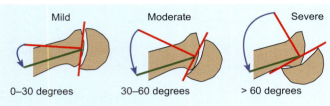

Mild   Moderate   Severe

0–30 degrees   30–60 degrees   > 60 degrees

shaft-epiphysis angle (lateral projection)

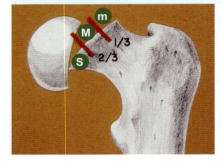

F   Severity of deformity in SCFE   Severity may be expressed as the slip angle, measured between shaft and epiphysis, or as translation of the epiphysis on the neck. m: mild. M: moderate. S: severe.

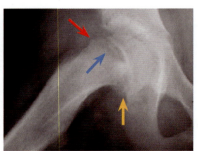

G   Remodeling in SCFE
The neck is heaped up (red), there is resorption of the metaphysis (blue), and projection of a rounding epiphysis beyond the neck (orange) has been likened to a "crow's beak."

- Evaluate the physis. A "preslip" [D] represents early presentation before deformity. Signs include widening of the physis, which may appear bounded by sclerotic margins, and rarefaction of the subjacent metaphysis.
- Evaluate the relationship of epiphysis and the neck of the femur [E]. The epiphysis appears slipped medial (anteroposterior projection) and posterior (lateral projection) to a line (Klein) drawn along the lateral and anterior margin of the neck.
- Determine severity of deformity [F]. This is measured as the shaft–epiphysis angle on the lateral view. The shaft is used due to version of the neck, which will vary its axis according to rotation of the hip. The direction of epiphysis is taken as a perpendicular to a line that marks its base. An alternate method is based upon translation of the epiphysis on the neck of the femur. This is less reliable because the epiphysis may obscure the neck, and remodeling may distort the neck.
- Observe signs of osseous reaction to chronic disease [G]. These may be useful when displacement is subtle.

SCINTIGRAMME   This may show increased uptake in a typical clinical presentation without clear röntgenographic signs. It also enables assessment of epiphysial perfusion in acute, severe, unstable SCFE, where risk of osteonecrosis is highest.

ULTRASONOGRAMME   This may show effusion early in the course of disease, including when röntgenogrammes are inconclusive. It also permits measurement of "step off" of epiphysis relative to the neck of the femur.

MAGNETIC RESONANCE IMAGING   This has become the second line of imaging after röntgenogramme, because it provides most information. It may detect an inflamed physis and a reactive joint effusion in the preslip state. It evaluates perfusion of the epiphysis and aids in ruling out other causes of hip pain where there is diagnostic dilemma.

Natural History

Outcomes after SCFE may be divided into early and late.

Early   Avascular necrosis results from tear or compression of the epiphysial blood supply. It is associated with acute, severe, unstable SCFE. Acuity does not allow vascular remodeling. Severe slip may stretch vessels to failure or lead to kinking and compression under a slipped epiphysis. Ischæmic bone is so painful that the child will not bear weight upon or move the affected hip: this is defined as an unstable presentation. Avascular necrosis has been associated with closed reduction, which historically was imprecise and too forceful. Gentle, controlled, open reduction may reduce osteonecrosis by unkinking and restoring proper orientation and patency of blood vessels supplying the epiphysis, in the same way as open reduction for neck of femur fracture.

Chondrolysis is rarer and more obscure than avascular necrosis. It is defined as a joint width ≤ 3 mm, or < 50% of the unaffected side. Pathogenesis after SCFE is unknown. It is more common in girls and African Americans. It tracks with avascular necrosis, being more common in acute, severe presentation and after closed reduction. The only known cause is mechanical, due to permanent articular implant penetration. The hip becomes stiff. Anti-inflammatory medications may relieve pain but do not alter natural history. The benefits of protected weight bearing, traction, continuous passive motion, and capsulectomy are uncertain. Recovery is variable and typically incomplete.

Late   Osteoarthritis is related to deformity. Mild SCFE may go undetected until presentation for arthroplasty as an adult, when a "tilt" or "pistol grip" deformity of the proximal femur may be seen on röntgenogramme. The grip represents the rounded and varus head and the neck of the femur, the cylinder, hammer, and trigger represent the trochanteric region, and the barrel represents the shaft. Mild deformity is accepted. Severe deformity is morbid from the outset of disease, beginning with restricted hip motion, proceeding to labrum and anterior acetabular cartilage injury, and ending in global joint degeneration. Deformity correction, by reduction or osteotomy, is indicated to alter this natural history. There is no consensus on moderate deformity.

Management

Objectives of treatment are stabilization of proximal physis of the femur without or with restoration of anatomy.

Stabilization of physis This is indicated for mild slips. It is urgent, in order to mitigate risk of further slip or transformation of a stable presentation to an unstable one, with its attendant risk of osteonecrosis. Protect weight bearing on the affected limb with crutches or a wheelchair, if the patient is at risk for fall with the former.

Immobilization in a hip spica cast was advocated to avoid operative complications and to simultaneously treat both hips; however, it has been associated with further slip and chondrolysis.

Open physeodesis with a bone peg under direct vision avoids articular or cervical penetration, effects more rapid physeal closure and therefore stability, allows osteoplasty in severe deformity, and requires no implant; however, it is invasive (long incision, bloody, increased operative time) and requires postoperative immobilization in hip spica cast until union.

The standard of care is *in situ* screw fixation [A]. This is cannulated and performed under image intensification, making it rapid through a small incision.

- A fracture table allows simultaneous use of two image intensifiers for anteroposterior and lateral imaging without manipulation of the hip. On a regular radiolucent table, lateral view is obtained by rotating the image intensifier and flexing the hip.
- Draw lines perpendicular to physis and centered in epiphysis on both projections: the incision is 1 cm at the intersection of the lines on the anterolateral thigh skin.
- Insert a terminally threaded guide wire perpendicular to the physis into the center of the epiphysis using the cutaneous lines as directional aids.
- Ream the cortex without or with the subphyseal hard bone, leaving the epiphysis in order not to dislodge the guide wire and not to risk articular penetration.
- Insert an appropriate length cannulated screw. Don't bury the screw lest it need be removed later. A titanium screw will allow MRI imaging, in the event of osteonecrosis. Use full threads: compression across the physis is not indicated, and risks insufficient threads in the epiphysis, where five threads are the minimum for stability. In addition, a partially threaded screw may not be able to back cut through a long column of bone during removal, if this be necessary. Using more than one implant increases the risk of articular or extraosseous penetration.
- Balance placing as many threads as possible in the epiphysis for stability with not penetrating the joint. The latter may be assessed by watching the screw tip approach then withdraw from the articular margin of the head of the femur during hip rotation under continuous image intensification. The rationale for continuous imaging of approach withdraw is the blind spots in static orthogonal imaging [B]. Alternatively, inject contrast into the screw: if the contrast fills and flows back out of the screw without an arthrogramme, the screw tip is safe [C]. This is a functional test, subject to less interpretation and less dependent upon limb position, and as such is more reliable.

After operation, the patient may walk *ad libitum*. There is no fracture to unite, so crutches or a walker with protected weight bearing are for comfort, and a 6-week time period is arbitrary. The physis fuses after a mean of 18 months, during which time axial loading activity, including jumping and running, should be avoided. Focus the patient, who typically is overweight, on swimming and closed chain kinetic activity. After physeal fusion, liberate the patient to activity *ad libitum*.

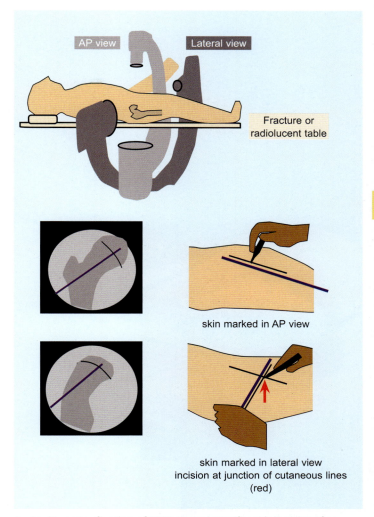

A In situ screw fixation of SCFE Image intensifier aids insertion of a cannulated screw perpendicular to physis into center of epiphysis (without reference to the neck).

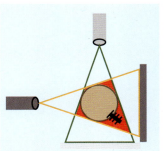

B Blind spot during imaging of SCFE Placement of the tip (*black*) of a screw beyond the subchondral margin of the head of the femur may escape detection due to the blind spots (*red*) of static imaging, despite orthogonal views.

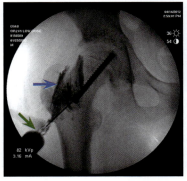

C Implantography Injection (*green*) of contrast reagent fills lumen and flows back out (*blue*) of fixation screw. Absence of a hip arthrogramme means the cannulated tip of the screw has not penetrated the joint.

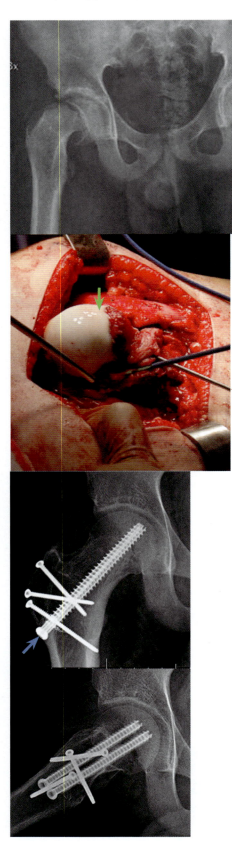

Reduction and stabilization of physis This is indicated for acute severe slips. A closed partial reduction may occur spontaneously with placement of patient on an operative table. Do not perform a forcible closed reduction: this is associated with osteonecrosis.

OPEN REDUCTION VIA ANTERIOR APPROACH Perform an anterior approach after Smith-Petersen in supine position. Open the joint to decompress a hæmatoma, and apply digital force at the apex of deformity. Use moderate force to move the epiphysis from an acute to a chronic position; pushing beyond the acute position risks injury to the retinacular vessels, which have shortened to accommodate the chronic position. Fix the epiphysis.

OPEN REDUCTION VIA HIP DISLOCATION This allows controlled maximal reduction under complete view. It is safe, actively avoiding the early complication of osteonecrosis, and allows restoration of anatomy to avoid late complications of coxarthritis.

- Position the patient lateral for a posterior approach through gluteus maximus.
- Cut the trochanter major lateral to piriformis, in order to avoid medial femoral circumflex artery.
- Elevate trochanter major with glutei medius et minimus off hip joint capsule, leaving piriformis and subjacent blood supply undisturbed.
- Cut capsule along the axis of the neck, extending a posterior limb parallel to acetabulum (away from retinacula of Weitbrecht) and an anterior limb parallel to base of the neck.
- Expose neck subperiosteally. Cut the posterior margin of trochanter major to take retinacula of Weitbrecht with medial circumflex vessels away from area of dissection to protect them.
- Stabilize the epiphysis in place with a temporary threaded wire, in order that it not displace during hip dislocation.
- Cut ligamentum teres to allow dislocation of the hip anteriorward by adducting the lower limb across the body. The retinacula of Weitbrecht may be demonstrated in continuity with epiphysis after dislocation.
- Mobilize the epiphysis through the physis. Trim callus from the anterior epiphysis–neck junction. Shorten the neck as necessary to reduce the epiphysis without tension.
- Fix the epiphysis antegrade by passing a guide wire through the fovea centralis to emerge from the lateral cortex of the femur subjacent to trochanter major. Withdraw guide wire to articular margin of the femur, and select a 5-mm shorter cannulated screw. Place a second guide wire retrograde parallel to the first guide wire. Place a cannulated screw retrograde over each wire. An ACL guide may improve accuracy of guide wire placement.
- Oozing of blood through epiphysial bone during physeal débridement and guide wire hole demonstrate preservation of blood flow.
- Reduce the hip, repair periosteum and close the capsule.
- Fix trochanter major at its original site around the epiphysial screws, adding washers or cutting a semitubular plate to enhance stability.

After operation, protect weight bearing with crutches or walker until union of trochanter major. Because this treatment is indicated for acute severe SCFE, avascular necrosis is a significant risk (*vide infra*).

D   Open reduction and internal fixation of SCFE Acute or chronic, severe, unstable SCFE (1) underwent open reduction and internal fixation (2) with cannulated full thread titanium screws and small fragment fixation of trochanter major. Temporary threaded fixation wire of epiphysis before dislocation (*red*). Epiphysis shows chronic changes (*green*). Cannulated screws placed immediately distal to trochanter major (*blue*).

Osteotomy This is indicated for chronic severe SCFE. In the chronic state, the epiphysial vasculature has shortened to accommodate for deformity of the proximal femur. As a result, an acute correction risks injury to this blood supply unless accompanied by sufficient shortening, which may be difficult to judge. This differs from the acute presentation, where reduction is indicated. A safer approach is osteotomy in the intertrochanteric region of the femur, remote from the epiphysial blood supply. Olisthy occurs along the plane of the proximal physis of the femur, principally in the sagittal plane to produce an extension (apex anterior) deformity, accompanied by a lesser degree of lateral rotation. Osteotomy that places emphasis on the apparent varus in the coronal plane, focusing on valgus realignment (Southwick), will not correct the deformity sufficiently. Osteotomy that primarily addresses the extension deformity, adding medial rotation of the distal fragment as necessary (Imhäuser), is more anatomic [E, F].

- Perform an anterolateral approach to the hip is utilized through a straight lateral incision.
- If the SCFE has been stabilized previously in an acute setting, the angle of the fixation screw, placed perpendicular to the physis, serves as a guide to correction as it is equal to the angle of posterior inclination of the epiphysis: this represents the degree of flexion of the distal fragment that is necessary to restore a normal relationship between epiphysis and diaphysis of the femur.
- A slotted chisel for a 90-degree blade plate is placed at the base of the trochanter major and is rotated until the anticipated anteriorward inclination of the side plate matches the direction of the fixation screw, or the desired degree of flexion based upon preoperative CT. Because no valgus is required, the chisel is placed perpendicular to the long axis of the shaft of the femur in the coronal plane. Once the chisel is started, remove any fixation screw, lest it get in the way.
- A transverse osteotomy is performed immediately proximal to trochanter minor.
- Insert the blade into the proximal fragment. Flex the distal fragment to the plate. Release adherent posterior soft tissues, including periosteum. Flexion of the distal fragment will be accompanied by obligate anterior translation, of which the amount is proportional to the degree of correction. In this way, the axis of the diaphysis will move toward the axis of the head of the femur, thereby compensating for osteotomy away from the site of deformity.
- Rotate the distal fragment medialward to match the uninvolved femur, and fix the distal fragment to the plate.
- Cut the anterior hip joint capsule to reduce contracture, which will allow the head of the femur to return to its normal position within the acetabulum as the thigh is extended back to the operative table.

Cheilectomy This is indicated for femoroacetabular impingement due to SCFE deformity in a patient in whom a more extensive reconstruction is not acceptable to the patient or surgeon [G]. This may be performed through an anterior approach, or a hip dislocation approach. Because the "lip" or head–neck prominence to be removed is anterior and lateral, the former approach is sufficient with less morbidity. The image intensifier may serve as an aid. The hip is flexed as a functional test to guide amount of resection. While this procedure may provide relief from impingement, it does not restore the correct relationship of articular surfaces of the head of the femur and acetabulum.

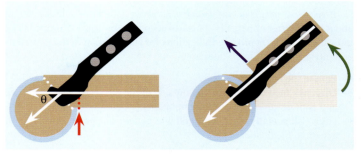

E Technique of flexion intertrochanteric osteotomy (Imhäuser) for SCFE A transverse intertrochanteric osteotomy is performed (*red*). The blade is inserted so that its plate is in line with the epiphysis (*white*). The distal fragment is flexed (*green*) and translated anteriorward (*blue*) to the plate.

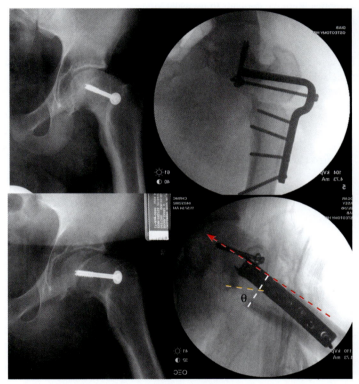

F Flexion intertrochanteric osteotomy (Imhäuser) of SCFE In the anteroposterior projection, the apparent varus is corrected, increasing the articulotrochanteric distance, offset, and neck–shaft angle, as well as bringing the trochanteric fossa into profile. The correction is highlighted by change in screw direction clockwise (valgus) without valgus displacement at osteotomy. The lateral projection shows that epiphysis is aligned with shaft of the femur (*red*). Correction is measured as θ. The corner of the proximal fragment (*orange*) sits inside the medulla of the distal fragment (*white*), which translates anteriorward with increasing flexion to compensate for a Z-shaped correction remote from locus of deformity.

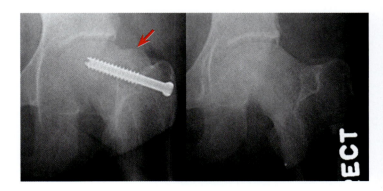

G Cheilectomy for SCFE A large prominence at superior corner of the neck of the femur (*red*), exposed by slip of epiphysis away posterior and medial, was débrided by an anterior approach. The screw head was prominent, contributing to the cam femoroacetabular impingement.

Prophylactic stabilization of contralateral physis Bilateral SCFE occurs in about one-quarter of patients. This has been used by some (Europe) as an indication for this approach. Indications for stabilization of the contralateral physis in the United States are:

- Pain in the contralateral hip
- High risk medically, including outside of the 10- to 16-year age range and comorbidity such as endocrinopathy
- High risk socially, such as unreliable patient or family, and difficult access to medical care

Complications of SCFE Treatment

Avascular necrosis In SCFE, avascular necrosis is not transient and tends to affect the entire epiphysis. Hip pain and stiffness set in within a year of injury or treatment. MRI may detect changes before collapse on röntgenogrammes. Remove implants to improve MRI evaluation of extent of head involvement and to avoid protrusion and injury to acetabulum in case avascular necrosis is partial, and the hip may be salvaged by redirectional osteotomy of the femur to move dead bone away from weight bearing. If osteonecrosis is extensive, consider hip arthrodesis in a young patient with isolated joint disease who will be unrestrained by other joint disease in systemic illness (e.g., juvenile inflammatory arthritis).

Primary
Termed "congenital" or "Development."
Acquired–local
Congenital deficiency of the femur.
Trauma   - malunion.
Avascular necrosis - management of developmental dysplasia of the hip.
- Legg-Calvé-Perthes disease
Slipped capital femoral epiphysis.
Tumor   - Bone cyst
- Fibrous dysplasia (Shepherd's crook deformity)

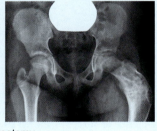

Iatrogenic   - postvarus osteotomy
Acquired—general
Skeletal dysplasia e.g., spondyloepiphysial dysplasia.

A   Classification of coxa vara There are three categories.

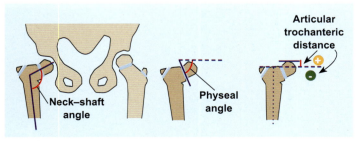

B   Measurements of the proximal femur Neck–shaft angle is most familiar, including from templating for adult reconstruction, but least precise. The articulotrochanteric distance is a functional measure.

Femoroacetabular impingement As deformity becomes more severe, apex anterior deformity at the head and neck junction produces cam impingement. This is an indication for reduction or osteotomy. Impingement may be exacerbated by implant prominence: as deformity becomes more severe, implant entry site migrates anteriorward and proximal on the neck of the femur, where a prominent head of screw *per se* may collide with acetabulum during hip flexion. This is an indication for implant removal once physis has closed if a severe SCFE is treated with *in situ* screw fixation. Implant removal is unnecessary for mild deformity.

COXA VARA

The proximal femur (despite the Latin *coxa*: "hip") may have a varus shape primarily in isolation, known as congenital or developmental coxa vara, as part of a localized or regional disease process, for example, Legg-Calvé-Perthes disease, or secondary to a generalized disorder, for example, in skeletal dysplasia [A].

Pathoanatomy

Varus of the proximal femur may be defined as [B]:

- Negative articulotrochanteric distance. This measurement becomes negative when the top of trochanter major (normally level with the center of the head of the femur) is proximal to the articular surface of the head of the femur.
- Physeal angle >30 degrees. This angle is subtended by a line drawn through proximal physis of the femur and the horizontal. Normal range is 0 to 30 degrees, mean 15 degrees. Physeal angle 30 to 60 degrees, while abnormal, may spontaneously improve or progress unpredictably; as a result, this is followed closely lest there be progression.
- Neck–shaft angle < 120 degrees, for relative varus, or < 90 degrees, for absolute varus. Normal development of neck–shaft angle is 150 degrees at birth to 125 degrees by maturity. Measurement is sensitive to femur rotation. The axis of the neck may be difficult to determine when incompletely grown early in life or when distorted by disease.

Primary coxa vara represents a focal growth disturbance of endochondral ossification in the medial inferior physis of the proximal femur. The defect is characterized by delayed chondral calcification and fibrous replacement. Coxa vara disadvantages the hip abductor muscles. Relative proximal location results in abutment of trochanter major against acetabulum and lateral ilium, limiting hip abduction. Reduction of the neck–shaft angle, associated with shortening of the neck of the femur (coxa brevis), shortens the affected lower limb and leads to length discrepancy.

Evaluation

History and physical examination History aids identification of acquired coxa vara. The condition typically manifests after walking. Abductor weakness results in a Trendelenburg gait. Hip abduction is limited. Trochanter major is prominent. The affected limb is short, with associated genu valgum. The older patient complains of lateral hip pain, in the region of trochanter major and in the buttock due to abductor muscle fatigue. A broad physical examination may show signs of a generalized disorder.

Imaging Röntgenogrammes are fundamental. They define the deformity and elucidate whether the presentation is primary or acquired. In primary coxa vara, an anomalous radiolucent line diverging from the inferior medial proximal physis of the femur forms an inverted Y and outlines a triangular island of bone having its base at the inferior contour of the neck [C]. Scintigraphy measures metabolic activity of primary osseous disease. MRI provides detail of the proximal physis of the femur and of a morbid process affecting bone. CT defines structure of the proximal femur, including in three-dimensions in preparation for operative treatment.

Management

Symptoms and signs may be managed medically, for example, nonnarcotic analgesics for hip pain. Osteotomy is indicated for:

- Unacceptable symptoms or signs, including hip pain from abductor fatigue or Trendelenburg gait
- Severe deformity, including negative articulotrochanteric distance, physeal angle >60 degrees, neck–shaft angle < 90 degrees
- Progressive deformity

Intertrochanteric osteotomy Perform a transverse osteotomy, and fix with a blade or plate placed into the epiphysis if necessary [C]. More complex osteotomies (e.g., Pauwels) or less secure fixation (e.g., smooth wires or cable) may jeopardize stability of construct, in particular in a young child. In primary coxa vara, reduce the physeal angle to < 30 degrees. Counsel parents that, like tibia vara (Blount), this is a growth disturbance, and as such, there may be recurrence of deformity despite correction. Whether the result of this osteotomy is improved, including reduction of recurrence, by concurrent physeodesis of the trochanter major, is debatable. This latter procedure is reserved for a child toward the end of the first decade.

Trochanteric transfer This is indicated in the second decade, after acetabulum has remodeled in response to the deformed femur, and for secondary coxa vara, as a less morbid alternative to intertrochanteric osteotomy. The trochanter major is transferred distal and lateral, to bring its top to the level of the center of the head of the femur.

SNAPPING HIP

This term encompasses extra-articular causes, in contrast with intra-articular causes such as disease of labrum [D]. It also is known as *coxa saltans*, from Latin *saltare*: "to jump." A snap may be heard or felt from the hip when a tight tendon or band shifts abruptly over an osseous prominence, such as when arising from a chair or changing direction of walking. Snapping may be accompanied by pain and a sense of hip instability. The iliopsoa may subluxate over the iliopectineal eminence during hip flexion–extension and medial–lateral rotation. The rectus femoris conjoined tendon may catch at the head of the femur during flexion. The iliotibial tract may subluxated over the trochanter major during walking.

Evaluation Presentation typically is in the second decade, when growth becomes rapid and sports become more demanding. Simulate the motion that produces snapping by physical examination, in order to localize the structure responsible. The Ober test reveals contracture of iliotibial tract. Crepitus may be palpated at the groin during extension and lateral rotation of the hip from a flexed, adducted, and medially rotated position, as the iliopsoa subluxates. Dynamic ultrasonography may show iliopsoa subluxation at the brim of the pelvis [A].

Management The foundation of management is stretching. This may be guided by a physiotherapist, who also may train the dancer who most commonly presents with a snapping iliopsoa, or the runner with an iliotibial tract contracture. For cases refractory to stretching, in addition to nonsteroidal anti-inflammatory agents and activity modification and progression, operative treatment is indicated. The iliopsoa may be lengthened open at the brim of the pelvis, or arthroscopically transcapsular or at trochanter minor. The latter may be associated with weakness of hip flexion. The iliotibial tract may be partially sectioned, ellipsed over the trochanter major or lengthened, open or arthroscopically.

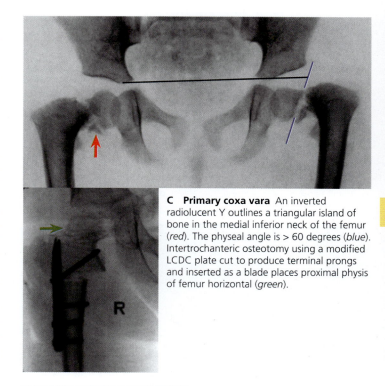

C Primary coxa vara An inverted radiolucent Y outlines a triangular island of bone in the medial inferior neck of the femur (*red*). The physeal angle is > 60 degrees (*blue*). Intertrochanteric osteotomy using a modified LCDC plate cut to produce terminal prongs and inserted as a blade places proximal physis of femur horizontal (*green*).

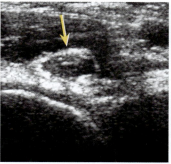

D Snapping hip Ultrasonogramme shows subluxation of the iliopsoa tendon (*yellow*) at the brim of the pelvis. Röntgenogrammes are normal.

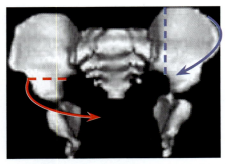

A Osteotomy for exstrophy of the bladder Site of osteotomy may be posterior, parallel to the sacroiliac joint (*blue*), or anterior, proximal to the acetabulum (*red*).

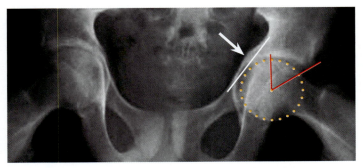

B Deepening of acetabulum In coxa profunda, the floor of the acetabulum thrusts medialward beyond ilioischial line (*white*). When the head of the femur (*orange*) crosses the ilioischial line, this is distinguished as protrusio acetabuli. Note that as the acetabulum deepens, center–edge angle (*red*) increases (in this case, 60 degrees), producing pincer impingement.

EXSTROPHY OF THE BLADDER

This also is known *ectopia vesicæ*. Anterior rupture of the cloacal membrane during the embryonic period with failure of midline closure of the pelvis results in eversion of the urinary bladder, genital anomalies, and diastasis of the innominate bones.

Evaluation This may be diagnosed by fœtal ultrasonogramme. The diagnosis is clear on physical examination of the neonate.

Management Surgical reconstruction and midline closure of the bladder, genitalia, and abdominal wall are aided by innominate osteotomy with medial rotation of anterior ring of the osseous pelvis [A]. Site of osteotomy may be posterior, parallel to the sacroiliac joint, or anterior, proximal to the acetabulum. Both osteotomies pass through the greater sciatic notch. Posterior osteotomy is performed in the prone position, requiring turning of the patient supine for bladder repair. Postoperative care includes suspension with lower limbs adducted together until stable callus, after which a cast or brace is applied until healing. Anterior osteotomy is performed in the supine position. It is fixed with wires, which are supplemented with cast or brace that features sufficient space for postoperative care of bladder repair. External fixation in older patients obviates the need for immobilization, which facilitates postoperative care.

Despite innominate osteotomy, pubic diastasis persists, as do retroversion of the acetabulum and out-toeing gait. Persistent acetabular deformity may be addressed at maturity with reverse peri-acetabular osteotomy, which may reduce potential for femoro-acetabular impingement, improve hip motion and reduce out-toeing gait.

PROTRUSIO ACETABULI

Evaluation Presentation is hip pain without or with stiffness in a patient at risk, including Marfan syndrome, seronegative spondyloarthropathy, and conditions that weaken bone. The condition is defined radiographically [B]. Displacement of the floor of acetabulum medial to the ilioischial line (of Köhler) is defined as *coxa profunda*: "deep hip." "Thrusting forward" of the head of the femur medialward beyond the ilioischial line is defined as *protrusio acetabuli*. Center–edge angle is > 45 degrees. MRI shows pincer morphology of acetabulum.

Idiopathic or primary protrusio acetabuli typically affecting middle-aged women, of whom 1/2 will have a bilateral presentation, first was described by the German surgeon A.W. Otto, whence the eponym Otto pelvis. It also is known by the Greek term arthrokatadysis: "joint sinking".

Management Treat an underlying arthropathy. Relieve symptoms with rest, activity modification, and nonsteroidal anti-inflammatory medications. Operate rarely. While physeodesis of the triradiate during childhood may slow deepening of the acetabulum, there are no reliable long-term studies of the procedure. Débridement of the anterior wall of acetabulum, or reverse periacetabular osteotomy, may relieve anterior femoroacetabular impingement.

FEMOROACETABULAR IMPINGEMENT

This relatively new concept fills a void heretofore unrecognized or deemed "overuse" hip pain. It depends on imaging, projection, and patient position. The natural history suggests premature coxarthritis.

Pathoanatomy

There are two types [A].

- In cam impingement, relative posterior displacement of the head of the femur brings the neck into premature contact with the acetabulum, thereby leading to osteophyte formation with or without cystic change. This is characteristic of deformity after slipped capital femoral epiphysis and of implant prominence after its surgical treatment [B]. It may be measured by the a angle between axis of the neck and junction of the neck and head. Cam impingement has been shown to increase risk of coxarthritis by more than twofold
- In pincer impingement, an acetabulum that is deep and excessively covers the head of the femur "pinches" the neck and thereby restricts motion. This is seen radiographically as an increased center–edge angle and as a retroverted acetabulum with a crossover sign [C].

Evaluation

Abnormal contact between the neck of the femur and edge of acetabulum produces a spectrum of disease.

- There is groin pain with terminal flexion, which is reduced. This differs from the pain of DDH, which is associated with normal or increased motion due to deficiency of the anterior acetabulum.
- Disease of labrum includes hypermobility, cyst, and tear. This may manifest as crepitus during activity and during physical examination.
- Articular cartilage of acetabulum degenerates.
- Neck of the femur reacts as a result of stress concentration.

Neck morphology is apparent on röntgenogrammes. Articular disease may be seen on MRI and arthroscopy. Diagnostic uncertainty may be addressed by adding anæsthetic to arthrography during MRI.

Management

Arthroscopy Absent significant underlying deformity, this is the most benign method. A diseased labrum may be débrided or repaired. A neck osteophyte or a prominent edge of acetabulum may be débrided, although the adequacy of these may be difficult to determine, for example, excessive bone removal from the neck of the femur risks fracture.

Open surgical treatment For osseous work, this offers greater control and allows dynamic testing to calibrate extent. Through a small incision anterior approach and exposure, labrum, neck osteophyte, and edge of acetabulum may be addressed. Through a hip dislocation technique, all may be addressed in addition to evaluation and management of acetabular cartilage. The severity of disease must justify the morbidity of the latter treatment method.

Primarily treat significant underlying osseous deformity. Correct the deformity of the proximal femur after severe slipped capital femoral epiphysis, as well as the labral tear it has produced. Reorient an acetabulum that is retroverted but not too large, rather than trimming the anterior rim, lest a deficiency state be created [D].

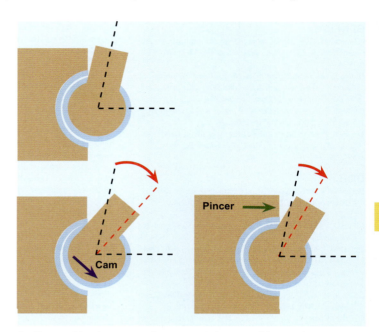

A   Types of impingement Cam type may be seen with posterior displacement of the head on the neck of the femur (*blue*). Pincer type occurs when acetabulum is deep and excessively covers the head of the femur (*green*). Femur contacts acetabulum at earlier flexion (*red*).

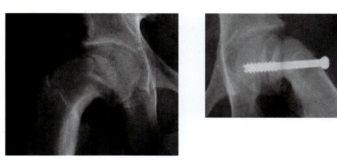

B   Cam impingement In slipped capital femoral epiphysis, this may be due to posterior displacement of the head on the neck, or to implant prominence on anterior neck with increasing olisthy.

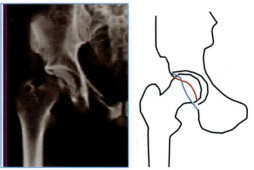

C   Acetabular retroversion Anterior wall (*red*) crosses posterior wall (*blue*) to impinge on the neck of the femur.

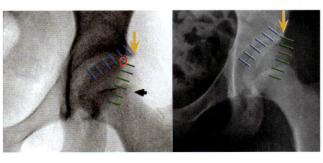

D   Open treatment of impingement The anterior wall (*blue*) of acetabulum, which crosses (*red*) posterior wall, was trimmed by an anterior approach, exposing acetabular deficiency (*orange*).

GENERAL

Chung SMK. The arterial supply of the developing proximal end of the femur. *J. Bone Joint Surg. Am.* 58(7):961–970, 1976.

Hilton J. *On the Influence of Mechanical and Physiological Rest in the Treatment of Accidents and Surgical Diseases, and the Diagnostic Value of Pain.* London: Bell and Daldy, 1863.

Pauwels F. *Biomechanics of the Normal and Diseased Hip.* New York: Springer-Verlag, 1976.

Trueta J. The normal vascular anatomy of the human femoral head during growth. *J. Bone Joint Surg. Br* 39(2):358–394, 1957.

DDH

Barlow TG. Early diagnosis and treatment of congenital dislocation of the hip. *J. Bone Joint Surg. Br.* 44(2):292–301, 1962.

Chiari K. Medial displacement osteotomy of the pelvis. *Clin. Orthop.* 98:55–71, 1974.

Dunn PM. Clicking hips should be ignored. *Lancet* 1:846, 1984.

Ferguson AB Jr. Primary open reduction of congenital dislocation using a median adductor approach. *J. Bone Joint Surg. Am.* 55(4):671–689, 1973.

Galeazzi R. *Il Pio Istituto Rachitici di Milano.* Milan, Italy: Bergamo, 1874–1913.

Ganz R, Klaue K, Vinh TS, Mast JW. New periacetabular osteotomy for treatment of hip dysplasias. Technique and preliminary results. *Clin. Orthop.* 232:26–36, 1988.

Graf R. Classification of hip joint dysplasia by means of sonography. *Arch. Orthop. Trauma Surg.* 102(4):248–255, 1984.

Harcke HT, Kumar SJ. The rôle of ultrasound in the diagnosis and management of congenital dislocation and dysplasia of the hip. *J. Bone Joint Surg. Am.* 73(4):622–628, 1991.

Harris WH. Etiology of osteoarthritis of the hip. *Clin. Orthop.* 213:20–33, 1986.

Hilgenreiner H. Zur frühdiagnose und frühbehandlung der angeborenen huftgelenkuerrenkung. *Med. Klin.* 21:1385, 1925.

Le Damany P. *La Luxation Congénitale de la Hanche; Études d'Anatomie Comparée, d'Anthropogénie Normale et Pathologique, Déductions Thérapeutiques.* Paris: F. Alçan, 1912.

Lequesne M, de Séze S. Le faux profil du bassin. Nouvelle incidence radiographique pour l'étude de la hanche. Son utilité dans les dysplasies et les différentes coxopathies. *Rev. Rhum. Mal. Osteoartic.* 28:643, 1961.

Lorenz A. The operative treatment of congenital dislocation of the hip. *Trans. Am. Orthop. Assoc.* 7:99, 1895.

Ludloff K. Open reduction of the congenital hip dislocation by anterior incision. *Am. J. Orthop. Surg.* 10(3):438–454, 1913.

Ortolani M. Un segno poco noto e sua importanza per la diagnosi precoce di prelussazione congenita dell'anca. *Pediatria.* 45:129–137, 1937.

Pavlik A. Stirrups as an aid in the treatment of congenital dysplasias of the hip in children. *J. Pediat. Orthop.* 9(2):157–159, 1989. Translated by V. Bialik & N.D. Reis.

Pemberton PA. Pericapsular osteotomy of the ilium for treatment of congenital subluxation and dislocation of the hip. *J. Bone Joint Surg. Am.* 47(1):65–86, 1965.

Perkins G. Signs by which to diagnose congenital dislocation of the hip. 1928. *Clin. Orthop.* 274:3–5, 1992.

Rosen S von. Early diagnosis and treatment of congenital dislocation of the hip joint. *Acta Orthop. Scand.* 26(2):136–155, 1956.

Salter RB. Innominate osteotomy in the treatment of congenital dislocation of the hip. *J. Bone Joint Surg. Br.* 43(3):518–539, 1961.

Sharp IK. Acetabular dysplasia. The acetabular angle. *J. Bone Joint Surg. Br.* 43(2):268–272, 1961.

Shenton EWH. *Disease in Bones and its Detection by X-Rays.* London: Macmillan, 1911.

Smith-Petersen MN. A new supra-articular subperiosteal approach to the hip joint. *Am. J. Orthop. Surg.* 15:592–595, 1917.

Staheli LT. Slotted acetabular augmentation. *J. Pediatr. Orthop.* 1(3):321–327, 1981.

Steel HH. Triple osteotomy of the innominate bone. *J. Bone Joint Surg. Am.* 55(2):343–350, 1973.

Sutherland D, Greenfield, R. Double innominate osteotomy. *J. Bone Joint Surg. Am.* 59(8):1082–1091, 1977.

Tönnis D. Normal values of the hip joint for the evaluation of X-rays in children and adults. *Clin. Orthop.* 119:39–47, 1976.

Tönnis D, Behrens K, Tscharani F. A modified technique of the triple pelvic osteotomy: early results. *J. Pediat. Orthop.* 1(3):241–249, 1981.

Trendelenburg F. *Dtsch. Med. Wschr.* 21:21, 1895.

Wagner, H. Osteotomies for congenital hip dislocation. In: *Proceeding of the Fourth Open Scientific Meeting of the Hip Society.* St. Louis, MO; 1976.

Wiberg G. Studies on dysplastic acetabula and congenital subluxation of the hip joint. *Acta Chirurg. Scand.* 83(Suppl. 58):1, 1939.

LCP

Calvé J. Sur une forme particulière de pseudo-coxalgie-Greffée sur des déformations charactéristiques de l'extrémité supérieure du fémur. *Rev. Chir.* 42:54–84, 1910.

Catterall A. The natural history of Perthes' disease. *J. Bone Joint Surg. Br.* 53(1):37–53, 1971.

Gage HC. A possible early sign of Perthes' disease. *Brit. J. Radiol.* 6:295–297, 1933.

Herring JA, Neustadt JB, Williams JJ, Early JS, Browne RH. The lateral pillar classification of Legg Calvé Perthes disease. *J. Pediatr. Orthop.* 12(2):143–150, 1992.

Köhler A. *Die Normale und Pathologische Anatomie des Hüftgelenkes und Oberschenkels in Röntgenographischer Darstellung.* Hamburg, Germany; 1905.

Legg AT. An obscure affection of the hip-joint. *Boston Med. Surg. J.* 162:202–204, 1910.

Little DG, Kim HKW. Potential for bisphosphonate treatment in Legg-Calvé-Perthes disease. *J. Pediatr. Orthop.* 31(2 Suppl):S182–S188, 2011.

Meyer J. Dysplasia epiphysealis capitis femoris. A clinical-radiological syndrome and its relationship to Legg-Calvé-Perthes disease. *Acta Orthop. Scand.* 34:183–197, 1964.

Miyamoto Y, Matsuda T, Kitoh H, Haga N, Ohashi H, Nishimura G, Ikegawa S. A recurrent mutation in type II collagen gene causes Legg-Calvé-Perthes disease in a Japanese family. *Hum. Genet.* 121(5):625–629, 2007.

Mose K. *Legg-Calvé-Perthes disease. A comparison among three methods of conservative treatment.* Thesis at Universitesforlaget, Arthus, Denmark, 1964.

Perthes GC. Über arthritis deformans juvenilis. *Deutsch. Ztschr. Chir.* 107:111–159, 1910.

Petrie JG, Bitenc I. The abduction weight bearing treatment in Legg-Perthes disease. *J. Bone Joint Surg. Br.* 53(1):54–62, 1971.

Rowe SM, Kim HS, Yoon TR. Osteochondritis dissecans in Perthes' disease. Report of 7 cases. *Acta Orthop. Scand.* 60(5):545–547, 1989.

Salter RB, Thompson GH. Legg-Calvé-Perthes disease. The prognostic significance of the subchondral fracture and a two group classification of the femoral head involvement. *J. Bone Joint Surg. Am* 66(4):479–489, 1984.

Stulberg SD, Cooperman DR, Wallensten R. The natural history of Legg-Calvé-Perthes disease. *J. Bone Joint Surg. Am.* 63(7):1095–1108, 1981.

Waldenström H. Der obere tuberkulöse collumherd. *Ztschr. Orthop. Chir.* 24:487–498, 1909.

Waldenström H. The first stages of coxa plana. *Acta Orthop. Scand.* 5:1–34, 1934.

SCFE

Boyer DW, Mickelson MR, Ponseti IV. Slipped capital femoral epiphysis. Long-term follow-up of 121 patients. *J. Bone Joint Surg. Am.* 63(1):85–95, 1981.

Carney BT, Weinstein SL, Noble J. Long-term follow-up of slipped capital femoral epiphysis. *J. Bone Joint Surg. Am.* 73(5):667–674, 1991.

Diab M, Hresko MT, Millis MB. Intertrochanteric versus subcapital osteotomy in slipped capital femoral epiphysis. *Clin. Orthop.* 427:204–212, 2004.

Dunn DM. Treatment of adolescent slipping of the upper femoral epiphysis. *J. Bone Joint Surg. Br.* 46:621–629, 1964.

Fahey JJ, O'Brien ET. Acute slipped capital femoral epiphysis. *J. Bone Joint Surg. Am.* 47(6):1105–1122, 1965.

Fröhlich A. Ein fall von tumor der hypophysis cerebri ohne akromegalie. *Wein. Klin. Rdsch.* 15:883–906, 1901.

Ganz R, Gill TJ, Müller ME, Gautier E, Ganz K, Krügel N, Berlemann U. Surgical dislocation of the adult hip. A technique with full access to the femoral head and acetabulum without the risk of avascular necrosis. *J. Bone Joint Surg. Br.* 83(8):1119–1124, 2001.

Hall JE. The results of treatment of slipped femoral epiphysis. *J. Bone Joint Surg. Br.* 39(4):659–673, 1957.

Harris WR. The endocrine basis for slipping of the femoral epiphysis. *J. Bone Joint Surg. Br.* 32(1):5–11, 1950.

Heyman CH, Herndon CH, Strong JM. Slipped femoral epiphysis with severe displacement. A conservative operative treatment. *J. Bone Joint Surg. Am.* 39(2):293–303, 1957.

Imhäuser G. Spätergebnisse der sog. Imhäuser-osteotomie bei der epiphysenlösung. Zugleich ein beitrag zum problem der hüftarthrose. *Z. Orthop.* 115:716–725, 1977.

Ingram AJ, Clarke MS, Clarke CS, Marshall RW. Chondrolysis complicating slipped capital femoral epiphysis. *Clin. Orthop.* 165:99–109, 1982.

Ippolito E, Mickelson MR, Ponseti IV. A histochemical study of slipped capital femoral epiphysis. *J. Bone Joint Surg. Am.* 63(7):1109–1113, 1981.

Jerre T. A study of slipped capital femoral epiphysis with special reference to late functional and roentgenological results and the value of closed reduction. *Acta Orthop. Scand.* (Suppl 6):3–15, 1950.

Key JA. Epiphyseal coxa vara or displacement of the capital epiphysis of the femur in adolescence. *J. Bone Joint Surg.* 8:53–117, 1926.

Klein A, Joplin RJ Reidy JA. Treatment in cases of slipped capital femoral epiphysis at Massachusetts General Hospital. *Arch. Surg.* 46(5):681, 1943.

Lacroix P, Verbrugge J. Slipping of the upper femoral epiphysis. A pathological study. *J. Bone Joint Surg. Am.* 33(2):371–381, 1951.

Lehman WB, Grant A, Rose D, Pugh J, Norman A. A method of evaluating possible pin penetration in slipped capital femoral epiphysis using a cannulated internal fixation device. *Clin. Orthop.* 186:65–70, 1984.

Loder RT, Richards BS, Shapiro PS, Reznick LR, Aronson DD. Acute slipped capital femoral epiphysis. The importance of physeal stability. *J. Bone Joint Surg. Am.* 75(8):1134–1140, 1993.

Moseley C. The "approach-withdraw phenomenon" in the pinning of slipped capital femoral epiphysis. *Orthop. Trans.* 9:497, 1985.

Murray RO. The etiology of primary osteoarthritis of the hip. *Brit. J. Radiol.* 38(455):810–824, 1965.

Resnick D. The "tilt deformity" of the femoral head in osteoarthritis of the hip, a poor indicator of previous epiphysiolysis. *Clin. Radiol.* 27(3):355–363, 1976.

Waldenström H. On necrosis of the joint cartilage by epiphysiolysis capitis femoris. *Acta Chir. Scand.* 67:936–941, 1930.

Weiner DS, Weiner S, Melby A, Hoyt WA Jr. A 30-year experience with bone graft epiphysiodesis in the treatment of slipped capital femoral epiphysis. *J. Pediatr. Orthop.* 4(2):145–152, 1984.

Wilson PD, Jacobs R, Schector L. Slipped upper femoral epiphysis. An end result study. *J. Bone Joint Surg. Am.* 47:1128–1145, 1965.

OTHER

Khan M, Adamich J, Simunovic N, Philippon MJ, Bhandari M, Ayeni O. Surgical management of internal snapping hip syndrome: a systematic review evaluating open and arthroscopic approaches. *J. Arthroscop.* 29(5):942–948, 2013.

Klaue K, Durnin CW, Ganz R. The acetabular rim syndrome. A clinical presentation of dysplasia of the hip. *J. Bone Joint Surg. Br.* 73(3):423–429, 1991.

Wild AT, Sponseller PD, Stec AA, Gearhart JP. The rôle of osteotomy in surgical repair of bladder exstrophy. *Sem. Pediatr. Surg.* 20(2):71–78, 2011.

ANATOMY

The lower limb spans the head of the femur to the toes. The leg lies between knee joint and ankle joint. Structures of the thigh are referred to as "femoral," from Latin *femur*: "thigh," such as fascia lata femoris: "broad fascia of the thigh," and os femoris: "bone of the thigh," or simply "femur." Because two bones occupy the leg, its structures are referred to as "crural," from Latin *crus*: "shank, leg," such as crural fascia.

Unlike the hip, which commands its own treatise, the knee is difficult to extricate from the lower limb, save by an arthroscope (*cf.* Sports chapter).

The patella is conferred autonomy due to its size and functional importance. Hence, the term "ligamentum patellæ" when convention dictates "quadriceps tendon," since the patella is lodged in this muscle as a sesamoid. The patella has a proximal base and a distal apex, referred to as superior and inferior poles. The anatomic terms aid understanding why children complain of pain rarely at the broad end (base) but frequently at the pointed end (apex), at which stress is concentrated. Anatomic terminology similarly aids remembering that the site of attachment of the lateral collateral ligament, known as fibular collateral ligament, differs from that of the medial collateral ligament, known as tibial collateral ligament.

Like the femur at the knee, the tibia has two condyles, which by being less rounded are less distinct. The raised space surrendered between the condyles for the cruciate ligaments is the "intercondylar eminence," commonly referred to as "tibial spine" due to its sharp terminus. Like the proximal femur, with its trochanters, the proximal tibia has an apophysis termed "tubercle." Unlike the femur, tibial apophysitis is common during growth.

Knee angle is defined between thigh and leg, or between femur and tibia. Popliteal angle (Latin *poples*: "ham, hollow of the knee") specifies the angle subtended by the leg relative to thigh in the sagittal plane [C], where it is a measure of "hamstring" tension. Full extension is defined as 0 degree, while hyperextension is defined as negative.

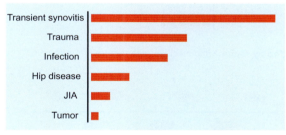

A Causes of limp by frequency Infection includes bone and joint, abscess, and diskitis. Hip disease excludes infection.

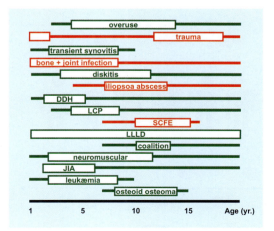

B Causes of limp by age Box is peak of presentation. Note that trauma is bimodal, including "toddler" fracture around 2 years. DDH: developmental dysplasia of the hip. (LCP, Legg-Calvé-Perthes; SCFE, slipped capital femoral epiphysis; LLLD, lower limb length discrepancy; JIA, juvenile idiopathic arthritis.) *Red* indicates urgent or emergent condition.

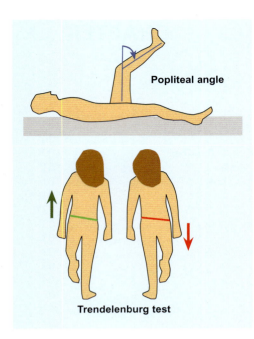

C Popliteal angle and Trendelenburg test.

Popliteal angle

Trendelenburg test

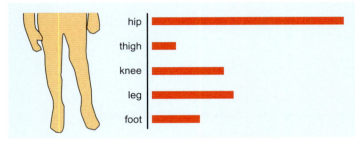

hip
thigh
knee
leg
foot

D Origin of limp by region Thigh includes pain referred from the hip.

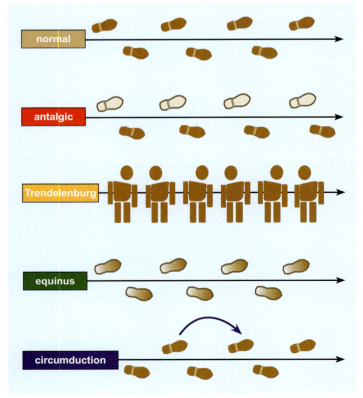

normal

antalgic

Trendelenburg

equinus

circumduction

E Types of gait.

LIMP

A limp signifies abnormal gait, which may be due to pain (conscious or subconscious), deformity, or neuromuscular imbalance. The limping child need not be a diagnostic "black box." It requires a thorough history and physical examination, which may be supplemented by laboratory and imaging studies. Transient synovitis is the most common cause [A]. The condition may be divided according to age and urgency. Different causes occur with different frequencies in different age groups [B]. Some are characteristic of certain ages (e.g., slipped capital femoral epiphysis circa puberty), while others are broadly distributed (e.g., lower limb length discrepancy). The varying causes may be divided into those that require urgent treatment (e.g., hip pyarthritis) and those that may be managed electively (e.g., developmental dysplasia of the hip). The hip dominates anatomically [D].

Gait Antalgic gait is defined by a shortened stance phase, of which the extreme is a refusal to walk [E]. A common theme in hip deformities producing limp is a Trendelenburg gait [C]. This results from a shift of the body over the affected hip in order to reduce the moment arm exerted on weak abductor muscles, which aids them in maintaining a horizontal pelvis during stance phase. In milder deformities, the gait may be apparent only after several cycles and may give way to pain as the hip abductors increasingly fatigue. This may be distinguished by its more lateral location from painful hip disorders, in which the pain is anterior in the region of the groin. Neuromuscular patients may exhibit an equinus gait, such as a hemiplegic who walks toe–toe. Equinus may drive the knee into recurvatum to plant the foot flat. Circumduction gait is characterized by incomplete knee flexion, actively (e.g., due to pain) or passively (e.g., due to contracture), which functionally lengthens the limb requiring swinging around the direction of walking to clear the ground.

Evaluation Age is the single most important discriminator of disease. Obtain a complete history. Is this acute, intermittent, or chronic? Are there associated symptoms (e.g., bruisability on leukæmia)? Is the limp local or a manifestation of a generalized condition (e.g., preceding illness)? Ask about milestones: delay may be an early tip-off of subtle neuromuscular disease [F]. Does the child complain of the limp? Long-standing, intermittent, milder pain may be suppressed in a child's consciousness producing the so-called "painless" limp (e.g., established Legg-Calvé-Perthes disease).

Look at the whole child. Does she or he seem in distress (which may differentiate synovitis from infection), suggesting an urgent presentation? Are the upper limbs (e.g., hemiplegia) or back (e.g., diskitis) affected? Before examining where it hurts, go to the other side to gain the child's confidence. The physical examination should be performed in both supine and prone positions. The supine position may show hip obligate lateral rotation with flexion as seen in slipped capital femoral epiphysis. The prone position has the distinct advantage of allowing uncoupling of the knee from the hip, which may masquerade one for the other. The knee may be ranged from extension to flexion without moving the hip. In the supine position, moving the knee requires flexion of the hip, making it difficult at times to tell which joint is the offender. In addition, as in examination for torsion, the prone position allows simultaneous comparison of hip rotation (especially medial), which is the most sensitive to disease. Finally, the prone position will reveal a hip flexion contracture that may be concealed by lumbar hyperlordosis without the physician manipulating the child. No room is big enough to evaluate gait in detail. In addition, running amplifies gait disturbances and impedes compensatory mechanisms.

Management This is in accordance with condition, of which the different types are discussed independently elsewhere. Röntgenogrammes are readily available, low morbidity, inexpensive, and useful for general screening. Ultrasonography is noninvasive. By contrast, needle aspiration is invasive and stressful to child and parent; however, it is of high diagnostic value. Do not let timidity or logistics delay or dissuade—the emergency setting offers the best opportunity. Specialized imaging focuses and elucidates, such as scintigraphy in radio negative case where occult fracture is

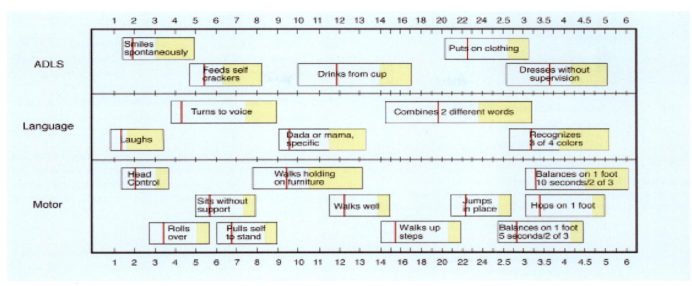

F Denver developmental screening test.

suspected. Obtain laboratory tests judiciously. C-reactive protein is more specific and sensitive for infection than is leukocyte count. Observation is an acceptable and prudent form of management. Before requesting a complex test, which may require anæsthesia or may be expensive, evaluate the child on another day if the presentation is not urgent. A final diagnosis may elude the most thorough investigator in up to 25% of cases.

LEG ACHES

Leg aches are "growing pains." This may be explained as overuse in a child who lacks judgment to avoid repetitive injury and lacks consequence when injured (due to rapid recovery). Other mechanisms implicated include rapid, episodic skeletal growth stretching surrounding soft tissues, increasing body weight, participation in sports at higher levels with escalating expectations, and developing body mechanics. One-third of children experience leg aches, in addition to headaches and stomach aches. All of these may be stressful to the family but are physiologically benign, resolving without sequelæ. Extensive evaluation, including MRI of the brain, gastrointestinal contrast study, and multiple röntgenogrammes of the lower limbs, is negative. Recognize and reassure.

Evaluation Leg aches usually affect both legs, though one side may predominate [A]. If they produce limp, it is intermittent. They are worst at the end of a busy day or at night, interfering with falling asleep but not awakening from sleep. Long duration presents a paradox: while trying for a family, this lowers the physician's concern (bad things do not linger without causing further trouble). They are not associated with other symptoms. They are poorly localized and may migrate from part to part within a limb or from side to side. This is consistent with benignity, but also calls for a broad physical examination. There are no "hard" objective signs, such as deformity, stiffness, swelling, discoloration.

Management Establish this diagnosis of exclusion, in order not to request unnecessary tests or tests that yield equivocal results, which may alarm a family and trigger further testing.

TORSION

This presents the greatest disparity between familial concern and disease.

Nomenclature

Version refers to normal axial rotation of a long bone. In the femur, this is the angle subtended between the neck and condyles, normally anteriorward 30 degrees at birth declining to 12 degrees at maturity. In the tibia, it is measured as the transmalleolar axis, with the knee as a neutral

History	
Geography	Non focal
Limp	Occasional, intermittent
Timing	End of day
	Interferes with falling asleep
	Long duration
Associated symptoms	None
Physical examination	
Tenderness	No
Deformity	No
Stiffness	No
Other soft tissue change	No
Tests	
Imaging	Normal
Laboratory	Normal

A Leg aches Distinguishing characteristics.

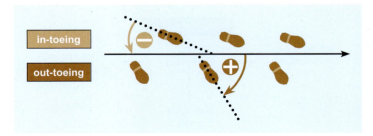

A Foot progression angle.

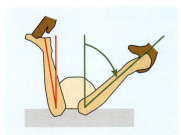

B Hip rotation test Prone position allows simultaneous evaluation to expose asymmetry from side to side and of all sites (hip, transmalleolar axis, and foot) of rotation. Asymmetric loss of medial rotation of the hip (*red*) is a concerning sign. In the patient pictured below, the feet easily rest on the table due to severe antetorsion (90 degrees+)

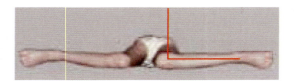

Site	Range of Rotation	Age
Hip	Medial: 30–70 degrees	▼
	Lateral: 30–70 degrees	▲
Transmalleolar axis	0–30 degrees	

C Range of rotation for hip and leg Ranges by the end of the first decade. Total arc at the hip is 100 degrees. Medial rotation of the hip declines while lateral rotation increases with age, as degenerative disease contracts the capsular fibers.

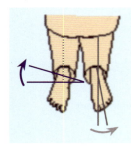

D Measurement of tibial rotation Thigh–foot angle is subtended between the long axis of the thigh and of the foot (*gray*). Transmalleolar axis is the angle subtended by a line drawn through the malleoli and a line drawn perpendicular to the axis of the thigh (*blue*).

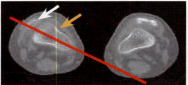
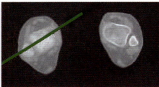

E CT in preparation for operative correction of torsion Rotational malalignment results in lateral patellar dislocations. The femora are rotated medialward (*red*), while the tibiae rotate lateralward (*green*). The opposite rotation wrings the lower limb to drive the patella (*white*) out of the trochlea (*orange*).

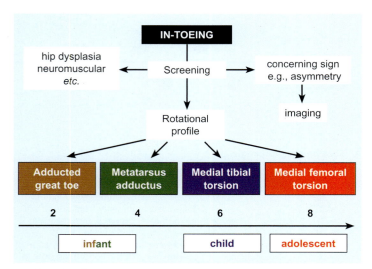

F Algorithm for in-toeing Numbers indicate age in years by which component of in-toeing resolves spontaneously in most cases. Boxes below abscissa indicated period of treatment if indicated.

reference: normal is 5 degrees at birth increasing to 15 degrees lateralward at maturity.

Torsion refers to abnormal version, > or < 2 standard deviations from the mean. For example, in the proximal femur, "antetorsion" is preferable to "excessive anteversion." "Retrotorsion" signifies neck inclination 15 degrees to 0 degree. Retroversion is abnormal *per se*.

Rotation may be described as medial and lateral, or internal and external. The latter distinguishes rotation as a movement.

Development

In the fetus, the lower limb rotates medialward to bring the apex of the knee anterior and the hallux medial. With growth, the lower limb unwinds lateralward, with declining femoral anteversion and increasing transmalleolar axis. Thus, in-toeing tends to resolve with growth, whereas out-toeing may worsen.

Evaluation

History This is essential to acknowledge the concerns of the family.

Physical examination Determine the rotational profile, which has the following components.

FOOT PROGRESSION ANGLE This is the angular difference between the axis of the foot and line of progression walking [A].

FEMORAL VERSION Measure hip rotation prone [B]. Significant asymmetry may be a sign of focal disease (e.g., slipped capital femoral epiphysis). Identify the midpoint between medial and lateral rotation, a measure of resting rotation. Normal medial rotation is <70 degrees; >90 degrees, which requires moving the limb off the side of the table, is considered severe [C]. A child with femoral antetorsion sits in a W position. The patellæ "squint" or "kiss" in the standing position. Running is characterized by an "eggbeater" pattern, as the legs flip out during swing phase.

ANGLE OF TIBIAL ROTATION This may be determined by thigh–foot angle or transmalleolar axis [D]. Thigh–foot angle is a measure of both leg (ankle) and foot (subtalar) rotation, whereas transmalleolar axis isolates the leg. In an infant, thigh–foot angle has wide variation due to ligamentous laxity: minimize this by guiding the foot to its neutral position rather than manipulating it into position. In an older child, it may be compared with transmalleolar axis to estimate contribution of hind foot rotation.

FOOT Examine the lateral border of the foot. This may be convex in metatarsus adductus, thereby producing in-toeing. It may be concave in forefoot abductus, as in flatfoot or overcorrected clubfoot. An adducted hallux, dynamic or static, may give the appearance of in-toeing.

Imaging Consider imaging for concerning sign, such as asymmetry of hip rotation, or as part of operative planning. For the former, start with screening röntgenogrammes. For the latter, CT measures rotation [E].

Management The natural history of torsion is unaffected by manipulative therapy or bracing. Sitting in the W position is OK. Twister cables are not OK. Each component of torsion resolves spontaneously in the majority of patients with growth over the first decade [F]. In the young child, it is difficult to determine the functional impact of torsion, for example, frequent falling is more likely due to judgment and development of gait mechanics than to torsion, unless severe. In fact, medial torsion may be advantageous in rectifying the course of tibialis posterior and poising the subtalar joint to lock, thereby expediting push-off. Conversely, increasing lateral rotation reduces lever arm of the foot, thereby weakening push-off. Appearance is determined by the family and often is a significant cause for consultation.

There is no evidence that persistent femoral antetorsion accounts for long-term morbidity such as osteoarthritis. Femoral retroversion is abnormal and is associated with slipped capital femoral epiphysis and femoroacetabular impingement.

Only operation can change long bone torsion. This is indicated in < 1% of patients, and after 8 years of age. Torsion must be severe, clearly a cause of dysfunction, and natural history must be allowed to complete its course. This is most likely in opposing or "miserable" malalignment [E], which is deleterious to the patellofemoral articulation, accounting for pain and patellar instability.

FEMORAL OSTEOTOMY This may be performed proximal or distal. Proximal incision may be covered more readily by clothing. Intertrochanteric osteotomy allows level proximal to trochanter minor, which heals readily and takes advantage of iliopsoas to add compression. Operation in the prone position, while requiring familiarity ("upside down"), allows comparison of both lower limbs for symmetry. Use a high angle plate (120 to 130 degrees) with longest blade into the head of the femur. This will provide an internal strut in the neck as protection against future osteoporosis.

TIBIAL OSTEOTOMY This is performed proximal to the tibial tubercle to correct patellofemoral malalignment. Distal metaphyseal osteotomy is easier [G]. Cut the fibula for severe deformity. Add fasciotomy of the anterior crural muscle compartment to reduce risk of compartment syndrome. Plate fixation forgoes cast. Wire fixation allows more distal osteotomy for healing, and implant removal in clinic.

GENU VALGUM AND GENU VARUM

Anatomic description of angulation at a joint or fracture addresses the distal skeletal element. Genu valgum refers to pointing of the leg away from the midline, or apex medial angulation of the knee, in the coronal plane. Genu varum is the opposite. Genu valgum is known as "knee-knee," due to overlap of the joints during walking. Genu varum is known as "bowlegs," after the arc formed by the lower limb.

Evaluation

There is a normal evolution with age, and a normal range, of knee shape [A]. Knee shape may be measured as an angle or indirectly by distance between the ankles (genu valgum) or knees (genu varum).

History Is this acute (e.g., after fracture) or chronic (e.g., in rickets)? Does it disturb the child, such as pain or limp, or is it primarily a parental concern?

Physical examination Look at the entire child: is this focal, regional, or part of a generalized condition [B]? Short stature is common in rickets and various syndromes, which also may be characterized by other deformities, cutaneous stigmata, or dysmorphic features. Is it symmetric? Asymmetric deformity is likely morbid and not a physiologic variant. Determine the rotational profile, and neutralize this to isolate the coronal plane. Measure knee angulation with the patellæ pointing straight forward, by turning the hips as necessary. Most infants referred for genu varum have medial tibial torsion instead. In order to compensate for in-toeing, such children rotate the hips lateralward, presenting an oblique view of the knee. This will display a normal bend as the knee flexes during walking, which is interpreted as bowing by an observer who assumes an anteroposterior view of the knee. A goniometer aids angular measurement. Intermalleolar and intercondylar distance may be an easier measurement. Obesity influences measurements. Examine the child supine (static), as well as standing and walking (dynamic), which may expose soft tissue laxity.

Laboratory analysis This is indicated for a metabolic disorder, such as rickets.

Imaging Röntgenogrammes are indicated if disease is suspected. Weight-bearing views simulate the functional position. Educate the technician to obtain a relaxed view with the feet or knees together. Do not distort the image by forcing the limbs together. Include hips to ankles, in order to view mechanical as well as anatomic axes [C]. Mechanical axis identifies deformity: in genu valgum, the axis passes lateral to the knee or medial to the ankle, and genu varum is characterized by the reverse. Anatomic axis identifies site of deformity, for

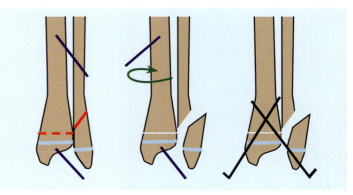

G Osteotomy of the tibia and fibula Wires are placed (*blue*) remote from osteotomy of the tibia (*red*) to facilitate measurement of derotation, in this case medialward (*green*) for lateral torsion. For large derotation, cut fibula and consider fixation if fragments are widely displaced.

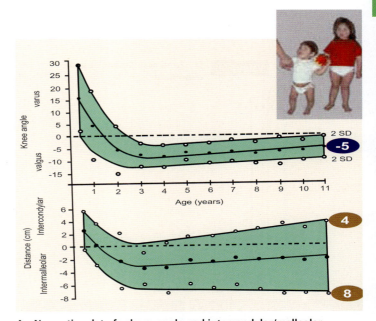

A Normative data for knee angle and intercondylar/malleolar distance Children are born bowlegged, becoming maximally knock-kneed at 3 years before ending at mild knock-knee by the end of the first decade. The siblings pictured show genua vara (12 months) evolving to genua valga (3 years).

Type		Sub-type
Physiologic		Normal developmental variation
P	Focal growth disturbance (over-/undergrowth)	Blount
a		Trauma
t		Infection
h		Inflammatory arthritis
o	Regional growth disturbance	Limb deficiency
l		
o	Primary bone disease	For example, osteogenesis imperfecta
g		
i	Other syndrome	For example, achondroplasia
c		

B Classification of knee angle Be systematic in approach.

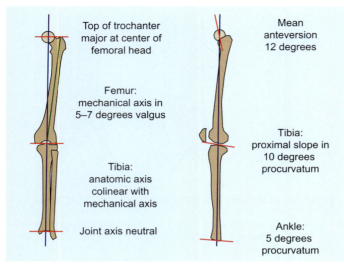

C   Mechanical and anatomic axes of the lower limb Mechanical axis passes through joint centers, a measure of bones in combination. Anatomic axis is bone centered.

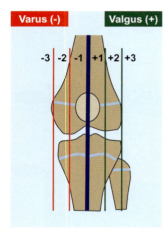

D   Zone assessment of knee alignment.

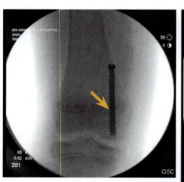

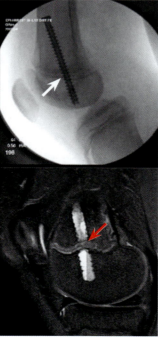

E   Screw physeodesis Cannulated (for percutaneous use) full thread (to ease extraction) transphyseal screw is placed in the medial physis (*orange*) of the distal femur for genu valgum and centrally in the lateral plane to avoid pro- or recurvatum deformation. MRI after implant removal shows intact physis with no osseous bridge.

example, hypoplasia of lateral condyle of the femur producing genu valgum, or growth disturbance of medial condyle of the tibia producing genu varum. Coronal deformity also may be assessed by noting through which zone of the knee the mechanical axis travels [D]. Eliminate anisomelia, so that the child does not bend the knee, by a block under the foot of the short limb. What is the quality of bone? Is deformity diffuse or focal? Are the physes normal? Is there evidence of previous injury or disease? Focus the assessment with CT or MRI as indicated, to provide greater detail and for operative planning. Consider obtaining serial photographs.

Management

Treat the primary disorder first in generalized conditions, for example, vitamin D for rickets (*cf.* Syndromes chapter). Treat the primary musculoskeletal cause of knee deformity as indicated, for example, Blount disease (*q.v.*). For physiologic knee (mal)alignment, consider natural history during growth. Because children are maximally knock-kneed at 3 years and stabilize to mild knock-knees toward the end of the first decade, that is the time to intervene. Management earlier consists of education and reassurance. Because children become maximally knock-kneed at 3 years never to return to bowlegs, bowlegs at this age are abnormal and should be treated.

Like torsion, nothing influences natural history of genu valgum or genu varum except surgery. Determine the site of deformity by complete imaging. Harness the physis to guide growth: tether the medial physis in genu valgum and the lateral in genu varum, until correction, at which point remove the tether. Temporary hemiphyseodesis may be achieved by staples, plate, or transphyseal screw [E]. Staples are the original. Early bending failure under force of growth has been addressed by corner reinforcement. They may dislodge due to smoothness of the tines. Plate and screws are more stable than staples, and span the physis. Screws may be placed percutaneously, are most stable, but are transphyseal; however, removal after correction has not been associated with permanent growth disturbance. This approach is low morbidity, ambulatory, and predictable. For angular correction, remove implants within 2 years, before a physis gives up growth completely.

Deformity in the mature child, in whom growth modulation is not possible, or deformity that is not focal or uniplanar, occurring in the setting of broader complex deformity such as limb length discrepancy, requires more powerful reconstruction. Plan an osteotomy, including making cutouts or with graphics that allow operative simulation. The closer the osteotomy to the site of deformity, the less the requirement for translation to compensate for distance away from the center of rotation. Be prepared to perform an osteotomy at more than one level. Primary bone disease can deform the entire structure. Plan the fixation, internal or external, and location. External fixators are more potent in allowing three-dimensional correction. They enable gradual correction, which reduces the need for reconstruction of, and injury to, surrounding soft tissues. They are more forgiving because they may be manipulated after operation.

BLOUNT DISEASE

Blount called this "tibia vara." It represents a growth disturbance of the posteromedial proximal physis of the tibia. The growing tibia spirals into varus (medial tether) as well as medial rotation and procurvatum (posterior tether), thereby forming a complex multiplanar deformity. While the condition originates in the tibia, where signs are most striking, it also may involve the distal femur.

Cause

Familial clustering suggests a genetic predisposition. Race is confusing: it has been reported most in Black Americans [A] and Scandinavians, with a worse prognosis in the former. A mechanical cause is suggested by association with early walking and obesity: a heavy child whose physiologic genu varum is greater the earlier is walking and who does not fully extend the knees during gait concentrates load at the posteromedial physis of the proximal tibia. Compression retards or arrests growth according to the Hueter-Volkmann principle. Wide gait due to obesity increases the varus moment at the knee, squeezing the medial physis. Asymmetric or unilateral disease suggests that other, local factors may play a rôle.

Evaluation

Classification Like idiopathic scoliosis, Blount disease may be divided by age into infantile (<4 years), juvenile (4 to 10 years), and adolescent (>10 years). Severity is inversely proportional to age of onset.

The condition also has been classified according to progressive physeal irregularity [B]. However, this system has high interobserver variability, in part due to variable ossification over a wide age range and to segmentation of a continuous process. As a result, it may be simplified into I-III and IV-VI, based upon likelihood of spontaneous recovery and bridge formation, which impacts operation and outcomes.

Natural history The most important predictor of severity and poor outcomes is age of onset: early in growth, the more cartilaginous proximal tibia is more fragile. Knee degeneration is proportional to severity of deformity. Body weight is an independent predictor of outcome, with body mass index >40 kg/m² being a critical value for severity.

History Ask about walking age. Also enquire about nutrition and exercise, as well as efforts at weight reduction.

Physical examination It often is difficult to distinguish physiologic varus from Blount disease before 2 years of age: bring such patients back at 3 years of age. Calculate body mass index. Measure the intercondylar distance standing. Examine the knee dynamically: is there lateral thrust at the knee during walking? The lateral soft tissue become so attenuated over time that they are unable to support fully the knee during stance phase, allowing the tibia to be displaced lateralward. The deformity may be exaggerated, associated with a clunk, by varus stress of the attenuated lateral soft tissues. Determine the rotational profile of the tibia, which produces in-toeing and must be addressed by osteotomy.

Imaging Obtain röntgenogrammes standing with the ankles together and the patellæ forward to obtain orthogonal views of the knees. Alert the technician to allow the feet to turn inward as much as necessary. Projection is critical to isolating the coronal plane. Röntgenogrammes may be challenging in the adolescent due to obesity and size, including getting

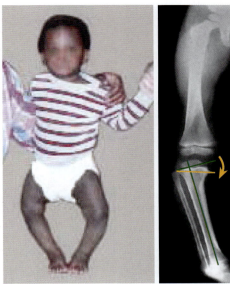
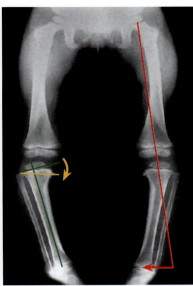

A Infantile tibia vara *Mechanical axis misses the ankle laterally (red). Beaking of medial metaphysis indicates growth disturbance. Its effect is measured as the metaphyseal–diaphyseal angle.*

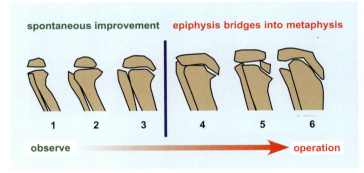

spontaneous improvement   epiphysis bridges into metaphysis

1   2   3   4   5   6

observe   operation

B Langenskiöld classification of Blount disease *This classification is commonly used but sometimes difficult to apply.*

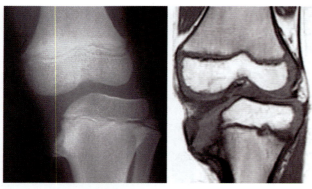

C MRI in Blount disease The medial condyle, absent on röntgenogramme, is visible on MRI, where depression explains medial subluxation of the femur.

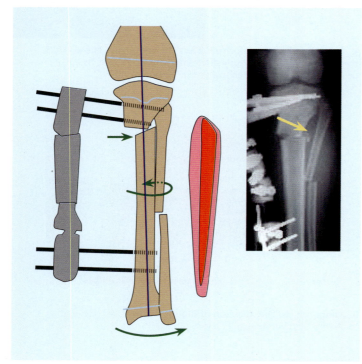

D Osteotomy of the tibia and fibula with external fixation Transverse osteotomy distal to tibial tubercle and more distal to fibula. Correction includes valgus, lateral rotation, and lateral displacement to bring ankle into line with mechanical axis (*blue*). Deformity reduced and osteotomy fixed with external fixator (*gray*). Anterior crural compartment fasciotomy (*red*) to reduce the risk of compartment syndrome.

the width of the knees on a single view. The earliest sign is varus with metaphyseal beaking [A]. Growth disturbance of the proximal physis of the tibia may be characterized according to the Langenskiöld classification. In long-standing disease, a significant (i.e., worthy of inclusion as part of surgical correction) proportion of the coronal deformity in adolescent presentation arises from the distal femur.

METAPHYSEAL–DIAPHYSEAL ANGLE This is the most established and useful measurement, formed by a line drawn through the metaphysis and one drawn orthogonal to the anatomic axis of the tibia in the coronal plane [A]. Substitute the axis of the fibula if the tibia is too deformed. In the incompletely ossified skeleton, a critical value is >15 degrees.

Arthrography outlines articular surfaces, often showing development of the medial condyle of the tibia invisible to röntgenogrammes because of a delay in ossification. MRI gives details of delayed ossification and deformation; articular changes, such as medial meniscal hypertrophy; and physeal changes, such as bridge formation [C].

Management

Do not forget the child: make sure a specialist is in charge of weight control. Orthopædic management is observation or surgical. Initially observe Langenskiöld I-III, as many improve spontaneously.

Osteotomy (infantile) Consider realignment osteotomy of the proximal tibia at 3 years of age [D]. Include osteotomy of the fibula distal to its proximal third to reduce risk of common fibular nerve injury. Factors associated with recurrence of deformity after operation include the following:

- Age >4 years
- Langenskiöld > III
- Body mass index >40 kg/m^2

Osteotomy realigns the tibia, unloading and protecting the knee. It decompresses the proximal physis but does not change the fundamental growth disturbance directly; as a result, the tibia may grow back into deformity. Inform the patient and family that index operation may be the first stage in treatment: potential for recurrence is part of preoperative expectations. Prolong interval to recurrence by measured overcorrection to 10-degree valgus. Fixation is by wires supplemented with cast, or a blade plate with offset applied medially to displace the distal fragment lateralward, which has the advantage of no external immobilization.

Growth modulation (juvenile) Lateral physeal tethering is indicated for:

- Juvenile onset, in which there is significant growth remaining.
- Mild deformity, which does not expect big correction. This is defined as Langenskiöld I-III, where the medial physis has reasonable growth potential, and a mechanical axis that traverses the medial condyle of the femur (does not miss medially).
- Body mass index <40 kg/m^2.

Confirm that there is no physeal bridge by MRI: if there is, lateral tether will arrest growth, achieving an even shorter limb.

Osteotomy (adolescent) If MRI shows a discreet physeal bridge in the adolescent, this may be resected with placement of a fat graft before performing an osteotomy. External fixation has advantages.

- Because of long-standing growth disturbance, and because of patient size, it allows stable correction of coronal (varus), transverse (medial torsion), as well as sagittal (procurvatum) deformities.

- Gradual rather than acute correction is possible, which may reduce neurovascular risk. Postoperative adjustment of correction compensates for any limitations of intraoperative imaging (e.g., not weight bearing, not full length).
- A limb shortened by severe disease may be lengthened in addition to corrected by distraction osteogenesis.

Level of osteotomy is distal to tibial tubercle: because this is remote from the site of deformity, the distal fragment must be translated lateralward as well as into valgus to compensate. Other osteotomy techniques include opening *versus* closing wedge and transverse *versus* oblique *versus* dome cuts. Opening lengthens the tibia, which partially addresses limb length discrepancy. Closing wedge may be safer by relaxing the common fibular nerve. Oblique and dome cuts increase surface area for union. Other fixation techniques include blade plate. The irregular shape of the tibia makes fitting this implant difficult if derotation and extension are included in correction. The subcutaneous medial face of the tibia makes implants prominent in this location. Add fasciotomy of the anterior crural muscle compartment by long scissors inserted through a small proximal incision and passed along the subcutaneous crest of the tibia to the extensor retinaculum.

Articular reconstruction For severe dysplasia of the medial condyle of the tibia in the adolescent, in whom remodeling potential is limited, an osteotomy may be performed to elevate the medial articular surface of the tibia to restore a horizontal joint line. Supplement the open procedure with arthroscopy to evaluate articular surface and guard against disruption or step-off [E].

ANTERIOR KNEE PAIN

This is one of the common "growing pains." Some call it the "headache of the knee." Do not attach the word "syndrome." There are similarities with the Minnesota Multiphasic Personality Inventory for back pain.

Evaluation

This is a diagnosis of exclusion. Pain may be projected to the anteromedial knee from a condition of the hip, after the law of Hilton (John Hilton, surgeon at Guy's Hospital London, 1860), which states that "a nerve which innervates a muscle that acts on a joint will innervate that joint and the skin overlying the muscle's insertion." Examine the hips, in particular rotation. Knee examination does not suggest focal disease [A]. The pain is associated with a period of rapid growth and certain activities such as walking on an incline, sitting, and squatting. It is poorly localized: the patient cups the knee cap in the hand or circles the front of the knee when asked to point to the locus of pain. There are no "hard" objective signs such as swelling or persistent gait disturbance and no specific antecedent event such as trauma.

Management

Educate the patient and family that this is a normal albeit frustrating occurrence in childhood, with a natural history of spontaneous resolution without sequelæ over months or even years. The patellofemoral articulation and core strength are the focus, without or with the aid of a physiotherapist, in order to address subclinical instability of weakness. Include a coach or athletic trainer for proper sports mechanics. Do not neglect general health measures such as stretching, activity modification, and weight reduction if indicated.

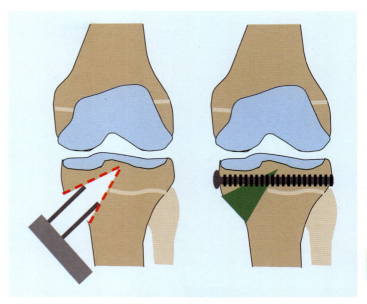

E Articular reconstruction of medial condyle of the tibia
Osteotomy is opened (*red*) to elevate the medial plateau. The gap is filled with a structural tricortical osseous graft (*green*) and fixed with cannulated screw(s).

Examination	Finding
Gait	Normal, including no limp
Deformity	Normal alignment
Inflammatory signs	None, including no swelling, warmth
Pain	Diffuse; no focal tenderness
Knee motion	Full, supple
Patella motion	Normal stable tracking
Crepitus	Patellofemoral in some
Stability	Normal
Rotational profile	Normal
Muscle tightness	Hamstring, quadriceps
Single limb deep bend	Valgus may expose core weakness
Hip	Full supple motion, no pain

A Checklist for evaluation of anterior knee pain There are no focal signs of disease.

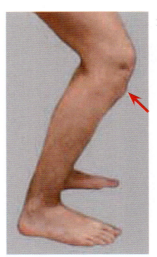

A Osgood-Schlatter condition
The presentation is classic.

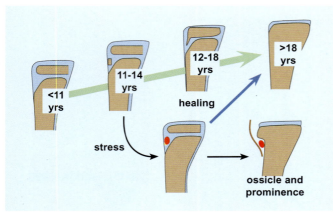

B Natural history of Osgood-Schlatter condition. Normal development of the apophysis (*green*) may be interrupted by excessive traction (*red*). Most heal and normalize (*blue*), but some remain as a separate ossicle or a prominence, which may be symptomatic.

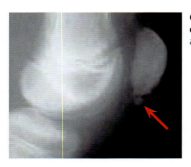

C Sinding-Larsen-Johansson condition Separate ossicle at the apex of patella (*red*).

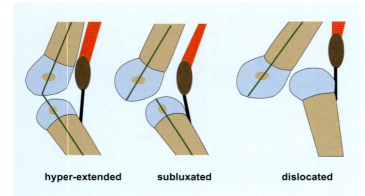

A Congenital dislocation of the knee.

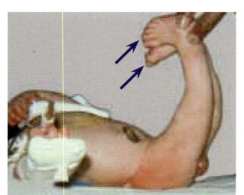

B Congenital knee dislocation Hyperextension of the knees was accompanied by postural clubfoot due to packaging pressure.

OSTEOCHONDROSIS OF THE KNEE

Osgood-Schlatter Condition

This represents a traction apophysitis of the tibial tubercle due to repetitive tensile microtrauma. It presents early in the second decade, during the period of prepubertal growth acceleration. The natural history is resolution with growth deceleration or cessation. In 10% of patients, a residual prominence or ununited ossicle may remain after maturity. The condition may result in a site of weakness that predisposes to fracture of the tibial tubercle.

Evaluation There is swelling and focal tenderness over the tibial tubercle [A]. The symptoms and signs are so classic that no imaging is necessary. Röntgenogrammes may not show the apophysis before ossification in a young child, or they may show normal fragmentation that becomes a cause of concern for the family. Röntgenogrammes also may show elongation of the patella, consistent with traction on the anterior knee during rapid growth.

Management Take the time to reassure the patient, as pain may be disabling. Modify activities. The patient may take anti-inflammatory agents *pro re nata*. Stretching of quadriceps femoris will reduce traction on tibial apophysis.

In the event of a healed though prominent tibial tubercle, which may be traumatized or hurt when pressed such as in kneeling, or an ununited ossicle in the ligamentum patellæ [B], operative treatment is an option. This consists of simple excision of ossicle(s) and shaving of the tibial tubercle.

Sinding-Larsen–Johansson Condition

This is a traction apophysitis at the other end of ligamentum patellæ, at the apex of the patella [C]. There is activity-related pain that correlates with tenderness at the apex of the patella. It is the ossified end of a spectrum that includes quadriceps tendinitis or "jumper's knee."

Evaluation and management resemble Osgood-Schlatter condition, with the exception that persistence beyond maturity does not occur.

DISLOCATION OF THE KNEE

Congenital Dislocation of the Knee

This may occur in isolation, or it may be associated with other condition, such as Larsen syndrome. It is divided into three types [A]:

- Hyperextension, which is characterized by recurvatum with normal contact of distal femoral and proximal tibial epiphyses
- Subluxation, where articular surfaces are partially in contact
- Dislocation, in which the articular surfaces are not in contact

The condition is caused by extrinsic *in utero* pressure, which also increases the risk of hip dysplasia.

Evaluation The physical appearance is classic [B]. Look for signs of a generalized disorder or for other packaging signs. Because the proximal epiphysis of the tibia is unossified at birth, röntgenogrammes may be difficult to interpret. Ultrasonography will better reveal the knee epiphyses and is useful to screen for hip dysplasia. Determine passive flexion of the knees: fixed subluxation or dislocation is a sign of quadriceps fibrosis, which has a poor prognosis for resolution with closed methods, and is more likely to be associated dislocation of the hips.

Management For supple hyperextension, defined as the ability to flex the knee, allow passive stretching by parents for the first 2 weeks because often this suffices. Serial casting accelerates resolution. For a stiff knee that cannot be flexed, surgical lengthening of the extensor mechanism may be necessary. Include lysis of adhesions to achieve unencumbered glide of the muscle. Aim for flexion to 45 degrees followed by postoperative manipulation to recover more motion, rather than overlengthening, in order to avoid weakness of the quadriceps femoris. Operation at 3 months is within the window for closed management of hip dysplasia, and postoperative spica cast cares for both problems.

Dislocation of the Patella

There are two types [A].

Congenital. While named for the patella, the bone is a passenger in congenital dislocation of the quadriceps femoris muscle.

Habitual. The fundamental abnormality is osseous deformity, including dysplasia of the femoral trochlea and genu valgum.

Evaluation Congenital may be isolated or associated with other condition, such as Rubinstein-Taybi syndrome or nail–patella syndrome. It presents after walking due to gait disturbance. The quadriceps is short and dislocated lateralward posterior to the center of rotation of the knee, where it acts as a flexor and pulls the tibia into valgus and lateral rotation. The patella cannot be reduced. Röntgenogrammes are helpful after ossification of the patella (4 to 6 years of age). Ultrasonography reveals a cartilaginous dislocated patella.

Habitual presents later and throughout childhood. There is tenderness around the patella with apprehension to lateral force. In knee extension, the patella may be laterally subluxated such that, when reduced abruptly with knee flexion the patella traces a J track into and along the femoral trochlea. The lateral margin of patella may resist elevation due to retinacular contracture. The medial soft tissues may be attenuated. The knee may be in excessive valgus. There may be flattening or even a medial scoop of the medial soft tissues at the patella, suggesting hypotrophy of vastus medialis. Röntgenogrammes may show a shallow or flat femoral trochlea, lateral displacement of patella in trochlea, lateral patellar tilt, and a patella that is proximally displaced (where it does not engage the trochlea). Obtain full length lower limb standing röntgenogrammes if there is significant valgus, to evaluate the mechanical axis.

Management Congenital dislocation of the patella is a surgical problem: the entire quadriceps femoris must be reduced (Stanisavljevic) [B].

- The incision extends from trochanter major to apophysis of the tibia.
- Mobilize the quadriceps from lateral intermuscular septum and subjacent femur.
- Release the lateral retinaculum.
- Advance vastus medialis to the lateral margin of patella.
- Imbricate the medial soft tissues.
- Medialize the lateral half of ligamentum patellæ to periosteum (Roux-Goldthwaite). Transfer of tibial tubercle violates the physis, risking recurvatum deformity.
- Support the reduction by semitendinosus tenodesis through an osseous tunnel in patella drilled form distal medial to proximal lateral (Galeazzi). An alternative medial support for reduction is the adductor magnus terminal tendon, which is harvested at the musculotendinous junction and sewn to the patellar retinaculum adjacent the medial patellofemoral ligament.

Management of habitual dislocation of the patella is discussed in Sports chapter.

OTHER CONDITIONS OF THE KNEE

Popliteal Cyst

The term refers to a "fluid-filled mass" (Greek κυστις: "bladder, fluid-filled sack") that appears in the posterior knee (Latin *poples*). This more properly should be referred to as a popliteal bursa (Greek βυρσα: "sack, *purse*"): it occurs subjacent to semimembranosus or medial head of gastrocnemius (or both) and fills with fluid in response to overuse. As a bursa, it is related to the joint by geography but not function. Language is important to distinguish this from other juxta-articular cysts (Baker), which communicate with the joint from which they originate, and represent a sign of internal derangement.

Evaluation Presentation is classic: location in medial popliteal fossa, fusiform shape, firm but not hard, nonreactive surrounding tissues, nontender [A]. Transillumination confirms that the mass is cystic and not

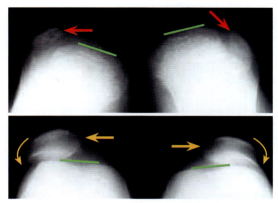

A Dislocation of patella Merchant views. In congenital dislocation (*red*), patella rests against the lateral surface of the lateral femoral condyle and does not engage the trochlea (*green*), due to a dislocation of the entire quadriceps mechanism. In habitual dislocation (*orange*), the patella rests laterally displaced, due to hypoplasia of the trochlea, without or with (*orange*) lateral tilt, due to contracture of the lateral retinaculum. In both, the trochlea is hypoplastic.

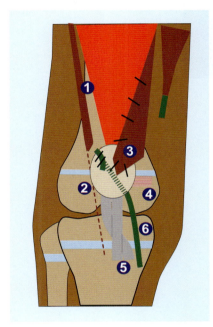

B Reconstruction for dislocation of patella.
1. Release and mobilization of quadriceps
2. Release of lateral retinaculum
3. Advancement of vastus medialis
4. Imbrication of medial soft tissues
5. Medialization of lateral half of ligamentum patellæ
6. Semitendinosus tenodesis

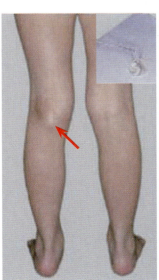

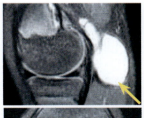

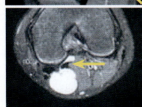

A Popliteal cyst This is located in the medial popliteal fossa (*red*). It is filled with clear gelatinous fluid **(inset)**. MRI shows no communication with the joint (*yellow*).

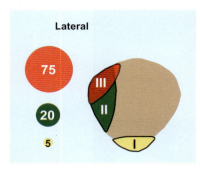

B Classification of bipartite patella Secondary ossification of the patella takes place from superolateral to inferior. Numbers represent % of total.

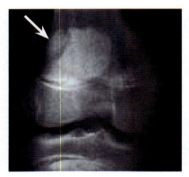

C Bipartite patella Superolateral (*white*) is the most common site.

solid. The mass disappears with knee flexion, as it has more room to flatten. Gait is normal. There is no deformity, crepitus, or other knee abnormality. Although unnecessary for diagnosis or treatment, aspiration yields clear gelatinous material. While ultrasonography and MRI will show the mass, they add little and may tempt intervention.

Management The child has no symptoms and normal function. Natural history is spontaneous resolution over months with no sequelæ. It may recur but remains benign. Because of such benignity, no active treatment is indicated. Focus on education of parents, who may worry about a pernicious process.

Bipartite Patella

The primary ossification center of patella appears at 4 to 6 years of age. Failure of coalescence of a secondary ossification center, which appears at the turn of the decades, results in a bipartite patella. Incidence is 2%, and bilaterality is 50%, with no gender predilection. Three types have been distinguished [B]. Significant trauma, or repetitive microtrauma, may disturb a quiescent synchondrosis to elicit pain, akin to a traction osteochondrosis. Watershed blood supply to the (supero)lateral patella impedes healing once injured.

Evaluation Most are asymptomatic, found incidentally on röntgenogramme [C]. Smooth borders and typical location distinguish this from fracture. In symptomatic bipartite patella, there is focal tenderness and enlargement of the patella. A cleft may be palpable due to the subcutaneous nature of the bone. A stress manœuvre in the squatting position may show separation compared with anteroposterior röntgenogramme. Scintigraphy, by showing increased uptake, and MRI, by showing œdema, may be useful to confirm the diagnosis.

Management Most respond to conservative measures, including activity modification, quadriceps stretching, anti-inflammatory agents, and if necessary a short course of bracing (30-degree knee flexion). This approach may be supplemented with steroid injection.

For intractable pain >6 months, consider operation.

- Fragment excision. This may be open or arthroscopic. While definitive, there is no consensus on fragment size limit.
- Vastus lateralis release, open or arthroscopic. This relieves pain by removing traction forces on the part. This is simplest, but quadriceps weakness is a concern.
- Débridement of the synchondrosis, followed by open reduction and internal fixation, is indicated for large fragments or when it is difficult to distinguish an acute fracture.

LOWER LIMB LENGTH DISCREPANCY

Lower limb length discrepancy (LLLD), or *anisomelia*, may be structural [A] or apparent. Contracture, dynamic asymmetry in function or remote deformity may produce an apparent discrepancy in limb length. Structural discrepancy may occur at the pelvis, femur, tibia, and foot, all of which should be included for complete assessment.

Cause

The fundamental basis for hypertrophy is hyperperfusion [B]. The causes of limb shortening are diverse. They may be primary osseous, or secondary, such as limb shortening in hemiplegic cerebral palsy.

Natural History

LLLD may be constant, such as shortening after malunion of femur fracture, or variable. Variable LLLD may be temporary, such as while a disease is uncontrolled (e.g., hyperaemia of inflammatory arthritis) or constant, as in limb deficiency. Constant LLLD is measured in millimeters or inches. Constantly variable LLLD is measured in % of limb length.

Up to 1/2″ LLLD is normal in the general population. Between 1/2″ and 1″ is a gray zone. Work of gait (joules) increases significantly for LLLD >5%, while oxygen consumption (ml/kg/min) has been shown to increase significantly beyond 1″ LLLD. Both result in visible alteration of gait. Mechanisms to compensate for LLLD include circumduction of the long limb, vaulting over the long limb, and equinus of the short limb. Children adapt to LLLD when adults are unable; hence, a 10-mm difference after arthroplasty may be a source of consternation.

It is impossible to arrive at consensus on relationship of LLLD to back pain. Similarly, reduction of center–edge angle secondary to titling of the pelvis has not been linked to hip degeneration. Pelvic obliquity may produce scoliosis, which is compensatory and remains supple and stable because time spent *per diem* standing erect with hips and knees extended represents such a small proportion of the day.

Evaluation

History Does the patient complain of pain, of inability to play or participate in sports, of appearance? Most patients will elucidate most primary disease, such as prior infection. How mature is the child? The primary physician can provide Tanner stage. Ask about familial stature. Discuss minimal acceptable height, starting at range for the population: women 4′11″ to 5′9″ (150 to 175 cm) and men 5′5″ to 6′4″ (165 to 193 cm). This may be influenced by multiple factors, including culture and surgical tolerance.

Physical examination Examine the whole child, in order to rule out primary disease, including musculoskeletal, neural, vascular, cutaneous, and abdominal examinations, for example, vascular malformation may manifest at the skin by discoloration or warmth. Take the height and plot it serially to calculate growth velocity. Upper and lower segment lengths aid in distinguishing hyper- from hypotrophy. Analyze gait, including walking and running.

The clinical discrepancy is the height of a block under the foot that levels the iliac crests. Pay attention to the height of tibial malleolus off the floor, which is a reflection of foot height. The supine position is necessary before the age of standing and allows differentiation of the femur and tibia [C]. Iliac spine to tibial malleolus, while technical in depending on a tape measure, is prone to inaccuracy due to difficulty in normalizing the pelvis and obscurity of its landmarks.

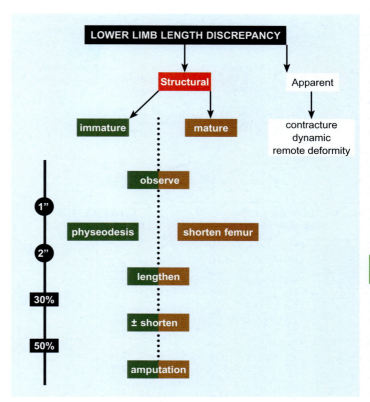

A Algorithm for lower limb length discrepancy (LLLD) Ordinate indicates the calculated amount of LLLD at maturity.

Type	Short	Long
Congenital	*Mild*: Hip dysplasia Clubfoot	Vascular anomaly
	Severe: limb deficiency skeletal dysplasia	
Other musculoskeletal	LCP SCFE	
Neural	Imbalance Paralysis	
Tumor	Physeal injury	Physeal hyperaemia
Infection	Physeal injury	Physeal hyperaemia
Trauma	Physeal injury Malunion	Physeal hyperaemia
Arthritis	Physeal maturation	Physeal hyperaemia

B Causes of lower limb length discrepancy Causes are varied.

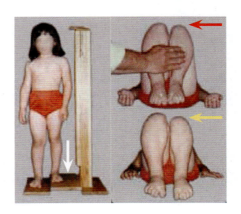

C Clinical assessment of LLLD Comparison of upper:lower segment lengths reveals right lower limb hypertrophy. The pelvis is leveled by standing on a lift (*white*), calculating total discrepancy. Femoral component of the discrepancy (*red*) is determined by comparing knee heights with hips flexed to 90 degrees and feet off table. Tibial component (*yellow*) is determined by comparing knee heights with hips flexed to 45 degrees and knees flexed to 90 degrees.

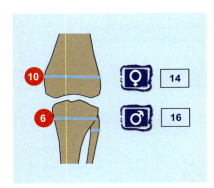

D Arithmetic method Distal femoral physis contributes 10 mm/year to growth, while the proximal tibia contributes 6 mm/year. Girls stop growing at 14 years, while boys stop at 16 years.

LOWER LIMB Multiplier for BOYS				LOWER LIMB Multiplier for GIRLS			
Age (yr + mo)	M	Age (yr + mo)	M	Age (yr + mo)	M	Age (yr + mo)	M
Birth	5.080	7 + 6	1.520	Birth	4.630	6 + 0	1.510
0 + 3	4.550	8 + 0	1.470	0 + 3	4.155	6 + 6	1.460
0 + 6	4.050	8 + 6	1.420	0 + 6	3.725	7 + 0	1.430
0 + 9	3.600	9 + 0	1.380	0 + 9	3.300	7 + 6	1.370
1 + 0	3.240	9 + 6	1.340	1 + 0	2.970	8 + 0	1.330
1 + 3	2.975	10 + 0	1.310	1 + 3	2.750	8 + 6	1.290
1 + 6	2.825	10 + 6	1.280	1 + 6	2.600	9 + 0	1.260
1 + 9	2.700	11 + 0	1.240	1 + 9	2.490	9 + 6	1.220
2 + 0	2.590	11 + 6	1.220	2 + 0	2.390	10 + 0	1.190
2 + 3	2.480	12 + 0	1.180	2 + 3	2.295	10 + 6	1.160
2 + 6	2.385	12 + 6	1.160	2 + 6	2.200	11 + 0	1.130
2 + 9	2.300	13 + 0	1.130	2 + 9	2.125	11 + 6	1.100
3 + 0	2.230	13 + 6	1.100	3 + 0	2.050	12 + 0	1.070
3 + 6	2.110	14 + 0	1.080	3 + 6	1.925	12 + 6	1.050
4 + 0	2.000	14 + 6	1.060	4 + 0	1.830	13 + 0	1.030
4 + 6	1.890	15 + 0	1.040	4 + 6	1.740	13 + 6	1.010
5 + 0	1.820	15 + 6	1.020	5 + 0	1.660	14 + 0	1.000
5 + 6	1.740	16 + 0	1.010	5 + 6	1.580		
6 + 0	1.670	16 + 6	1.010				
6 + 6	1.620	17 + 0	1.000				
7 + 0	1.570	Mature Length = L ¥ M		Modified from Dror Paley et al., *JBJS Am* 2000			

E Multiplier method The multiplier varies by age and by gender.

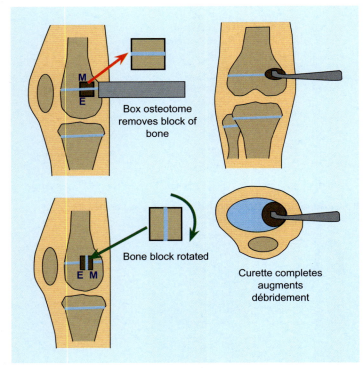

Box osteotome removes block of bone

Bone block rotated

Curette completes augments débridement

F Open physeodesis The distal femur (or proximal tibia) is exposed, a block of bone and physis is excised (*red*), rotated 90 degrees (*green*), and replaced, thereby forming a bridge of metaphyseal (M) and a bridge of epiphysial (E) bone across the physis.

Imaging

ULTRASONOGRAPHY Start with ultrasonographic screening of the abdomen to rule out Wilms tumor in the setting of hemihypertrophy.

RÖNTGENOGRAPHY Röntgenogrammes may be generalized or focused. Generalized röntgenogrammes are used to calculate discrepancy. Teleröntgenogrammes (from Greek τηλε: "at a distance, far off"), which represents a single exposure on a long film, risk inaccuracy due to parallax. Orthoteleröntgenogrammes (green) are a synthesis of separate orthogonal exposures of the hip, knee, and ankle (emitter moves) on a single film, giving a full view of the lower limbs to permit complete assessment of coronal alignment without terminal distortion. Scanogrammes are focused views of the hip, knee, and ankle (small cassette moves) with a ruler for reference but with intervening segments excluded; as a result, they are useful for length but not deformity. With computed röntgenography, teleröntgenogrammes have become standard. Focused röntgenogrammes are requested to view site of deformity and for operative planning.

Röntgenogrammes aid maturity assessment, including left hand–wrist films (Greulich and Pyle atlas), as well as physeal appearance. The latter has a practical influence on operative options.

OTHER MODALITIES CT (scout view to limit radiation exposure) and MRI may be used in cases where computed röntgenography is difficult or confusing.

Management

Balance the broad target of <1″ and the lack of clarity regarding long-term outcomes against treatments of questionable benefit and significant risk.

Orthotics Do not underestimate the costs of orthotics. The obvious cost is pecuniary, from "custom" fabrication, from the need for multiple orthotics for different shoes and occasions, as well as when an orthotic is lost. A more insidious cost is the definition of a problem for a child who may have no complaint or disability. Furthermore, what is the end point if the discrepancy will not resolve? A lifelong intervention is a formidable prospect.

INTERNAL LIFTS These may be placed in the shoe, where they are discreet. However, not more than 10 mm can be placed before the heel will slip out of the cup, and this is within the normal range for the population.

EXTERNAL LIFTS These may compensate for a large discrepancy. They are benign in avoiding surgery. They are not benign in their conspicuity and become less functional with increasing height. They may be combined with internal lifts to mitigate these negatives.

Physeodesis Obliteration of the growth plate is indicated in the immature child for LLLD 1″ to 2″. It is performed at the distal femur and proximal tibia, where physes are most rapidly growing and accessible. Timing is essential to ensure a discrepancy at maturity <1″. Longitudinal data reduce error. Physeodesis of the proximal tibia should be accompanied by physeodesis of the proximal fibula before age 10 years, to avoid relative overgrowth of the fibula.

SIMPLE METHOD This is applied to congenital discrepancy in the perinatal period or in infancy. Begin a conversation about amputation for a limb that is <50% the length of the contralateral side at birth. Final discrepancy may be estimated as double the discrepancy in the 3rd year of life, when half of adult height has been reached.

ARITHMETIC METHOD This makes the assumptions that growth is linear and that girls and boys cease growth consistently [D]. It has the advantages of practicality with the recognition that the goal is a broad target.

MULTIPLIER METHOD This is complex for the promise of greater accuracy [E]. It is based upon normative data for femoral and tibial lengths during growth as well as for growth remaining (Anderson).

- LLLD:
  Dm [limb length discrepancy at skeletal maturity] = D [current limb length discrepancy] × M [multiplier].
- Length at Skeletal Maturity (Lm):
  Lm = L [current length of long limb] × M.

- Timing of Epiphysiodesis:
  Le [desired length of bone to undergo epiphysiodesis at time of epiphysiodesis] = Lm − Ge [amount of femoral or tibial growth remaining at age of epiphysiodesis]. Ge = e/0.71 for femur and e/0.57 for tibia.

There are three principal techniques of epiphysiodesis. A cube of bone centered on the physis may be excised, rotated 90 degrees, and reinserted, disrupting the physis and creating two bridges of bone between metaphysis and epiphysis (Phemister) [F]. The physis is identified by direct visualization and needle palpation.

The physis may be drilled and débrided percutaneously with the aid of image intensification (Canale) [G]. Use of cannulation allows accurate placement of wires: these are overdrilled, and intervening physis may be excised with curette and rongeur. This is effective and requires less exposure.

Because of the inherent inaccuracies of predicting growth and discrepancy, the physis may be fixed to arrest growth. If limb equalization occurs before maturity, the implants may be removed to prevent overcorrection and shortening of the longer limb. Implants are the same as for angular correction, including staple, plate, and cannulated screw.

Shortening In the mature patient with LLLD 1″ to 2″, an equivalent segment of the longer femur may be excised open or closed. Blade plate fixation allows the most proximal shortening in the subtrochanteric region, which has less impact on quadriceps femoris and hamstring strength than diaphyseal level. In the closed method [H], two cuts are made in the diaphysis separated by a distance equivalent to the desired discrepancy by a circular saw blade that moves eccentrically as the axis is turned. A fragmenter splits the ring of bone and a hook pushes the fragments out, after which the femur is shortened and nailed. This technique has not received wide adoption.

Shortening will relax the muscle envelope of the thigh, which cannot adapt to reduction beyond 10% of the total length of the femur, resulting in weakness.

Lengthening This is indicated for LLLD >2″, which is too much to lose functionally due to distortion of the surrounding soft tissue, and socially, including body proportions.

Lengthening device may be external or internal. External fixator may be unilateral [I] or circular (e.g., Ilizarov). It may be supplemented with a medullary nail or a plate, which reduce time of external fixator, obviate the need for casting after external fixator removal, and support the lengthening. The most recent internal device is a medullary nail controlled with an external magnet. This eliminates pin site care and complications and may be more comfortable because it does not tether the surrounding skin and muscle. However, in the femur such lengthening occurs along the mechanical axis, driving the knee medial, increasing lateral compartment stress. Previous devices, such as the ratchet nail, have been problematic, including binding limiting lengthening. "Run away" or over lengthening also is a potential complication of a remotely controlled device.

Operative principles to enhance bone regeneration include the following:

- Metaphyseal osteotomy
- Protection of the soft tissue envelope, including minimizing incision, dissection, periosteal stripping
- Corticotomy to leave the medulla in continuity
- Osteotomy with a mechanical device such as Gigli saw rather than a motorized device, which may burn the bone

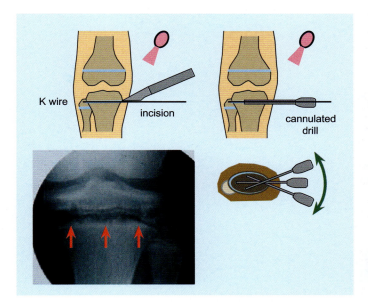

G Percutaneous physeodesis Under image intensification (*pink*), cannulated drill is fanned (*green*), leaving a shadow across the proximal physis of the tibia (*red*).

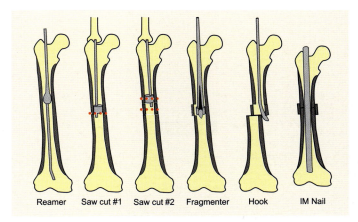

Reamer   Saw cut #1   Saw cut #2   Fragmenter   Hook   IM Nail

H Closed femoral shortening A segment of medulla is cut (*red*) by an eccentric saw blade. Once the ring of bone is driven out, the femur is shortened and nailed.

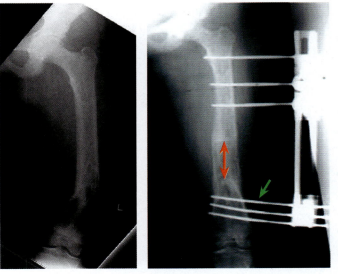

I Lengthening + deformity correction Unilateral external fixator corrected deformity immediately at index operation for a 15-year-old girl with Ollier disease. Forces generated by lengthening bend distal pins (*green*).

After operation, a 1-week latency period is observed to allow the bone to mount a healing response. Distraction begins at a rhythm of 1/4 mm four times *per diem* for a rate of 1 mm/day. This is followed by serial röntgenogrammes: the rate may be adjusted based upon quality of regenerate, for example, slowed or even reversed temporarily in the event of discontinuity. After the desired lengthening or deformity correction, distraction stops and consolidation begins. Consolidation is twice the length of distraction; hence, the estimate that total time of lengthening is 1 cm/month (10-mm distraction for 10 days, 20 days for consolidation). If external fixation is used alone, the barrel is removed at the end of consolidation, leaving the pins in place, to allow a period of dynamization (2 to 4 weeks): problems can be rectified by reapplying the barrel. Finally, pins are removed, in office if the patient can tolerate this and if cone shaped, which become loose after the first revolution.

Lengthening is complicated.

- Pin site infection. Educate patients and parents about pin care, including mobilization and prevention of sealing of skin around pins. Superficial infections may be treated by ambulatory oral antibiotics. Less often, incision and drainage are necessary.
- Delayed union may require arrest or compression of lengthening device, or lengthening of the consolidation phase. Nonunion may require grafting.
- Premature consolidation is treated by accelerating the rate of lengthening; rarely, osteotomy is required.
- Deformity of the callus. This is a reflection of soft tissue forces. It may be corrected by adjusting the frame during or at the end of distraction.
- Muscle contracture. These include triceps suræ and toe flexors in tibial lengthening, and rectus femoris and hamstrings for femoral lengthening. Instruct patients about daily stretching exercises. Other modalities include static or dynamic splints.
- Nerve injury. This is more frequent in tibial than femoral lengthening. Flex the knee for peroneal nerve symptoms. Reduce the rate of distraction. Occasionally, nerve decompression may be necessary.
- Arthritis. Lengthening increases joint forces. Joint stability, bony and soft tissue, is a prerequisite to successful lengthening. The effects of prolonged joint compression remain unclear.

LOWER LIMB DEFICIENCIES

Congenital limb deficiencies occur in about 1 in 10,000 children, or about one-tenth the frequency of clubfoot or hip dysplasia. Boys outnumber girls (3:2), the lower limb is twice as affected as the upper limb, and >80% of cases are single limb.

Limb deficiencies may be congenital or acquired. Most congenital deficiencies are sporadic, occurring in children who are otherwise normal, and they have no genetic basis. Other causes include syndromic, for example, thrombocytopenia-absent radius (TAR) syndrome, and environmental, such as thalidomide phocomelia. Acquired limb deficiency may result from injury, as in trauma, or disease treatment, such as tumors.

Congenital limb deficiencies generally may be divided into terminal, in which all distal elements are absent, or intercalary, in which a segment between others is absent [A]. Deficiencies may be transverse, crossing the entire limb, or paraxial, affecting one side of the longitudinal axis of a limb.

Involve others early, including geneticist, orthotist–prosthetist, occupational and physical therapists, social worker, psychologist, patient support groups. Recognize the rôle of culture, in particular with regard to amputation. Remember that children can adapt. Save the knee whenever possible. Transarticular amputations are preferable, in order to avoid osseous overgrowth and subsequent stump problems. Prepare the patient and family for staged procedures. Align expectations and incentives so that the correct balance struck between risks of multiple and complex procedure and rewards of function and appearance.

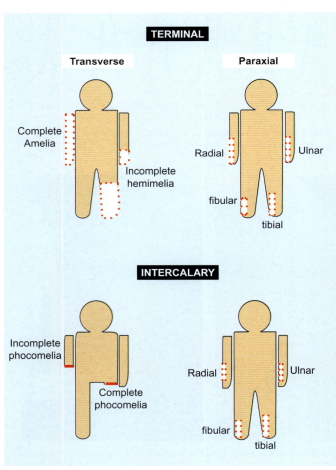

A   Classification of congenital limb deficiencies.

Femoral Deficiency

"Proximal femoral focal deficiency" (PFFD) focuses on deformity of the hip. "Congenital short femur" represents a milder form on a continuum of femoral deficiency (Hamanishi). The spectrum of disease may be divided into:

- Presence or absence of a hip joint (Aitken) [B]. This influences salvage. Hip deformity correlates with femoral shortening.
- A femur that is too short or long enough for salvage (Gillespie).
- Associated fibular deficiency (*q.v.*).

Evaluation A limb >50% length of contralateral side may be salvageable. On röntgenogrammes, there appears to be discontinuity between proximal epiphysis and rest of femur. A femur <50% length of contralateral side, with a tapering proximal end and no epiphysis or acetabulum, is too short and lacks a hip joint to salvage. Arthrography may be necessary to determine hip integrity [C]. How unstable is the knee? Cruciate absence requires spanning of the knee during lengthening of the femur.

Management Have a clear treatment plan by the end of the first year, to allow prosthetic fitting by walking age if indicated.

Absent hip, femur < 50% Convert the limb to above-knee amputation. Syme amputation to improve prosthetic fitting. Fuse the knee, without or with excision of the distal epiphysis. The former addresses the fact that with growth the residual stump will become too long for an above-knee prosthetic. The latter addresses that issue by a delayed timed amputation. Leave the proximal femur free against ilium, where it will provide three-dimensional motion.

An alternative approach for very short femora involves fusing the hip and leaving the knee free to function as a hinge hip joint.

An alternative approach is to convert to a below-knee amputation. This requires a good ankle. Instead of Syme amputation, perform a Van Nes rotationplasty [D]. This is complex to perform and complicated for the patient. It substitutes the hinged ankle for the hinged knee, which is significantly more functional than an above-knee amputation. It requires fortitude to become accustomed to the appearance of a foot pointing backward.

Present though deformed hip, femur > 50% Reconstruct the hip, including valgus osteotomy for coxa vara. This will stabilize the hip and add length in anticipation of lengthening. It also may accelerate ossification, thereby limiting deformity.

Good hip, femur > 50% Lengthen and correct deformity as necessary.

Fibular Hemimelia

This postaxial longitudinal deficiency is the most common lower limb deficiency. There is shortening or partial or complete absence of the fibula [E]. A fibrous analogue may replace the osseous fibula. The tibia, tethered by the short fibula, is short and bowed anteromedially. Ankle deformities include ball and socket in milder cases, and increasing valgus with instability and equinus as the fibula shortens taking with it the lateral malleolus. The foot shows loss of postaxial rays and talocalcaneal coalition. Hypoplasia of the femur and lateral condyle together with absent anterior cruciate ligament complete the spectrum. Deformity is proportional to amount of shortening.

Like tibial hemimelia (*q.v.*), most cases are sporadic. It has been reported in association with varus femur, hip dislocation, tarsal coalition, and digital anomalies as Fuhrmann syndrome, and linked to a mutation in WNT7A gene on 3p25.1.

Evaluation How many rays are present? How deformed is the ankle? Is the foot displaced proximalward such that it rests against the distal lateral leg? These will determine whether the foot is salvageable. Is the

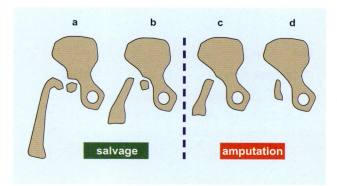

B Classification of femoral deficiency Like other classifications, this may be grouped into two (a + b; c + d), based upon outcomes.

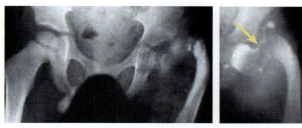

C Imaging Arthrography clarifies what röntgenogrammes suggested. There is severe coxa vara, still unossified.

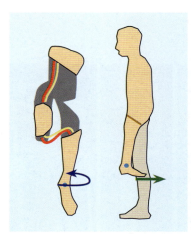

D van Nes rotationplasty The leg is rotated 180 degrees (*blue*), converting the ankle into an active knee joint. A below-knee prosthetic is applied to the foot, which is turned backward.

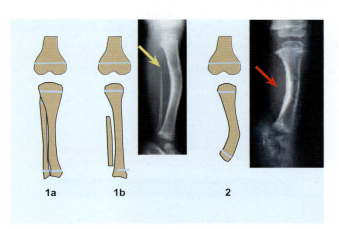

E Fibular deficiency classification The fibula may be short, very short (*yellow*), or absent (*red*). A system based upon fibula has limitations in not taking into account the ankle and foot or the femur.

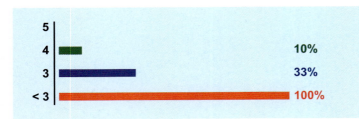

F Amputation for fibular hemimelia Amputation is correlates with number (ordinate) of rays of the foot.

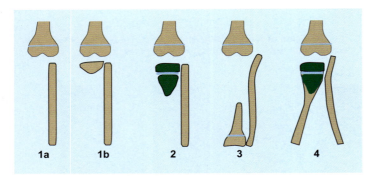

G Classification of tibial hemimelia The presence of proximal tibia (*green*) correlates with quadriceps function, which improves outcomes of reconstruction.

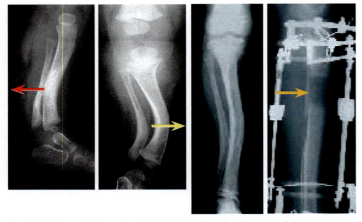

A Posteromedial bowing This is defined by the direction of the apex posterior (*red*) and medial (*yellow*). In the second decade, persistent bowing and shortening (4.5 cm) was treated by correction and lengthening with circular external fixator (*orange*).

B Anterolateral bowing This may be associated with neurofibromatosis type I. Ψ: pseudarthrosis.

fibula palpable, including malleolus? Is there a cutaneous dimple overlying anteromedial bowing of the tibia? Examine the entire limb to determine the width of the spectrum. Is the knee stable to cruciate ligament testing? This impacts lengthening.

Röntgenogrammes elucidate shortening of the fibula, bowing of the tibia, architecture of the ankle, condition of subtalar joint, and number and anomalies of rays in the foot.

Management Amount of shortening of the fibula does not correlate with foot salvage. The two principal questions are as follows:

- Can the foot be saved? A foot with less than three rays will be too thin to support weight effectively [F]. Severe valgus and equinus deformity of the ankle will be too unstable and may become stiff and painful even if reconstructable. In such cases, Syme amputation is indicated.
- How is knee stability? For salvageable limbs, deformity correction of the tibia followed by lengthening requires external fixator spanning of the unstable knee to the femur.
- A stable ankle in the setting of mild shortening may require no treatment (≤5% shortening of lower limb) or lower limb length equalization by timed contralateral physeodesis (≤10% shortening of lower limb).

Tibial Hemimelia

Tibial hemimelia is a preaxial longitudinal deficiency classified based upon the extent of loss, without or with fibular deformity [G]. In type 1, the tibia is absent or demonstrates a nonfunctional remnant. I type 2, the proximal epiphysis and tibial tubercle are present, predictive of growth and preservation of knee function. Type 3 is rare and lacks a functional quadriceps mechanism. While type 4 has a complete tibia, distal divergence from the fibula results in proximal migration of the talus, which impacts ankle function.

Most cases are sporadic. Autosomal dominant and recessive transmissions have been described. Association with Langer-Giedion syndrome and evidence from a murine model suggest that tibial hemimelia may be caused by deletion of a gene involved in limb development contiguous with the gene for Langer-Giedion syndrome at 8q24.1.

Evaluation History will reveal other syndrome. Determine how much tibia is present. Ultrasonography may be helpful at birth when röntgenogrammes are negative. Is quadriceps femoris function present? This is essential to preservation of the knee. Is the ankle salvageable in a type 4?

Management Surgical decision is based principally around quadriceps function and secondarily upon ankle stability.

ABSENT TIBIA, ABSENT QUADRICEPS Transgenual amputation with shortening of the femur by timed physeodesis to prepare for an above knee prosthetic.

ABSENT TIBIA, PRESENT QUADRICEPS Centralization of the fibula (Brown procedure) with Syme amputation. The fibula may be stable enough, and the quadriceps may be functional enough, that the patient may function like a below-knee amputee.

PROXIMAL TIBIA, ACTIVE QUADRICEPS Synostosis of the tibia and fibula with Syme amputation is highly functional and durable.

TIBIOFIBULAR DIASTASIS, PRESENT QUADRICEPS Consider reconstruction of the ankle to stabilize talus and preserve foot. The rarity of type 4 precludes consensus.

TIBIAL BOWING

There are three types, named according to the apex of the tibia:

- Anteromedial. This results from fibular hemimelia (*q.v.*), in which the short fibula tethers the tibia like a string on a bow.
- Posteromedial.
- Anterolateral.

There is no bowing posterolaterally, where the fibula lies to obstruct this direction.

Posteromedial Bowing

Because the deformity improves with time, because intrauterine position has been implicated as a cause rather than intrinsic disease, and because outcomes are favorable, it may be referred to as "physiologic." However, it is not entirely benign, potentially ending with shortening (2 to 7 cm) requiring limb equalization [A], mild bowing, and calcaneovalgus foot deformity that may require reconstruction.

Evaluation Recognize it so that you may recommend to the family observation for spontaneous improvement. Degree of bowing correlates with amount of shortening. Röntgenogrammes quantify bowing (up to 70 degrees) and percentage of shortening, which remains constant throughout growth and allows prognostication.

Management Observe for improvement. Stretching of the foot by parents is benign. Treat lower limb length discrepancy according to general principles, including shoe lift if mild, contralateral physeodesis if moderate, and lengthening—with deformity correction if there is residual posteromedial bowing—for a discrepancy >2″.

Anterolateral Bowing

This may progress to a fracture at the apex of the bow that tends not to heal, hence the term "pseudarthrosis of the tibia." In 60% of cases, this is a sign of neurofibromatosis [B]. Of all patients with neurofibromatosis, 10% will develop pseudarthrosis of the tibia.

Pseudarthrosis of the tibia has been classified [C], based upon radiographic changes at the apex, presence or absence of a pseudarthrosis of the fibula, and associated deformity of the foot.

Evaluation Enquire about a family history of neurofibromatosis. Examine the whole child, including the skin for café au lait markings. Most pseudarthroses develop by 3 years of age; later onset is less severe and associated with more favorable prognosis. Röntgenogrammes show primary osseous changes that distinguish an acute traumatic fracture. Distinguish focal fibrocartilaginous dysplasia by its milder deformity, more benign radiographic appearance, lack of fibular involvement, and spontaneous improvement.

Management

No FRACTURE The first goal is to prevent fracture. Once anterolateral bowing has been identified, apply a brace, which is worn for all weight-bearing activity throughout childhood.

FRACTURE There is no consensus. The pseudarthrosis does not want to heal, so simple fixation without or with bone grafting is insufficient. The pseudarthrosis is surrounded by a cuff of hamartomatous tissue, including fibroblasts and osteoclasts but lacking neural elements. This soft tissue must be excised in addition to all abnormal bone, in order to maximize the environment for healing. The residual defect may be filled with autogenous bone graft, a free vascularized fibula, or by transporting bone from the proximal healthy tibia [D]. Fixation may be internal, such as a medullary nail passed from proximal epiphysis to calcaneus for stability [E], or external, which though difficult in the younger child has the added benefit of allowing compression at the pseudarthrosis docking site. Radical resection with internal fixation and interposition of a cement spacer for to induce a foreign body reactive membrane (Masquelet), followed by removal of the cement and autogenous osseous grafting of the cavity, has shown early success in the same manner as with large osseous defects from trauma or débridement of infected nonunion. Supplementation with recombinant human bone morphogenetic protein-2 (rhBMP-2) is clinically controversial. While this may not increase the rate of union (quantitative), it may reduce the rate of refracture, suggesting a better qualitative response to treatment. Combining rhBMP-2 with bisphosphonate increases union rate while reducing callus fibrosis in a murine model of neurofibromatosis with pseudarthrosis.

Despite union (mean time 15 months), some refracture, such that only half of cases heal long term. Union that survives into the second decade is durable. For nonunion, perform a Syme amputation and fit the patient with a below-knee prosthetic. It is a painful irony that some nonunions unite once amputation is performed.

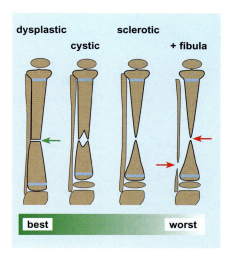

C Classification of tibial pseudarthrosis Prognosis is best for simple type (*orange*) and worst when there is a pseudarthrosis of the fibula (*red*).

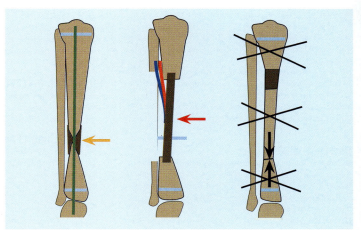

D Surgical options for pseudarthrosis of the tibia These include medullary nail and autogenous bone graft (*green*), free vascularized fibula (*red*), or bone transport by external fixator (*black*).

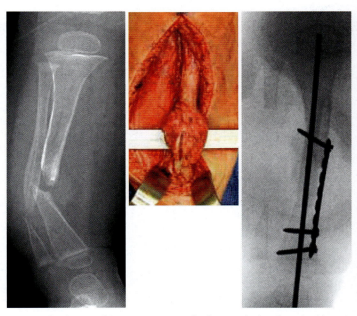

E Pseudarthrosis tibia treatment methods Pseudarthrosis excised *in toto*, including surrounding soft tissue mass leaving muscle and wide segment of bone leaving a gap. A vascularized fibula was transferred into gap and secured by medullary interference fit in proximal and distal tibia fragments. Construct was fixed with medullary nail from proximal epiphysis to calcaneus, as well as plate for rotational control.

LIMP

Sutherland DH, Olshen R, Cooper L, Woo SL. The development of mature gait. *J. Bone Joint Surg. Am.* 62(3):336–353, 1980.

LEG ACHES

Naish JM, Apley J. Growing pains: a clinical study of non-arthritic limb pain in children. *Arch. Dis. Child.* 26(126):134–140, 1951.

TORSION

Delgado ED, Schoenecker PL, Rich MM, Capelli AM. Treatment of severe torsional malalignment syndrome. *J. Pediatr. Orthop.* 16(4):484–488, 1996.

Fuchs R, Staheli LT. Sprinting and intoeing. *J. Pediatr. Orthop.* 16(4):489–491, 1996.

Staheli LT, Corbett M, Wyss C, King H. Lower-extremity rotational problems in children. Normal values to guide management. *J. Bone Joint Surg. Am.* 67(1):39–47, 1985.

GENU VALGUM AND VARUM

Davids JR, Blackhurst DW, Allen BL. Radiographic evaluation of bowed legs in children. *J. Pediatr. Orthop.* 21(2):257–263, 2001.

Davids JR, Blackhurst DW, Allen BL Jr. Clinical evaluation of bowed legs in children. *J. Pediatr. Orthop. B.* 9(4):278–284, 2000.

Heath CH, Staheli LT. Normal limits of knee angle in white children—genu varum and genu valgum. *J. Pediatr. Orthop.* 13(2):259–262, 1993.

Vankka E, Salenius P. Spontaneous correction of severe tibiofemoral deformity in children. *Acta Orthop. Scand.* 53(4):567–570, 1982.

BLOUNT DISEASE

Blount WP. Tibia vara. Osteochondrosis deformans tibiae. *J. Bone Joint Surg.* 19:1–29, 1937.

Blount WP, Clarke GR. Control of bone growth by epiphyseal stapling; a preliminary report. *J. Bone Joint Surg. Am.* 31(3):464–478, 1949.

Gushue DL, Houck J, Lerner AL. Effects of childhood obesity on three dimensional knee joint biomechanics during walking. *J. Pediatr. Orthop.* 25(6):763–768, 2005.

Langenskiöld A. Tibia vara; (osteochondrosis deformans tibiae); a survey of 23 cases. *Acta Chir. Scand.* 103(1):1–22, 1952.

Levine AM, Drennan JC. Physiological bowing and tibia vara. The metaphyseal-diaphyseal angle in the measurement of bowleg deformities. *J. Bone Joint Surg. Am.* 64(8):1158–1163, 1982.

Rab GT. Oblique tibial osteotomy revisited. *J. Child. Orthop.* 4(2):169–172, 2010.

Smith SL, Beckish ML, Winters SC, Pugh LI, Bray EW. Treatment of late-onset tibia vara using Afghan percutaneous osteotomy and Orthofix external fixation. *J. Pediatr. Orthop.* 20(5):606–610, 2000.

Thompson GH, Carter JR. Late-onset tibia vara (Blount's disease). Current concepts. *Clin. Orthop.* 255:24–35, 1990.

van Huyssteen A, Hastings C, Olesak M, Hoffman E. Double-elevating osteotomy for late-presenting infantile Blount's disease. *J. Bone Joint Surg. Br.* 87(5):710–715, 2005.

Westberry DE, Davids JR, Pugh LI, Blackhurst D. Tibia vara: results of hemiepiphysiodesis. *J. Pediatr. Orthop. B.* 13(6):374–378, 2004.

OSTEOCHONDROSIS

Osgood R. Lesions of the tibial tubercle occurring during adolescence. *Boston Med. Surg. J.* 148:114–117, 1903.

Schlatter C. Verletzungen des schnabelförmigen Fortsatzes der oberen Tibiaepiphyse. *Beitr. Klin. Chir.* 38:874–887, 1903.

CONGENITAL DISLOCATION OF THE KNEE

Curtis B, Fisher RL. Congenital hyperextension with anterior subluxation of the knee: surgical management and long term observations. *J. Bone Joint Surg. Am.* 51(2):255–269, 1969.

CONGENITAL DISLOCATION OF THE PATELLA

Galeazzi R. New tendonous and muscular transplant applications. *Archivio di Ortopedia.* 38:315–325, 1922.

Stanisavljevic S, Zemenick G, Miller D. Congenital, irreducible, permanent lateral dislocation of the patella. *Clin. Orthop.* 116:190–199, 1976.

POPLITEAL CYST

Wilson PD, Eyre-Brook AL, Francis JD. A clinical and anatomical study of the semimembranosus bursa in relation to popliteal cyst. *J. Bone Joint Surg. Am.* 20(4):963–984, 1938.

BIPARTITE PATELLA

Scapinelli R. Blood supply of the human patella: its relation to ischaemic necrosis after fracture. *J. Bone Joint Surg. Br.* 49(3):563–570, 1967.

LOWER LIMB LENGTH DISCREPANCY

Anderson M, Messner MB, Green WT. Distribution of lengths of the normal femur and tibia in children from one to eighteen years of age. *J. Bone Joint Surg. Am.* 46:1197–1202, 1964.

Canale ST, Russell TA, Holcomb RL. Percutaneous epiphysiodesis: experimental study and preliminary clinical results. *J. Pediatr. Orthop.* 6(2):150–156, 1986.

Green WT, Wyatt GM, Anderson M. Orthoroentgenography as a method of measuring the bones of the lower extremities. *J. Bone Joint Surg.* 28:60–65, 1946.

Greulich WW, Pyle SI. *Radiographic Atlas of Skeletal Development of the Hand and Wrist.* 2nd ed. Stanford, CA: Stanford University Press; 1959.

Gross RH. Leg length discrepancy: how much is too much? *Orthopedics.* 1(4):307–310, 1978.

Gurney B, Mermier C, Robergs R, Gibson A, Rivero D. Effects of limb-length discrepancy on gait economy and lower-extremity muscle activity in older adults. *J. Bone Joint Surg. Am.* 83(6):907–915, 2001.

Ilizarov GA. *Transosseous Osteosynthesis. Theoretical and Clinical Aspects of the Regeneration and Growth of Tissue.* Berlin, Germany: Springer-Verlag; 1992.

Little DG, Nigo L, Aiona MD. Deficiencies of current methods for the timing of epiphysiodesis. *J. Pediatr. Orthop.* 16(2):173–179, 1996.

Moseley CF. A straight-line graph for leg-length discrepancies. *J. Bone Joint Surg. Am.* 59(2):174–179, 1977.

Nordsletten L, Holm I, Steen H, Bjerkreim I. Muscle function after femoral shortening osteotomies at the subtrochanteric and mid-diaphyseal level. A follow-up study. *Arch. Orthop. Trauma Surg.* 114(1):37–39, 1994.

Paley D, Bhave A, Herzenberg JE, Bowen JR. Multiplier method for predicting limb-length discrepancy. *J. Bone Joint Surg. Am.* 82(10):1432–1446, 2000.

Phemister DB. Operative arrestment of longitudinal growth of bones in the treatment of deformities. *J. Bone Joint Surg.* 15:1–13, 1933.

Song KM, Halliday SE, Little DG. The effect of limb-length discrepancy on gait. *J. Bone Joint Surg. Am.* 79(11):1690–1698, 1997.

Westh RN, Menelaus MB. A simple calculation for the timing of epiphyseal arrest: a further report. *J. Bone Joint Surg. Br.* 63(1)-B:117–119, 1981.

Winquist RA. Closed intramedullary osteotomies of the femur. *Clin. Orthop.* 212:155–164, 1986.

HEMIMELIA

Achterman C, Kalamchi A. Congenital deficiency of the fibula. *J. Bone Joint Surg. Br.* 61(2):133–137, 1979.

Aitken GT. Proximal femoral focal deficiency – definition, classification and management. In: *Proximal Femoral Focal Deficiency: A Congenital Anomaly: Symposium held at the National Academy of Sciences, Washington, D.C.* 1968:1–22.

Frantz CH, O'Rahilly R. Congenital skeletal limb deficiencies. *J. Bone Joint Surg. Am.* 43(8):1202–1224, 1961.

Jones D, Barnes J, Lloyd-Roberts GC. Congenital aplasia and dysplasia of the tibia with intact fibula. *J. Bone Joint Surg. Br.* 60(1):31–39, 1978.

Gillespie R, Torode IP. Classification and management of congenital abnormalities of the femur. *J. Bone Joint Surg. Br.* 65(5):557–568, 1983.

Stevens CA, Moore CA. Tibial hemimelia in Langer-Giedion syndrome—possible gene location for tibial hemimelia at 8q. *Am. J. Med. Genet.* 85(4):409–412, 1999.

BOWING

Andersen KS. Congenital pseudarthrosis of the leg. Late results. *J. Bone Joint Surg. Am.* 58(5):657–662, 1976.

Ghanem I, Damsin JP, Carlioz H. Ilizarov technique in the treatment of congenital pseudarthrosis of the tibia. *J. Pediatr. Orthop.* 17(5):685–690, 1997.

Johnston CE. Congenital pseudarthrosis of the tibia: results of technical variations in the Charnley-Williams procedure. *J. Bone Joint Surg. Am.* 84(10):1799–1810, 2002.

Keret D, Bollini G, Dungl P, Fixsen J, Grill F, Hefti F, Ippolito E, Romanus B, Tudisco C, Wientroub S. The fibula in congenital pseudarthrosis of the tibia: the EPOS multicenter study. European Paediatric Orthopaedic Society (EPOS). *J. Pediatr. Orthop. B.* 9(2):69–74, 2000.

Ohnishi I, Sato W, Matsuyama J, Yajima H, Haga N, Kamegaya M, Minami A, Sato M, Yoshino S, Oki T, Nakamura K. Treatment of congenital pseudarthrosis of the tibia: a multicenter study in Japan. *J. Pediatr. Orthop.* 25:219–224, 2005.

Pannier S, Pejin Z, Dana C, Masquelet AC, Glorion C. Induced membrane technique for the treatment of congenital pseudarthrosis of the tibia: preliminary results of five cases. *J. Child. Orthop.* 7(6):477–485, 2013.

Pappas AM. Congenital posteromedial bowing of the tibia and fibula. *J. Pediatr. Orthop.* 4(5):525–531, 1984.

Romanus B, Bollini G, Dungl P, Fixsen J, Grill F, Hefti F, Ippolito E, Tudisco C, Wientroub S. Free vascular fibular transfer in congenital pseudoarthrosis of the tibia: results of the EPOS multicenter study. European Paediatric Orthopaedic Society (EPOS). *J. Pediatr. Orthop. B.* 9(2):90–93, 2000.

FOOT AND ANKLE

ANATOMY

Greek πους (root ποδ-) is Latin *pes* (root ped-): "foot", which gives the root –ped- in English. Do not confuse Greek παις (root παιδ-): "child", which is represented in American usage as -ped- after the custom of simplifying diphthongs, as in Pediatrics. The only exception in American usage is the term Orthopædic, which retains the diphthong to avoid limitation of scope to the foot.

The foot may be divided into hindfoot, midfoot, and forefoot [A]. The hindfoot consists of the talus and calcaneus. Latin *talus* is Greek αστραγαλος: *astragalus*. The midfoot is made up of cuboid bone, navicular bone, and the three cuneiform bones (medial, intermediate, and lateral, or numbered). Latin *navicula* is Greek σκαφη: "small boat, *skiff*," to describe the bone's shape; hence the distinction "tarsal navicular or scaphoid." The forefoot includes metatarsal bones and phalanges. Hindfoot and midfoot correspond to the galenic concept of ταρσοσ: "*tarsus*," as the equivalent in the foot of καρποσ: "*carpus*" in the hand. The mid- or transverse tarsal joint, through which the French surgeon François Chopart (1743–1795) recommended amputation, consists of talonavicular and calcaneocuboid articulations. The French surgeon Jacques Lisfranc de St. Martin (1790–1847) favored amputation at the junction of tarsus and metatarsus, from Greek μετα-: "next".

A Nomenclature for normal function and disease The two entities are named independently.

Site	Motion	Deformity
Ankle	Plantar flexion (extension) / Dorsiflexion (flexion)	Equinus / Calcaneus
Subtalar joint	Inversion / Eversion	Varus / Valgus
Heel	Dorsad *pitch* at rest	↑ Calcaneus / ↓ Equinus
Midfoot	Coronal plane	Adductus / Abductus
Midfoot	Sagittal plane	Cavus / Planus
Forefoot	Axial plane	Pronation / Supination
Toes	Distal interphalangeal flexion	Mallet
Toes	Intermediate phalangeal flexion	Hammer
Toes	Interphalangeal flexion + metatarsophalangeal extension	Claw
Hallux	Adduction / Abduction	Valgus / Varus

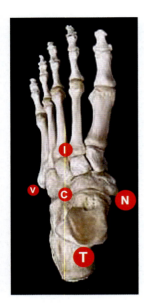

B   Accessoria of the foot T: os trigonum (15%). N: naviculare accessorium (15%). C: calcaneus secundarius (5%). I: os intermetatarseum (5%). V: os vesalianum (rare).

Distinguish normal motion from morbid deformity [A]. This resembles the distinction of version (normal "turning" of a part of a long bone) from torsion (abnormal or "excessive") for long bones of the lower limb. When ankle plantar flexion exceeds the normal range or is fixed (eliminating dorsiflexion) due to disease, this is known as equinus, from Latin *equus*: "horse," after the posture of a horse's foot. The opposite is known as calcaneus, after the bone that is most distinctive in the deformity. The midfoot and forefoot do not move actively but may be deformed. Adductus describes "direction toward" and abductus "direction away" from the midaxis of the foot. Cavus describes a medial plantar longitudinal arch that is "scooped out" higher than normal, whereas in planus, the arch is "flat." In pronation, the forefoot appears rotated toward the midline due to flexion or depression of the first ray; elevation or extension of the first ray rotates the forefoot away from the midline into supination. Toe deformities are distinguished according to the joint affected. Flexion of the distal interphalangeal joint likens the toe to a diminutive mallet on account of a smaller distal skeletal element than is presented with flexion of the intermediate interphalangeal joint, which is likened to a hammer. Interphalangeal flexion with metatarsophalangeal extension gives the toe a claw appearance.

Anatomists and surgeons differ at the ankle. The former group's flexion, following the convention that applies this term to reduction of angle in the direction of motion at a joint, is the latter's dorsiflexion. The opposite motion is termed extension by the anatomist and plantar flexion by the surgeon.

Anatomists and surgeons also differ at the foot (and the hand). Normal motion is described relative to the foot, whereas the midaxis of the body is used to define deformity. *Valgus* refers to pointing of the hallux (the distal skeletal element) "away" from the body midaxis at the metatarsophalangeal joint. The equivalent active motion is under the action of *adductor* hallucis muscle, which pulls the great toe away from the midaxis of the body but "toward" the midline of the foot.

The foot may be divided into columns. Medial includes the talus and first ray. Lateral includes the calcaneus and fifth ray. This concept is fundamental to an understanding of foot mechanics (*q.v.*).

The foot is replete with accessory ossicles [B]. Some have fanciful names, such as os vesalianum at the base of the 5th metatarsal bone, after the Barbantian "Father of Anatomy" Andreas Vesalius (1514–1564). Others may be sufficiently common and sufficiently noisome to be worthy of a classification (*cf.* Accessory Navicular Bone). The malleoli may present separate ossification centers, of which appearance peaks between 6 and 9 years and which fuse with remainder of bone 1 to 2 years later. Distinguish these normal variants from avulsion fracture or other disease.

MECHANICS

Two models aid understanding of normal function and disease of the foot.

Tripod

This highlights the interconnectedness of the foot in bearing weight [C]. The legs of the tripod are the first and fifth rays, as well as the calcaneus. In a supinated forefoot with a hypermobile first ray, the calcaneus tips into valgus at the subtalar joint as the medial longitudinal arch reduces to produce a flatfoot. Correction of a flatfoot by calcaneal lengthening without correction of forefoot supination will fail as the first ray returns to the ground by hindfoot eversion

Acetabulum Pedis

Calcaneus and navicular bone (with remainder of foot) form a cup that rotates around a ball formed by the head of the talus [D]. In clubfoot, the acetabulum is displaced plantad and medialward, such that navicular bone abuts tibial malleolus and the head of the talus becomes palpable at lateral proximal dorsum of the foot. The acetabulum moves in an opposite direction in flatfoot. This concept underpins casting for clubfoot, which is rotated out of adductus and varus *via* the acetabulum. In flatfoot, cutting the calcaneus and lengthening the lateral column swings the foot around the head of the talus to reduce hindfoot valgus and restore normal alignment of the first ray with the talus.

EVALUATION

History

The foot has been a source of complaint and concern in every culture and in every age. A dichotomy may exist between child and parent, and between parent and physician. A parent may regard flexible flatfoot as an abnormality worthy of treatment when the child has no concerns and to the surgeon it is a normal variant. The foot may be the focus of a remote condition, either benign such as in-toeing due to tibial torsion or grave such as cavus as a sign of neural disease.

Physical Examination

Global Perform a complete assessment. The foot may manifest a sign of primary neural disease, such as dysrrhaphism, or hereditary motor and sensory neuropathy. Ask the patient to walk and run. Which way do the feet point? Do they appear symmetric, or does asymmetry betray a problem remote from the feet such as at the hip? Is there a normal progression of heel–flat-toe in stance and ankle flexion in swing?

Focal The foot is a dynamic structure [E]. Start viewing the foot from the back. What is the position of the hindfoot standing and when the patient is up on the metatarsal heads? Add a block to support the lateral border of the foot: does the hindfoot evert as the medial front leg of the tripod sinks to the floor? These are tests of flexibility of the subtalar joint. Are "too many toes" visible beyond either malleolus in the standing position? How much space is there under the medial longitudinal arch in the lateral position? Evaluate the foot in weight-bearing and unloaded positions. Does the arch shape vary between the two?

Evaluate the skin, which tells a story. Callus is a response to abnormal pressure, which provides a functional outcome of deformity. Ulcer may have an exogenous cause, such as constrictive shoe wear, or endogenous cause, such as sensory loss. A single deep furrow is a sign of reduced skin motion over a joint with fixed deformity, such as posterior to an equinus ankle in structural clubfoot. A primary physician may rely on the observation that multiple fine creases suggest stretching and relaxation of skin over a mobile ankle to distinguish metatarsus adductus, a benign condition, from clubfoot.

Pain varies according to age [F]. Most disorders and complaints concentrate around the turn of the decade. Palpate for tenderness: the foot is geographic and will reveal the source of pain [G].

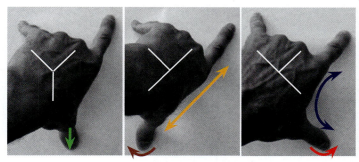

C The foot as tripod Thumb represents calcaneus. As a neutral calcaneus (*green*) rotates into valgus (*brown*), the medial longitudinal arch diminishes (*orange*) to keep ground contact with the first ray, which is relatively extended bringing the forefoot into supination. By contrast, when the calcaneus assumes a varus inclination (*red*), the arch elevates (*blue*) and the forefoot pronates as the first ray flexes to maintain contact with the ground.

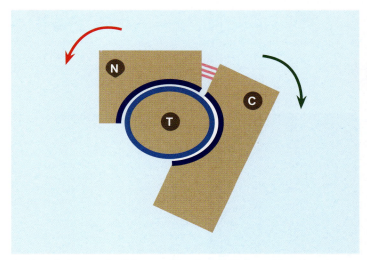

D Acetabulum pedis Calcaneus (C) and navicular bone (N), with intervening ligaments (*pink*), may rotate around talus (T) plantad and medialward (*red*), for example, in clubfoot, or lateralward and dorsad (*green*), for example, in flatfoot.

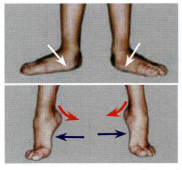

E Dynamic examination of the foot In standing, weight-bearing position, the foot is flat (*white*). Upon standing on the metatarsal heads, the hindfoot inverts (*red*) and the medial longitudinal arch reconstitutes (*blue*), demonstrating that the deformity is flexible.

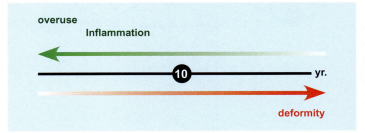

F Foot pain Foot pain varies according to age.

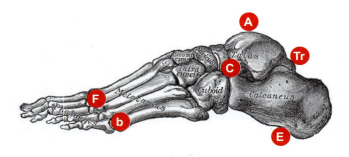

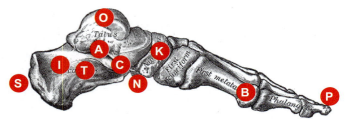

G   Foot pain Foot pain is geographic. A: arthritis. B: bunion. b: bunionette. C: coalition. E: enthesitis. F: Freiberg infraction. I: osteomyelitis. K: Köhler condition. N: accessory navicular. O: osteochondritis dissecans. P: paronychia. S: Sever apophysitis. T: trauma. Tr: os trigonum.

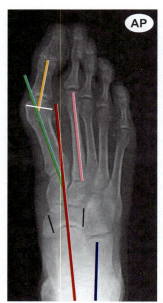

H   Radiographic examination of the foot Measure relationships in anteroposterior (AP) and lateral (L) projections between the talus (*red*), calcaneus (*blue*), first metatarsal bone (*green*), navicular bone (*black*), proximal phalanx of hallux (*orange*), and second metatarsal bone (*pink*). Some relationships vary with age, such as the talocalcaneal angle, which declines from 30 to 50 degrees at birth to 15 to 30 degrees by age 5 years. Other angles are stable, such as the pitch of the calcaneus at 20 to 30 degrees. *Subtalar joint incompetence, such as after overcorrection of clubfoot, may allow the calcaneus to slide lateralward from under the talus to produce hindfoot valgus while maintaining parallelism of the bones and thereby a reduced talocalcaneal angle.

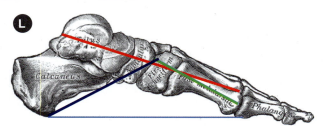

Uncouple ankle and subtalar joints when determining motion. Invert the hindfoot to bring calcaneus directly under talus and thereby lock the subtalar joint before flexing the ankle. Patients with contracture of triceps suræ will compensate for limited ankle flexion by swiveling through subtalar joint to place the foot flat on the ground. Flex and extend knee joint to isolate gastrocnemius muscle from soleus muscle. Ankle flexion >30 degrees is one criterion of ligamentous laxity. Flexibility of subtalar joint impacts deformity reconstruction. Deformity correction in the setting of a rigid joint is addressed by a compensating osteotomy or transarticularly by arthrodesis.

Imaging

While the foot lends itself to (hyper) analysis radiographically, there remains debate regarding applicability of metrics to functional outcome.

Röntgenogramme This is the mainstay [H]. Obtain views of weight bearing, because this is the functional position of the foot and foot shape varies significantly according to loading. There will be imprecision when drawing the longitudinal axis of irregular bones, such as the talus and calcaneus, and during growth with incomplete ossification.

Distinguish lateral view of the foot from lateral view of the ankle, which differs in the setting of deformity. Mortise view of the ankle delineates trochlea of the talus. Special views include oblique of the foot to view sinus tarsi and calcaneonavicular relationship and Harris view, which projects along the posterior facet of subtalar joint orthogonal to long axis of the calcaneus. Stress views may be useful in deformity, such as to distinguish oblique from vertical talus, and in trauma, such as Lisfranc injury.

Measurement	Normal	Abnormal
Talus–calcaneus	AP: 15–30 degrees	▼ Varus
	L: 15–30 degrees	▲ Valgus*
Talus–1st metatarsal (Méary)	AP: 0 degrees	Medial: metatarsus adductus
		Lateral: abductus
	L: 5 degrees	▲ Flatfoot
		▼ Cavus
Talus–navicular	joint neutral	Medial: clubfoot
		Lateral: flatfoot
Talus inclination	10–35 degrees	▼ Cavus
		▲ Flatfoot
Calcaneus (Campbell)	L: 20–30 degrees	▼ Equinus
		▲ Calcaneus
Calcaneus–1st metatarsal (Hibbs)	L: 120–150 degrees	> 150 degrees: flatfoot
		< 120 degrees: cavus
Intermetatarsal	< 10 degrees	> 15 degrees: Bunion
Hallux valgus	< 15 degrees	> 30 degrees: Bunion

Other modalities Scintigramme reveals occult bone lesions, as in early osteomyelitis. Ultrasonography is useful for foreign body that may be radiolucent, such as glass, or operatively to aid and limit dissection. Computed tomography (CT) gives the finest bone detail, as in determining location and extent of tarsal coalition, and aids surgical planning, in particular with three-dimensional reconstruction. Magnetic resonance imaging (MRI) provides the best view of soft tissue, as in tumor; can expose osseous reaction to disease; and aids in the evaluation of mixed lesions, such as osteochondritis dissecans.

TOE DISORDERS

Toe anomaly may be isolated or part of a generalized disorder [A]. They hurt, can be unsightly, and interfere with shoe wear.

Syndactyly

This affects the 2nd to 3rd more than the 4th to 5th toes and often is bilateral. The skin bridge may be complete, involving the nails, or incomplete, receding variably from the nails. Isolated toe syndactyly is benign: it is asymptomatic and poses no dysfunction. Educate parents that release to improve appearance is outweighed by surgical risk and scar. The condition may be part of polydactyly.

Polydactyly

This is summarized in [B]. Familial form follows autosomal dominant inheritance with variable penetrance.

Postaxial polydactyly is subclassified into type A, in which a well-formed extra digit articulates with the 5th or a 6th metacarpal, and type B, characterized a rudimentary extra digit (pedunculated postminimi). A heterozygous mutation in the GLI3 gene on 7p14.1 has been found in both type A and type B. Autosomal dominant inheritance type A has been mapped to 7q22, 13q21, and 19p13. An autosomal recessive type A has been mapped to 13q13. Postaxial polydactyly is a feature of three-fourths of patients with trisomy 13.

In preaxial polydactyly, the metatarsal bone may be duplicated or widened to present a partial or separate condyle for the supernumerary digit. Mutation of the binding sites for transcription factors SOX9 and PAX3 in the LMBR1 gene (sonic hedgehog family) on 7q36.3 has been found in preaxial polydactyly. Preaxial hallucal polydactyly is a feature of diabetic embryopathy.

Operation is indicated toward the end of the first year, as a balance between osseous development and independent walking. Excise the less developed supernumerary digit, which may be determined by the nail, overall toe size, or radiographic appearance. Include partial or complete metatarsal resection to avoid prominence laterally or a wide web space centrally. The latter also may be ameliorated by reconstruction of the intermetatarsal ligament. Plan flap(s) or skin graft for associated syndactyly.

Bracket epiphysis This represents medial extension of the physis of hallucal phalanx or metatarsal to give origin to a preaxial polydactyly [C]. Growth of the epiphysis results in a broad-based bone that resembles a "triangle," hence the original name "delta phalanx," after the Greek letter Δ.

The epiphysis and physis are radiolucent but may be seen on MRI. Excision includes proximal extension to resect the physeal bracket, along with release and reconstruction of remaining hallux to avoid varus deformity.

Curly Toe

The toe is flexed and rotated along its longitudinal axis under the next medial toe due to flexor contracture. This affects the lesser toes and often is bilateral. Half resolve spontaneously with walking. Deformity persistent beyond age 4 years is treated by flexor tenotomy at proximal cutaneous crease.

Presentation in the second decade may require complex reconstruction due to secondary contracture, including capsulotomy without or with flexor to extensor transfer. In the Girdlestone-Taylor procedure, the flexor is harvested *via* distal and proximal interphalangeal incisions, retrieved through a dorsal incision, through which a capsulotomy may be performed and where the tendon is sewn to the extensor.

Claw Toe

This is defined as metatarsophalangeal hyperextension with interphalangeal flexion [D]. It is a feature of extensor recruitment alone or in the setting of neural disease, where flexors are unopposed. Evaluation and management do not occur in isolation but are directed at the primary cause, such as cavovarus foot.

Toe Deformity	Disorders
Polydactyly	Bardet-Biedl syndrome Chondroectodermal dysplasia Carpenter syndrome Cephalopolysyndactyly syndrome (Greig) Femoral-facial syndrome
Syndactyly	Apert syndrome Oculodentodigital syndrome Pterygium syndrome
Metatarsal dysplasia	Achondrogenesis Brachydactyly syndrome Otopalatodigital syndrome
Broad toe	Acromesomelic dysplasia Rubinstein-Taybi syndrome
Macrodactyly	Proteus syndrome Neurofibromatosis Vascular malformation
Deficiency or absence	Amniotic band syndrome (Streeter)

A Select syndromes associated with toe deformities.

Feature		Rate
Axis	Pre-	15%
	Post-	85%
Familial	30%	
Blacks	10 X Whites	
Syndactyly	10%	
Hand	30%	
Generalized disorder	Pre-	20%
	Post-	10%
Genetics	Pre-:	LMBR1 mutation on 7q36.3
	Post-	GL13 mutation on 7p14.1. 7q22, 13q13, 13q21, 19p13 trisomy 13

B Polydactyly Features that distinguish polydactyly include genetic mapping.

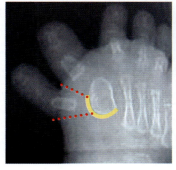

C Bracket epiphysis This rare form of preaxial polydactyly requires recognition, complete resection (*red*) to include part of the U-shaped physis and epiphysis (*yellow*), and reconstruction to avoid hallux varus.

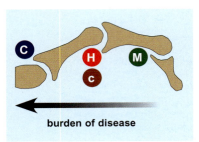

D   Defining deformity
C: claw. H: hammer. c: curly. M: mallet. Note that a curly toe, in addition to interphalangeal flexion like a hammer toe, adds an axial deformity.

burden of disease

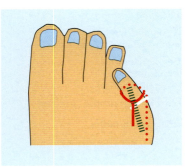

E   Butler procedure Incision (*red*) allows for derotation and plantad displacement of the toe. Extensor tendon (*green*) is sectioned, as is the dorsal MP capsule (*white*).

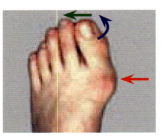

F   Bunion Hallux is deviated away from midline (*green*) and rotated (*blue*) against the second toe. The metatarsal head is prominent, and overlying soft tissues are reactive (*red*).

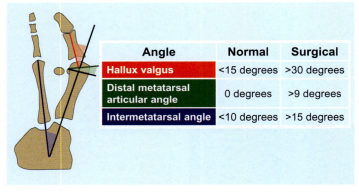

Angle	Normal	Surgical
Hallux valgus	<15 degrees	>30 degrees
Distal metatarsal articular angle	0 degrees	>9 degrees
Intermetatarsal angle	<10 degrees	>15 degrees

G   Radiographic assessment of bunion Note obliquity of metatarsocuneiform articulation.

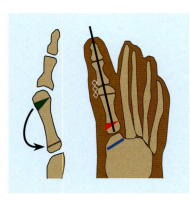

H   Osteotomies for bunion Distal osteotomy to correct DMAA is combined with medial soft tissue reconstruction. Opening wedge proximal osteotomy addresses increased IMA. While the distal exsected bone (*green*) may be transferred as shown on left, allograft (*red*) is more stable and can be tailored given that distal and proximal deformities rarely are equivalent. Alternatively, the proximal osteotomy may be made in the medial cuneiform (*blue*) if this is trapezoidal and the metatarsocuneiform articulation is inclined. The correction is fixed with a medullary wire that may be supplemented with a crossed wire for rotational control.

Hammer Toe

This is defined as flexion deformity of the proximal interphalangeal joint (PIP). Metatarsophalangeal and distal interphalangeal (DIP) joints are obligatorily extended to contact the ground. Second toe is most affected. Presentation includes callus over dorsum of PIP joint and tends to be delayed into the second decade, when rigid deformity necessitates Girdlestone-Taylor procedure or PIP arthrodesis.

Mallet Toe

The essential lesion is fixed flexion deformity of the DIP joint. Presentation and treatment are similar to those of hammer toe

Overlapping Toe

Overlapping of the 2nd to 4th toes are benign and resolve spontaneously in infancy.

Digitus minimus varus Proximal and dorsal migration, with adduction and rotation to present the nail lateralward, of the 5th toe to overlap with the 4th typically is fixed. Operative correction (Butler) includes the following [E]:

- Circumferential incision (be careful of neurovascular bundles!) at base of toe with dorsal limb centered on metatarsal and longer plantar limb at border of glabrous skin
- Section of extensor tendon
- Section dorsal metatarsophalangeal capsule
- Rotation of cutaneous flaps to reinforce and maintain reduction of the toe

Bunion

Greek βουνιον: "small hill, tumulus," whence "*bunny*," describes the prominence of the head of metatarsal bone [F]. Childhood bunion represents a primary growth disturbance of the hallucal metatarsal, reflected in the appellation metatarsus primus varus. This may be quantified by the distal metatarsal articular angle (DMAA) and further revealed by trapezoidal deformity of the medial cuneiform. In neuromuscular patients, bunion may result from imbalance of muscle forces. In adult bunion, exogenous factors conspire to deform and destabilize the static and dynamic metatarsophalangeal soft tissues.

Evaluation The ratio of girls:boys is 5:1. A family history in half of patients suggests mendelian inheritance with variable penetrance. The hallux deviates away from midline and rotates such that the nail inclines medialward, eventually lying under or over the second toe. Soft tissue over the exposed and prominent head of metatarsal is callused, red, and sore. Pain also may be felt over displaced plantar sesamoids. Assess hypermobility of the first ray at the metatarsocuneiform articulation. Patients may present in the absence of pain or dysfunction due to cultural disapprobation.

Röntgenogrammes quantify deformity, form the basis for surgical indications, and guide operation [G].

Management Education is fundamental, including wearing of shoes with a sufficiently wide toe box and minimizing heel height. Orthotics do not provide a durable result.

Surgical treatment may be divided into four according to site and aspect of deformity corrected. There are numerous techniques and combinations, which betrays the facts that bunion is not homogeneous and that no single procedure is universally effective [H].

- Soft tissue. This includes plication of medial capsule and release of adductor hallucis laterally. The former may be performed through drill holes for security. Beware of the first dorsal metatarsal artery, which enters the head on the lateral side. Following the principle that soft tissue reconstruction will fail in the setting of osseous deformity, combine this with osteotomy.
- Osteotomy—distal. This is indicated when there is no proximal deformity. It corrects the DMAA and hallux valgus when the intermetatarsal angle (IMA) is normal.

- Osteotomy—proximal. Indication is abnormal IMA. Opening wedge adds length to a short 1st metatarsal.

Base of metatarsal to medial cuneiform arthrodesis. This allows plantar flexion (in addition to coronal correction) of the metatarsal to address hypermobility of the first ray, in order to stabilize the medial limb of the tripod in flatfoot.

The principal complications are avascular necrosis of the head of metatarsal and over-/undercorrection. The former is related to lateral dissection. The latter are related to maturity in the uninvolved child, in whom operation should be delayed until physeal closure. In neuromuscular disease, metatarsophalangeal arthrodesis balances control of correction against reduced physical demand.

Bunionette

This also is known as tailor's bunion, after repetitive pressure and rubbing at the dorsal aspect of the 5th metatarsal head in the cross-legged position on an unyielding surface. The deformities mirror bunion on the opposite side of the foot. The disorder is less common and less troubling than is bunion in children. As a result, it rarely comes to surgery, which consists of the 5th metatarsal osteotomy to reduce prominence of the head.

Dorsal Bunion

The head of the 1st metatarsal is prominent at the dorsum, with associated flexion contracture of the metatarsophalangeal joint. An imbalance between a stronger tibialis anterior muscle than peroneus longus muscle lifts the 1st metatarsal. It may be a consequence of operative release of clubfoot, in which tibialis anterior may be hyperactive and a weakened triceps suræ is compensated for by flexor recruitment. Surgical management includes the following:

- Flexion osteotomy of the 1st metatarsal or medial cuneiform, to correct deformity
- Plantar metatarsophalangeal joint capsular release
- Transfer of flexor hallucis longus to the neck of the 1st metatarsal (reverse Jones), to support correction and to reduce metatarsophalangeal joint flexion
- Transfer of tibialis anterior to lateral cuneiform bone

Hallux Rigidus

The hallux does not move due to arthritis of the metatarsophalangeal joint. Dorsiflexion is lost first. Presentation is in the second decade. Repetitive trauma, osteochondritis dissecans (OCD), and hypermobile first ray have been implicated. Pain may be elicited with motion under resistance, in particular during standing on the metatarsal heads. Röntgenogrammes show signs of degeneration, including reduction in joint width, osteophyte, and possible OCD of the metatarsal head.

Initial treatment is supportive, including stiff shank or insert to limit metatarsophalangeal joint motion. Surgical options include the following:

- Joint débridement, including cheilectomy, to alleviate pain and improve motion.
- Metatarsophalangeal arthrodesis. This eliminates pain, is durable, and allows a high level of function in an active adolescent.

Hallux Varus

The hallux points medialward. Acquired deformity results from overcorrection of bunion. Congenital hallux varus may be dynamic or static. The former is due to overactivity of abductor hallucis muscle and is self-limited in infancy. In the latter, a palpable contracture of the muscle may become visible under the medial skin with abduction of the forefoot (Lichtblau test). Surgical release of abductor hallucis may be reinforced by lateral transfer of extensor brevis tendon.

Macrodactyly

This may be isolated [I] or associated with other condition, including Proteus syndrome, neurofibromatosis, or vascular malformation. It interferes with shoe wear, is readily traumatized, and is unsightly. Accommodate by modifying shoe wear. Physeodesis has limited utility, for example, it limits length but does not address width. Debulking is ineffective. Consider amputation of metatarsal as well as affected toe, in order to avoid a wide web space for adjacent toes to incline toward and create secondary deformity.

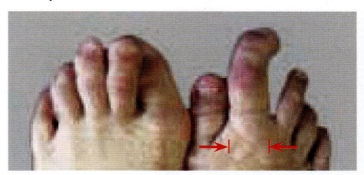

I **Macrodactyly** There is hypertrophy of the entire second ray (*red*), which should be included in a resection.

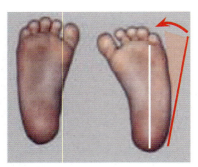

A Metatarsus adductus Lateral border of the foot is curved (*red*). Heel bisector passes through the fourth web space

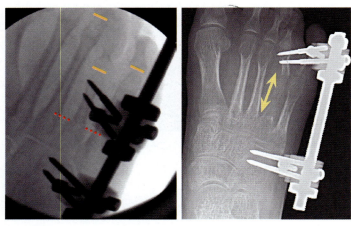

B Lengthening of brachymetatarsia The 4th metatarsal is short (*orange*). An external fixator is placed, the bone is cut at proximal metaphysis (*red*), and lengthened (*yellow*) with intervening callus.

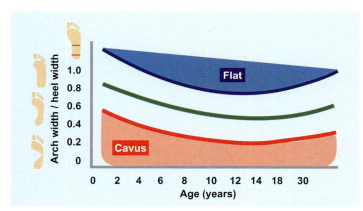

A Midfoot:heel contact area Ratio of the arch width to the heel width varies with age. Normal mean is 0.5, and range is 0.25 to 0.75. Below this range is cavus (*red*). Above this range is flat (*blue*).

Type	Hindfoot	Cause
Physiologic	Normal	Idiopathic
Pathologic	Cavovarus	Neural—central e.g., Friedreich ataxia Neural—peripheral e.g., Charcot-Marie-Tooth Muscular e.g., Duchenne
	Calcaneocavus	Spinal cord disease e.g., poliomyelitis

B Classification of cavus This classification includes the majority of causes of cavus feet. Pathologic cavus is often associated with neurologic disorders.

FOREFOOT

Metatarsus Adductus

The metatarsus is "directed" (Latin *ducere*) "to(ward)" (Latin *ad-*) the midline. This is one cause of in-toeing. It may be a "packaging sign" of uterine crowding, in association with plagiocephaly, torticollis, and hip dysplasia.

Evaluation The lateral border of the foot is curved [A]. The heel bisector, which normally passes through the second toe, is displaced lateralward with increasing severity. The deformity may be flexible or rigid, which some distinguished by the appellation *metatarsus varus*. Flexible metatarsus adductus is divided into active, which corrects with stimulation of the foot, and passive, in which the lateral border may be straightened and made concave by displacing the forefoot lateralward with one hand while securing the heel in the other hand. The hindfoot and ankle are supple.

The natural history is spontaneous resolution in > 90%. Rigid or persistent metatarsus adductus may interfere with shoe wear.

Management Education about the benignity of the condition is the cornerstone. Modalities such as stretching exercises in the first year and reversing shoes after walking age do not adversely impact the child and give parents some agency.

Rigid deformity is treated according to age.

- Under 5 years, serial casting. A sequela is recurrence.
- After 5 years, opening wedge cuneiform osteotomy with structural allograft and closing wedge cuboid osteotomy (bone is too cancellous to be structurally effective) with internal fixation. Tarsometatarsal capsulotomies with metatarsal osteotomies (Heyman-Herndon) is an unnecessarily complex procedure fraught with complications.

Brachymetatarsia

This may affect the hallucal metatarsal, as an atavic trait representing regression from a structure adapted for terrestrial erect weight bearing and locomotion to one adapted for arboreal life, in which the hallux more closely resembles an opposable thumb in relative size, position, and mobility (Morton foot).

Lesser brachymetatarsia typically affects the 4th toe, which is displaced proximalward and dorsad, furrowing the web space. Severe deformity is characterized by transfer metatarsalgia and pressure against the upper toe box. Two surgical techniques have been advocated:

- Osteotomy and acute lengthening over a medullary wire, with intercalary bone graft. Autograft necessitates a second incision; allograft may not unite. Length is limited by soft tissue envelope, including toe ischaemia.
- Osteotomy and callus distraction by external fixator [B]. This carries pin-site risks but, because it is gradual, it is more potent and less threatening to the adjacent neurovascular structures.

MIDFOOT

Cavus

Latin *cavus* describes a medial longitudinal arch that is "hollowed out," as a "*cave*" is in the earth. While arch height is difficult to measure, the reduction in contact area that follows may be measured in the ratio of midfoot width:heel width [A]. Cavus may be divided into physiologic and pathologic. Physiologic is an isolated finding at one end or 2.5% above the Gaussian distribution for the general population. Pathologic is neuromuscular or syndromic [B].

Evaluation The essential problem in cavus is reduction of contact area (A), which increases pressure (P) for the same force (F) of body weight after the formula $P = F/A$. The foot hurts and reacts by forming calluses to increase the contact area [C].

In isolated cavus, the hindfoot is uninvolved. Determine flexibility of cavus, toes, subtalar, and ankle joints. Triceps suræ contracture may result in recruitment of the long digital extensors, which are visible under the dorsal skin, leading to flexible claw toes. Hindfoot varus displaces callus lateralward. It also stresses the ankle, including episodes of instability. Callus also appears over the dorsa of the clawed toes. Severe and rigid deformity is difficult to shoe.

Rule out other disease. The history may be obvious in an established diagnosis such as cerebral palsy. A family history may reveal a peripheral neuropathy. The child should be undressed and in a gown. Examine all systems, in particular the rest of the skeleton (e.g., other deformity), nervous (e.g., diminished deep tendon reflexes in peripheral neuropathy), muscular (e.g., weakness or wasting), and cutaneous (e.g., sign of dysrrhaphism). Unilateral deformity and hindfoot deformity are abnormal. Clawing of the toes may be a sign of intrinsic muscle disease.

Röntgenogrammes aid the determination of site(s) and severity of deformity, and operative planning. Consider other testing based upon index of suspicion. MRI may reveal a spinal cord tumor. Electrodiagnostic and gene testing are indicated for Charcot-Marie-Tooth diseases and muscular dystrophies (*cf.* Neuromuscular Diseases). Appropriate referral, for example, to a neurologist, completes the evaluation.

Management Arch supports increase contact area, thereby reducing pressure. Orthotic for the hindfoot restores normal distribution of force at subtalar and ankle joints. Ankle–foot orthotics may aid clearance of the floor during swing phase of gait.

Because the natural history of significant deformity is poor, surgical treatment is common. The causes and presentations are diverse. Learn principles and tailor methods.

- Timing balances size of the foot—to allow for sufficient ossification—versus joint motion—which declines with age and as such will limit surgical options [D].
- Determine whether deformity is flexible or rigid [E]. Flexibility allows correction *via* joint motion rather than by excision and fusion: this will preserve function and improve outcomes. Casting is nonoperative soft tissue release. Osteotomy for the rigid foot creates a secondary osseous deformity to compensate for the primary articular deformity.
- Examine every muscle for strength and contracture [F]. Transfer strong muscles to recover motion lost to neural imbalance or myopathy. Split transfers guard against opposite deformity in unpredictable disease. Avoid transfer of weak muscles or muscles out of phase, except in a supportive rôle. Lengthen contracted muscles to reduce their deforming force.

Surgery may be divided into several components.

SOFT TISSUE Plantar release may be isolated or inclusive. The former is performed at the medial midfoot, where the edge of plantar aponeurosis is readily palpable. The latter (Steindler) is performed through a medial approach to the hindfoot, which allows identification of neurovascular structures and section (or "stripping") of plantar aponeurosis and deep muscles of the foot off the tuber of calcaneus, as well as the talonavicular capsule. The first two address cavus, while the third component aids hindfoot correction *via* the acetabulum pedis.

Plantar release usually is the first stage of care. Casting may correct remaining, more global contracture, preparing the flexible foot for second stage surgery, which will include muscle work. Cast until a plateau is reached, which determines whether osteotomy will be necessary if deformity remains.

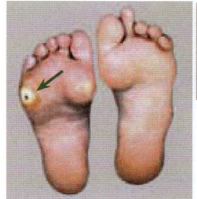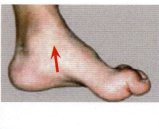

C Physical examination of cavus The deformity increases load on the metatarsal heads. If sensation is poor, for example, spina bifida, skin breakdown (*green*) is not uncommon. The arch points to the locus of disease (*red*), in this case, the spine.

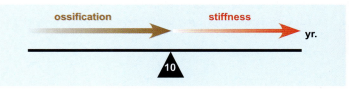

D Timing of operation Balance ossification against stiffness.

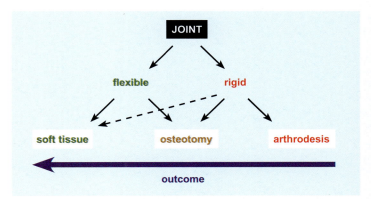

E Surgical principles: joint Joint integrity influences type of procedure.

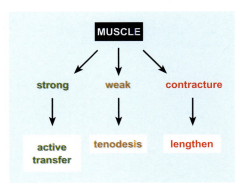

F Surgical principles: muscle Muscle strength and excursion influence type of procedure.

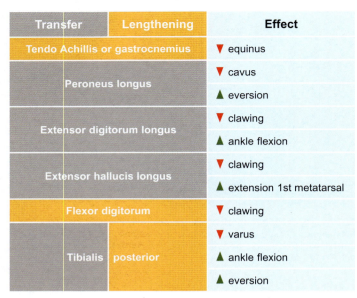

Transfer	Lengthening	Effect
Tendo Achillis or gastrocnemius		▼ equinus
Peroneus longus		▼ cavus
		▲ eversion
Extensor digitorum longus		▼ clawing
		▲ ankle flexion
Extensor hallucis longus		▼ clawing
		▲ extension 1st metatarsal
	Flexor digitorum	▼ clawing
Tibialis	posterior	▼ varus
		▲ ankle flexion
		▲ eversion

G Muscle surgery for cavus Lengthening or transfer reduces deforming forces and augments motion.

MUSCLE TRANSFER OR LENGTHENING Triceps suræ release is postponed until after casting [G]. Gastrocnemius recession is indicated when Silfverskiöld sign is present: ankle flexion improves sufficiently with knee flexion, when the gastrocnemius is relaxed. Tendo Achillis lengthening may be percutaneous or open: the former is less invasive, the latter more controlled.

The goal of muscle transfer is balanced function after, not to effect, deformity correction.

Peroneus longus flexes the first ray. Releasing this muscle removes its deforming force. Transferring the muscle to peroneus brevis, which everts the hindfoot, allows it to counteract varus.

The digital extensors, recruited against overpowering posterior crural muscles, exacerbate claw deformity. Their power of ankle flexion is dissipated at the metatarsophalangeal joints. Transfer removes a deforming force and enables the muscles to be more effective. Extensor hallucis longus may be transferred to the neck of the 1st metatarsal, to aid its extension. Extensor digitorum longus may be transferred to lateral cuneiform, to augment ankle flexion, or to cuboid (peroneus tertius, if present, may be a more secure anchor point) to add eversion.

Lengthening of the plantar aspect of the foot, along with improved ankle flexion, stretches the digital flexors, which are unopposed after extensor transfer. This may be addressed by percutaneous flexor release at the proximal cutaneous crease of the toes, which is simpler than multiple phalangeal arthrodeses.

Tibialis posterior, the principal agent of varus, may be lengthened above the tibial malleolus, where the tendinous fraction is sectioned, or by a Z-manner in the midfoot during plantar release. The tendon may be transferred to aid ankle flexion or eversion, but this takes the muscle out of phase and is reserved for the neuromuscular, paralytic foot, where it acts as a passive transfer. It may be rerouted *in toto* through the interosseous membrane to the lateral cuneiform, or it be split behind the foot to the peroneus brevis.

OSTEOTOMY The forefoot may be elevated by midfoot osteotomy. Mildest is medial cuneiform osteotomy to elevate the 1st metatarsal. Osteotomy proceeds lateralward with increasing deformity. Osteotomy may be opening of closing wedge: the former lengthens a short foot, while the latter is less resisted by overall contracture and thereby may afford greater correction. Translational osteotomies, which correct cavus by dorsad displacement of the distal foot, are more limited and create a secondary deformity. Midfoot osteotomies are fixed with wires.

Osteotomy of the calcaneus may compensate for rigid hindfoot varus. Valgus osteotomy resects a lateral closing wedge. Because the center of deformity is the subtalar joint, lateral displacement of the calcaneus fragment is necessary to bring the tuber in line with the mechanical axis. Superior displacement of the calcaneus fragment is indicated when pitch is increased, as in calcaneocavus. Screw fixation is more stable.

ARTHRODESIS This is indicated for deformity that is rigid—when the foot cannot be corrected by harnessing joint motion—and severe—when compensating osteotomy is insufficient. A dorsal wedge resected through the transverse tarsal joint corrects cavus. A lateral wedge resected through the subtalar joint corrects varus. Fix with staples or plates.

Accessory Navicular Bone

This accessorium also is known as os tibiale externum or os naviculare secundarium. It represents a "secondary" center of ossification that is lodged as a sesamoid in the tibialis posterior tendon. It affects 15% of the population. Three types are distinguished [H]. The cornuate type has fused late to elongate the navicular like a "horn" (Latin *cornu*).

I independent ossicle **II** apophysis **III** cornuate

hypermobility synchondrosis injury mass effect

H Classification of accessory navicular Pain (*red*) is most associated with type II, where the synchondrosis (*blue*) is stressed repeatedly by the pull of the tibialis posterior tendon (*orange*).

Evaluation Presentation is toward the inflection of the decades. Chronic inflammation from repetitive stress, microfracture of synchondrosis, and/or direct trauma to an osseous prominence conspires to produce pain that is focal and reproducible by palpation. The navicular is prominent. Overlying skin is reactive, typically red and thick.

Röntgenogrammes are the standard and sufficient in the classic presentation. While it may be visible on anteroposterior and lateral projection, an external oblique projection is tangent to the navicular and remainder of the foot, thereby exposing the accessorium *en profil*. Although the navicular ossifies by 5 years, the accessorium ossifies later. Other imaging modalities are reserved for special circumstances. Scintigramme may focus vague foot pain. MRI gives detail of the tibialis posterior tendon, before and after operation.

Management Initial treatment is symptomatic and supportive. Modify shoe wear to decompress the accessorium. University of California Biomechanics Laboratory orthotic inverts a valgus hindfoot to reduce pressure on the navicular. Rest the foot in a cast. Persistent pain may be addressed by patience for fusion with the main bone, or simple excision [I]. Make a linear incision centered on the bone. Divide tibialis posterior sharply in line with its fibers. Identify the gap, synchondrosis, or scar between the two bones, through which the accessorium may be shelled out least traumatically. Blunt remaining prominence or edge. Do not defy Ockham's razor: broad excision and advancement of tibialis posterior (Kidner procedure) lest the it be attenuated by the accessorium and in order to support the medial longitudinal arch is unnecessarily complicated and risks the tendon's function.

Flatfoot

The condition is discussed here even though the principal problem is proximal to the midfoot because the name describes the medial longitudinal arch. This also is known in Latin as *pes planovalgus*, to encompass deformity of the hindfoot.

There are three types of flatfoot [J]. The components of flexibility are change of shape of the medial longitudinal arch with loading and supple subtalar joint motion. Flexible flatfoot may be divided into without and with triceps suræ contracture. The former is a normal variant and accounts for no symptoms or dysfunction. The latter may cause pain as decreased excursion of the calcaneus, tethered by the heel cord, restricts ankle motion and transfers force to the subtalar joint, at which the calcaneus swivels out leaving the head of the talus unsupported to drop to the ground. Rigid flatfoot has an immutable shape and a stiff subtalar joint: the foot hurts, interferes with shoe wear, and often requires treatment. It is typified by tarsal coalition and vertical talus (*q.v.*).

The essential pathomechanical features of flexible flatfoot are as follows [K]:

- Calcaneus may be equinus or plantar flexed relative to the tibia.
- Calcaneus rotates lateralward at subtalar joint into the valgus.
- Talus falls into equinus, plantar flexed relative to the tibia and calcaneus.
- Navicular is abducted and dorsiflexed relative to the talus.
- The 1st metatarsal is extended, supinating the forefoot.

Flexible flatfoot distributes *Force* of weight bearing over a large surface *Area*, reducing *Pressure* after the formula $P = F/A$ (*cf.* Cavus). This is advantageous, as manifest by reduced stress fractures in the flatfooted. An unyielding foot (tight heel cord or rigid) concentrates force over a small area (e.g., head of the talus) [L].

Secondary deformities may be divided into osseous and soft tissue. The lateral column is relatively short. The tibialis posterior tendon is attenuated. The plantar and medial talonavicular joint capsule is lax.

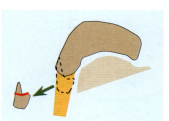

I Excision of accessory navicular Shell the accessorium sharply out of the tibialis posterior tendon. Blunt remaining prominence or edge.

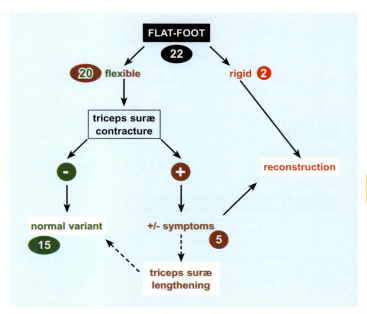

J Algorithm for flatfoot Numbers represent % of white population affected.

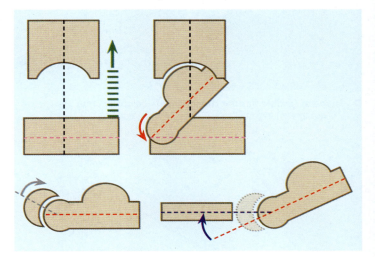

K Pathomechanics of flatfoot.

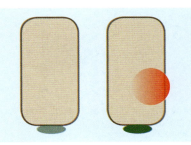

L Stiffness concentrates force A flexible flatfoot without tether distributes force over a large surface area. Tight heel cord (*dark green*) prevents the head of the talus (*red*) from accommodating during weight bearing, thereby concentrating force.

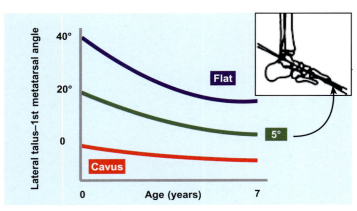

M Development of the medial longitudinal arch The arch stabilizes at mean slight plantar sag (*green*) by age 7 years.

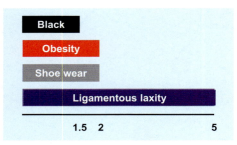

N Associations with flatfoot Numbers represent multiples of the general population. Obesity suggests a mechanical factor, as does exogenous force from shoes. Laxity points to ligament and not muscle as primary tissue site.

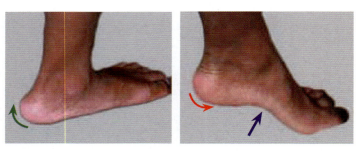

O Shape of flexible flatfoot changes with weight bearing Heel moves from valgus (*green*) to varus (*red*), no arch to arch (*blue*).

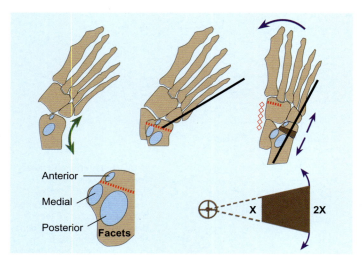

P Lateral column lengthening Lateral column is short (*green*). Wire (*black*) stabilizes calcaneocuboid joint, graft, and osteotomy (*red*). Osteotomy is extra-articular between calcaneal facets. Trapezoid graft for medial center of rotation (*brown*).

Evaluation Flexible flatfoot is normal in infancy ("fat foot") and reduces with growth [M]. Several characteristics are associated with flexible flatfoot [N]. While flatfoot and bunion are independent, the two conditions are influenced by shoe wear. Is there a toe–toe gait, suggesting triceps suræ contracture? Examine the foot standing flat, standing on the metatarsal heads and unweighted. Does extension of the hallux restore an arch by tightening the plantar aponeurosis *via* a windlass mechanism (Jack)? Determine subtalar flexibility, and whether the medial longitudinal arch reconstitutes [O]. Examine the skin for signs of decompensation, such as callus or sore, which reflect force concentration. Move the subtalar joint. Lock the subtalar joint and flex the ankle, with the knee extended and flexed, to determine whether the tendo Achillis is tight or whether there is an isolated contracture of the gastrocnemius muscle. Is there tenderness, such as over a prominent head of the talus, along tibialis posterior tendon or peroneal tendons, or at the insertion of tendo Achillis? Distinguish hindfoot valgus from ankle valgus, which may be seen in neuromuscular disease such as spina bifida.

Imaging Röntgenogrammes are the standard and sufficient. Evaluate relationship of the talus and calcaneus in the anteroposterior projection: divergence with overlap suggests a competent subtalar joint; lateral displacement of the calcaneus without concomitant divergence suggests joint incompetence, as after excessive clubfoot release. The lateral projection exposes extent of equinus. The metatarsals are evaluated for overlap or divergence, to aid assessment of forefoot supination. Röntgenogrammes may reveal other cause of flatfoot, such as tarsal coalition.

Management Perhaps the most important component of management is education. Flexible flatfoot is normal. Orthotics are unnecessary. They do not alter foot shape. That an "arch support" can harm the foot is a paradox to many patients: there is no room, and jamming something against the medial foot hurts. Do not underestimate cost, including of "custom" fabrication and psychic for the child.

Address a tight heel cord either by compensating for it, for example, with a heel lift, or by stretching it, with exercises. The latter is ambitious for a small muscle group, because it requires isolating the ankle joint by locking the subtalar joint (with which the public is unfamiliar), and in a child who may be otherwise distracted.

Operation Lengthen the triceps suræ, either at tendo Achillis or at gastrocnemius muscle, to decompress the subtalar joint. Because surgical intervention is reserved for significant primary deformity that typically presents in company of secondary deformities, this usually is combined with reconstruction.

Arthroereisis (Greek ερεισις: "pushing against"), in which a block to subtalar eversion is inserted into the calcaneus at the sinus tarsi to actively or passively counteract hindfoot valgus, may improve foot posture early but will degrade the subtalar joint long term.

Lateral column lengthening is indicated for a reducible and competent subtalar joint [P, Q]. This is anatomic, harnessing the acetabulum pedis and addressing secondary deformity, and physiologic, avoiding arthrodesis.

- Lengthen the heel cord or the triceps aponeurosis, depending upon the site of contracture.
- Oblique incision in lines of von Langer over sinus tarsi.
- Expose dorsal distal calcaneus preserving calcaneocuboid joint.
- Lengthen peroneus brevis and cut aponeurosis of abductor digital minimi, which become contracted in a short lateral column.
- Identify site of osteotomy between anterior and middle facets of calcaneus. Some patients have no distinction between these, in which case select 10 to 15 mm proximal to calcaneocuboid joint.
- Expose plantar surface of calcaneus and divide periosteum and lateral plantar aponeurosis.
- Cut the calcaneus with osteotome or saw.
- Drive a smooth wire retrograde across the calcaneocuboid joint (to stabilize it) into the osteotomy.

- Prepare a trapezoid allograft or autogenous corticocancellous graft from the ilium. Lateral side is 2× medial side of graft. This accounts for the center of rotation of acetabulum pedis remote at the center of the head of the talus.
- Distract osteotomy and place graft, securing both by advancing wire retrograde.
- By a medial longitudinal incision, expose and plicate the talonavicular joint and tibialis posterior tendon.
- Flex the ankle and evaluate metatarsal heads. If supination, perform a closing wedge osteotomy of the medial cuneiform. Leaving a supinated forefoot risks recurrence as the medial limb of tripod ultimately will reach the ground by driving the hindfoot back into the valgus.

Medial displacement osteotomy of the calcaneus is indicated for lateral translation of the calcaneus and remainder of the foot at an incompetent subtalar joint, or when subtalar joint is stiff such that acetabulum pedis cannot be reduced around the head of the talus. It is a compensating osteotomy that brings ground contact point in line with mechanical axis (*cf.* Cavus).

Skewfoot

This also is known as Z-foot, which describes the appearance of the three parts of the foot as limbs of the letter [R]. It is a combination of metatarsus adductus and flatfoot, with hindfoot valgus and midfoot adductus, and should be managed according to the same principles.

Surgical correction includes *both* medial column lengthening and lateral column lengthening. These do not counteract each other, but rather address the two deformities at different sites in the foot: midfoot where there is adductus, and hindfoot where there is valgus.

Calcaneovalgus

This is a benign condition produced by uterine crowding [A]. It is striking to parents and primary physicians. The natural history is spontaneous resolution without sequelæ over the first few months of life. There is no association with long-term deformity.

Evaluation The ankle is hyperflexed, and the hindfoot is in valgus, plastering the foot against the anterior distal leg, which may be indented. Distinguish flexibility of talonavicular joint and dorsiflexion of calcaneus from vertical talus, in which the former is stiff and the calcaneus is in equinus. Palpate the subcutaneous border of the tibia and malleoli to rule out posteromedial bowing (*q.v.*). Look for other packaging signs, such as plagiocephaly, torticollis, and hip dysplasia.

Management Stretching by parents does not harm the child and gives them agency.

HINDFOOT

Clubfoot

This also is known as Latin *tali-pes equino-cavo-varus*, a term that describes the "talus" serving as "foot" to be walked on in the severe untreated form, and the deformities of the ankle, midfoot, and hindfoot. The name does not include the leg, which also is involved. It has been recognized since ancient times. Hephæstus, god of blacksmiths, fire, and volcanoes (Roman Vulcan), was called "lame" due to deformity of the feet [A]. The Hippocratic Corpus discusses the condition at length, including manipulative correction.

Clubfoot may be divided postural, which is extrinsic related to *in utero* position and resolves spontaneously, and structural, which is an intrinsic defect [B]. Structural clubfoot may be divided into idiopathic and associated with generalized condition, which includes neuromuscular disease (e.g., spina bifida) and syndromes (e.g., arthrogryposis). Idiopathic clubfoot is bilateral in half the cases and affects boys more. The cause is unknown and multifactorial, including genetics (it is familial) and encompassing all tissues (soft and hard) [C]. A base substitution in the highly conserved homeodomain of paired-like homeodomain transcription factor

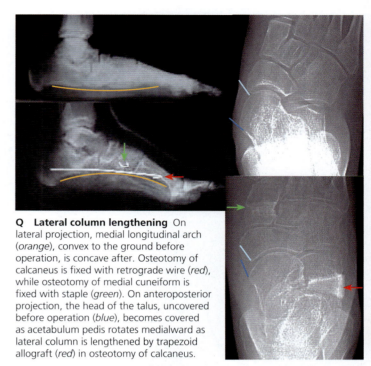

Q Lateral column lengthening On lateral projection, medial longitudinal arch (*orange*), convex to the ground before operation, is concave after. Osteotomy of calcaneus is fixed with retrograde wire (*red*), while osteotomy of medial cuneiform is fixed with staple (*green*). On anteroposterior projection, the head of the talus, uncovered before operation (*blue*), becomes covered as acetabulum pedis rotates medialward as lateral column is lengthened by trapezoid allograft (*red*) in osteotomy of calcaneus.

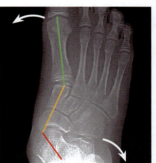

R Skewfoot The first metatarsal (*green*) and forefoot are adducted relative to midfoot (*orange*). The hindfoot is valgus, with an exposed head of talus (*red*) as navicular is abducted.

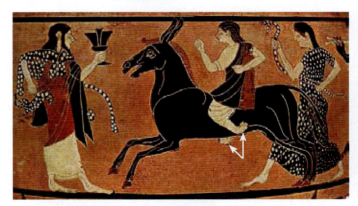

A Clubfoot is ancient Hephæstus, with clubfeet (*white*), led to Olympus by Dionysus (chalice).

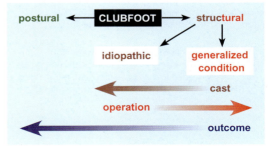

B Algorithm for clubfoot Treatment and outcome vary according to subtype.

Cause	Finding
Genetic	Mutation in PITX1 gene (5q31.1). Pairwise concordance in twins.
Bone	Medial and plantar declination of neck of talus. Delayed ossification of talus.
Capsule/ligament	Contracture of plantar aponeurosis, tibionavicular ligament.
Muscle	Shortening of myotendinous junctions in tibialis posterior, triceps suræ, digital flexors.
Vascular	Hypoplasia of tibialis anterior, peroneal arteries.
Nerve	Feature of neural diseases

C   Cause of clubfoot is multifactorial.

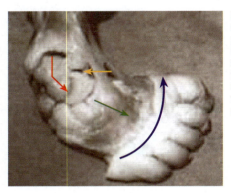

D   Pathomechanics Neck of the talus is declined plantad and medialward (*red*). Acetabulum pedis swings around the head of the talus (*blue*). Navicular is apposed to malleolus of the tibia (*orange*). Forefoot is adducted (*green*).

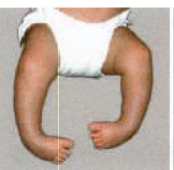
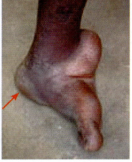

E   Natural history of clubfoot Left will progress to right. Note heel pad over the head of the talus (*red*).

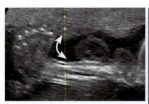

F   Imaging of clubfoot Ultrasonography offers an opportunity for education in preparation for treatment in the immediate neonatal period (*white*). Röntgenogrammes show parallelism of the talus (*red*) and calcaneus (*yellow*), a sign of hindfoot varus, and adductus of forefoot (*green*).

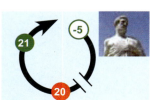

G   Evolution of treatment The dominance of operation (20th century) has ceded to manipulation (21st), returning to what was advocated by Hippocrates (5th BC).

1 (Pitx1) has been found in affected members of a five-generation family. Pitx1 has been found to direct hindlimb morphology and can effect forelimb to hindlimb transformation. In a mouse model, PITX1 deletion results in clubfoot, peroneal artery hypoplasia, and spatially corresponding muscle hypoplasia. PITX1 haploinsufficiency may cause a developmental field defect of the leg, of which clubfoot is the most striking feature.

Pathomechanics

There are several components of clubfoot deformity [D].

- Ankle is *equinus*.
- Neck of the talus is short, plantar flexed and rotated medialward, down to 90 degree (normal 150 degrees).
- Acetabulum pedis is plantar flexed and rotated medialward into hindfoot *varus*, while the trochlea of the talus is retained in ankle mortise. This brings calcaneus parallel to the talus in both sagittal and coronal planes. It swings navicular to appose malleolus of the tibia.
- The forefoot is flexed, producing *cavus*, and deviates medialward into *adductus*.
- Hypoplasia of the limb distal to the knee produces a thin calf and a small foot.

Natural history Untreated disability results from functional reduction of the foot to a single bone [E]. Treatment improves outcome but not always. Casting may lead to no or incomplete correction, and surgery may lead to a stiff foot or an overcorrected foot.

Evaluation Postural clubfoot is supple, and the skin has multiple creases. Exclude other conditions by taking a complete history and examining the entire child. In metatarsal adductus, the heel can be placed into valgus and the ankle has unrestricted motion.

There are many clinical classifications based upon multiple components with variable reproducibility and prognostic utility. Their principal benefit is to focus the physical examination.

- Equinus
- Varus
- Cavus
- Adductus
- Flexibility
- Head of the talus, which is exposed dorsolateral
- Cutaneous creases, posterior and medial
- Stigmata of decompensation, such as callus
- Foot size and stiffness, which are proportional to severity

IMAGING Clubfoot may be diagnosed *in utero* starting at 12 weeks [F]. The finding should persist over time and despite movement. Three-dimensional ultrasonography does not add value. Complete survey for fetal compression (e.g., fibroids) and for other anomalies: false-positive rate is up to 40%. While deformity may be seen on röntgenogrammes [F], because management begins soon postpartum, and because radiographic correlations with outcomes are unclear, this modality is reserved for the older child, in particular as part of operative preparation.

Management The clubfoot is intrinsically diseased and never will be normal. The calf always will be thin, the foot always small and different in appearance. Management has evolved in a circle [G]. The goals of treatment are to do no harm and to achieve normal function [H].

CASTING (PONSETI) This is effective for >90% of cases begun in the first few weeks of life. It also is effective, or at least an aid, for patients in the first few years of life. Fundamental is an understanding of the acetabulum pedis.

- An above-knee cast is applied every week for 6 weeks.
- The deformity is approached sequentially according to the acronym CAVE (*C*avus, *A*dductus, *V*arus, *E*quinus).
- The first cast pushes up against the first ray to reduce cavus, supinating the forefoot and exaggerating the deformity.

- The forefoot is pushed to swing the acetabulum pedis around the head of the talus.
- Counterpressure is applied against the head of the talus or against the malleolus of the fibula [I]. The former is more effective by being at the center of rotation but risks pressure phenomenon where the skin is thinnest. The latter relies on securing the talus in ankle mortise, which is supported against lateral distortion.
- Do not address equinus until other components of deformity are corrected. The tendo Achillis is t he tether, securing the ankle, against which the subtalar joint is manipulated.

Tendo Achillis section This is indicated for equinus, in 90% of case. Zealous ankle flexion against an unyielding tendo Achillis risks dorsiflexion at the midfoot, creating a rocker-bottom deformity.

- A percutaneous heel cord tenotomy is performed in office or in operating room.
- Topical cream provides only cutaneous anæsthesia. Injection of anæsthetic may distort anatomy and risk posteromedial neurovascular bundle.
- Insert scalpel parallel to medial border of tendo Achillis 1 cm proximal to calcaneus.
- Advance blade into space anterior to tendon (which may be developed by a clamp), turn 90 degree, and cut posteriorward.
- Apply final cast in hypercorrected position.

Bracing This is indicated for all patients (J).

- The brace consists of firm above-ankle boots connected by a metal bar, set at shoulder width. A pad above the heel prevents the foot from slipping out of the shoe. There have been multiple modifications.
- The original concept was "to control the position of one foot by means of the other" (Browne). Extension of one limb during spontaneous kicking drives the subtalar joint of the flexed limb into eversion.
- The brace is worn full time until standing, after which it is applied during sleep until 3 years of age.
- Recurrence is indirectly proportional to compliance with bracing. While the design is simple, application can be challenging over time and as the child becomes older.

Tibialis anterior transfer After 3 years of age, this is indicated for residual dynamic supination. Perform after structural (static) deformity, which a tendon transfer cannot overcome, has been corrected. The tendon is moved *in toto* (not split as in neuromuscular disease) to lateral cuneiform [K].

For idiopathic clubfoot resistant to the above approach, or in clubfoot associated with other condition, a formal surgical correction may be indicated, starting at 6 months of age. Do not offer a "blue plate special" to every patient; rather, follow an "a la carte" approach according to location and severity of deformity [L].

Posterior release

- Prone position is easier because the limb needs no manipulation but less familiar.
- A variety of incisions have been advocated, including circumferential (Cincinnati) from base of 1st metatarsal medial passing 1 cm proximal to posterior ankle crease to tip of fibular malleolus lateral.
- Mobilize neurovascular bundle.
- Z-lengthen tendo Achillis, starting medial at calcaneus.
- Trace flexor hallucis longus, which has a distal muscle belly, to the posterior capsule of the subtalar joint, which is opened circumferentially. Preserve the talocalcaneal and deep deltoid ligaments.
- Section calcaneofibular ligament deep to peroneal tendons.

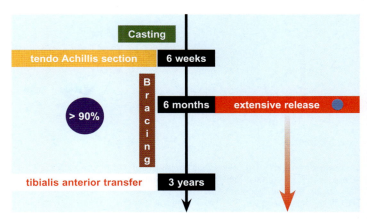

H   Algorithm for treatment of clubfoot.

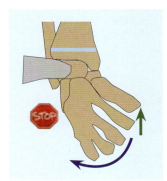

I   Casting technique (Ponseti) Start by elevating the first ray to correct cavus (*green*). Swing acetabulum pedis (*blue*) around the talus, which is stabilized by pressure at the exposed head (*grey*) or at malleolus of fibula. Do not correct the midfoot and forefoot distal to acetabulum pedis (STOP), for example, about a fulcrum at calcaneocuboid joint (Kite).

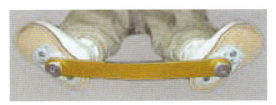

J   Browne brace Firm ankle boots are screwed to a metal bar at shoulder width in abduction that may be bent for eversion.

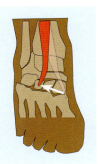

K   Tibialis anterior transfer The tendon is moved *in toto* to lateral cuneiform.

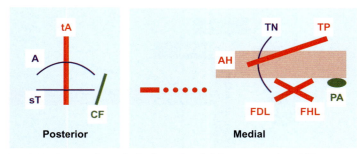

L   Components of surgical release for clubfoot tA: tendo Achillis. A: ankle joint. sT: subtalar joint. CF: calcaneofibular ligament. AH: abductor hallucis. PA: plantar aponeurosis. TP: tibialis posterior. TN: talonavicular joint. FHL: flexor hallucis longus. FDL: flexor digitorum longus. The flexors may be distally at the toes (*dotted*).

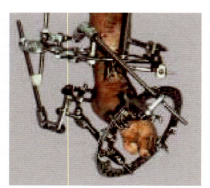

M   Ilizarov frame Complex procedure for complex deformity.

MEDIAL RELEASE

- Release the three origins of the abductor hallucis muscle distal, between medial and lateral plantar nerves, and proximal at tuber of calcaneus, thereby opening the "door to the cage" (Henry)
- Perform a plantar release (*cf.* Cavus)
- Z-lengthen tibialis posterior tendon
- Perform a capsulotomy of talonavicular joint

DIVISION OF TOE FLEXORS

- This may be performed through the medial approach or fractionally posterior to the tibial malleolus.
- Alternatively, it may be performed distally. With dorsiflexion tension applied to the ankle, insert a scalpel in the midline of the base of the each toe, cutting flexor tendon by a narrow arc windscreen wiper action. Division at this level preserves the tendon sheath, allowing rapid tendon regeneration without adhesion formation.

OSTEOTOMY This is indicated as a supplement to soft tissue work, or in case of undercorrection. Persistent deformity impairs outcome.

- Persistent adductus interferes with shoe wear. This may be addressed by medial column lengthening through medial cuneiform, or lateral column shortening. The former may be more effective as it is accommodating to overall contracture rather than pushing against it. Partial resection of cuboid is joint sparing compared with calcaneocuboid arthrodesis (Evans) or arthroplasty (Lichtblau).
- Persistent varus leads to excessive plantar pressure over the lateral border of the foot. It may be improved by lateral displacement of calcaneus. Wedge osteotomies stretch the medial soft tissues if open and may result in lateral impingement if closing.

EXTERNAL FIXATION Advanced deformity in older children may be managed with an Ilizarov frame [M], which allows gradual stretch of severe contracture and when extensive scarring precludes internal reconstruction. Orthotic support after removal of frame guards against recurrence of deformity.

SALVAGE For uncorrectable clubfoot, talectomy provides enough room in the ankle to position the foot plantigrade. The same may be achieved by wide resection and arthrodesis. These procedures are appropriate for patients with limited physical demand.

Complications

RECURRENCE This is most common. It is inversely proportional to compliance with nonoperative management, including bracing. Manage with education, repeat casting, and bracing.

STIFFNESS This may result from excessive articular pressure during casting, compartment syndrome complicating surgery, avascular necrosis of the talus, and operative scarring.

OVERCORRECTION This includes opposite deformity and weakness. Excessive hindfoot valgus from enthusiastic release, in particular of talocalcaneal and deltoid ligaments, results in incompetence of subtalar joint. Calcaneus and remainder of foot displace lateralward out from under talus. Triceps suræ may be weakened by overlengthening or repeated lengthenings. Flexor recruitment in this setting, exacerbated by hyperactive tibialis anterior, may lead to dorsal bunion (*q.v.*). Unlike casting, where overcorrection is the goal, err on the side of undercorrection at surgery. Overcorrection is difficult to rectify.

Vertical Talus

While it may be regarded as the most severe rigid flatfoot, it also is known as rocker-bottom foot, for the convexity of the plantar surface [N]. Half of cases are bilateral. It is distinguished by its rigidity from *oblique talus*, which is abnormally plantar flexed but which may be reduced manually and on stress röntgenogrammes.

Cause More than half of cases are associated with other conditions, which may be divided into central nervous system (e.g., spina bifida), neuromuscular (e.g., arthrogryposis), and syndromes (e.g., Costello, deBarsy). Fifteen percent of cases have a family history. A mutation in HOXD10 gene (2q31.1) has been implicated, which also is associated with foot deformity typical of Charcot-Marie-Tooth disease. HOX gene mutations have been found in radioulnar synostosis and hand–foot–genital syndrome.

Pathomechanics

- The essential lesion is in the midfoot: talonavicular dislocation. This displaces the remainder of the distal foot toward dorsad and lateralward, where a soft tissue contracture develops, including the tendons of the anterior and lateral crural compartment muscles.
- In the hindfoot, the calcaneus is plantar flexed into equinus and rotated lateralward, with concomitant contracture of triceps suræ.
- In severe cases, subluxation of tibialis posterior–anterior to tibial malleolus and peroneals over the fibular malleolus converts these into dorsiflexors, exacerbating deformity.

Evaluation Even more importantly than clubfoot, exclude other condition by taking a complete history and examining the entire child. Head of the talus projects into the plantar aspect of the foot, producing a convex sole. Hindfoot is in equinus and valgus, which aids distinction from calcaneovalgus. The forefoot is dorsiflexed and abducted. There are simultaneous contractures of dorsiflexors and plantar flexors. There is a deep dorsal cutaneous crease, in which a gap is noted where the head of the talus is absent.

IMAGING Lateral projection röntgenogramme demonstrates a talus that is vertical, in line with the tibia [O]. Dorsiflexion and plantar flexion stress views show no change in orientation of the talus and no change in its relationship with navicular or the 1st metatarsal (if navicular is not ossified in the infant), suggesting fixed dislocation of talonavicular joint [P]. The calcaneus is plantar flexed into equinus.

Management Akin to clubfoot, surgical management of vertical talus has evolved from extensive and complex to directed and less invasive.

CASTING Six serial weekly casts are applied as the forefoot is manipulated into plantar flexion and inversion against counterpressure applied to the head of the talus. Confirm talonavicular reduction by röntgenogramme. The foot now resembles a clubfoot in equinus.

TENDO ACHILLIS SECTION This is performed like clubfoot.

DORSAL WITHOUT OR WITH POSTERIOR RELEASE Indication is failure of talonavicular reduction by casting.

- A transverse incision is made over talonavicular joint. Extensor tendons are fractionally lengthened in the distal leg. Perform capsulotomies of the ankle, talonavicular, and calcaneocuboid joints. Use a blunt elevator as a shoehorn to reduce talonavicular joint, which is held with a wire.
- Perform a percutaneous tendo Achillis section to correct equinus.
- In an older patient, consider open Z-lengthening of tendo Achillis, as well as ankle and subtalar capsulotomies.

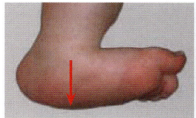
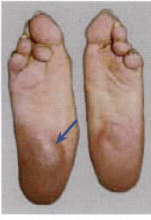

N   Vertical talus Vertical talus (*red*) gives the foot a rocker-bottom appearance. Untreated, it will produce significant disability in the parent, who bears weight on the head of the talus (*blue*).

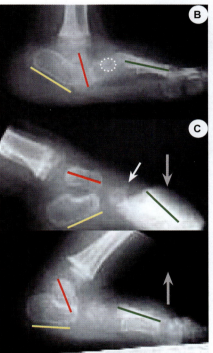

O, P   Imaging Vertical talus (*red*) is plantar flexed vertical, calcaneus is plantar flexed into equinus (*yellow*), navicular (*white*) is dislocated dorsad on the talus, and talo–first metatarsal relationship shows increased angulation and dorsad displacement. An oblique talus, the talus moves from vertical position, calcaneus from equinus, navicular from a reduced position, and the 1st metatarsal from alignment with the talus in plantar flexion stress view to oblique position, normal pitch, and dorsad displacement of navicular and 1st metatarsal, respectively, under dorsiflexion stress.

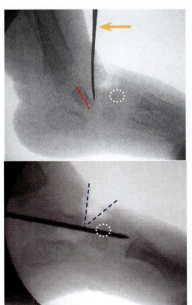

Q   Operation for vertical talus Dislocation of navicular (*white*) on the talus is approached directly *via* a dorsal incision (*blue*), through which soft tissue contractures also may be addressed. It is reduced (*orange*) and fixed with a wire.

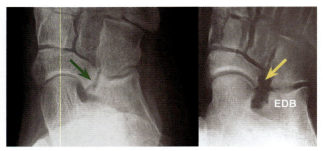

R Calcaneonavicular coalition A nonossified coalition (*green*) is resected to talonavicular and calcaneocuboid margins, leaving a gap (*yellow*), which may be filled with extensor digitorum brevis (EDB) or fat.

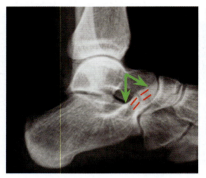

S Anteater sign Anterior process of calcaneus is long, gracile, and curved (*green*) as it extends into navicular, with which it forms a coalition (*red*). The dorsal margin of the talus does not show beaking, which in children is a traction phenomenon secondary to stress transfer, while in adults, it may be a degenerative sign.

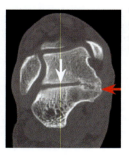

T Talocalcaneal coalition CT axial view shows the middle facet compartment is irregular (*red*), while the posterior is preserved (*white*). This is definitive and quantifiable.

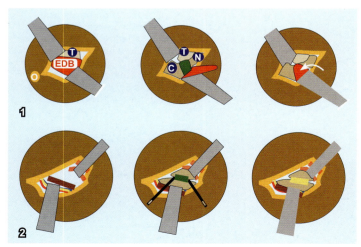

U Excision of calcaneonavicular (1) and talocalcaneal (2) coalitions
1. T: talus. EDB: extensor digitorum brevis. C: calcaneus. N: navicular. O: Ollier.
2. Neurovascular bundle and flexor hallucis longus retracted plantarward. Keith needles (*black*) delimit coalition. Fat graft (*yellow*).

Tarsal Coalition

The term may be misleading: this is not an active process of coalescence but a failure of segmentation. Two types represent the majority: talocalcaneal and calcaneonavicular. They may be familial, bilateral, and multiple. One percent incidence suggests that most coalitions are silent. However, coalition reduces motion, may produce a rigid deformity of the foot, and imposes increased stress on adjacent joints, which may elicit pain, muscle spasm, and risks degenerative arthritis. Coalitions may be present in other disorders, such as clubfoot and limb deficiency, in which there also may be a ball and socket ankle.

Evaluation Presentation is early second decade. Obtain a family history: autosomal dominant inheritance has been demonstrated. This is the most common cause of rigid flatfoot, although half of coalitions do not produce this deformity. Rule out other cause of restricted joint motion in the foot, such as juvenile idiopathic arthritis. Coalitions may be fibrous or cartilaginous, which manifest as irregular narrowing on imaging, or osseous, which accounts for the greatest stiffness but may be least symptomatic because of their stability. Röntgenogrammes usually suffice for diagnosis. CT defines anatomy for operative planning and screens for other coalition. CT and MRI aid mapping of articular coalitions; the latter also evaluates soft tissues for other lesion. Scintigraphy may illuminate an atypical clinical presentation.

Management Initial management is symptomatic and supportive, including with orthotic or 6-week cast. Operative treatment is indicated for persistent unacceptable pain and significant foot deformity [Q].

Calcaneonavicular Coalition This is extra-articular: as such, there is less stiffness and deformity, and outcomes of resection are better. Locus of pain is sinus tarsi. It is seen *en profil* by oblique projection röntgenogramme [R]. Lateral projection may show extension of anterior process of calcaneus to navicular, resembling the snout of an anteater [S].

Resection is performed through an oblique incision over sinus tarsi [U]. Extensor digitorum brevis (EDB) is elevated from its origin at the anterior calcaneus. The coalition is resected to the borders of talonavicular and calcaneocuboid joints. The resultant gap may be filled with EDB, pulled in by sutures drawn through the sole and tied over a button, or with fat harvested from the area of the natal crease, which by sparing EDB does not distort the dorsal contour of the foot.

Talocalcaneal Coalition This is articular: it tends to create more stiffness and deformity and to have poorer outcomes. Locus of pain is medial hindfoot. The coalition begins at the middle facet, from which it may reach into the posterior facet. It is seen best on a Harris axial view: the middle facet joint is irregular, fused or invisible, or it may be inclined >20 degrees. Other signs, such as C margin of the talus on lateral projection, are debatable. CT [T] and MRI are essential to map the extent of articular involvement: any significant invasion of the posterior facet precludes resection.

Surgery must address both coalition, as source of pain, and deformity, against worsening of which the coalition may be a final tether. A calcaneus in valgus (>15 degrees) may be liberated to decline further by resection of a medial coalition. Such operation should include resection of coalition and lateral column lengthening. Approach coalition *via* a linear incision from anterior margin of tendo Achillis to navicular. Take down abductor hallucis, retract neurovascular bundle, and develop interval between flexor digitorum longus and flexor hallucis longus, which courses under sustentaculum tali. Identify normal posterior and anterior subtalar compartments to delimit the middle facet coalition. Define the plane of nonosseous coalition bluntly to guide excision, which continues until normal cartilage surfaces are visible and there is unrestricted subtalar motion. Repair the flexor retinaculum to retain the fat graft.

Consider talocalcaneal arthrodesis for coalition of >50% of total subtalar surface area, as excision leaves insufficient articular surface for reasonable joint function. Correct deformity by appropriate angulation of joint resection and fusion planes.

ANKLE

Toe Walking

This may be idiopathic or associated with other condition, including clubfoot, cerebral palsy, spina bifida, muscular dystrophy, arthrogryposis [A]. Contracture may involve a short triceps suræ *in toto*, gastrocnemius muscle, or accessory soleus muscle. In the uninvolved child, it may be an atavic trait.

Natural history Most idiopathic toe walking resolves in the first few years, though residual triceps suræ may persist. Morbid toe walking does not improve.

Evaluation Exclude other disease by taking a complete history and examining the entire child [B]. Is gait equinus, flatfoot, or normal heel-toe? Is the shape of the foot triangular, reflecting osseous reaction to differential force? Are the toes splayed? Check the skin for callus, suggesting decompensation. Determine site of contracture by performing Silfverskiöld test: lock subtalar joint by inverting the heel, and flex the ankle with knee flexed and knee extended [C]. Significant difference in ankle motion suggests selective contracture of gastrocnemius muscle.

Management There are no long-term functional outcome studies. Toe walking is unsightly for many. It interferes with shoe wear. Shifting force distal in the foot theoretically risks deformity, pain, and overuse injury such as stress fracture.

Stretching, including with a physiotherapist, is difficult in this age group. Serial casting takes control but may not provide a durable result. Orthotics, such as an articulated ankle–foot having a plantar flexion block, with no end point may be a greater treatment burden than surgery.

Because most improve spontaneously, and because recurrence is greater before 4 years, do not operate before that age. For persistent toe walking, surgical lengthening is low morbidity and effective.

Gastrocnemius recession This is indicated in the presence of a Silfverskiöld sign. The incision is linear at the myotendinous junction midline or along medial border of gastrocnemius. Sural nerve may enter surgical field, often heralded by accompanying vein. Divide plantaris. Separate widely gastrocnemius aponeurosis from that of subjacent soleus: this allows selective section of the former and free retraction of its edges with ankle flexion in knee extension. The aponeurotomy may be chevron (Vulpius), tongue-in-groove (Baker), or transverse (Strayer). While there is no risk of overcorrection, undercorrection is possible: preoperative ankle flexion must be >10 degrees with the knee flexed, which simulates operative result.

Heel cord lengthening Indication is triceps suræ contracture, or insufficient ankle flexion (<10 degrees) with the knee flexed. This may be percutaneous or open. The former may be two anatomic cuts (*white*), rotated 45 degrees to account for the normal rotation of the tendo Achillis fibers [D]. Alternatively, three cuts (Hoke) may be performed in the same plane, to cut enough fibers to effect a lengthening. Open Z-lengthening, *via* a linear incision parallel but off the medial margin of the tendon, leaves a visible scar but offers more control. Repair the tendon under moderate tension in neutral ankle position to avoid excessive lengthening, which will lead to weak push-off and is difficult to salvage.

Ball and Socket Ankle

This is an acquired deformity secondary to extensive osseous tarsal coalition, which is congenital [E], in particular in association with limb deficiency. The ankle is molded into a socket that allows inversion–eversion in addition to flexion–extension, to compensate for loss of subtalar motion. The tarsal coalition is too extensive to take down: it may be completed if symptomatic. Ball and socket is not addressed per se; rather, treatment focuses on limb deficiency.

Tarsal Tunnel Syndrome

The passage of tibial nerve, posterior tibial artery, tibialis posterior, and long digital flexor tendons from the leg into foot is converted into

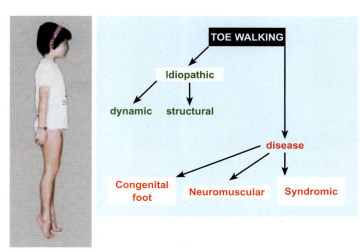

A   Algorithm for toe walking.

Feature	Idiopathic	Disease
Geography	Localized	General
	Bilateral	Bilateral
Development	Normal mile-stones	Delayed, including walking > 18 months
Timing	Walking age	Independent
Natural history	Most improve	Static or progressive

B   Features of idiopathic versus morbid toe walking.

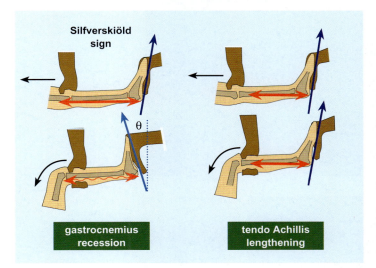

C   Locus of contracture This influences operation. Perform a tendo Achillis lengthening if θ < 10 degrees.

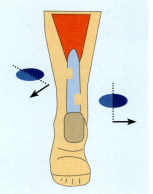

D   Tendo Achillis lengthening The anatomic percutaneous technique adjusts the angle of two step-cuts according to the normal rotation of the tendon's fibers.

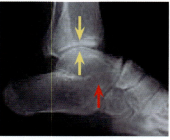
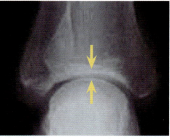

E Ball and socket ankle There is an extensive talocalcaneal coalition (*red*) subjacent to a spherical talar trochlea articulating with a spherical ankle socket, rounded in orthogonal planes (*yellow*).

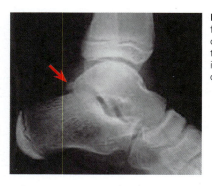

F Os trigonum Incidental finding of a secondary ossification center separate from the talus. The regular appearance is consistent with an accessory ossicle in an asymptomatic child.

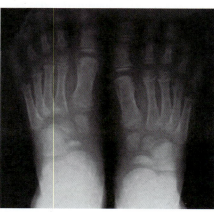

G Köhler disease The navicular is small, collapsed and hyperdense (*red*), and the site of tenderness.

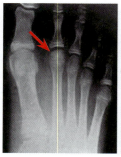
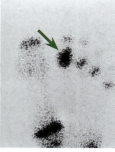

H Freiberg infraction The 2nd metatarsal head shows sclerosis but no collapse or other irregularity (*red*). Scintigramme shows increased uptake (*green*).

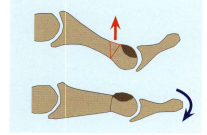

I Metatarsal osteotomy for Freiberg infraction Realignment of the avascular segment (*brown*).

the tarsal tunnel extension of the flexor retinaculum (laciniate ligament) from malleolus of the tibia to calcaneus and plantar aponeurosis.

Evaluation Rarity in children results in delayed diagnosis. Insidious onset medial ankle pain, including at night, together with plantar dysæsthesia in adolescent girls more than boys. Tinel sign is pathognomonic on physical examination, which also reveals inversion of the hindfoot to relax tibial nerve such that the patient walks on the lateral border of the foot. Dorsiflexion–eversion is a provocative test to stretch tibial nerve. Delayed tibial nerve conduction confirms the diagnosis. A local anæsthetic block aids prediction of operative result.

Management Rest the ankle by modifying activity and with an orthotic as necessary. Decompression of the tarsal tunnel is indicated for persistent symptoms and disability. Include the flexor retinaculum, and the origins of abductor hallucis muscle from calcaneus and plantar aponeurosis proximally as well as from between medial and lateral plantar nerves.

Os Trigonum

This secondary ossification center may remain separate from the posterior lateral rim of the talus as a silent accessorium [F]. Such an ossicle has smooth borders without sclerosis. If the bone is fractured off the talus during forced ankle extension under load, such as *en pointe*, it will hurt and will continue to do when this action is repeated.

Evaluation Dancers are most affected. Pain is localized to the posterior ankle with stress manœuvre. Röntgenogrammes show the bone, which may move on flexion and extension lateral views of the ankle. Scintigraphy shows focal increased uptake. MRI will show inflammatory changes in the bone and surrounding soft tissue, including flexor hallucis longus tenosynovitis.

Management Symptom control and activity modification may not be practicable in an active child, such as a ballerina. If unacceptable pain persists, excise the ossicle and decompress the flexor hallucis longus *via* an incision off the lateral border of tendo Achillis or with the assistance of an endoscope.

Osteochondrosis

Sever and Köhler conditions (not "diseases," not "syndromes") are relatively common and benign, having a natural history characterized by spontaneous resolution with supportive care for pain. Freiberg infraction is rare and obscure, with grave potential.

Sever

This represents apophysitis of the calcaneus. Traction by the tendo Achillis, developmentally short or tightened by growth acceleration, results in micromotion between apophysis and remainder of bone.

Evaluation Presentation is at the turn of the decades. There is tenderness over the apophysis. There is contracture of triceps suræ, which reproduces the pain upon stretching and may elicit posterior knee pain at the origin of gastrocnemius. Imaging is negative; in fact, röntgenogrammes may raise unnecessary concern about the normal fragmented and sclerotic appearance of the apophysis.

Management Address the tight triceps suræ either by compensating for it, for example, with a heel lift, or by stretching it, with exercises. Educate the patient and family that this will resolve but may take months.

Köhler

Collapse, sclerosis, and fragmentation of the navicular [G]. A propensity for boys, in whom the bone ossifies 1 to 2 years later (by 5 years of age) and therefore may be mechanically vulnerable to repetitive injury, the radiographic appearance, and histologic studies showing necrotic bone suggest a vascular insult. This insult is transient and reversible, because the bone recovers completely.

Evaluation Presentation is in the middle of the 1st decade. There is focal tenderness at navicular, which may be prominent and red due to inflammation. Röntgenogrammes confirm the diagnosis and alarm the parents; they also demonstrate reconstitution over 1 to 3 years.

Management Educate parents that this looks worse than it is, including a > 30-year follow-up study showing no sequelæ in adulthood. Modify activity. For significant pain, for example, limp, unable to play, or participate in sports, apply a below-knee walking cast for 6 weeks.

Freiberg Infraction

Infraction reflects avascular necrosis, affecting the 2nd metatarsal head. Implicated causative factors include repetitive trauma, tenuity of blood supply, and abnormal loading of a prolonged 2nd metatarsal.

Evaluation Presentation is in the second decade, more often in girls. There is focal tenderness, limp, and poor push-off. Röntgenogrammes show collapse and irregularity of the 2nd metatarsal head. Scintigraphy may establish the diagnosis before radiographic change [H].

Management Educate the patient and parents that this may not resolve completely. Administer anti-inflammatory agents for a scheduled short course or *pro re nata*. Rest the foot in a cast for 6 weeks and follow with a custom orthotic to unload the 2nd metatarsal head or a firm sole shoe. Modify activity to minimize foot trauma.

Operative treatment is indicated for residual articular incongruity and overgrowth leading to persistent pain and degenerative changes.

- Joint débridement alleviates pain but may not be durable.
- Excisional arthroplasty of the proximal 2nd phalanx with interposition of the tendon of extensor digitorum longus decompresses the 2nd metatarsal head.
- Dorsiflexion osteotomy of the 2nd metatarsal may redirect a geographic lesion away from the weight bearing or joint loading [I].

TUMORS

The foot makes up 3% of body mass but 6% of musculoskeletal tumors. Weight bearing and exposure of the foot accelerate diagnosis. Indistinct fascial boundaries in mid- and hindfoot do not permit radical resection, by contrast with the forefoot, where ray resection permits salvage. Prosthetic replacement is compatible with good function.

Soft Tissue

Ganglion (Greek γαγγλιον: "knot, tumor, cyst") is most common and most benign. It is associated with joint or tendon and may be mistaken for an osseous excrescence, which may be ruled out by röntgenogramme. Treat symptomatically and accommodate to it, including by shoe and activity modification. Lesions responsible for unacceptable pain or dysfunction may be excised. Remain extracapsular to trace the stalk to its origin. Perform a capsulectomy to prevent reaccumulation by a one-way valve mechanism.

The benign tumors plantar fibromatosis and pigmented villonodular synovitis, as well as the malignant synovial cell sarcoma, are discussed in Tumors (*q.v.*).

Bone

Subungual exostosis arises frequently from the hallux [A]. The tumor displaces and distorts the nail plate and wall. As a result, it often is misdiagnosed as an infection or soft tissue excrescence and treated by other health care providers as such. Lack of success ultimately prompts referral or röntgenogrammes, which reveal the osseous lesion arising from the distal phalanx. Excise the lateral border of the nail plate for exposure. Sharply dissect the disrupted matrix to allow the most anatomic repair. Resect the entire osteochondroma flush with normal phalangeal cortex. Sew wall to plate to close the space.

The benign tumor cysts and chondroblastoma, as well as the malignant osteosarcoma, are discussed in Tumors (*q.v.*).

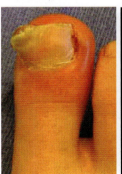 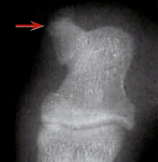

A Subungal exostosis This may be mistaken for infection or soft tissue excrescence. Röntgenogrammes confirm the diagnosis (*red*).

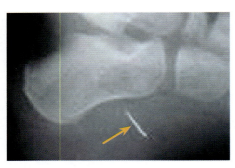

A Needle penetration into heel Site of entry and surrounding inflammation (*red*) correspond with röntgenogrammes showing a broken tip (*orange*).

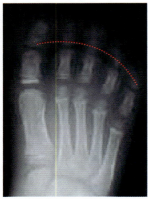
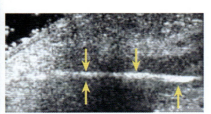

B Wood puncture The foot is swollen (*red*). Ultrasonogramme reveals a wood fragment (*yellow*) when röntgenogrammes show no foreign body.

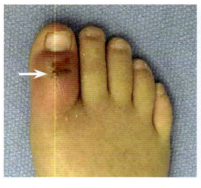
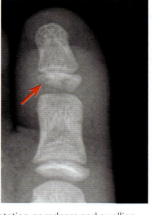

C Pseudomonas infection Delayed presentation or redness and swelling around a puncture wound (*white*) correlated with epiphysial erosion (*red*) suggestive of interphalangeal pyarthritis.

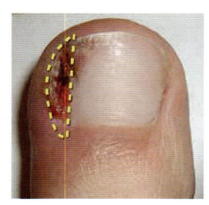

D Winograd operation for infected ingrown toenail Excises granulation tissue, lateral margin of plate, and germinal as well as sterile matrices (*yellow*).

INFECTION

Puncture Wounds

Most are plantar. Most infections are by *Staphylococcus aureus*. In shoes, *Pseudomonas æruginosa* becomes a significant though still secondary agent.

Evaluation Rule out retained foreign body. Röntgenogrammes show metal [A] and some glass according to lead content. They also show soft tissue swelling, obscuration of fascial planes, gas, and osteomyelitis. Ultrasonography is useful for wood and other radiolucent material [B]. Time to presentation of associated infection suggests the organism: 1 to 3 days *S. aureus*, 7 to 10 days *P. æruginosa*. Site also is suggestive: *P. æruginosa* is unlikely remote from a joint, such as the heel pad. Delayed presentation of redness and swelling is typical of pyarthritis by *P. æruginosa*, which is chondrophilic and slow growing [C].

Management Update tetanus immunization. Wound exploration in the emergency setting is too much for the child and often for the surgeon: do this in the operating room, where a thorough irrigation can be performed. For clean wounds, administer a antibiotic *per venam* to cover gram-positive organisms and follow within the week. Operative treatment is indicated for a dirty contamination, such as from a farm, together with expanded coverage for gram-negative and anaerobic organisms. Educate parents to return for any sign of delayed infection, including pain, redness, swelling, and fever over the subsequent 7 to 10 days, the temporal window for *Pseudomonas* pyarthritis. This is a surgical emergency.

Paronychia

Infected ingrown toenails [D] result from anatomical predisposition, improper nail trimming, and repetitive trauma in a shoe. There is a greater lateral curvature of the nail plate into the nail wall. Nails are trimmed too proximal, such that during growth, the corner of the plate drives into rather than clear of the distal extension of the nail wall. Shoe preference is tight with a narrow toe box. The most common pathogen is *S. aureus*.

Evaluation Granulation tissue overlies the junction of the nail plate and wall, which is swollen and tender.

Management Educate the patient on proper nail trimming, which includes leaving the corners of the plate clear of the walls rather than continuing in a smooth round contour. Institute warm dilute soap water soaks twice daily. Insert a cotton wisp under corner of plate twice daily to provide a ramp that separates the plate from the wall during growth. Antibiotics accelerate recovery.

For persistent or recurrent infection, matricectomy is indicated (C). Débride granulation tissue gently, in order not to damage nail wall for later repair. Excise the lateral edge of the nail plate. Curette away subjacent germinal and sterile matrices to bone of phalanx. Repair of wall to remaining plate narrows the nail.

TOE DEFORMITY

Aikin OF. The treatment of hallux valgus: a new operative procedure and its results. *Med. Sentinel* 33:678–679, 1925.

Albuisson J, Isidor B, Giraud M, Pichon O, Marsaud T, David A, Le Caignec C, Bezieau S. Identification of two novel mutations in Shh long-range regulator associated with familial pre-axial polydactyly. *Clin. Genet.* 79(4):371–377, 2011.

Chang CH, Kumar SJ, Riddle EC, Glutting J. Macrodactyly of the foot. *J. Bone Joint Surg.* 84-A:1189–1194, 2002.

Cockin J. Butler's operation for an over-riding fifth toe. *J. Bone Joint Surg.* 50-B(1):78–81, 1968.

Furniss D, Critchley P, Giele H, Wilkie AOM. Nonsense-mediated decay and the molecular pathogenesis of mutations in SALL1 and GLI3. *Am. J. Med. Genet.* 143A(24):3150–3160, 2007.

Girdlestone GR. *J. Chartered Soc. Physiotherapy* 32:167, 1947.

Lichtblau S. Section of the abductor hallucis tendon for correction of metatarsus adductus varus deformity. *Clin. Orthop.* 110:227–232, 1975.

M[c]Bride ED. A conservative approach to bunions. *J. Bone Joint Surg.* 10:735–739, 1928.

Peterson HA, Newman SR. Adolescent bunion deformity treated with double osteotomy and longitudinal pin fixation of the first ray. *J. Pediatr. Orthop.* 13(1):80–84, 1993.

Radhakrishna U, Blouin J-L, Mehenni H, Patel UC, Patel MN, Solanki JV, Antonarakis SE. Mapping one form of autosomal dominant postaxial polydactyly type A to chromosome 7p15-q11.23 by linkage analysis. *Am. J. Hum. Genet.* 60(3):597–604, 1997.

Shea KG, Mubarak SJ, Alamin T. Preossified longitudinal epiphyseal bracket of the foot: treatment by partial bracket excision before ossification. *J. Pediatr. Orthop.* 21(3):360–365, 2001.

Taylor RG. The treatment of claw toes by multiple transfers if flexor into extensor tendons. *J. Bone Joint Surg.* 33-B(4):539–542, 1951.

Umm-e-Kalsoom BS, Kamran-ul-Hassan NS, Ansar M, Ahmad W. Genetic mapping of an autosomal recessive postaxial polydactyly type A to chromosome 13q13.3-q21.2 and screening of the candidate genes. *Hum. Genet.* 131(3):415–422, 2012.

FOREFOOT

Kite JH. Congenital metatarsus varus: report of 300 cases. *J. Bone Joint Surg.* 32(3)-A:500–506, 1950.

HINDFOOT

Alvarado DM, M[c]Call K, Aferol H, Silva MJ, Garbow JR, Spees WM, Patel T, Siegel M, Dobbs MB, Gurnett CA. Pitx1 haploinsufficiency causes clubfoot in humans and a clubfoot-like phenotype in mice. *Hum. Mol. Genet.* 20(20):3943–3952, 2011.

Anderson RJ. The presence of an astragaloschaphoid bone in man. *J. Anat. Physiol.* 14:452–455, 1879.

Browne D. Modern methods of treatment of club-foot. *Br. Med. J.* Sep:570–572, 1937.

Cowell HR. Extensor brevis arthroplasty. *J. Bone Joint Surg.* 52-A:820, 1970.

Crim J, Kjeldsberg K. Radiographic diagnosis of tarsal coalition. *Am. J. Roentgenol.* 182(2):323–328, 2004.

Evans D. Relapsed clubfoot. *J. Bone Joint Surg.* 43-B:722–733, 1961.

Ezra E, Hayek S, Gilai AN, Khermosh O, Wientroub S. Tibialis anterior tendon transfer for residual dynamic supination deformity in treated club feet. *J. Pediatr. Orthop.* 9(3)-B:207–211, 2000.

Giannini S, Ceccarelli F, Vannini F, Baldi E. Operative treatment of flatfoot with talocalcaneal coalition. *Clin Orthop.* 411:178–187, 2003.

Grogan DP, Gasser SI, Ogden JA. The painful accessory navicular: a clinical and histopathological study. *Foot Ankle* 10(3):164–169, 1989.

Kite JH. *The Clubfoot.* New York, NY: Grune & Stratton; 1964.

Leonard MA. The inheritance of tarsal coalition and its relationship to spastic flat foot. *J. Bone Joint Surg.* 56(3)-B:520–526, 1974.

Lichtblau S. A medial and lateral release operation for clubfoot: a preliminary report. *J. Bone Joint Surg.* 55(7)-A:1377–1384, 1973.

M[c]Kay DW. New concept of and approach to clubfoot treatment. Section II. Correction of the clubfoot. *J. Pediatr. Orthop.* 3(1):10–21, 1983.

Ponseti IV. Congenital club foot: the results of treatment. *J. Bone Joint Surg.* 45(2)-A:261–344, 1963.

Raikin S, Cooperman DR, Thompson GH. Interposition of the split flexor hallucis longus tendon after resection of a coalition of the middle facet of the talocalcaneal joint. *J. Bone Joint Surg.* 81(1)-A:11–19, 1999.

Swiontkowski MF, Scranton PE, Hansen S. Tarsal coalitions: long-term results of surgical treatment. *J. Pediatr. Orthop.* 3(3):287–292, 1983.

Turco VJ. Surgical correction of the resistant clubfoot: one stage posteromedial release with internal fixation. *J. Bone Joint Surg.* 53(3)-A:477–497, 1971.

Wilde PH, Torode IP, Dickens DR, Cole WG. Resection for symptomatic talocalcaneal coalition. *J. Bone Joint Surg.* 76(5)-B:797–801, 1994.

Zadek J, Gold AM. The accessory tarsal scaphoid. *J. Bone Joint Surg.* 30(4)-A:957–968, 1948.

MIDFOOT

Dwyer FC. Osteotomy of the calcaneum for pes cavus. *J. Bone Joint Surg.* 41-B:80–86, 1959.

Echarri JJ, Forriol F. The development in footprint morphology in 1851 Congolese children from urban and rural areas, and the relationship between this and wearing shoes. *J. Pediatr. Orthop.* 12(2)-B:141–146, 2003.

Harris RI, Beath T. Etiology of peroneal spastic flat foot. *J. Bone Joint Surg.* 30(4)-B:624–634, 1948.

Harris RI, Beath T. Hypermobile flat-foot with short tendo achillis. *J. Bone Joint Surg.* 30(1)-A:116–140, 1948.

Hibbs RA. An operation for "clawfoot". *JAMA* 73:1583–1585, 1919.

Jahss MH. Tarsometatarsal truncated-wedge arthrodesis for pes cavus and equinovarus deformity of the fore part of the foot. *J. Bone Joint Surg.* 62(5)-A:713–722, 1980.

Japas LM. Surgical treatment of pes cavus by V-osteotomy: preliminary report. *J. Bone Joint Surg.* 50(5)-A:927–944, 1968.

Lamy L, Weissman L. Congenital convex pes planus. *J. Bone Joint Surg.* 21(1):79–91, 1939.

Mazzocca AD, Thomson JD, Deluca PA, Romness MJ. Comparison of the posterior approach versus the dorsal approach in the treatment of congenital vertical talus. *J. Pediatr. Orthop.* 21(2):212–217, 2001.

Méary R. Symposium sur le pied creux essentiel. *Rev. Chir. Orthop.* 53:390–466, 1967.

Mosca VS. Calcaneal lengthening for valgus deformity of the hindfoot. Results in children who had severe, symptomatic flatfoot and skewfoot. *J. Bone Joint Surg.* 77(4)-A:500–512, 1995.

Peterson HA. Skewfoot (forefoot adduction with heel valgus). *J. Pediatr Orthop.* 6(1):24–30, 1986.

Ragab AA, Stewart SL, Cooperman DR. Implications of subtalar joint anatomic variation in calcaneal lengthening osteotomy. *J. Pediatr. Orthop.* 23(1):79–83, 2003.

Staheli LT, Chew DE, Corbett M. The longitudinal arch: A survey of eight hundred and eighty-two feet in normal children and adults. *J. Bone Joint Surg.* 69(3)-A:426–428, 1987.

Steindler A. Stripping of the os calcis. *J. Orthop. Surg.* 2(1):8–12, 1920.

van der Wilde R, Staheli LT, Chew DE, Malagon V. Measurements on radiographs of the foot in normal infants and children. *J. Bone Joint Surg.* 70(3)-A:407–415, 1988.

Ward CM, Dolan LA, Bennett DL, Morcuende JA, Cooper RR. Long-term results of reconstruction for treatment of a flexible cavovarus foot in Charcot-Marie-Tooth disease. *J. Bone Joint Surg.* 90(12)-A:2631–2642, 2008.

Wenger DR, Leach J. Corrective shoes and inserts as treatment for flexible flatfoot in infants and children. *J. Bone Joint Surg.* 71(6)-A:800–810, 1989.

ANKLE

Alberktsson B, Rydholm A, Rydholm U. The tarsal tunnel syndrome in children. *J. Bone Joint Surg.* 64(2)-B:215–217, 1982.

Grogan DP, Walling AK, Ogden JA. Anatomy of the os trigonum. *J. Pediatr. Orthop.* 10(5):618–622, 1990.

Lamb D. The ball and socket ankle joint; a congenital abnormality. *J. Bone Joint Surg.* 40(2)-B:240–243, 1958.

Silfverskiöld N. Reduction of the uncrossed two-joints muscles of the leg to one-joint muscles in spastic conditions. *Acta Chir. Scand.* 56:315–330, 1924.

Strayer LM. Recession of the gastrocnemius; an operation to relieve spastic contracture of the calf muscles. *J. Bone Joint Surg.* 32(3)-A:671–676, 1950.

OSTEOCHONDROSIS

Borges JL, Guille JT, Bowen JR. Köhler's bone disease of the tarsal navicular. *J. Pediatr. Orthop.* 15(5):596–598, 1995.

Freiberg AH. Infraction of the second metatarsal bone. A typical injury. *Surg. Gynecol. Obstetr.* 19:191–193, 1914.

Köhler A. Über eine haufige bisher anscheinend unbekannte Erkrankung einzelner kindlicher Knowchen. *Munchen Med. Wochenschr.* 55:1923, 1908.

Sever JW. Apophysitis of the os calcis. *NY State J. Med.* 95:1025–1029, 1912.

Waugh W. The ossification and vascularization of the tarsal navicular and their relation to Köhler's disease. *J. Bone Joint Surg.* 40(4)-B:765–777, 1958.

TUMOR

Landon GC, Johnson KA, Dahlin DC. Subungual exostosis. *J. Bone Joint Surg.* 61(2)-A:256–259, 1979.

INFECTION

Jacobs RF, M[c]Carthy RE, Elser JM. Pseudomonas osteochondritis complicating puncture wounds of the foot in children: a 10-year evaluation. *J. Infect. Dis.* 160(4):657–661, 1989.

Winograd AM: Modification in the technic of operation for ingrown toe-nail. *JAMA* 92:229–230, 1929.

TRAUMA

Trauma is the leading cause of death in children. It is second to infection as a cause of morbidity. Fractures peak during lunch play in school and in late afternoon during sports. Three-fourths of fractures occur outdoors. One-fourth of fractures are of the radius [A]. The most common operated fracture is of the supracondylar humeral region. The school playground is the richest source of fractures. Boys sustain more fractures than do girls [B]. Annual fracture incidence in children is 2%. Refracture rate averages 0.5%, higher for some (e.g., of radius and ulna), and lower for others

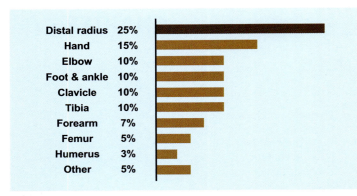

A Distribution of fractures by location Numbers have been simplified to aid comparisons.

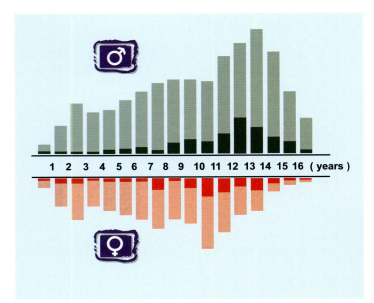

B Distribution of fractures by gender and age Boys (*green*) have a peak 3 years after girls (*red*). Physeal fractures (*dark*) represent 1/5 of children's fractures.

Feature	Management
Chondral model	Less visible on röntgenogramme
Peri-osteum	Healing Internal stability
Bone	Less mineral, more cancellous: ductile—yield not break less comminution
Physis	Point of weakness Growth disturbance Remodeling
Ligaments	Last to fail Joint stability Fracture before ligament tear

C Structural features of a child's bone The distinctive features significantly affect management.

and lower for others. Increasing sports participation is shifting the number of fractures to younger patients. Most pædiatric fractures are isolated and of the appendicular skeleton, which form the subject of this chapter.

PHYSIOLOGY

Children's bones differ from those of adults [C]. The differences and consequences diminish with age, so that during adolescence, treatment approaches that of the adult.

Growth Plate

The growth plate, or physis, is the most distinctive feature of a child's skeleton. It adds to the risk of growth disturbance. It is weaker than bone, which is weaker than ligament [D]. It is most vulnerable during periods of growth acceleration, such as puberty. It enables remodeling [E].

Remodeling This refers to correction of a malaligned bone with growth [E]. This consists of two principal components:

- Differential growth at the physis, which accelerates on the concave side
- Differential growth at the fracture, which shows periosteal laying down of bone by apposition in the concavity and bone resorption on the convexity of the apex of deformity

Remodeling rectifies epiphysial and articular orientation, as well as the mechanical axis. Several factors influence remodeling:

- Growth of the child. This is determined by maturity, which may be measured by Tanner stage or years of growth remaining based upon the arithmetic method that states girls stop growing significantly around 14 years and boys around 16 years.

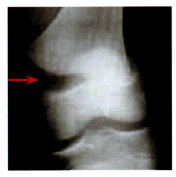

D The physis is weak Force of fracture travels along the path of least resistance, the distal femoral physis (*red*).

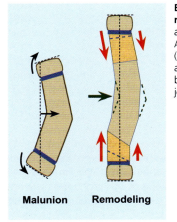

E Mechanism for remodeling Differential growth occurs at physis (*red*) and periosteum (*green*). As remodeling proceeds, mechanical axis (*black*) centers toward the longitudinal axis of the bone, and the epiphyses become horizontal to rectify the adjacent joints.

Malunion   Remodeling

While 2 years of growth remaining may be regarded as a requirement for remodeling, the process is more predictable for fractures occurring in the first decade than in the second decade.

- Growth of the bone. Physes that are more active are more potent. The greatest percent growth of bone occurs at proximal humerus more than distal radius more than distal femur [F]. As a result, greater displacement of fractures of proximal humerus and distal radius may be accepted: remodeling substitutes for reduction [G].
- Location of fracture within a bone. More remodeling is required in the diaphysis than in the metaphysis [H]
- Plane of joint motion. Forces that stimulate new bone formation are greatest in the plane of motion (Wolff law). In addition, an enarthrodial joint can accommodate greater residual deformity than a more restricted joint, such as a ginglymus, which can accommodate only in the sagittal plane of motion.

Duration of acute remodeling, which is the period of observation before intervention for malunion, is typically 1 year but occasionally up to 2 years, for example, proximal metaphysis of tibia fracture.

Injury Physes are located adjacent to an epiphysis, which is a secondary ossification center that forms the articular surface of a bone "on top" (Greek επι−) of the physis, and an apophysis, which grows "away" (Greek απο−) from the physis to serve as a site of attachment of a muscle. Injuries to and displacement of the former are less tolerated than are the latter. Ligaments attach to epiphyses, thereby concentrating force during joint motion at the physis, which increases risk of injury.

Growth disturbance occurs most frequently from trauma and infection. Infection typically results in a diffuse zone of injury. Trauma may do the same, as in a crush mechanism, or it may produce a discrete bridge of bone: displacement brings metaphysis from one side into contact with epiphysis on the other side, which unite. Injury also may stimulate a growth plate to overgrow. This is most striking in the femur and may be related to hyperæmia.

Force of fracture travels through the hypertrophic zone, because this is the level of highest stress concentration between the zone of provisional calcification adjacent to metaphysis and the proliferative and germinal zones adjacent to epiphysis. Growth will resume after fracture provided the blood supply is preserved, and there is no mechanical disruption of the rest of the physis. The latter may occur at an undulating or otherwise irregular physis, such as the distal femur or distal tibia, where "Poland hump" may act as a spike to tear across the proliferative and germinal zones. The distal physis of tibia also is vulnerable due to force concentration of body weight over a relatively small area. This may explain injury to the tibial apophysis, where force of quadriceps is concentrated.

Injury may be marked on bone by a growth arrest line (Harris) [I]. This represents condensation of mineral due to temporary growth arrest locally after fracture or diffusely after a generalized severe illness. Date of injury may be calculated based upon distance from physis and physeal rate of growth. Slowing or arrest of growth is indicated by a reduction of distance. Partial growth disturbance is suggested by obliquity of the line relative to the physis, suggesting asymmetric growth by an unhealthy physis.

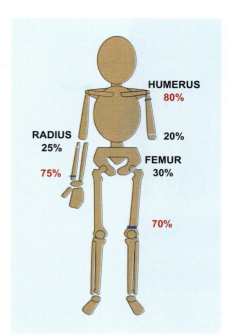

F Remodeling at physis This is proportional to % of total bone growth. Proximal humerus, distal radius, and distal femur have best remodeling potential.

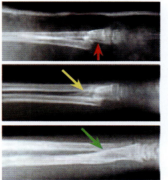

G Remodeling of forearm In the radius, the distal fragment is apposed to the proximal fragment like a bayonet on the barrel of a rifle. Callus is laid down in the concavity on the dorsum, thereby straightening the fracture over several months (*green*). In the proximal humerus, a completely displaced fracture (*red*), including angulation >60 degrees and significant shortening, remodels completely (*green*). Both children are <10 years.

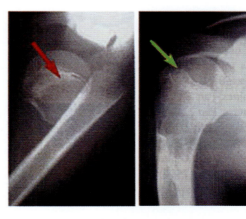

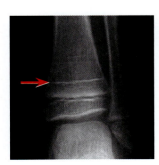

I Growth arrest line This (*red*) is parallel to the distal physis of tibia, suggesting symmetric growth. The distance of 5 mm after 1 year is consistent with normal growth rate of an uninjured physis.

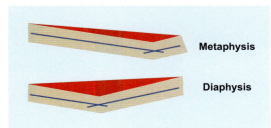

H Remodeling according to site For the same angular deformity, more correction (area in *red*) is required for midshaft than distal deformity.

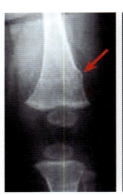
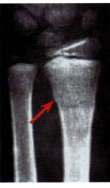

J Buckle fracture This is characteristic of immature bone.

Bone

Reduction in mineralization with a more collagenous extracellular matrix, and a larger proportion of cellular component, result in a more ductile material that can buckle when stressed [J] or plastically deform [K] and that resists fragmenting into multiple pieces. The lag in mineralization behind longitudinal growth renders immature bone more porous and thereby more susceptible to injury.

Periosteum

This is more metabolically active in the child than in the adult. It does not tear as readily, leaving continuity for new bone formation. This explains the exuberant callus seen in the infant and the rapid union and increased potential for remodeling seen throughout childhood. The periosteum is thick. The structural integrity of a child's periosteum adds internal stability to fractures. However, it also may interfere with reduction and growth if it becomes entrapped within a fracture.

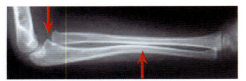

K Plastic deformation The fixed deformity drives the head of radius out of joint and prevents it from relocating. A more brittle bone would break, which would increase displacement and the chance of spontaneous reduction of radial head.

Ligaments

In a child, ligament is stronger than bone, which is stronger than physis [L]. Ligaments, and perichondrium, protect a physis they span from displacement. Ligaments resist failure such that they do not tear but rather transmit force to dissipate in an avulsion fracture [M].

Chondral Model

An increasing proportion of the skeleton, growing by endochondral ossification, is invisible on röntgenogramme with decreasing age. Early on, landmarks may be absent. Later, articular fragment size may be underestimated, as typified by the patellar sleeve fracture [M].

CLASSIFICATION

There are several classifications of pædiatric fractures. In the most accepted system [A], fractures are divided into five categories based upon pattern and mechanism, as evaluated by röntgenogramme. Type V is rare and identifiable only in retrospect, when compression of the physis has led to growth disturbance. The first four types may be divided into two groups, extra-articular or articular, thereby dividing fractures into those which risk growth and those which risk growth and osteoarthritis. The two groups also may be distinguished by operative rate. Physeal fractures are managed according to criteria for acceptable displacement that vary according to site; most are treated nonoperatively. Articular fractures are treated according to universal principles, which do not accept >2-mm step-off in order to minimize risk of osteoarthritis; as a result, most are treated operatively.

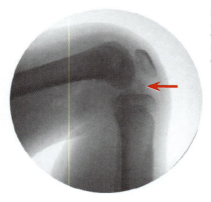

L Ligament avulsion The intercondylar eminence of tibia fails before the anterior cruciate ligament, which may stretch but does not tear.

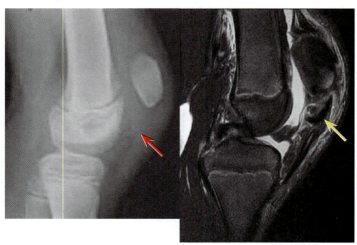

M Chondral model The apex of patella pulls off with a sleeve of cartilage that is barely visible on röntgenogramme (*red*) yet represents a large semilunar fragment when viewed by MRI (*yellow*).

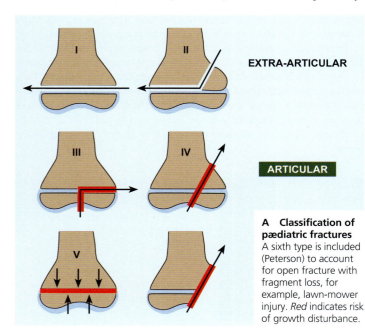

EXTRA-ARTICULAR

ARTICULAR

A Classification of pædiatric fractures A sixth type is included (Peterson) to account for open fracture with fragment loss, for example, lawn-mower injury. *Red* indicates risk of growth disturbance.

EVALUATION

Up to 15% of fractures in children are missed or misdiagnosed at first evaluation. Individual fractures will be addressed separately.

History

Infants do not speak. Falls and other mechanisms may be unwitnessed. Children, who are in pain and scared, may not be able or willing to answer questions. Caregivers of abused children will be evasive or lie.

Physical Examination

Pseudoparalysis refers to refusal to use a limb because of pain. The upper limb is held suspended as if paralyzed. The child refuses to bear weight on the lower limb. Because the child comes with parents, and both may be distressed, there is pressure not to disturb the child any more than already has been done, by injury, by those enlisted to help at the scene, by transportation to a medical facility, and by others who already have examined the child. Be thorough, for example, do not miss an open wound covered by a splint. Be persistent: management of a postoperative neural deficit after reduction and fixation of a supracondylar humerus fracture is predicated on knowledge of the preoperative function.

Divide type I open fractures into outside-in and inside-out [A]. The latter is produced by the osseous fragment pushing through the skin from a clean environment, rather than in the former case, where contamination from the outside may be introduced into the fracture. Inside-out open fractures may be washed in the emergency setting, treated with a single dose of antibiotics, and treated as though closed with close observation. After cast application, cut a window in the cast to make the lesion visible for follow-up. All other open fractures are managed according to general principles. The window for surgical débridement may be opened to 24 hours in children.

Compartment syndrome in children is not as fulminant as in adults. Bleeding raises compartment pressure, producing a tense limb that hurts. Increasing pressure, exacerbated by capillary leaking, first occludes venous outflow and only later occludes arterial flow to produce pallor, pulselessness, and paræsthesias. Have a high index of suspicion, for example, after supracondylar humerus fracture. While this is a clinical diagnosis first and foremost, data may be necessary in children when their presentation may be mild [B]. Delay in diagnosis is not unusual, but this is mitigated by the fact that full recovery may be expected up to 36 hours after injury. Distinguish exertional compartment syndrome (*cf.* Sports chapter).

Imaging

Röntgenogramme This is the mainstay of trauma imaging. In addition to anteroposterior and lateral projections, special views may be helpful, for example, oblique for condylar fractures [C] and mortise of the ankle. Beware of TRASH: The Radiologic Appearance Seemed Harmless. The term encompasses osteochondral lesions that may be incompletely visible on this imaging modality. These typically occur in the first decade. The elbow is a rich source, due to the multiple ossification centers with varying appearance, such as an epiphysial separation in the infant, a displaced intra-articular medial condyle fracture, or radiocapitular subluxation. Occult injuries may manifest secondarily in soft tissue, for example, the sail sign at the elbow [D]. Imaging the contralateral uninjured side may be helpful in the setting of atypia, such as a skeletal dysplasia.

Arthrogram This outlines the articular surface when affected by fracture and unossified [E]. In addition to aiding diagnosis, this modality may influence operative decision making and may be used to confirm acceptability of reduction of articular fractures, for example, of the lateral condyle of humerus (*q.v.*).

Scintigramme This also is useful for röntgenographically occult injury. In a child who refuses to bear weight on the lower limb or in whom the physical examination is nonlocalizing, scintigramme may reveal an injury and focus the evaluation.

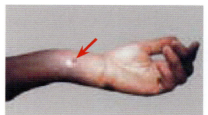

A Type I open fracture This inside-out subtype, resulting from a "poke" through the skin (*red*) by a bone fragment, may be treated with local care at initial encounter, after which it is managed as a closed fracture with close follow-up.

Pressure

Diastolic pressure—compartmental pressure ≤30 mm Hg

Compartment pressure ≥30 mm Hg

Mean arterial pressure—compartment pressure ≤40 mm Hg

B Compartment syndrome These data have been suggested to support the clinical diagnosis of compartment syndrome.

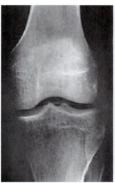
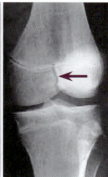

C Special views on röntgenogramme Oblique projection (*blue*) uncovers a condylar fracture invisible on standard anteroposterior projection.

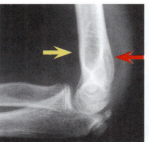

D Soft tissue on röntgenogramme Bleeding from an occult fracture elevates the joint capsule, creating a contrast in density. The sign is significant posteriorly (*red*) when the elbow is at 90 degrees of flexion because the capsule is draped tightly over the back of the joint, requiring significant fluid under pressure to elevate it. An anterior sign (*yellow*) is inconclusive as the capsule is relaxed off the distal humerus in this elbow position.

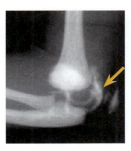

E Arthrogram for radionegative injury The distal epiphysis of humerus is unossified in the 1st year of life. Thus, an epiphysial separation (*orange*) is invisible on röntgenogramme, where the secondary signs of abnormal relationships of radius and ulna with humerus raise suspicion that is confirmed by arthrogram.

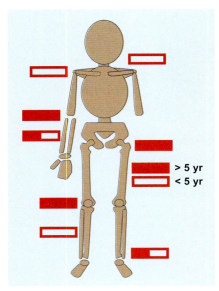

A Operative treatment In the immature child, the rate (*red*) varies by site. Overall rate is increasing, the forearm having the greatest flux.

> 5 yr
< 5 yr

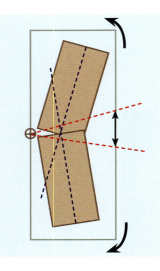

B Cast wedging If fragments drift in a cast, cut it at the level of the fracture. The center of rotation for correction is not the apex of fracture but the edge of the cast. Draw lines perpendicular to the fragments (*red*), intersect them at the edge of the cast at the level of the fracture, and measure the distance (*black*) on the opposite side of the cast to determine the size of dowel to be inserted. Cut the dowel to have flanges that are applied to the outside surface of the cast where they prevent migration inward to pressure the skin.

Computed Tomography This is most useful to evaluate an articular fracture, to most accurately measure interruption of the surface. While outcome studies have suggested that >2 mm of articular step-off on röntgenogramme significantly increases the risk of posttraumatic arthritis in certain joints, for example, wrist and ankle, this rule has been extrapolated widely to all joints and to CT, which is a more sensitive modality. There is no consensus on diastasis without step-off. CT also aids preoperative planning, for example, to determine location of fixation in a triplane ankle fracture.

Magnetic Resonance Imaging Use judiciously, as this modality requires sedation of a first-decade child. MRI is most useful to evaluate associated soft tissue injury, such as in the setting of spine fracture in order to evaluate the neural elements, or at the knee in order to rule out meniscal tear in the setting of intercondylar eminence of tibia fracture. MRI often is utilized for complications and preparation for reconstruction, for example, mapping of a physeal bridge or determination of presence and extent of osteonecrosis of the head of femur.

Ultrasonogramme This is inexpensive, nonradiating, portable, and facile in the outpatient or emergency setting where it may be performed by the surgeon; is not stressful; and asks little of the child. It is useful for diaphyseal fractures, where its specificity may be relied upon in decision to image further. The imprecision of ultrasonogramme around physes and joints limits its utility and influence on management.

MANAGEMENT

Cast

This is safe and inexpensive and has long experience to support it. Not as relevant to children as they are in adults are concerns about joint stiffness and interference with activities such as mobility and work. Despite this, operative treatment for children's fractures is on the rise [A]. Fiberglass is becoming the standard because it is less messy and lighter.

A splint may be applied at the initial encounter, for example, emergency department, if operation is anticipated or if the limb must remain accessible for observation, for example, swelling.

Position the patient, and assistant, appropriately. A stockinette may be folded to soften cast edges. For width of padding, balance risk of pressure sore against loss of reduction. Focus padding over prominences, for example, malleolus; over other areas of stress concentration, for example, cast edges; and where a saw will cut the cast, for example, "racing strips" along anticipated path of saw, at time of cast removal. Extensor transitions may be angled, to limit sliding of the limb in cast, for example, right angle at posterior elbow; by contrast, flexor transitions must be smooth, for example, in the antecubital fossa, to avoid soft tissue injury.

Roll—do not stretch—cast material, in order not to compress the muscle compartments. Open casts, for example, "bivalve," if swelling is anticipated. Cut the padding as well if bleeding is anticipated, as blood will harden padding risking a circumferential constriction.

A waterproof cast is attractive to patients: it allows bathing but requires care to dry. It may give a conflicting signal to a child who has been instructed in protected weight bearing yet is allowed to swim with a cast.

Wedge a cast for fragment drift [B].

A plaster cast may be soaked off. Plaster and fiberglass casts typically are sawed off. The saw has a blunt blade that breaks a cast and as such will not cut skin it touches transiently. Gain the child (and the parent's) confidence by demonstrating on your finger and inviting the child to try. The blade heats as it works, thereby risking skin burns that may leave a permanent scar. Insert plastic strips where there is access to protect the skin. Stop periodically and cool the blade. Renew the blade regularly. Do not dwell: push in, pull out, and keep moving.

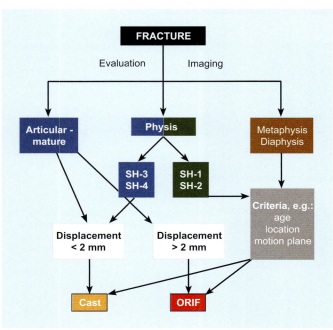

C Algorithm for management of children's fractures.

FRACTURE

Evaluation   Imaging

Articular - mature   Physis   Metaphysis Diaphysis

SH-3 SH-4   SH-1 SH-2

Criteria, e.g.: age location motion plane

Displacement < 2 mm   Displacement > 2 mm

Cast   ORIF

Fixation

Use enough fixation. If mobilization is not imperative, supplement with a cast, which may allow simpler and less morbid fixation, for example, inserted percutaneously and removed in the clinic. The soft tissue envelope, including periosteum, is robust, and the energy of injury is more likely low compared with adults. As a result, children's fractures have inherent stability, which, along with more rapid and reliable healing, allows for less invasive and less rigid fixation, for example, elastic nails instead of plates.

The articular surface is more important than the physis: do not sacrifice reduction and stability for concerns about growth disturbance. Osteoarthritis has no simple solution, whereas much can be done about growth disturbance. Furthermore, implants (even threaded) may be placed across a physis so long as their cross-sectional area is small, the physis is not dissected (extraperiosteal, extrachondral), and they are removed within 2 years (before the physis gives up growth).

Remove plates applied in the first decade. Periosteal appositional growth will make them intraosseous by maturity. Do not remove before 6 months, in order to minimize refracture. External fixators produce ugly scars. Their rigidity and any distraction at the fracture may delay union: do not remove them before there are at least three continuous cortices of bone. As with frames for lengthening, remove the barrel and let the child bear weight, with or without a cast, for 2 to 4 weeks. In the event of a refracture, the barrel may be applied in a reduced position.

Bend smooth wires with a long tail over the skin; otherwise, the skin will overgrow them. Save a child an anæsthetic by pulling wires in the clinic, even those placed medullary in the forearm. Deep infection is rare: irritated entry sites usually recover after wire removal.

Figure C represents an algorithm for management.

PHYSEAL BRIDGE

Growth disturbance after fracture may be due to chondrocyte injury in germinal or proliferative zones of the physis, or it may be due to a bridge (or bar) of bone forming across and tethering the physis. The former is remediable by secondary reconstruction, such as limb lengthening to compensate for growth arrest. The latter may be treated directly by bridge resection.

Small bridges may lyse spontaneously. Central bridges are more likely to lyse and less likely to cause deformity than peripheral ones. Central bridges may cause a fishtail deformity, which is better tolerated in the distal femur [A], where it results in a lower limb-length discrepancy, than in the distal humerus, where it is associated with elbow stiffness. Peripheral bridges produce angular deformity [B].

Time for growth is necessary for a disturbance to manifest. Educate patients about alignment of limb or joint, and follow up patients at risk through the anniversary of fracture. Röntgenographic findings include angulation after healing, asymmetric Harris growth arrest line, and limb-length discrepancy. MRI maps the physis to localize and aid determination of the extent of a bridge [C]. This modality may reduce zeal for resection, and thereby improve outcomes of resection, by giving a more accurate (and realistic) representation of the physis.

Resect bridges that occupy <25% to 50% of the physis and in a child with ≥2 years of growth remaining [D]. Outcomes are related to the size of the bridge and the health of the adjacent physis. Growth acceleration after peripheral bridge resection may correct angular deformity ≤10 degrees [E]. For greater angular deformity associated with a bridge, combine with a corrective osteotomy, which facilitates access to the bridge for resection.

If the physeal bridge exceeds 50%, complete physeodesis is indicated. For angular deformity, osteotomy may be performed through the physis, where a structural graft may be placed to accomplish both goals of physeodesis and correction. Residual limb-length discrepancy is managed according to general principles (*cf.* Limb chapter).

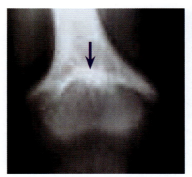

A Fishtail deformity This is produced by a central bridge, as seen on tomogram (*blue*).

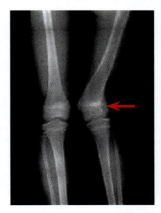

B Angular deformity This resulted from a Salter-Harris II fracture of the lateral distal femur (*red*).

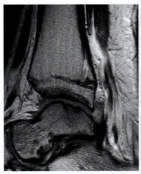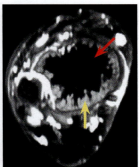

C Physeal bridge mapping MRI shows that the bridge is extensive, as evidenced by a ring of cartilage signal (*yellow*) surrounding a >50% center of bone (*red*) occupying the distal physis of tibia.

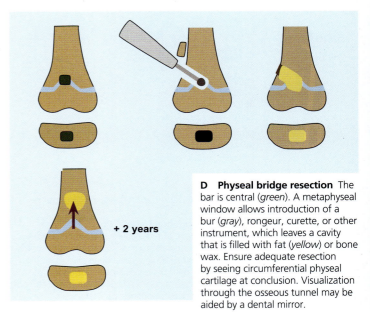

+ 2 years

D Physeal bridge resection The bar is central (*green*). A metaphyseal window allows introduction of a bur (*gray*), rongeur, curette, or other instrument, which leaves a cavity that is filled with fat (*yellow*) or bone wax. Ensure adequate resection by seeing circumferential physeal cartilage at conclusion. Visualization through the osseous tunnel may be aided by a dental mirror.

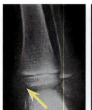
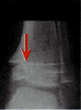
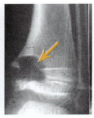
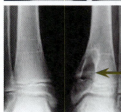

E   Resection of physeal bridge Salter-Harris III fracture (*yellow*) resulted in peripheral bridge (*red*). The bridge was resected leaving a hole that was filled with fat (*orange*). Growth resumed and function was normal despite the osseous scar (*green*).

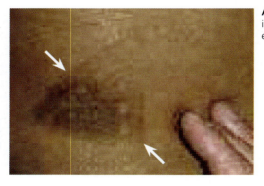

A   Skin stigma This iron mark is most eloquent.

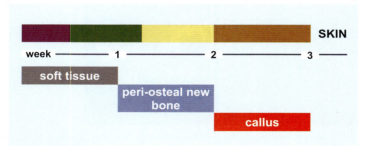

B   Corner fracture Timeline of changes in skin and bone after injury. Evidence of remodeling continues for months.

Specificity	Fracture
High	Corner, bucket handle Femur before walking age Posterior rib Scapula Spinous process Sternum
Medium	Multiple Bilateral Different stages of healing Skull
Low	Clavicle Long bone—pattern (transverse, spiral) nonspecific

C   Specificity of fractures for nonaccidental trauma. The activity level of an infant who does not walk is inconsistent with the energy necessary to break a femur. The thorax is flexible, making ribs and sternum difficult to break. Posterior rib fractures suggest a child running away. Scapula is embedded in muscle and takes considerable violence to break. Spinous processes break under vigorous traction. Multiple fractures in various stages of healing (15% of total presentations) are only medium in specificity, in part due to osteogenesis imperfecta.

NONACCIDENTAL TRAUMA

The original report emphasized skull fracture and multiple fractures in various stages of healing (Caffey). The New York Society for the Prevention of Cruelty to Children was founded in 1874 as the world's first child protective agency. The Federal Child Abuse Prevention and Treatment Act was established in 1974. One-third of abuse is neglect and 1/3 is physical injury, with the final 1/3 including sexual, emotional, and other causes.

The magnitude of the problem is arresting. Prevalence is 1%. Most abuse occurs in the first 3 years of life: 1/2 are <1 year and 1/4 are 1 to 3 years. Abuse accounts for 3/4 of fractures <2 years. After initial presentation, risk of repeat abuse (morbidity) is 1/3, while risk of death (mortality) is up to 10%.

Evaluation

Have a high index of suspicion, and be swayed only by objective findings, for example, not by socioeconomic level. Note that an abuser will seek attention at different facilities for repeat events. Infant prematurity, parental youth, and unmarried status are risks factors. The skin tells the story: cutaneous lesion is the most common finding [A], including burns and bruises. Bruises turn purple (0 to 3 days), then green-yellow (3 to 7 days), and then yellow-brown (after 1 week) [B]. Scalds spare inguinal and popliteal regions due to reflex flexion of hips and knees. One-third of children will have head injury.

Fractures may be categorized according to specificity for nonaccidental trauma [C]. The corner fracture is nonaccidental *a priori*. The differential diagnosis list includes osteogenesis imperfecta (in particular type IV, which does not have the distinctive blue sclerae), osteomyelitis, infantile cortical hyperostosis, leukæmia, hypervitaminosis A, and rickets.

Imaging

Röntgenogrammes are the standard, ordered *per* protocol: both views of chest and skull; anteroposterior views of arms, forearms, hands, pelvis, thighs, and legs; and lateral view of spine [D]. Scintigramme surveys the skeleton and may expose fractures in difficult to image locations in a young child with incomplete ossification. False-negative rate for röntgenogramme approaches 10%, whereas for scintigramme, it is 1%.

Management

Most important is safety of the child: consult other providers, including pædiatricians, who may admit a child to complete an evaluation, and social workers, who understand how to interface with governmental agencies.

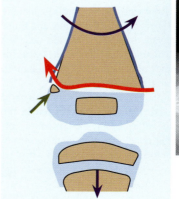
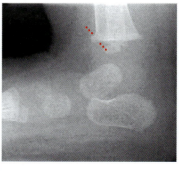

D   Corner fracture This is pathognomonic of nonaccidental trauma. The perichondrium holds on to a piece of bone at the corner of the metaphysis (*green*). Mechanism of injury is torsion under traction (*blue*). If the force (*red*) travels more proximal through metaphysis and breaks out at both metaphyseal corners, the curvilinear appearance has been likened to a "bucket handle."

FOOT

Foot fractures account for 5% of children's fractures, yet rarely is there an indication for operation. Half involve the metatarsal bones.

Toe

Hallux fracture may involve avulsion of the nail plate and injury to the nail matrix, which may be flipped into a physeal separation as indicated by persistent displacement despite reduction. Treat this open injury with irrigation, open reduction, and smooth wire fixation. Lesser toe injuries may be displaced such that they require reduction and buddy-tape immobilization.

Metatarsal

Fall from a height, such as a bunk bed, may result in a pædiatric equivalent of Lisfranc injury. This is characterized by a flexion and axial force that drives the medial cuneiform into the first metatarsal to second metatarsal interspace, creating a lateral proximal Salter-Harris IV fracture of the first metatarsal [A]. Reduce if necessary, fix with wires, and immobilize in a cast.

Stress fractures in adolescents are diaphyseal and heal uneventfully with protection and immobilization [B].

The base of the fifth metatarsal presents several patterns:

- Apophysitis or avulsion. The radiolucent apophyseal cartilage is oriented longitudinally. This occurs under pull of peroneus brevis in a prepubescent child, who presents with tenderness and swelling. Protect weight bearing and immobilize in a cast.
- Accessory ossicle. Do not confuse this with fracture (*cf.* Foot chapter). This is rounded, with an orientation if determinable that is oblique.
- Metaphyseal–diaphyseal fracture [C]. Jones described this in himself after a night out dancing with his wife. Mechanism is inversion with abrupt traction by a peroneus brevis that attempts to rectify the foot. The fracture, which is transverse, occurs at a vascular watershed zone, hence the risk of delayed or nonunion. Most heal in a cast. Consider percutaneous screw fixation in a mature adolescent or for delayed union: use at least a 4.5-mm screw that fills the medulla to obtain internal cortical purchase.

Compartment Syndrome

A medial incision that takes down abductor hallucis, the "door to the cage" (Henry), gives access to the deep muscles of the foot. Add two longitudinal dorsal incisions.

Tarsus

Fractures in this region represent <5% of foot fractures in children. These are treated according to general principles. Complications, for example, of head of talus after neck fracture, and comminution, for example, of calcaneus fracture, are less frequent in children. Beware of an occult injury producing limp in the young child [D]. Scintigramme may reveal a stress fracture when physical examination demonstrates foot tenderness, yet röntgenogramme is normal.

Soft Tissue

The burden of soft tissue injury for fracture in the child's foot is relatively high due to mechanism of use of the foot, for example, running and jumping, on the ground, and due to mechanisms of injury, for example, lawn mower. Such injuries require complex reconstruction [E].

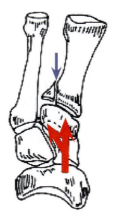

A **"Bunk bed" fracture** This Salter-Harris IV fracture of first metatarsal (*blue*), produced under the flexion and axial force transmitted by medial cuneiform bone, is a pædiatric equivalent of Lisfranc injury.

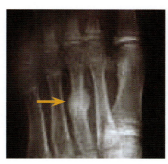

B **Metatarsal stress fracture** This heals with a circular radiodense blush of callus (*orange*).

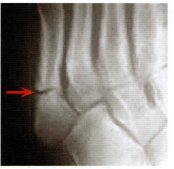

C **Jones fracture** This fracture occurs in the metadiaphyseal region, at a vascular watershed region (*red*). The transverse orientation distinguishes this from the longitudinal apophyseal cartilage.

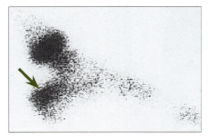

D **Occult fracture of calcaneus** Increased uptake (*green*) in a 5-year-old limping child with heel tenderness.

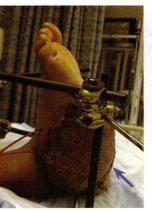

E **Open fracture of calcaneus** While this does not follow a physeal fracture classification, it captures the motivation for adding a sixth type that includes loss of a part (*white*). A lawn mower removed the anterior part of calcaneus (*red*) along with surrounding soft tissues. Because of the lateral location of the injury, perfusion and sensation to the distal foot were preserved. Reconstruction included internal fixation of calcaneus with extensive osseous graft as well as free flap coverage.

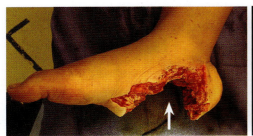
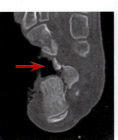

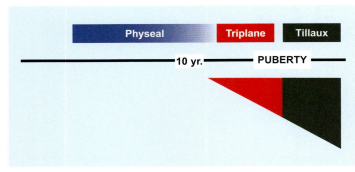

A   Categorization of ankle fractures in children Types reflect maturation of distal tibia.

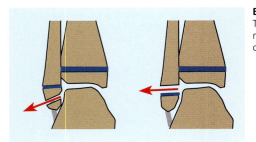

B   Fibula avulsion These typically are managed successfully closed.

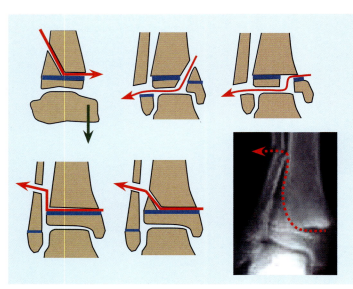

C   Salter-Harris fractures Patterns vary, as do the forces producing them, for example, ankle extension (*green*).

ANKLE

The distal physis of tibia closes by 15 years in girls and 17 years in boys. On mortise view röntgenogramme, there should be ≤8 mm clear space between tibia and fibula, and ≥1 mm overlap of tibia and fibula. Acceptable limits for talar position are <2 mm shift and <5 degrees tilt. The child is vulnerable to physeal fractures at the ankle because all the ligaments that bind the joint attach to the epiphyses. Ankle fractures in children may be divided into physeal and transitional [A].

Physeal Fracture

These occur before puberty, when physes are wide open. Avulsion fractures of fibula rarely require reduction and fixation [B]. Persistent fragments that do not unite may require delayed osteosynthesis if large, or excision. Do not confuse accesoria, for example, *os subtibiale* (up to 20% of children), with avulsions: the former are rounded with no matching surface on the main fibula fragment.

Salter-Harris I fractures of the distal fibula are a presumptive diagnosis based upon history of trauma, physical examination showing tenderness and swelling, and normal röntgenogrammes. They are overdiagnosed: most represent a bone contusion or ankle sprain. Immobilize without or with weight bearing until resolution of pain.

Several patterns are possible [C]. Salter-Harris II fractures may be displaced, for example, posterior with a metaphyseal fragment by an ankle extension force. Intact ankle ligaments secure the distal fragment. Rest the heel on a firm platform, and apply the reduction force to bring the leg to the distal fragment: this will permit greater force than can be applied by holding the heel, in order to effect a single and as complete as possible reduction. The broad physeal surface makes the reduction stable. Up to 10 degrees of residual angulation of tibia is acceptable if there is 2 years growth remaining. Associated fibula fractures may be left alone or stabilized with a percutaneously placed medullary wire, which acts as an internal splint. Residual gapping at the fracture represents soft tissue involution, in particular periosteum, which has been implicated in growth arrest. Educate the patient and family that, despite the apparent benignity of this type of fracture (including management by closed methods), growth arrest occurs in 1/4 of cases, exposing the fragility of this physis.

Salter-Harris III and IV are articular. If articular step-off is >2 mm, open reduction and internal fixation are indicated [D]. If the articular surface is not clearly delineated on röntgenogrammes (including oblique views), CT will allow accurate measurement. The surgical approach depends upon the fracture pattern. Plan incision(s) to include a direct view of the articular margin, for example, anteromedial approach to the tibial malleolar fragment. Irrigate the joint to wash out any osteochondral fragments too small to fix. Clean the fracture to remove débris that would obstruct anatomic reduction, including a periosteal flap. Palpate the articular surface with a blunt instrument to confirm that the marginal read is accurate. Fixation includes two screws in epiphysis to stably restore the joint. Excise the metaphyseal fragment and overlying periosteum. The fragment is not essential for stability or union, and its removal is an anticipatory bridge excision, which will develop in up to 1/3 of cases [E].

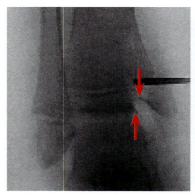
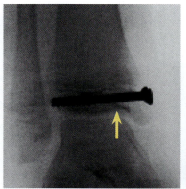
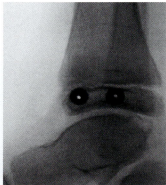

D   Salter-Harris IV fracture Articular surface is displaced >2 mm (*red*). Open reduction restores congruity of articular surface (*yellow*). Two epiphysial screws, inserted percutaneously, provide stability, including against rotation, that is supplemented by a cast. After fracture healing, remove epiphysial screws, because they increase peak contact pressure across the tibiotalar joint.

Transitional Fracture

This occurs during the transition between immaturity and mature child, as the distal physis of tibia undergoes the process of closure. As a result, growth disturbance is not a concern. This represents 10% to 15% of pædiatric ankle fractures.

Triplane This fracture is so named after the three planes through which force travels: sagittal disrupts the articular surface, transverse shears the physis, and coronal produces a posterior metaphyseal spike [F]. It may be medial or lateral, two-part, three-part, or four-part, presenting numerous patterns and variants that evade a useful classification. The fundamental mechanism is lateral rotation of the ankle, which may be divided into three stages: the first produces an ankle sprain or Tillaux fracture (vs.), the second produces a triplane fracture, and the third stage produces a fibula fracture in half of cases. Because of their complexity, CT is essential to plan fixation, including location of incisions and implant direction. Restore length to take advantage of desmotaxis by fixing the fibula if fractured [G]. Build the distal tibia by starting at the epiphysis. Add fixation, for example, anteroposterior screws, to capture the posterior metaphyseal spike, as necessary to reduce the epiphysis to the remainder of tibia. Add a screw to fix the syndesmosis if disrupted. Beware that soft tissue swelling may influence timing of operation.

Tillaux The pathogenesis reflects direction of closure of the distal physis of tibia: this begins central, proceeds medial, turns posterior, and ends at the anterolateral corner, which will be separate and due to stress concentration prone to avulsion under pull of anterior tibiofibular ligament during lateral rotation of the ankle [H]. Unlike the triplane fracture, which is characterized by significant deformity as the distal epiphysis of tibia breaks and separates from the rest of the bone taking with it the foot, a Tillaux fracture presents with no significant deformity and minimal swelling. Tillaux patients are 1- to 2-year older than triplane patients. Because ankle alignment is normal, this fracture may not be evident on röntgenogramme, in particular on anteroposterior projection, in which fibula obscures lateral corner of distal tibial physis. Because of this, and the fact that it is articular, CT is indicated. For displacement >2 mm, perform open reduction *via* an anterolateral approach that enables inspection of the articular surface. Reduction of the fragment requires simultaneous compression with pointed tenaculum and posteromedial translation with tamp. Fix with one screw parallel to the articular surface and one oblique for rotational control. Do not worry about the physis, which by definition is mostly closed.

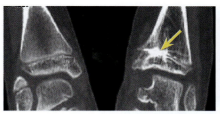

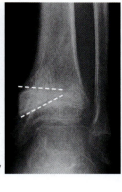

E Growth arrest after Salter-Harris II fracture Because of varus and bridge > 50% (*yellow*), complete physeodesis with corrective osteotomy was performed through the physis, where a tricortical allograft (*white*) was stabilized by an interference fit and two bioabsorbable wires.

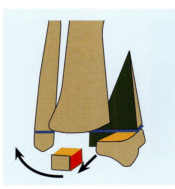

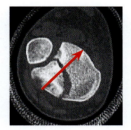

F Triplane fracture Force of fracture travels through three planes: sagittal (*red*), transverse (*orange*), and coronal (*green*). CT scan aids planning of fixation: *arrow* indicates path of anteroposterior screw (*yellow*).

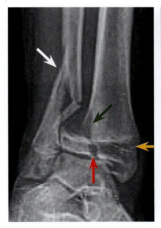

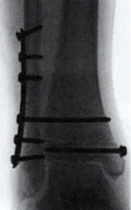

G Triplane fracture open reduction and internal fixation Plating of fibula proximal to its distal physis restored length. No anteroposterior implants were necessary to fix the posterior metaphyseal fragment, which was reduced anatomically by desmotaxis. Two screws fixed the epiphysis, and a screw through the plate stabilized the syndesmosis.

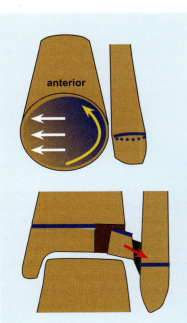

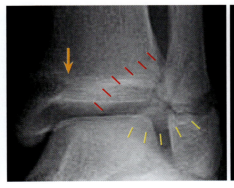

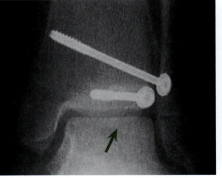

H Tillaux fracture Distal physis of tibia closes medialward (*white*) and then posterior to anterior (*yellow*). Fragment is avulsed under pull of anterior tibiofibular ligament (*green*). Fragment is difficult to see on AP röntgenogramme, which shows medial physeal closure (*orange*). It is managed by open reduction (*green*) and fixed.

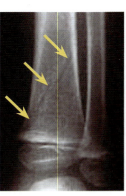
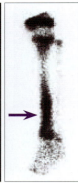

A   Toddler fracture The typical pattern is distal metaphyseal oblique proximal lateral to distal medial (*yellow*). Scintigramme shows increased uptake (*blue*).

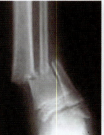
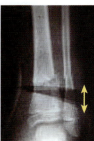

B   Tibia and fibula fractures These fractures may be treated effectively in cast, which was wedged for drift (*yellow*) noted at 1-week follow-up.

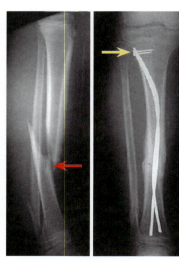

C   Operation for tibia fracture This unstable fracture (*red*) in an adolescent is best treated operatively. Flexible medullary nails avoid the physis, in particular the tibial apophysis, which is hypersensitive to growth disturbance, and may be placed through a lateral proximal window (*yellow*) where they will not be prominent under cover of the anterior crural muscles. Ender nails are secured in place by eyelet screws, controlling migration and facilitating removal if necessary.

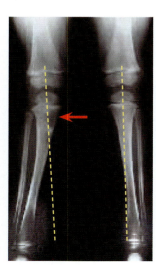

D   Valgus following proximal metaphysis of tibia fracture 5-year-old girl sustained an undisplaced right proximal tibial fracture (*red*), which was treated in an above-knee cast. Valgus deformity is evident at 1 year after injury.

TIBIA

The subcutaneous surface of the tibia makes it slow to heal and prominent when malunited. Unlike femur, overgrowth is insignificant: mean 5 mm up to 10 mm. The tibia bears 80% of body weight through the leg. Compartment syndrome is a real risk after this fracture.

Toddler Fracture

The name describes the age of presentation. Energy is low, for example, hyperextension of the knee when landing from a jump. The child may limp or refuse to walk. Physical examination shows tenderness but little else: no swelling and no deformity. Röntgenogrammes show a faint oblique line or may be negative. Scintigramme shows increased uptake [A]. Alternatively, a presumptive diagnosis may be made based upon the typical presentation. Treat with a walking cast: apply the cast above the knee, flexed to 60 degrees, for an older child in less controllable circumstances, to automatically limit activity.

Diaphyseal Fracture

In the first decade, most tibial diaphyseal fractures may be managed by reduction and above-knee cast. Flex the knee to at least 45 degrees to ease clearance of the floor with crutches. Include a valgus mold for an intact fibula, which pushes a broken tibia into varus. Follow with weekly röntgenogrammes until stable [B]. Modify ankle position to take advantage of tension produced through the posterior compartment muscles that may be harnessed to support a reduction in the sagittal plane, for example, extend the ankle and relax these muscles in an apex anterior fracture. Up to 10 degrees of residual valgus angulation and 5 degrees of varus are acceptable. Step-off is a concern at the subcutaneous border of the mid-diaphysis, though this will remodel in the first decade. Transverse plane deformity does not remodel significantly: be cognizant of transmalleolar axis relative to flexed knee during reduction and application of cast.

In the adolescent, surgical management reduces risk of malunion, lessens the burden of follow-up, and obviates the need for casting. Open diaphyseal fractures also are treated operatively for wound care and healing and because, often, soft tissue interposition prevents acceptable reduction. Flexible medullary nails [C] are benign, load sharing, and stable enough to effect and maintain reduction and to stand alone for most fractures. Exceptions include significant comminution and bone loss, where external fixation is indicated.

Stress Fracture

Ten percent of all stress fractures affect immature children, while 30% occur in the mature adolescent. The tibia is most affected, comprising 45% of all stress fractures. Sports are the most common cause. Girls are affected more than boys, in part due to a hypoœstrogenic state induced by activity. Röntgenogrammes may be negative: confirm diagnosis with scintigramme. Manage by immobilization, protected weight bearing, or activity modification. Monitor healing by symptoms and until scintigramme normalizes.

Proximal Metaphyseal Fracture

Greenstick fractures of the proximal metaphysis of tibia in the 3- to 7-year-old child (Cozen) may be followed by the development of valgus deformity [D]. Mechanism is valgus force. Medial overgrowth exacerbates normal development from varus to valgus in this age group. Röntgenogrammes show deviation of tibia away from mechanical axis and asymmetry of growth arrest line.

The natural history is spontaneous correction over a 2-year window. Educate family so that they may be patient during this period of observation. For persistent deformity, modulate growth by temporarily arresting the medial proximal physis with an implant that may be removed at correction.

Intercondylar Eminence Fracture

The intercondylar eminence also is referred to as the spine of the tibia. This fracture occurs around the turn from first to second decades. Mechanism is knee hyperextension and axial loading, as in sudden braking while riding a bicycle. The anterior cruciate ligament may stretch but does not fail, a fate that befalls the intercondylar eminence where the cruciates attach. While it is named after the nonarticular part of the knee, the fracture may extend to the articular surfaces of both condyles and may be associated with meniscal tear.

Evaluation The patient presents with knee pain that prevents weight bearing and effusion due to hæmarthrosis in fracture. Pain will not allow Lachman or pivot shift testing.

IMAGING The fracture may be classified on lateral view röntgenogramme [E]. CT allows accurate measurement of fragment displacement. Displacement >2 mm is unacceptable even though this is a nonarticular fracture, not because of concern for union or posttraumatic arthritis, but because this will introduce laxity in the anterior cruciate ligament that may destabilize the knee. MRI will show associated articular and ligamentous injury. Half of cases will show medial more than lateral meniscal or intermeniscal ligament entrapment, in type 3 more than type 2. Meniscal tear is rare (<5%).

Management In the emergency setting, aspirate the knee, inject a local anæsthetic, and apply a cast in full knee extension. In this position, the femoral condyles may compress any articular extension of the fracture to reduce the fragment. If there is meniscal entrapment, the reduction will be incomplete. If the fragment is solely nonarticular, it may be displaced by the extension manœuvre because the anterior cruciate ligament is taught. Confirm acceptable reduction with röntgenogrammes or CT.

Type I fractures are treated in an above-knee cast at 30 degrees flexion (relaxed anterior cruciate ligament).

Operative reduction and internal fixation is indicated for displaced fractures [F]. Articular structures may be explored and repaired by arthroscopy, by which the fracture also may be reduced and fixed. If MRI shows an isolated fracture, it may be treated *via* a linear incision parallel to the ligamentum patellæ starting at the apex of patella and continuing to the anterior articular margin. Because the anterior cruciate ligament is presumably stretched before the fracture occurs, débride the bed of the fracture in order to countersink the fragment and thereby tension the ligament. Fixation may be by suture passed through drill holes in the apophysis, for example, if fragment is small or comminuted, or a screw, which may be placed epiphysial or transphyseal and which may be metallic or bioabsorbable. Postoperative immobilization and weight bearing are tailored to union of fracture, meniscal repair if performed, and associated collateral ligament injury if present. Plan removal of transphyseal, to avoid growth disturbance, or metallic screws, which will overgrow.

Outcomes are obscure. Children may demonstrate persistent anterior cruciate ligamentous laxity on testing despite operative treatment yet have normal function, as determined by outcome instruments, for example, Lysholm knee score >90/100, and by return to preinjury level of activity. Educate patients and families that not uncommon after this injury are stiffness and prolonged knee pain, which will resolve with dedicated rehabilitation.

Proximal Physeal Fracture

The greatest importance of these fractures is potential for popliteal artery injury by posterior displacement of the proximal metaphysis, as the proximal fragment is retained by the ligaments of the knee. Knee hyperextension drives the distal fragment into the vessel, which may be occluded or torn as it is tethered at the soleus fascia and interosseous membrane. The fractures are treated according to general principles of Salter-Harris types.

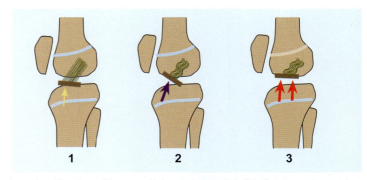

E Classification of intercondylar eminence of tibia fractures Type 1 is acceptably displaced and may be treated with cast: it will heal without anterior cruciate ligament (*green*) laxity. Type 2 may be reducible and, if so, may be treated closed in cast. Type 3 is surgical and may be whole or comminuted.

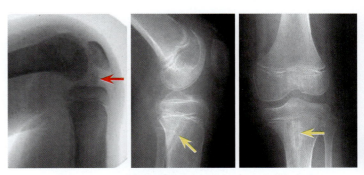

F Operative treatment of intercondylar eminence of tibia fractures This type 2 fracture (*red*) was irreducible. It was fixed with a bioabsorbable transphyseal screw (*yellow*), which loses purchase after union but before physeal arrest.

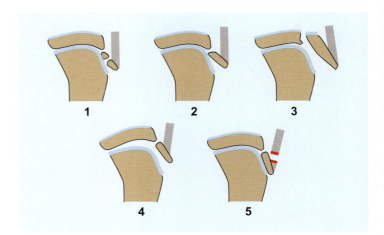

G Classification of tibial tubercle fractures Type 1 is a fracture within the tubercle. It may be minimally displaced, designated A, which is difficult to differentiate from chronic Osgood-Schlatter condition, or displaced, designated B. Types 2 and 3 may be subdivided into A without or B with fragmentation of the displaced fragment. In type 4, force lifts tibial tubercle then continues along the proximal physis of tibia. More than one variant are included in type 5, including avulsion of the ligamentum patellæ (*gray*) and a triplane pattern.

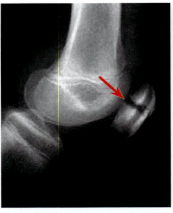
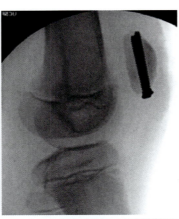
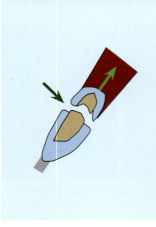
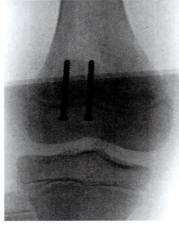

Tubercle Fractures

This fracture occurs during the pubertal growth acceleration. Mechanism is eccentric contraction of quadriceps femoris against flexion and axial loading of the knee, as in jumping during basketball.

Evaluation The patient presents with knee pain that prevents weight bearing and anterior knee swelling or articular effusion due to hæmarthrosis if the fracture extends through the epiphysis. Pain and avulsion of the tibial tubercle produce a knee extension lag. There may be a history of Osgood-Schlatter condition. Avulsion of the anterior tibial recurrent artery has been implicated in associated compartment syndrome.

IMAGING The fracture may be classified on lateral view röntgenogrammes [G].

Management Minimally displaced fractures are casted in knee extension, to relax quadriceps femoris. Displacement weakens quadriceps femoris, which is an indication for operative treatment. Articular extension risks posttraumatic arthritis and may include injury to intra-articular structures. Approach displaced fractures *via* a midline incision. Explore and irrigate the joint open through the type 3 fracture or by arthroscopy. Fix fragments by screws parallel to the joint contour placed in apophysis and epiphysis. Repair a torn patellar retinaculum to support internal fixation. Repair a torn ligamentum patellæ in type V by suture through drill holes or anchors. Add an anterior crural fasciotomy performed along tibial crest through same incision by long scissors, as prophylaxis against compartment syndrome.

Genu recurvatum does not complicate such fractures or their treatment because the fractures occur when the proximal tibial physis is closing. Screw prominence may be addressed by implant removal after union.

PATELLA

There are two principal types of patella fractures, which occur with similar frequency.

Transverse Fracture

These fractures resemble those in adults [H]. Mechanism includes a direct blow.

Marginal Fracture

These may be superior, involving the base of patella, or inferior, involving the apex [I]. They are named "sleeve" fractures after the long soft tissue covering of cartilage and periosteum that accompanies a relatively smaller fragment of bone. Mechanism is avulsion due to sudden eccentric contraction of quadriceps femoris.

Evaluation The patient presents with knee pain that prevents weight bearing, articular effusion due to hæmarthrosis from fracture, and loss of knee extension.

IMAGING Röntgenogrammes underestimate the injury: they may show only a fleck of bone, or they may be limited to soft tissue findings of swelling and hæmarthrosis outlining the ligamentum patellæ. Diagnostic aspiration will show blood and fat. MRI reveals the extent of cartilage and retinacular damage. Distinguish bipartite patella (*cf.* Lower Limb chapter).

Management Untreated, the periosteum heals to form an elongated patella. Long term, articular discontinuity and irregularity predispose to posttraumatic arthritis. Because these include a large articular component, open reduction and internal fixation are indicated. If the osseous margin in a sleeve fracture is too small to receive a screw, a tension band construct with wires and a heavy nonabsorbable suture, supplemented by a cast, will effectively stabilize the fragment.

H   Transverse patella fracture This may result from a direct blow as well as from sudden pull of quadriceps femoris (*green*). The fracture was fixed with cannulated screws augmented with heavy nonabsorbable suture. Screws were countersunk below the cartilage rim so that the suture creates a tension band construct.

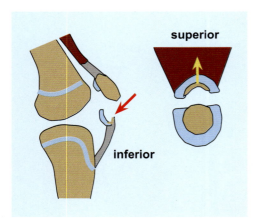

I   Marginal patella fractures A sleeve of cartilage may tear off along with a sliver of bone from the apex (*red*), or a rim may fracture off the base (*yellow*).

superior

inferior

FEMUR

Distal Physeal Fracture

These are classified by the Salter-Harris system.

Evaluation Consider nonaccidental trauma in an infant. The more typical presentation is an early second-decade child with pain and swelling, without or with knee deformity. There is tenderness at the distal femoral physis but not along the substance or distal attachments of the collateral ligaments. A knee effusion also differentiates physeal injury from collateral ligamentous injury.

IMAGING Röntgenogrammes may be negative in a nondisplaced type I fracture or show only subtle widening. Stress röntgenogrammes, which require sedation, may expose loss of physeal integrity [A]. However, this manœuver also further injures a physis prone to growth disturbance. Consider scintigramme or MRI, both of which will show altered signal at the distal physis, if history and physical examination do not provide a diagnosis with confidence. Articular extension is an indication for CT to determine surface step-off. While the knee is more forgiving of articular irregularity than are the wrist and ankle, most follow the 2-mm rule.

Management Apply an above-knee cast with protected weight bearing for nondisplaced fractures. For displaced Salter-Harris I fractures, close reduction and percutaneous crossed wire fixation, supplemented with a cast, are effective [B]. This also may be performed for Salter-Harris II types; alternatively, if the metaphyseal fragment is large, closed or open reduction and screw fixation may be more stable and avoid physis and articular surface. Salter-Harris III and IV require open reduction under direct visualization of the articular surface, to which access is obtained by a midaxial medial or lateral incision that is curved toward tibial tubercle to permit an arthrotomy. Fixation is by screws placed in epiphysis and in metaphysis, which are supplemented by a cast [C]. In the event that screws alone are not stable, for example, when there is extensive comminution, apply an extraperiosteal and extraperichondral plate that will be removed after union. Do not sacrifice restoration and stability of the joint for fear of growth disturbance.

Outcome Half of these physeal fractures will arrest, partially causing deformity and/or completely causing shortening. The undulating shape has been implicated in shearing of the columnar architecture of the physis during displacement. Educate the family of this risk at first encounter. Monitor actively: because of the rapid growth of the distal femoral physis, signs of growth disturbance will be evident by the anniversary of fracture. Consider resection of small, discrete bridges, or complete physeodesis for those that are unresectable, without or with corrective osteotomy as indicated.

Distal Metaphyseal Fracture

This is a site of torus fracture in a young child, which is managed by an above-knee cast [D]. In neuromuscular patients, osteopenia and a long lever arm in the setting of stiffness conspire to fracture this region. Limit casting in such a setting in order not to exacerbate osteopenia. The distal metaphysis of femur is a common location for benign tumors of bone, for example, nonosteogenic fibroma, which may lead to morbid fracture.

In the adolescent, sport is the most frequent culprit. The distal fragment tends to be pulled apex posterior by gastrocnemius and into varus by adductor magnus. Displaced fractures are treated by open reduction and internal fixation. A locking plate, as a fixed angle device, stabilizes distal fractures without the need to span the physis to anchor in the epiphysis. An external fixator is an alternate for distal fractures, as well as for open injuries and a floating knee.

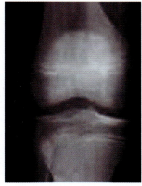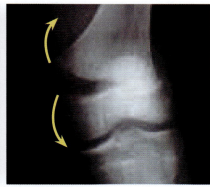

A   Salter-Harris I fracture The presenting röntgenogramme showed no abnormality. Because of clinical suspicion, stress manœuver was performed, revealing an unstable fracture of the physis (*yellow*).

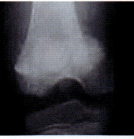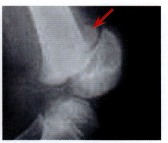

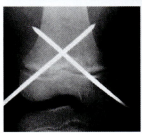

B   Displaced Salter-Harris II fracture There is an anterior metaphyseal fragment that is too small to receive an independent implant. The fracture was reduced and fixed with crossed wires passed percutaneously through each condyle. The procedure resembles that for the pædiatric supracondylar humerus fracture.

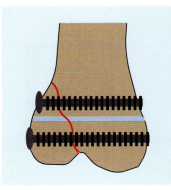

C   Salter-Harris III and IV fractures These are treated with open reduction and internal fixation with large screws placed extraphyseal and parallel to joint surface. Full thread facilitate extraction if necessary, for example, before corrective osteotomy for growth

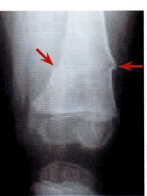

D   Distal metaphysis torus fracture This is a low-energy fracture managed in a cast.

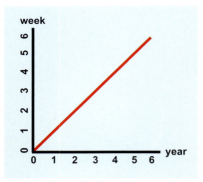

A   Healing of femur fracture Relationship between time of immobilization in weeks until stable callus and age in years is linear, reflecting rapidity of healing.

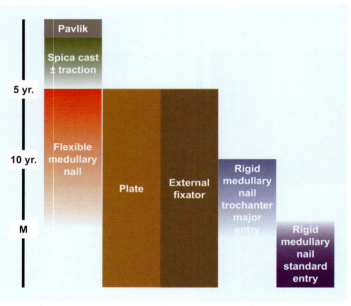

B   Management of femur fractures according to age Operative treatment begins with school. The cervicotrochanteric physis and the trochanter major apophysis influence choice of implant.

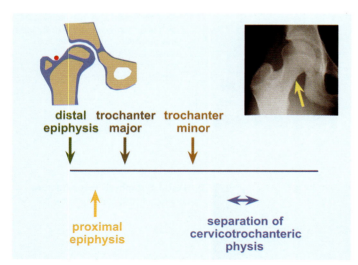

C   Ossification of proximal femur The cervicotrochanteric physis is continuous from trochanter major to neck of femur until early in the second decade, after which the two centers become independent. Injury to this physis may lead to a thin valgus neck (*yellow*), which may fracture more readily, and a small trochanter major, which may weaken the hip abductors. A trochanteric fossa starting point for antegrade nailing may injure the medial femoral circumflex artery entry (*red*) in an immature child with a small femur. The trochanter major apophysis grows longitudinally until the end of the first decade, after which appositional growth takes over.

Diaphyseal Fracture

Presentation is bimodal: 2 to 4 years, which tend to be low energy such as play, and adolescence, which include motor vehicle crash and other high-energy mechanisms. Due to its thick muscle envelope, the femur has an exceptional capacity to heal, to heal rapidly and to remodel [A]. Overgrowth is greatest for femoral diaphyseal fractures in the first decade: mean 1 cm up to 1″. As a result, shortening up to 1″ is acceptable and 1 cm is desirable. Unlike adults, hæmorrhage does not require replacement after this fracture in children.

Evaluation Investigate for nonaccidental trauma in an infant with a femur fracture before walking. The patient complains of pain immediately after a traumatic event and is unable to bear weight. The thigh is swollen and deformed, held in hip flexion and lateral rotation with knee flexion, a position aimed at relaxing deforming forces on the fracture to reduce pain.

Imaging Röntgenogrammes show fracture, pattern, alignment, and shortening.

Management This follows age [B].

Birth to school age Immobilize without and with reduction. A Pavlik harness suffices in the 1st year. Caution parents that, while time to stable callus is rapid, this time will be punctuated by pain as the child instinctively kicks with the lower limbs. For the older infant, apply a spica (Latin *spica*: "ear of grain," after the pattern of applying the strips of plaster or fiberglass) cast in the "human position" (Salter). This brings the distal fragment to the proximal fragment, in response to deforming muscular forces:

- Hip flexion to 90 degrees, because the proximal fragment is flexed by iliopsoa. This allows sitting, including transportation by car.
- Hip abduction 45 degrees, to counteract hip abductors. This gives access to the perineum for care.
- Gentle lateral hip rotation, for the lateral hip rotators.
- Apply a valgus mold against the varus force of adductor magnus on the distal fragment.
- Knee flexion >60 degrees, to reduce shortening by injured muscles in spasm. Compression of the popliteal fossa during application of traction in knee flexion risks compartment syndrome.

Even though the cast may be applied in an emergency setting, in the operating room, the child is reliably relaxed and imaging is optimal. Obtain röntgenogrammes at 1 week for alignment and shortening, and to make sure family is coping, because a spica cast is a heavy burden of care. Acceptable alignment is ≤30 degrees in sagittal plane, the plane of motion of the knee, and ≤10 degrees in the coronal plane. Even though little remodeling occurs in the transverse plane, the patient can compensate by hip rotation ≤30 degrees. Such numbers are guidelines, influenced by several factors and prone to measurement error. Factors include age–for example, more is accepted at a younger age due to greater remodeling potential–and location–for example, more may be acceptable closer to an enarthrodial joint that can compensate for residual deformity. Error may be intra- or inter-observer, as well as the result of parallax related to positioning.

Coming out of a spica cast is stressful for a child: prepare the family and offer a hip abduction brace as a weaning device. A limp will persist for weeks, reflecting in part the accompanying psychic injury. Obtain röntgenogrammes at anniversary of fracture to measure for overgrowth.

Traction Consider this for shortening >1″. Use a distal femoral pin, because the tibial apophysis is prone to growth disturbance. Apply weight until shortening becomes <1″, and continue until callus is stable enough to cast, which is confirmed by reduced pain on physical examination and radiographic appearance. As the age of operation declines, the indication for traction fades. Traction counteracts shortening, which correlates with energy of injury, which correlates with the age of the child, which correlates with operative treatment. Cost is equivalent to operative treatment, which allows a child to get out of bed and get back to a normal environment.

5 YEARS TO MATURITY Starting at school age, operative treatment is indicated. The standard treatment in adults is antegrade medullary nailing. The principal determinant of technique in a child is physis [C].

Flexible medullary nailing avoids the physes [D]. It may be antegrade, starting at lateral cortex distal to trochanter major, or retrograde, starting at lateral and medial cortices proximal to distal femoral physis. The technique has several advantages:

- It is safe, avoiding physes.
- It is load sharing, encouraging callus formation and union.
- It allows for controlled shortening, which counteracts the overgrowth phenomenon.
- Its lack of rigidity is an advantage when the soft tissue envelope has not been extensively disrupted. As the fracture heals, normalization and symmetry of muscle contraction allow spontaneous correction of rotational malalignment, which does not otherwise remodel significantly.
- It may be performed through discrete incisions.

Use same diameter nails, to avoid differential stress that risks fracture displacement. Select a nail that is 40% of isthmus diameter, so that 2 fill ≥ 80% of the canal. Nails may be C-shaped or S-shaped.

There are three types of flexible nails [E]. The original report by Rush described fixation of a proximal ulna fracture in an adult. Ender introduced his nails for periprosthetic fractures, after the concept of filling a vase with stems until they all stand straight, as proposed earlier by Rush. The original report from Nancy described fixation of both bone forearm fractures. Image intensification aids selection of extraphyseal entry site. There is no consensus on routine implant removal, although it may be necessary for tip prominence.

Contraindications for flexible medullary nailing are comminution and adult weight.

Bridge plating acts as an internal extramedullary splint, fixed proximal and distal to the fracture. It avoids physes and is rigid; as such, it may be used for all ages. It can span a region of comminution for length-unstable fractures. It may be performed by a less invasive submuscular technique. Locking screws add stability to very proximal or distal fractures. A plate fixes rotation (no spontaneous correction), is load bearing, does not allow "physiologic" shortening, and may be overgrown by a bone increasing in diameter *via* periosteal apposition, thereby necessitating removal.

External fixation has the same advantages as bridge plating. It has the additional advantage of allowing access to soft tissues in open fractures while staying remote from the zone of injury. Conical pins may be removed in clinic: they loosen after the first revolution. Because of the rigidity of the implant, and morbidity of pin sites, premature removal has resulted in refracture. Wait until there are at least three continuous cortices of callus, and dynamize the construct first by removing the barrel but leaving the pins in place for 2 to 4 weeks.

Beginning in the second decade, antegrade rigid nailing through trochanter major is safe and effective. It has the benefits that have made antegrade rigid nailing the standard for adult femur fractures. Because of appositional growth after 8 years, the trochanter major is durable, and it is remote from the lateral epiphysial vessels in the retinacula of Weitbrecht. Küntscher's original report of medullary nailing of femur fractures through a trochanter major starting site included a 10-year-old boy.

Implant choice [F] is secondary to the principal innovation in treatment of femur fractures, namely, the decision to operate in the skeletally immature.

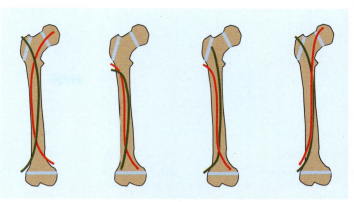

D Flexible nailing of femoral diaphyseal fracture Nails may be antegrade or retrograde, inserted lateral and medial. Retrograde allows more proximal fixation for more proximal fractures. Nails may be passed across physis, which will not be disturbed because nail is smooth and diameter is small compared with total cross-sectional area, and into epiphysis, which is hard and mechanically stable. Two lateral entry points are simpler and use a single incision.

Nail	Features
Rush	Steel Most rigid Sharp beveled tip to allow penetration of bone and deflection off cortical surface. Hooked end for steering and extraction Predetermined lengths
Ender	Steel Blunt beveled tip to allow deflection off cortex Prebent to ease passage through medulla Eyelets at end may receive cortical screws that allow nails to be inserted flush with cortex, prevent migration, and facilitate steering and extraction Predetermined lengths
Nancy (France)	Titanium or steel Most flexible makes them easiest to insert Bent keel tip facilitates passage through medulla and across fracture for reduction Memory metal results in three point contact in medulla Cut to length, which along with widest range of diameters makes this most versatile

E Flexible nails.

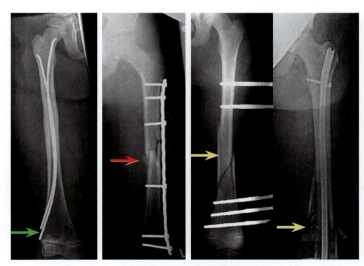

F Implant choices for femoral diaphyseal fractures Nancy nails were inserted through a single lateral incision (*orange*), which is easier and saves the child a scar. Plate bridges the fracture as an internal fixator (*red*). Indication for external fixator was comminution (*yellow*), which also may be treated effectively with a trochanter major nail in an adolescent.

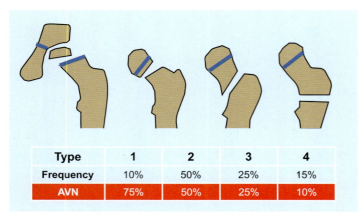

Type	1	2	3	4
Frequency	10%	50%	25%	15%
AVN	75%	50%	25%	10%

G   Delbet-Colonna classification of proximal femoral fractures AVN: avascular necrosis. AVN in intertrochanteric fractures is explained by injury to the retinacular vessels at the intertrochanteric notch, arising from the anastomotic ring between medial and lateral femoral circumflex arteries.

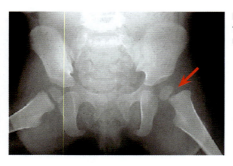

H   Transcervical femoral fracture Beware of nonaccidental trauma.

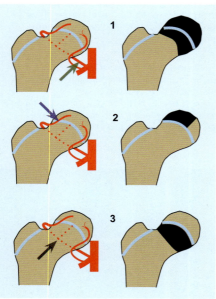

I   Patterns of avascular necrosis (Ratliff) Injury to medial femoral circumflex (*green*) results in head and neck necrosis. Injury to the lateral epiphysial artery (*blue*) kills the head. Injury to the ascending superior metaphyseal vessels (*gray*) leads to cervical necrosis with preservation of the epiphysis.

Proximal Fracture

These are so rare that no surgeon has substantial experience (Blount). They are classified by the Delbet-Colonna system [G].

Physeal

This Salter-Harris I type is most common in infancy and early childhood [H]. It has an association with nonaccidental trauma. The fracture is subtyped as A without or B with dislocation of the epiphysis, for example, hip dislocation followed by fracture during reduction leaving the epiphysis behind. Avascular necrosis is universal in B. Displaced fractures require open reduction *via* an anterior approach. Fix with smooth wires bent over lateral proximal metaphyseal cortex, and supplement with a hip spica cast in the "human position" (*v.s.*). Follow closely with röntgenogrammes for wire migration and avascular necrosis.

Cervical

This occurs in older children. MRI delineates minimally displaced fractures. Displaced fractures require open reduction *via* an anterior approach. Fix with screws: there is enough proximal fragment to benefit from the stability of this implant, which may be removed once healed if placed across the physis to avoid growth disturbance or in the event of osteonecrosis. Given the grave consequences of such fractures, reduction and stability are more important than the physis.

Cervicotrochanteric

This is managed like cervical fracture.

Intertrochanteric

This is managed by a fixed angle device, including blade plate and cephalomedullary nail.

Complications

Complications distinguish this fracture due to tenuity of the blood supply to the proximal femur. Patterns of avascular necrosis have been classified geographically [I], mapping according to location of vessel injury. While trauma is the principal agent, the effect may be mitigated by accurate reduction for vessels that are occluded by displacement but not torn. This necessitates open treatment with direct visualization, which also decompresses intracapsular hæmatoma. The window for presentation of avascular necrosis is up to 2 years after injury.

   Vascular insufficiency and instability, even with fixation, account for delayed or nonunion [J]. Malunion, typically coxa vara, has been associated with spica casting with incomplete reduction and with late displacement. Physeal arrest may lead to abnormal growth of the proximal femur or limb-length discrepancy, which increases in significance with decreasing age. Late displacement may occur for fractures treated in a hip spica cast: follow closely with serial röntgenogrammes.

J   Cervical nonunion Cervical fracture (*green*) was managed by closed reduction and two screw fixation. Cervical avascular necrosis (*red*) with preservation of the epiphysis resulted in nonunion (*yellow*), progressive collapse into coxa vara, and backing out of implants. This was treated by valgus osteotomy fixed with a blade plate. The neck was grafted through the osteotomy with autogenous bone graft obtained from the wedge exsected to put the proximal femur into valgus and thereby move the fracture from shear to compression.

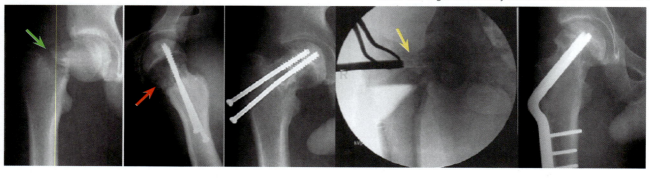

CLAVICLE

Clavicle fractures may occur through bone or through proximal or distal physes [A].

Physeal Fracture

This presents in the first decade; the second decade ushers in clavicular dislocation, which may be differentiated by ultrasonogramme or MRI. Physeal fractures remodel well due to the intact periosteal sleeve that is in continuity between bone and physis. Coracoclavicular and acromioclavicular ligaments remain intact. Manage with a shoulder sling until nontender and the patient is able to raise the upper limb above the horizon.

Diaphyseal Fracture

These may be divided into birth or other trauma. The neonate may present with pseudoparalysis. This may be distinguished from brachial plexopathy by presence of a Moro reflex, which the child will manifest despite pain of fracture. Most common mechanism is a direct blow during a fall. The patient presents with tenderness, inability to lift the upper limb, swelling, and often visible deformity of this subcutaneous bone.

Röntgenogrammes are sufficient to show the fracture. Thirty- to 40-degree cephalic tilt of the X-ray beam isolates the clavicle from the thorax. Distinguish pseudarthrosis of the clavicle (*cf.* Upper Limb chapter). Consider MRI if there is neurovascular compromise.

Closed management consists of a shoulder sling: the bone heals and remodels well. The absolute indication for operative treatment is injury to the surrounding soft tissues, which may be real in an open fracture or impending, as evidenced by blanching of the skin. Make a direct approach *via* an inferior incision along the long axis of clavicle, protecting rami of the supraclavicular nerve. A plate is the implant of choice, which may require removal for prominence if applied dorsal.

A relative indication extrapolated from the adult experience is shortening >2 cm, which is associated with muscle weakness. This may serve as a guideline for the adolescent. The benefit of operative treatment in adults rests in the prevention of nonunion, which is the dominant predictor of functional outcome. The number needed to treat to avoid nonunion is high (>5). Nonunion and malunion are not significant concerns in a child. These, along with earlier return to activity but no long-term difference in activity level, must be balanced by implant removal and postoperative infection.

HUMERUS

Proximal Fracture

Like clavicle fracture, proximal humerus fractures may be divided into birth or other trauma. Remodeling is excellent due to the highest differential in growth of the proximal physis (80%) and accommodation of the enarthrodial adjacent joint [A]. Even though the head is supplied primarily by the anterolateral ascending branch of the anterior circumflex artery, avascular necrosis is not the concern for the proximal femur.

Evaluation The neonate may present with pseudoparalysis. The older child presents with tenderness, without or with a palpable anterior apex, and with the arm rotated medialward to relax tension in the pectoralis major against the distal fragment.

IMAGING Röntgenogrammes should include an axillary view. Most fractures are Salter-Harris I (neonate), Salter-Harris II (older child), or transmetaphyseal at the surgical neck.

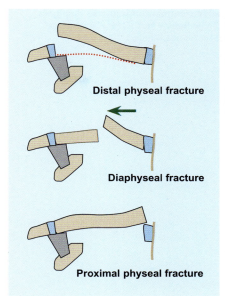

A Clavicle fracture types These may be physeal: the bone escapes through the periosteum, which remains in continuity (*red*) to aid remodeling and healing. A diaphyseal fracture may jeopardize the overlying skin (*green*).

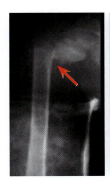
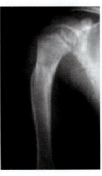

A Proximal humeral fracture The remodeling potential of the proximal humerus is excellent. This fracture was completely displaced and shortened in an 8-year-old girl. It had remodeled completely 2 years later.

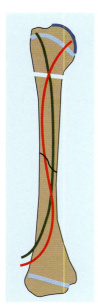

B Operative treatment of humerus diaphysis fracture Ender flexible medullary nailing may be performed retrograde through a small incision.

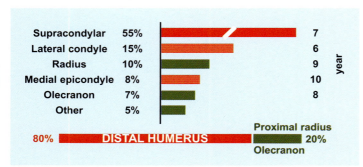

Supracondylar	55%		7
Lateral condyle	15%		6
Radius	10%		9
Medial epicondyle	8%		10
Olecranon	7%		8
Other	5%		

80% DISTAL HUMERUS　　　**Proximal radius 20% Olecranon**

A Elbow fractures in children Frequency and mean age of presentation.

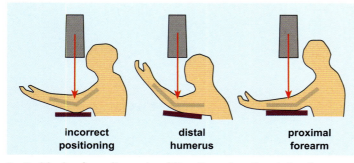

incorrect positioning　　distal humerus　　proximal forearm

B Positioning for radiographs of the elbow Even though the elbow hurts, take time in positioning the upper limb to obtain orthogonal, focused, and specific views to best see a fracture.

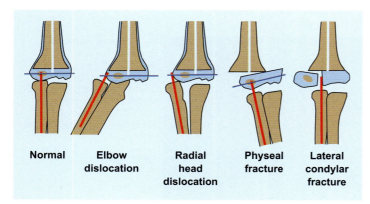

Normal　Elbow dislocation　Radial head dislocation　Physeal fracture　Lateral condylar fracture

C Radiographic alignment of elbow In the normal state, radius points to capitulum in every position and view, ulna is centered under humerus, and radius and ulna move together.

Management The proximal humerus can be expected to remodel ≤90 degrees in the first decade. As a result, most fractures are managed by a shoulder sling. In the second decade, acceptable angulation declines to 45 degrees at 2 years of growth remaining. Reduction is best in the operating room, where the patient is most effectively relaxed, imaging is best, and stability may be determined. Reduction may be hindered by buttonholing of the metaphysis into the deltoid or interposition of the biceps tendon between fracture fragments.

Indications for operative fixation include open fracture, neurovascular compromise, and unacceptable or unstable reduction. For unstable reduction, percutaneous wires may be placed retrograde without or with antegrade fixation through the greater tubercle. For the other indications, use a deltopectoral approach for complete access, followed by wire or screw fixation. Forgo anatomic reduction—this will heal and remodel well—for less dissection.

Diaphyseal Fracture

These may be associated with injury to the radial nerve (Holstein-Lewis), which is tethered as it pierces the lateral intermuscular septum traveling anterior to gain access to the surface of brachialis muscle.

Most fractures may be managed closed with a hanging arm cast or a functional brace. Acceptable displacement is ≤30 degrees angulation and bayonet apposition ≤ 2 cm. For fractures with neurovascular compromise, or unacceptable or unstable reduction, operative treatment is indicated. If the radial nerve is explored, the fracture may be plated. Alternatively, flexible medullary nails may be placed retrograde through a lateral approach, using an entry site posterior to the ridge where the implants may lie under cover of triceps with less prominence [B].

ELBOW

Pædiatric elbow fractures are common, complex, and often complicated [A]. Eighty percent occur at the distal humerus, 20% affecting the proximal radius and olecranon.

Evaluation

Fall from a play structure is the most common mechanism. The patient complains of elbow pain. Swelling may be diffuse, for example, supracondylar fracture, or unilateral, for example, lateral condyle fracture. The elbow may be well aligned or deformed. The skin may be unaffected, ecchymotic, puckered, or breached. Compartments may be soft, firm, or tense. Pulses may be normal, reduced, or absent. The hand may be warm and pink with brisk capillary refill or cool and blanched or blue. Neural function may be normal or compromised: because this requires cooperation of a child in pain and who is frightened, the examination may be inconclusive. There may be concomitant injuries, such as of wrist in addition to elbow.

Imaging

Order specific tests and specific views for specific problems.

Röntgenogramme This is the mainstay for imaging elbow fractures [B]. Obtain anteroposterior and lateral views of the distal humerus (not elbow) for supracondylar fracture. A radiocapitular view isolates head and neck of radius relative to capitulum, for fracture and dislocation. Medial oblique view may reveal a fracture of the lateral condyle of humerus invisible on anteroposterior and lateral projections.

In addition to the bone, look at the soft tissues, for example, sail sign of occult fracture. In addition to individual bones, look at the relationships between them [C].

Röntgenogramme assesses ossification of the distal humerus, which follows a predictable sequence [D]. Variant ossification may simulate fracture. Absent ossification may conceal fracture.

Arthrogramme This outlines the unossified cartilaginous distal humerus that surrounds the ossification centers. It distinguishes a physeal fracture from elbow dislocation. It shows the articular surface for fractures that extend into the joint, for example, lateral condyle fracture. It permits a dynamic examination of the elbow, for example, for radial head instability.

Ultrasonogramme This noninvasive, rapid, nonradiating, and non-stressful modality can detect an elbow effusion, including a lipohæmar-throsis elevating the posterior fat pad; soft tissue injury, for example, collateral ligament tear; and abnormal relationship of osseous landmarks, for example, increased radiocapitular distance in nursemaid's elbow.

Other MRI, CT, and scintigramme have indications that follow general principles, for example, MRI for soft tissue injury such as ligament tear or osteochondritis dissecans lesion.

Anatomy

A condyle is a rounded paired end of a long bone that is articular. In the distal humerus, the lateral condyle is called "capitulum," the medial "trochlea." Nonarticular apophyses positioned "on top of" (Greek επι–) each condyle are the medial and lateral epicondyles, which serve as sites of attachment for the flexor pronator mass and the mobile wad, respectively, as well as the collateral ligaments.

The vascular supply to the distal humerus is tenuous [E]. Lack of distal anastomoses and dependence of capitulum on one terminal branch and trochlea on two terminal branches of the brachial artery makes these osseous structures vulnerable to delayed union or nonunion or avascular necrosis after fracture.

The capitulum is flexed 40 degrees relative to the shaft of the humerus. A line drawn along the anterior surface of humerus bisects the capitulum. The physis of capitulum subtends a mean angle of 72 degrees (range 64 to 81 degrees) relative to the longitudinal axis of humerus (Baumann angle). The distal humerus is thinned in the sagittal plane to receive the olecranon into a fossa. This forms on lateral projection röntgenogramme an "hourglass," of which the humeral diaphysis forms the upper chamber and the trochlea forms the lower chamber. The tenuity of the olecranon fossa makes reduction and its maintenance difficult, akin to balancing two playing cards on edge.

The carrying angle (10 to 15 degrees, greater in girls than boys) is made up of the brachial angle, between long axis of humerus and transverse elbow axis, and the antebrachial angle, between long axis of ulna and transverse elbow axis.

Pulled Elbow

This may be produced when a nursemaid suddenly pulls a child by the arm away from danger [G]. Presentation is 1 to 5 years.

Evaluation Despite the name, half of cases have no history of a pull. Subluxation of radial head with interposition of annular ligament is sensed by the child as instability. The elbow is slightly flexed and the forearm is stuck in pronation. The child will not move the upper limb, even though play continues suggesting no pain at rest. There is no swelling or deformity. Röntgenogrammes screen for a fracture, and ultrasonogramme may show displacement of the radial head. Recurrence may occur in 15%: it correlates inversely with age but does not persist beyond the first decade.

Management The presentation tends to be characteristic, such that a reduction manœuver may be attempted without imaging. The palpable click when the head of radius centers unencumbered against the capitulum is both therapeutic and confirmatory of the diagnosis. Reduce by forceful forearm supination, in which position the annular ligament is taut, thumb pressure on the anterior head of the radius, and elbow flexion, followed by repeated pronation and supination. Alternatively, start with hyperpronation to reproduce the mechanism of injury. In the absence of a click, observation for half an hour will show the child beginning to use the upper limb again. Teach a parent the manœuver for

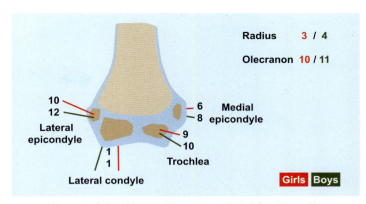

Radius   **3 / 4**

Olecranon **10 / 11**

10
12
Lateral epicondyle

6 Medial
8 epicondyle

9
10

1
1

Trochlea

Lateral condyle

Girls Boys

D Ossification of distal humerus Mean age (years) for girls and boys.

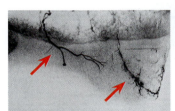

E Vascularity of distal humerus The trochlea is perfused by nonanastomotic end arterioles (*red*).

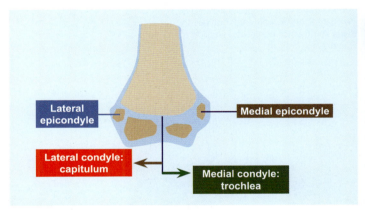

Lateral epicondyle

Medial epicondyle

Lateral condyle: capitulum

Medial condyle: trochlea

F Anatomic landmarks of the distal humerus The distal physis of humerus (*blue*) contributes to longitudinal growth and differs from the physes for the epicondylar apophyses.

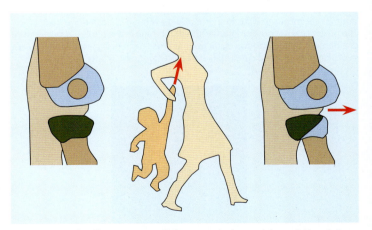

G Nursemaid's elbow Because of the eccentric shape of the radial head, the broadest part contacts the incisure on the ulna in supination, making this the most stable position for the proximal radioulnar articulation. In pronation, the annular ligament (*green*) is relaxed. With a pull on the elbow (*red*) with the forearm in pronation, the annular ligament slips in between capitulum and radial head, which subluxates to become partially uncovered.

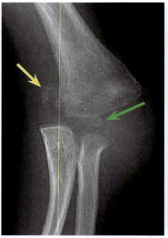
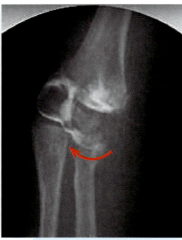

H   Distal physeal separation
Röntgenogrammes show malalignment of ulna–radius relative to humerus. Proximal radius is aligned with capitulum, which has moved from its normal location (*green*). Ulna is aligned with bone that represents healing around the trochlea (*yellow*). That radius and ulna are aligned with the bone of the distal humerus demonstrates that the elbow joint is not dislocated. Arthrogram (*red*) outlines the distal epiphysis of humerus, revealing the fracture.

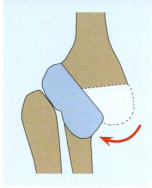

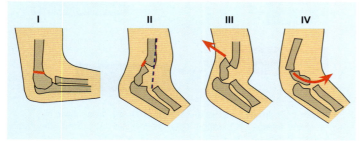

I   Classification of supracondylar humerus fractures (Gartland) I is non- or minimally displaced. II is displaced posterior to a line drawn along the anterior cortex of the distal humerus (*blue*), with intact posterior cortex. In III, the posterior cortex is disrupted as the distal fragment is displaced posterior to the humerus. Flexion of the distal fragment has been designated type IV. A designation of A indicates medial displacement, and B lateral.

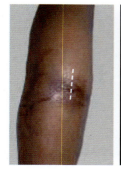
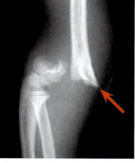

J   Cutaneous injury associated with supracondylar humerus fracture The proximal spike (*red*) tents and bruises and may perforate the antecubital skin. If closed reduction does not produce acceptable alignment, open reduction may be performed *via* an incision over the site of injury (*white*).

recurrent episodes. In uncertain cases, for example, after prior reduction attempts, place the patient in a sling and re-evaluate the next day. Consider MRI for persistent pain or lack of use.

Distal Humerus Physeal Separation

This fracture occurs in children <7 years, after which it cedes to supracondylar fracture as the physis stabilizes by the formation of a V-shaped cleft between the condyles.

Evaluation It is associated with birth trauma and nonaccidental trauma. The child presents with pain, swelling, and pseudoparalysis. The wide physeal surfaces limit deformity, in particular tilt, as compared with supracondylar fracture. Physical examination may reveal "muffled crepitus," as cartilage moves against cartilage. Röntgenogrammes show that the radius and capitulum (which appears at 1 year) are in line with each other, demonstrating that the elbow joint is not dislocated, but out of line from the remainder of the humerus, demonstrating that the elbow joint has shifted off the distal humerus. If röntgenogrammes are unclear, ultrasonogramme will show enough to decide management, without the need for sedation as would be required for MRI.

Management Cubitus varus is the most common complication of closed reduction and casting. Treat this like a supracondylar humerus fracture (*q.v.*). Perform an arthrogramme to ensure accurate visualization of the distal humerus, which will aid reduction and percutaneous wire fixation [H].

Supracondylar Humerus Fracture

This represents more than half of pædiatric elbow fractures. It is the most operated pædiatric fracture. Stress concentration as the distal metaphysis of humerus thins abruptly to the fossa of olecranon, which provides a fulcrum in the extended elbow of an outstretched upper limb planted to stop a fall, makes this site vulnerable to fracture.

Classification The fracture has been classified according to the direction and extent of sagittal displacement [I]. Extension types represent >95%. They are produced by a fall onto the outstretched upper limb, with the hand as the point of contact. Flexion type is produced by a fall onto the flexed elbow, with the olecranon as the point of contact. This is more unstable because the posterior soft tissue envelope, which acts as an internal tether for closed reduction, is disrupted to allow the distal fragment to flex and translate anteriorward. Of extension types, 2/3 are I, with equal distribution of the remainder among II and III.

Evaluation The elbow hurts, is swollen, and assumes a sinuous shape. In extension type, the antecubital skin may be bruised by the proximal spike, puckered when the proximal spike perforates the brachialis (indicating potential for difficult reduction), or breached [J]. The forearm compartments may be tense: pain with passive stretch may be difficult to assess in a child who is scared. Similarly, the child may not cooperate with motor and sensory testing of the hand: be patient and persist. It is essential to know the injury function, to ensure that no significant change occurred by operation. Are pulses palpable and comparable to the other side? Is the hand warm or cool, pink or dusky? Is capillary refill brisk, <2 seconds?

IMAGING Röntgenogrammes classify the fracture. They also assess reduction and fixation. Measure Baumann angle, an indirect measure of carrying angle. Pay attention to the medial cortex: do not accept shortening or overlap, because this risks cubitus varus. Restoration of the hourglass indicates correction of rotation. A lateral of the distal fragment and an oblique of the proximal fragment, which present a widening fracture surface, represent malrotation. In fact, this is the intended appearance of osteotomy to correct cubitus varus (*v.i.*). Make sure every implant captures enough of both fragments.

Management Type I is treated with above-elbow cast. Types II and III are treated by closed reduction and wire fixation, within 24 hours of injury. The technique originated in adults (Swenson). Reduction consists of several components.

- "Milk" the limb. This may be accomplished manually or by a von Esmarch rubber bandage. It reduces swelling, which facilitates manipulation of the fracture. Be gentle over the proximal spike, where the brachial artery is draped and where this manœuver may add injury.
- Traction. Take time to overcome muscles in spasm. Include varus and valgus, to disengage any cortical overlap, and medial and lateral rotation of the distal fragment.
- Anterior and distalward force on olecranon. This is akin to reduction of a distal radius fracture.
- Flex the elbow to lock the reduction against the intact soft tissue envelope. This may blanch the hand. Pronate and supinate the forearm to fine-tune the final position. Do not be so zealous with this step that the posterior soft tissues are torn and now the fracture is a less stable type IV.

If reduction is unacceptable closed, open the fracture. Make an incision over the proximal spike, long enough to bluntly dissect free entrapped brachialis and other soft tissues [J]. Insert into the fracture an elevator that may be used as a shoehorn to translate the distal fragment anteriorward. At this point, the reduction may be completed closed. Medial and lateral incisions are indirect and may destabilize the fracture. A formal exploratory anterior incision carries risk in a traumatized and distorted elbow.

Fixation is percutaneous with smooth Kirschner wires of diameter appropriate for age [K]. These may be inserted lateral, through capitulum, or medial, through medial epicondyle. Iatrogenic injury to the ulnar nerve by medial wire may be mitigated by inserting this after lateral fixation in elbow extension to relax the ulnar nerve posteriorward and by making a small incision to reflect the ulnar nerve. Medial and lateral wires are biomechanically most stable. Lateral wires are stable enough, if the count equals the type, for example, three wires for a type III.

Flexion type fractures are treated by closed reduction and wire fixation. Reduction is gentle and variable according to instability of distal fragment.

After operation, apply an above-elbow cast in 80 degrees of flexion. Increasing flexion increases risk of compartment syndrome. Bivalve the cast to allow for early swelling. Follow the patient within a week for röntgenogrammes and to overwrap the cast. Displacement is unlikely after 1 week, because this fracture heals rapidly. Remove wires and cast in the clinic at 3 to 4 weeks after operation.

Complications

NEURAPRAXIA This occurs in 10% to 15% of cases [L]. Nerves traversing the elbow are stretched and not cut by the fracture. When the distal fragment is displaced lateralward, the anterior interosseous nerve is tethered by the proximal spike. When displaced medialward, the radial nerve is draped over the spike. In flexion type, the ulnar nerve is injured as it travels posterior to the elbow.

Iatrogenic neurapraxia with medial wiring is 4%, > 90% ulnar. Iatrogenic neurapraxia of lateral-only wiring is 3%, half of the median nerve. Iatrogenic injury is understood by a medial wire to the ulnar nerve. Not clear are the contributions of reduction, including multiple attempts, and wire insertion, including multiple attempts and passage beyond the opposite cortex, all of which contribute regardless of insertion side.

The majority of nerve injuries are apraxias. Recovery may be long and follows a pattern expected of wallerian degeneration: ulnar nerve is last to recover, with a window up to 8 months. Educate the patient and family, who may witness a claw hand before function returns. Consider electromyography and nerve conduction studies at 6 months: if there is no evidence of significant recovery, neurolysis is indicated. Act upon a change in nerve function after operation. Exploration is immediate and direct. Consider removal of a medial wire for ulnar deficit. Check röntgenogrammes for a fracture gap suggesting nerve entrapment. An early MRI neurogram may be performed after wire removal.

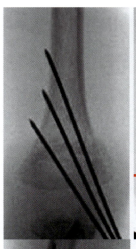
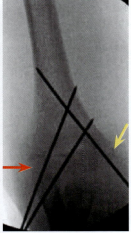
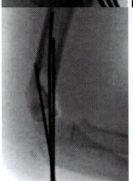

K   Fixation patterns Lateral through capitulum (*red*) avoids the ulnar nerve. Medial through the epicondyle (*yellow*) is made safer for ulnar nerve by extending the elbow and reflecting the nerve by a small incision. Diverge wires at the fracture in both planes. Do not cross at the fracture site. Start wires anterior in order to capture the capitulum and the bone of the olecranon fossa.

AIN	Radial	Median	Ulnar	PIN	Multiple	Total
5.5	4.5	3.5	2	1	1.5	12.5

L   Nerve injury % for extension type. AIN: anterior interosseous nerve. PIN: posterior interosseous nerve.

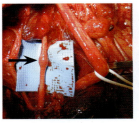

M   Vascular injury The brachial artery was explored for a dysvascular hand after fixation. The median nerve is retracted. The artery, thinned by spasm, was occluded by a thrombus (black). The artery was grafted due to an associated intimal tear.

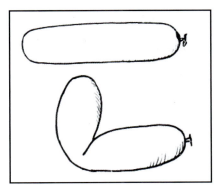

N   Swollen limb Bleeding into the limb has been likened to a balloon (Charnley). It will be constricted at the elbow with flexion, which is associated with compartment syndrome if > 90 degrees.

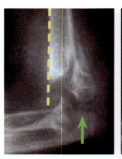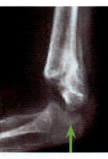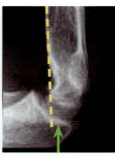

O   Remodeling in sagittal plane Remodeling is possible in the plane of elbow motion. The capitulum moves anteriorward to be crossed by the anterior humeral line over 3 years.

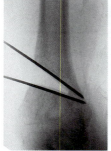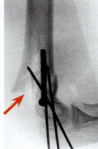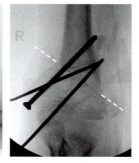

P   Osteotomy for cubitus varus There are many techniques. By a lateral approach, a wedge is resected. Osteotomy is closed and the distal fragment is rotated lateralward (mismatch between proximal and distal fragments on lateral) to correct varus and medial rotation. Osteotomy is fixed with a screw, which is retained, supplemented with percutaneous wires. The most common complication is displacement, hence the screw or alternately use of a plate or external fixator.

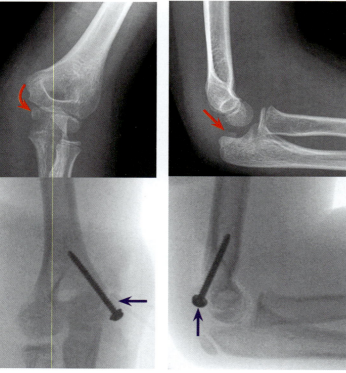

Q   ORIF of medial epicondyle fracture The epicondyle is incarcerated in a valgus elbow (*red*), leaving the donor site empty. It is reduced to its posterior location and fixed with a screw (*blue*).

VASCULOPATHY A change in circulation is noted in 5% of cases, most in type III, including reduction in temperature, reduced or absent pulse, change in cutaneous color, and slowed capillary refill. While bone and joint outcomes are unaffected by when the fracture is surgically treated within the first 24 hours, a dysvascular distal limb, characterized as cold, blanched, or dusky, with absent pulses and sluggish capillary refill, is an emergency.

Reduce and fix the fracture. If vascular status is normal, characterized by present pulses, observe. If the distal limb is dysvascular, explore the brachial artery and repair as indicated. There is no consensus on the pulseless limb (by Doppler), but well-perfused hand. Pulselessness may be regarded as an indication for vascular imaging or exploration of the brachial artery [M], which will show injury in more than half of cases. A well-perfused hand may be regarded as a sign of collateral flow that is sufficient until a brachial artery in spasm recovers or a thrombus recannulates, or even if the brachial artery remains occluded. The latter scenario cannot predict future vascular demand.

Less than 1% of cases are complicated by compartment syndrome. This has been related historically to closed reduction and casting in elbow flexion > 90 degrees [N]. This led to splinting in extension until swelling dissipated, followed by flexion for reduction while the fracture remains malleable (Egyptian method).

MALUNION This may be hyperextension or cubitus varus. A goal of reduction is to position the distal fragment so that the capitulum is crossed but not necessarily bisected by the anterior humeral line. The strict criteria for reduction of this fracture, which is nonarticular, are related to the small differential of growth at the distal humerus (20%) and the ginglymoid nature of the elbow joint. If the distal fragment is posterior to the anterior humeral line, remodeling may improve alignment in the plane of joint motion. This is variable, increasing with decreasing age [O].

Lack of coronal plane remodeling results in cubitus varus, as the distal fragment tends to displace to shorten the medial column. Despite the name, which emphasizes the coronal deformity, varus is accompanied by medial rotation, such that the clinical deformity is striking, as both the elbow (varus) and the forearm (medial rotation) are affected. Indication for operative treatment is unacceptable appearance [P]. Evidence of dysfunction, including ulnar neuritis, is limited. Wire fixation alone is associated with osteotomy displacement.

STIFFNESS Loss of >5 degrees occurs in <5% of cases. One factor is heterotopic ossification, as an aberrant response to muscle injury, in particular brachialis. Heterotopic ossification may be excised once motion has plateaued.

Medial Epicondyle Fracture

This is an avulsion, under pull of medial collateral ligament following a valgus stress sustained by a fall onto the outstretched upper limb. Half are associated with elbow dislocation.

Evaluation Dislocation results in an elbow that is diffusely swollen with medial ecchymosis, a presentation that is out of proportion with avulsion of a small osseous fragment. There may be a history of chronic elbow pain due to overuse. There may be ulnar neurapraxia, from stretch, entanglement around the epicondyle, or entrapment in the joint.

IMAGING When incarcerated, the fragment may be obscured on röntgenogrammes by overlap with the olecranon. In such a case, its absence from the normal site is a key sign.

Management Because the epicondyle is not articular and does not contribute to longitudinal growth of the humerus, significant displacement has been accepted historically. Apply an above-elbow cast with the forearm in pronation to relax the flexor–pronator mass. Mobilize the elbow early (3 weeks) because the global soft tissue injury to the joint will stiffen the elbow. Educate patient and family that recovery will be protracted, and consult a physiotherapist.

Absolute indication for intervention is incarceration in the joint of the epicondyle, which does not escape during spontaneous reduction [Q]. If the fragment cannot be extracted by a closed manœuvre consisting of elbow valgus, forearm supination, and wrist and finger extension (Roberts), which reproduces the mechanism and tensions the flexor–pronator mass, open reduction is indicated.

Operation for displacement, and how much, is debatable. Controversy swirls around elbow instability rather than mal- or nonunion. This is akin to fracture of the intercondylar eminence of tibia, where associated laxity of the anterior cruciate ligament may have the greater impact on functional outcome. As a result of this recognition, in particular for the throwing athlete who will apply extreme valgus stress during cocking and swing (e.g., baseball pitcher), millimeter displacement beyond single digits is an indication for reduction and fixation. First find and decompress the ulnar nerve. Fix the fragment with a screw and washer, or with two wires and a nonabsorbable suture in a tension band construct. Mobilize early to avoid elbow stiffness. Because of the subcutaneous nature of the epicondyle, implant removal is not uncommon.

Lateral Condyle Fracture

This is a challenging fracture because it is articular, it is bathed in synovial fluid, and it depends upon a posterior terminal nonanastomosing branch of the brachial artery. These factors conspire to delay or prevent union and to create growth disturbance.

The fracture originally was classified according to exit at the articular surface (Milch). In type I, the fracture travels through the capitulum. In type II, the fracture emerges between capitulum and trochlea, thereby separating radiocapitular from ulnohumeral joints to produce an unstable elbow. This recognition is the principal contribution of this system. Alternatively, the fracture may be classified according to articular breach and displacement [R, S], which guide treatment. The mechanism of injury combines avulsion under varus stress with axial loading through radius.

Evaluation The patient presents with pain, lateral swelling, ecchymosis, and crepitus without gross elbow deformity.

IMAGING Röntgenogrammes are the standard. Oblique views, in particular medially directed, may expose a fracture invisible on standard anteroposterior projection. Operative arthrogram aids assessment of fracture type and reduction of articular surface.

Management Less than 2 mm of diastasis of the metaphysis suggests an intact articular surface. This may be managed by above-elbow cast. Follow weekly with röntgenogrammes for late displacement.

For displacement > 2 mm, outline the articular surface with an arthrogram: if intact, fix with divergent percutaneous wires. If the articular surface is disrupted, and for widely displaced fractures, open reduction and internal fixation are indicated:

- Consider performing this in the prone position [T].
- Do not dissect the distal fragment, in particular posterior, where its tenuous blood supply enters. Excessive dissection for complete visualization risks osteonecrosis.
- Expose the anterior cortex of the proximal fragment and the anterior fracture edges.
- Clean the fracture to the trochlea.
- Reduce the distal fragment with a pointed tenaculum, applying medialward translation, flexion (the capitulum is flexed 40 degrees), and compression. Read the reduction anterior and lateral.
- Fix with divergent steel wires inserted percutaneously remote from incision. Bioabsorbable pins have been used for longer fixation without cutaneous exposure given that these fractures heal relatively slowly. A screw may be used if there is a large metaphyseal fragment.
- Excise the lateral periosteum at the fracture to reduce lateral overgrowth and spur formation.

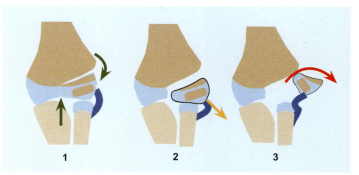

R Classification of lateral condylar fractures In type 1, the lateral condyle fragment hinges at an intact articular surface, opening at the metaphysis. This may be treated closed. In type 2, the fragment is completely separated and translated but not rotated (*orange*). In type 3, the fragment is widely rotated (*red*).

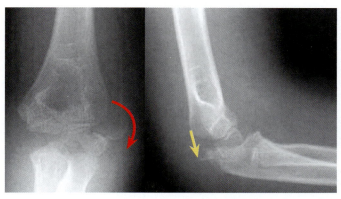

S Lateral condyle of humerus fracture The fracture passes through the capitulum (Milch I). The fragment is widely rotated (*red*) and displaced (*yellow*), making this a type III.

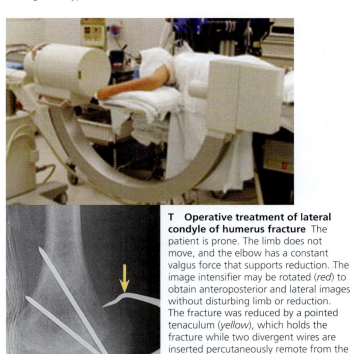

T Operative treatment of lateral condyle of humerus fracture The patient is prone. The limb does not move, and the elbow has a constant valgus force that supports reduction. The image intensifier may be rotated (*red*) to obtain anteroposterior and lateral images without disturbing limb or reduction. The fracture was reduced by a pointed tenaculum (*yellow*), which holds the fracture while two divergent wires are inserted percutaneously remote from the surgical incision.

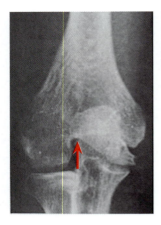

U Growth disturbance Fishtail deformity (*red*) represents focal osteonecrosis from injury to the lateral trochlear vessel. Distortion of the distal articular surface of humerus limits motion.

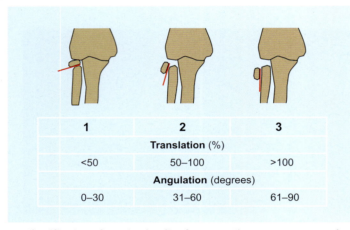

	1	2	3
Translation (%)			
	<50	50–100	>100
Angulation (degrees)			
	0–30	31–60	61–90

V Classification of proximal radius fractures The two components of displacement are translation and angulation.

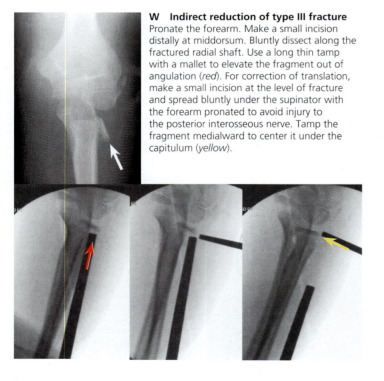

W Indirect reduction of type III fracture Pronate the forearm. Make a small incision distally at middorsum. Bluntly dissect along the fractured radial shaft. Use a long thin tamp with a mallet to elevate the fragment out of angulation (*red*). For correction of translation, make a small incision at the level of fracture and spread bluntly under the supinator with the forearm pronated to avoid injury to the posterior interosseous nerve. Tamp the fragment medialward to center it under the capitulum (*yellow*).

Medial Condyle Fracture

This represents <1% of elbow fractures in children. The approach to this resembles lateral condyle fracture. The following are distinctive features:

- The medial condyle fracture may be missed on röntgenogramme, due to the relatively late appearance of its ossification center, hence its inclusion in TRASH: The Radiological Appearance Seemed Harmless. Normal appearance of medial epicondyle when a medial fracture is suspected clinically is an indication for MRI of the elbow.
- Two independent branches of brachial artery supply the trochlea. Injury to the lateral ramus may lead to osteonecrosis of the lateral aspect of the trochlea, producing a fishtail deformity of the distal humerus [U].

Proximal Radius Fracture

More than 90% of proximal radius fractures are transmetaphyseal (neck) or involve the proximal physis (Salter-Harris II, or I). Radial head fracture is rare in a child. The radiocapitular joint stabilizes the elbow against valgus stress and provides longitudinal stability of the forearm and wrist during grip. Like condylar fractures, articular location slows union. Like medial epicondyle fractures, proximal radius fractures stiffen the elbow. Delay of open treatment > 48 hours increases the likelihood of stiffness.

Evaluation Pain is localized at the proximal radius and exacerbated by supination. There is associated swelling but no gross deformity of the elbow. The patient may complain of referred wrist pain.

IMAGING Radiocapitular view (45 degrees oblique with elbow flexed at 90 degrees) röntgenogramme isolates capitulum and proximal radius away from overlap by trochlea and ulna, respectively. Angulation may be easier to measure, but translation may be more important due to the cam effect of the proximal radius on ulna [V].

Management Apply an above-elbow cast for type 1 for 3 weeks.

Type 2 and 3 fractures are indications for operative treatment. Start with manipulation under anæsthesia, where the child is fully relaxed and imaging is good. Apply thumb pressure on the radial head with the elbow flexed at 90 degrees, with a varus force to open the radiocapitular joint and while repeatedly pronating and supinating the forearm. With pronation, advance the thumb, so that it blocks the radial head during supination.

Open treatment may be indirect or direct. Indirect approach *via* a small incision may reduce stiffness [W]. A flexible medullary nail inserted retrograde may hook the proximal fragment, reducing it by rotation of the nail [X]. A wire may be inserted into and in the plane of the fracture, after which it may be levered to elevate the proximal fragment and correct angulation, akin to the Sauve-Kapandji technique for the distal radius. For fractures irreducible by indirect methods, open reduction is performed *via* a Kocher approach.

This is an example where open reduction of a fracture need not be followed automatically by internal fixation. The fovea of radius stabilizes the fragment against the capitulum. Move the elbow and forearm to make sure the reduction is stable: if not, then fix it with 1 to 2 wires.

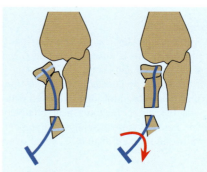

X Indirect reduction of type III fracture A flexible medullary nail (*blue*) is introduced retrograde across fracture into proximal fragment, which is reduced by rotation of the nail (*red*).

Olecranon Fracture

A unique feature of olecranon fracture in a child is apophyseal avulsion in type I osteogenesis imperfecta. This occurs at a younger age and may be bilateral. Because of reduced bone quality, treat with a tension band construct that uses long medullary wires, which are more stable due to bending and internal cortical contact.

Evaluation Pain is localized over the olecranon. Make sure that there is no pain over radial head and that forearm supination is supple, to rule out a Monteggia fracture (*v.i.*). There is associated swelling but no gross deformity of the elbow.

IMAGING Röntgenogrammes demonstrate articular extension, displacement, and comminution. CT is indicated to evaluate a fractured articular surface.

Management Displacement <2 mm may be managed in an above-elbow cast in 30 degrees of flexion, to relax the triceps brachii.

Surgical treatment is indicated for articular displacement >2 mm. Most pædiatric olecranon fractures are uncomminuted and can be effectively fixed with a tension band construct, using a nonabsorbable suture rather than wire.

FOREARM

Monteggia Fracture

Force applied to the forearm results in osseous failure of the ulna with ligamentous failure of the radius, including annular and quadrate ligaments. This may be missed in a young child before ossification of the proximal epiphysis of radius or when focus on an ulna fracture distracts from injury at the elbow.

Evaluation There is pain over ulna fracture and radiocapitular articulation, where head of radius may produce a fullness or may be palpable. There may be a posterior interosseous nerve deficit due to traction by the displaced radial head in the supinator.

The fracture has been classified by Bado [A, B].

IMAGING Röntgenogrammes may show fracture or plastic deformation of the ulna, with the apex into the interosseous space toward the radius. On lateral projection, ulnar border is normally straight: beware of an anterior convexity. Obtain dedicated elbow images, including radiocapitular view. CT and MRI may be necessary to confirm complete reduction of head of radius because its ossification center is small.

Management Even though the fracture is classified according to direction of radial head dislocation, and disability is related to radial head dislocation, the ulna fracture guides treatment.

- Plastic deformation or greenstick fracture of ulna. Perform a closed reduction, which both straightens ulna and reduces radial head. Follow with weekly röntgenogrammes to rule out late displacement.
- If closed reduction does not stabilize the radial head, and for complete fracture of ulna, which may drift despite reduction and result in late dislocation of radial head, place a percutaneous medullary wire into the ulna, which as it straightens and lengthens allows closed reduction of radial head. Use the largest diameter to engage isthmus because length is as important as alignment. Perform an arthrogram and put the elbow and forearm through full range of motion to make sure head of radius is anatomically located and stable.
- Comminuted or otherwise length-unstable ulna fracture. Open reduction and plate fixation of the ulna to restore length are necessary for a stable reduction of radial head.

For chronic presentation, defined as >3 months, consider reconstruction [C]. Anterior dislocation of radial head may hurt and limit motion of the elbow. Despite this, children are undeterred, which, together with variable results after late reconstruction, argue for observation. Balance this with deformation of proximal radius, elbow instability, and degenerative arthritis in the adult, which may be more persuasive.

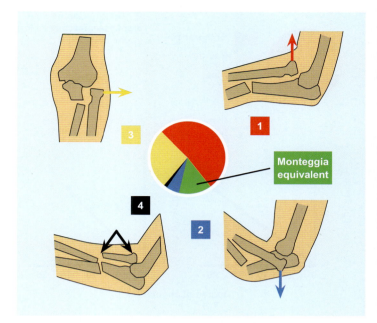

A Classification and distribution of Monteggia fracture The first three types are distinguished by direction of radial head dislocation. Type 4 includes fracture of both bones, in addition to radial head dislocation.

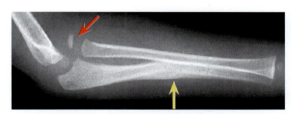

B Monteggia equivalent Bado recognized a further category of equivalent lesions. There is a fracture through the proximal physis of radius. The anterior apex of ulna fracture dislocated the head of radius at time of injury.

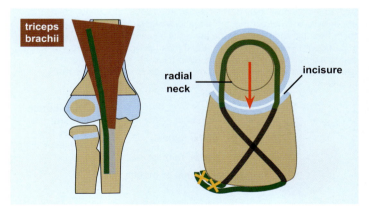

C Reconstruction of chronic Monteggia fracture Prerequisite is no dysplasia of the radial head. An extended Kocher incision allows access to triceps aponeurosis and proximal ulna for osteotomy. Position the patient prone with forearm supinated, and stay under supinator, in order to avoid posterior interosseous nerve. Open the radiocapitular joint and remove obstacles to reduction, including the torn and degenerated annular ligament. Cut the ulna and allow it to lengthen and realign with an apex dorsal bow. Drill two tunnels (*gray*) through the ulna to emerge on either side of radial incisure. Weave a slip of triceps aponeurosis (*green*), left attached at its distal insertion, through the tunnels around the neck of radius. Tension the reconstructed ligament while pronating and supinating the forearm, sewing free end of aponeurosis to insertion (*orange*). Fix the ulna with a plate in the position that achieves a radial head relocation without pressure. Tunnel architecture results in a net force (*red*) that is centered in incisure.

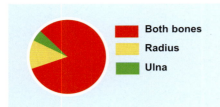

D Distribution of diaphyseal fractures Most involve both bones.

- Both bones
- Radius
- Ulna

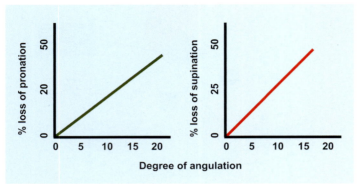

E Loss of motion with angulation of both bones of forearm 10 degrees of residual angulation in the midforearm produces a loss of rotation that approaches 20% of pronation (*green*) and 25% of supination (*red*). Due to its steeper curve, 40% of supination is lost by 15 degrees.

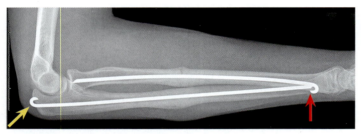

F Medullary nailing of both bone forearm fractures Rush rods are the original and continue to be effective. Their hooked ends may be sunk into olecranon (*yellow*) in a mature adolescent and lay flush at the radial entry site (*red*) to reduce prominence. The beveled end allows nails to glance off the opposite cortex. Retract the dorsal tendons of the distal forearm to protect them from the sharp edge at the tip of the nails. Steinmann pins are versatile, in particular for younger children. Bend their tip slightly to create a bevel and to aid traversal of the fracture. Bend the other end into a hook, which can engage the entry sites less prominently and which facilitates extraction if necessary.

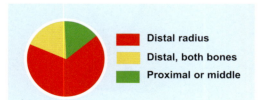

G Distribution of forearm fractures Distal radius predominates.

- Distal radius
- Distal, both bones
- Proximal or middle

Type	Displacement	Comment
Epiphysial	<50% translation	
Metaphyseal	≤ 30 degrees in 1st decade ≤ 20 degrees in 2nd decade Bayonet apposition in 1st decade	0.9 degrees/ month sagittal 0.8 degrees / month coronal

H Acceptable displacement in distal radius fractures Remodeling of distal radius is excellent given 75% growth at this end of the bone. Up to 10 degrees of angulation produces no dysfunction in the adult. For metaphyseal fractures, remodeling approaches 1 degree/month and is reliable up to 20 degrees, variable between 20 and 30 degrees.

Both Bone Fracture

Forearm fractures behave like intra-articular fractures: malunion restricts movement in the transverse plane. Most involve both bones [D]. The mechanism of injury is a fall onto an outstretched upper limb, planting of the hand, and supination of the distal forearm to produce an apex volar deformity or pronation of the distal forearm to produce an apex dorsal deformity.

Evaluation The forearm is deformed and swollen. Check the skin for breach. Rule out compartment syndrome. Examine the entire upper limb for another fracture, for example, supracondylar humerus fracture producing a "floating elbow."

IMAGING Röntgenogrammes show the following:

- Which bone is fractured
- Apex and degree of deformity
- Level of fracture—proximal, middle, and distal
- Fracture pattern—plastic deformation, greenstick, complete, and comminuted
- The bicipital tuberosity, which is the landmark for determining rotation. It is seen *en profil* medial at 90 degrees of supination and lateral at 90 degrees of pronation. In neutral, it is overlapped by the radius.

Management For uncomplicated fractures, including no significant cutaneous breach and no compartment syndrome, closed reduction is the initial approach. The manœuvre that distinguishes both bone forearm fracture reduction is rotation: two bones are being reduced simultaneously, and the mechanism of injury includes rotation. The direction of rotation of the distal forearm may be determined by the adage, "Turn the thumb toward the apex." Position the forearm in cast to counteract deforming forces on the distal elements. Supinate for proximal fractures in response to the action of supinator on the proximal fragment and pronator on the distal fragments. Harness the interosseous membrane when molding the cast to have the shortest anteroposterior diameter.

Acceptable residual angulation is determined by age, level of fracture, and anticipated loss of forearm rotation [E]. Residual angulation of 15 degrees leads to 25% loss of pronation. Supination is more sensitive, with 25% loss occurring at 10 degrees. As a result, a guideline is ≤20 degrees in the first decade, relying on remodeling for partial correction, which declines to 10 degrees in the adolescent. Bayonet apposition is acceptable in the first decade.

Operation is indicated for complicated fractures, unacceptable or unstable reduction, concomitant fractures, and refracture, which occur in 5% of cases. Flexible medullary nailing may be performed closed *via* entry points proximal to Lister tubercle after retraction of extensor pollicis longus and under anconeus to avoid proximal physis of ulna [F]. If closed reduction is difficult, open the fracture sites (dissected by the trauma) enough to admit tenacula safely. In the first-decade child, nailing of a single bone, often the ulna because it is easier, may be sufficient if the other bone is reduced thereby to an acceptable angle. In such a case, the nail acts as an internal splint for the uninstrumented bone. Plate fixation is indicated for comminuted fractures. Plates are more stable but require formal, more extensive dissection. In the first-decade child, potential for bone overgrowth is an indication for plate removal, which is not uncomplicated.

Distal Radius Fracture

This is the most common fracture in children [G]. Mechanism is a fall onto the outstretched upper limb. Greater than 95% are apex volar, as the child lands on the palm of the hand. This fracture may be transmetaphyseal, torus or complete, or a Salter-Harris type. The type II metaphyseal fragment is the original "Holland" fragment, after the first published röntgenogramme by the English radiologist Charles Thurston Holland (1863–1941).

Evaluation There is sinusoid deformation of the wrist associated with swelling. Examine the volar wrist, for example, for tense ecchymosis, and rule out carpal tunnel syndrome.

IMAGING Röntgenogrammes show the following:

- Fracture type
- Apex and amount of deformity

Management Because outcomes for torus fracture are predictably good, apply a below-elbow cast or splint and modify activity. In the distal radius, displacement may be divided into epiphysial and metaphyseal [H]. For Salter-Harris III or IV fractures, >2-mm displacement is unacceptable at the articular surface.

For uncomplicated fractures, including no carpal tunnel syndrome, that are displaced significantly, closed reduction is the initial approach:

- Apply traction. This may be prolonged before reduction to take advantage of viscoelasticity by hanging the limb by finger traps.
- Reproduce the mechanism of injury to aid unlocking fragments.
- Translation. This is distal followed by anterior. Do not flex the wrist to achieve the latter, because this will reduce the volume and compress the contents of the carpal tunnel.
- Apply an ulnar force to counteract with supination to relax the brachioradialis, which is a major deformer and which accounts for late displacement in cast [I].

Abide by the adage, "One reduction by one surgeon" (Blount), for physeal fractures, in order not to add to the risk of growth disturbance. Follow with röntgenogrammes because displacement occurs during the first 2 weeks in 5% of cases.

Indications for operation are as follows:

- Complicated fractures, for example, requiring carpal tunnel release, in order to avoid late displacement requiring repeat intervention
- Multiple fractures, for example, ipsilateral supracondylar humerus fracture
- Unacceptable or unstable reduction, for example, drift in cast

Fix with 1 to 2 percutaneous transphyseal wires passed retrograde through the styloid process of radius [J]. Bluntly dissect the soft tissues in this region, where rami of the superficial radial nerve course on their way to the dorsal hand.

Galeazzi Fracture

This represents fracture of the radius with disruption of the radioulnar joint. In children, soft tissue integrity leads to physeal variants [K]. Unlike Monteggia fracture, this is rare in children compared with adults, peaking during adolescence. The radius fracture may be apex volar with volar displacement of the ulna, which is produced by a supination force on the forearm. Alternatively, a pronation force results in an apex dorsal radius fracture with dorsal displacement of the ulna.

These are managed closed in most children. Indications for operation are unstable or irreducible distal ulna and unacceptable angulation of the radius. Plate the radius and cross pin the ulna.

WRIST AND HAND

Half of hand injuries have an osseous component. Incidence is bimodal: a peak occurs at preschool, consisting of a crush mechanism where soft tissue injury predominates, for example, a closing door, while a larger peak is seen in the second decade, when sports lead to fractures [L].

Scaphoid Fracture

While carpal fractures are rare in children, the scaphoid is most frequently broken. Peak incidence is in the teenage years. Because they are rare, scaphoid fractures may be missed in children.

Evaluation There is guarded wrist motion. Tenderness at the volar distal pole is more reliable than in the anatomic snuffbox, which may be uncomfortable in the normal state.

IMAGING Include an oblique scaphoid view röntgenogramme [M]. If röntgenogrammes are negative, consider scintigramme for detection

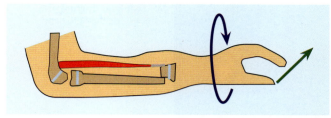

I Deforming force of brachioradialis To counteract brachioradialis (*red*) during reduction, apply an ulnar force to (*green*) and supinate (*blue*) the distal fragment.

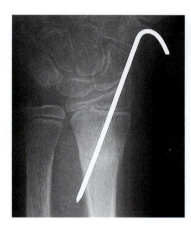

J Fixation of distal radius fracture A wire is passed percutaneously retrograde through styloid process of radius.

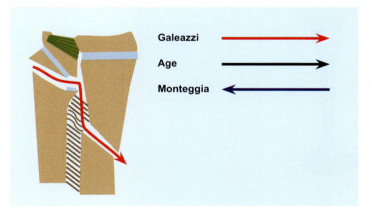

K Galeazzi equivalent Salter-Harris II of distal ulna with metaphysis of radius (*red*) The distal radioulnar joint and triangular fibrocartilaginous complex (*green*) that stabilizes it remain intact. The force parallels the direction of the fibers of the interosseous membrane (*brown*). Galeazzi fracture has been described as a reverse Monteggia fracture, based upon both the characteristics of the injury and the age of presentation.

Part	Most injured
Rays	Border
Digit	Smallest finger
Thumb	In adolescents
Phalanx	Proximal
	Base
Metacarpal	5th
	Shaft

L Distribution of hand fractures The smallest finger is most exposed and most injured.

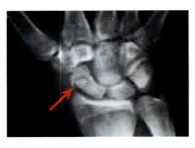

M Scaphoid fracture This is treated according to general principles.

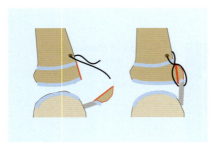

N Fixation of hand fractures Most are pinned. Large fragments may be fixed with screws. For small but critical fragments, tension band construct takes advantage of stout surrounding soft tissues, which are restored in the process.

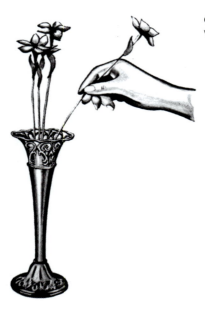

O Bouquet pinning As the vase is filled, the flowers rectify.

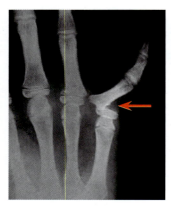

P "Extraoctave" fracture Despite displacement at presentation, this was readily reduced closed. The fracture of the fourth phalanx requires no reduction.

and CT or MRI for characterization. MRI also reveals associated triangular fibrocartilage complex tears.

Management Distal pole fractures heal in a thumb spica cast, as do nondisplaced waist fractures. Displaced waist fractures are at risk of osteonecrosis and are treated with open reduction and internal fixation. Open reduction and internal fixation, with autogenous bone grafting, are indicated for established nonunions. Wrist pain after successful treatment of scaphoid fractures may represent persistent triangular fibrocartilage complex tears, which may be addressed arthroscopically.

Metacarpal Fracture

Physeal Nonarticular types are managed by closed reduction and casting. Articular types require open reduction and wire internal fixation if displaced, to reduce risk of posttraumatic arthritis.

BENNETT FRACTURE Fractures of the base of first metacarpal include Salter-Harris III and IV types [N]. They often require operation for displacement, due to intrinsic mobility of the thumb and deforming forces of its muscular attachments, opponens pollicis for a radial epiphysial fragment and abductor pollicis longus for an ulnar fragment.

Neck

BRAWLER'S FRACTURE The most common metacarpal fracture in children is of the neck of fifth metacarpal. It is more fittingly called "brawler's fracture" because a boxer is trained to punch not swing, to not make contact with the most mobile metacarpal. This presents a flexion deformity, which should be reduced if the metacarpal head is prominent in the palm. Reduction also is indicated for associated rotational deformity of the smallest finger. Flex the metacarpophalangeal joint to 90 degrees and drive the proximal phalanx of the smallest finger dorsal to extend the distal metacarpal fragment (Jahss manœuvre).

Shaft These fractures are treated according to general principles. Acceptable alignment, from second to fifth metacarpals, is 20, 30, 40, and 50 degrees, respectively. Rotational deformity such that the finger crosses others during flexion is unacceptable. Unacceptable loss of length is >3 mm, which is associated with a decrease in extrinsic flexion and extension ratios as well as reduction in interosseous power for grip > 10%.

Operative treatment consists of closed or open reduction with transverse or medullary wire fixation or a combination of the two techniques. Medullary nailing has been described as bouquet pinning, after the universal concept (*cf.* flexible nailing of femur fractures) that filling the canal will simultaneously correct angulation and restore length [O]. The starting points for retrograde nailing are the radial and ulnar collateral recesses. Antegrade nailing, starting at the base of metacarpal and prebending the wire tips, may reduce neck fractures in the same manner as for proximal radius fractures (*q.v.*).

Phalangeal Fracture

Educate the patient and family that juxta- and intra-articular digital fractures are at risk for prolonged stiffness or permanent loss of motion and that associated swelling may persist for months.

Physeal The metacarpophalangeal collateral ligaments originate from the metacarpal epiphysis and insert onto the epiphysis of the proximal phalanx, which accounts for the high frequency of physeal fractures in this region.

SKIER'S, GAMEKEEPER'S THUMB Salter-Harris III fracture at the base of first metacarpal, including skier's (acute) or gamekeeper's (chronic) thumb, often requires surgical intervention due to intrinsic mobility of the thumb.

MIDDLE PHALANX Fractures of this epiphysis may result from hyperextension, during which the volar plate holds onto a fragment, or under eccentric load of the central slip, which avulses a dorsal fragment. Treat volar plate avulsions with a short period of immobilization and early motion, to avoid stiffness: a fibrous union is stable and does not interfere with function. Immobilize (in full extension) avulsions of the central slip longer to allow it to heal without a lag.

"EXTRAOCTAVE" FRACTURE Salter-Harris I or II fracture of the proximal phalanx of the smallest finger with abduction of the distal fragment may extend the reach of a pianist's hand [P]. Lever the smallest finger.

radiad over a pencil or other similarly shaped object placed deep into the fourth web space., This requires fortitude of both patient and surgeon. After reduction, buddy taping is as effective as a splint or cast.

Jersey fracture Eccentric load on flexor digitorum profundus, as when a finger is caught in a jersey during sports, may avulse a volar fragment off the distal phalangeal epiphysis. Since superficialis is intact, the child will be able to flex the proximal interphalangeal joint, leading to missed or delayed diagnosis if the distal joint is not isolated and tested. The fracture may be widely displaced proximalward in the tendon sheath. This is treated by open reduction, often over a dorsal button.

Mallet fracture In mallet fracture, a fragment of dorsal epiphysis of the distal phalanx is pulled off during eccentric loading of the extensor tendon. Splint this in extension. Counsel patient and parents that an extensor lag (<10 degrees) or a dorsal prominence may persist after healing, which does not impact function. Subluxation of the distal phalanx is an indication of extensive injury and an indication for operative treatment.

Seymour fracture This is an open Salter-Harris I or II physeal fracture of the terminal phalanx associated with avulsion of the base of the nail. Flexed posture of the finger may lead to confusion with a mallet injury. The infolded germinal matrix obstructs reduction and may lead to a pseudomallet deformity if not lifted out of the physeal region. Because of this, and because this is open with a risk of infection, open reduction and internal fixation are indicated. Repair the nail bed after careful extraction from the fracture. Fix the phalanx with a percutaneous wire passed retrograde and longitudinally across the interphalangeal joint, as much to protect the nail bed repair as to stabilize the fracture.

Shaft For nonarticular types, buddy taping suffices. Follow long oblique or spiral fractures closely for late displacement.

Tuft fracture The mechanism is a crush of the finger tip. Most significant is evaluation of the nail. For a subungual hæmatoma > 50%, remove the plate and explore and repair the nail bed as indicated. Place a spacer between bed and eponychium to facilitate regrowth of the plate.

Condyles The mechanism of condylar fracture is axial load with shear or impaction (akin to a pilon fracture). Pattern of fracture may be unicondylar, bicondylar, or comminuted. Röntgenogrammes may show a double shadow on lateral projection, reflecting displacement of one of the condyles relative to the other. CT may be necessary to measure accurately articular displacement. The level of fracture is at the opposite end of the physis, limiting remodeling. Because of this, along with the fact that it is an articular fracture of a small joint, little displacement is acceptable. Manage by closed reduction with a percutaneous wire used as a joystick. If open reduction is necessary, preserve the soft tissue envelope in order not to add to the risk of avascular necrosis. The long fracture surface may receive screws for fixation.

Dislocation

Most dislocations are uncomplicated and stable once reduced. Apply traction for reduction, which is followed by buddy tapping for 1 to 2 weeks with early mobilization to avoid stiffness.

Irreducible dislocations, more likely at the metacarpophalangeal joint, typically are due to volar plate entrapment [Q]. These are termed complex because an open reduction is necessary: a dorsal approach, while indirect from the volar plate, avoids the digital neurovascular bundle that is displaced into the dislocation.

Tendon Laceration

This is evaluated and managed according to general principles. A child with a deep wound will be more difficult to examine in an emergency setting than an adult: consider the operating room, including extension of the laceration [R]. Partial tendon laceration is more difficult to diagnose than complete laceration, which alters the resting position of the hand [S]. After tendon repair, cast immobilization (4 weeks) yields better results than protected mobilization, in part due to less tendency to stiffness and less cooperation in the child.

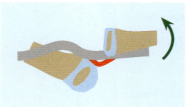

Q Complex dislocation Dorsal displacement (*green*) of proximal phalanx brings with it the volar plate (*red*), which becomes interposed to obstruct reduction.

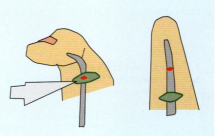

R Site of laceration A tendon laceration sustained in a flexed position may present a cutaneous wound (*green*) that is proximal to a partial injury (*red*) or that is distal to a complete injury.

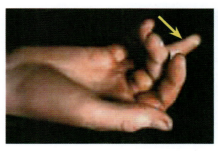

S Complete laceration There is no resting flexor tone.

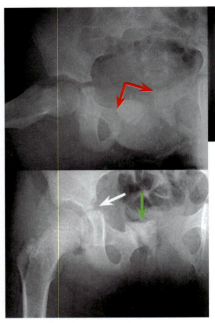
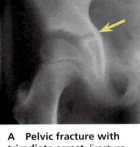

A Pelvic fracture with triradiate arrest Fracture with pubic diastasis (*red*) was treated with immobilization and protected weight bearing. Triradiate physeal bridge developed (*yellow*), which was excised (*white*) to restore growth and avoid posttraumatic hip dysplasia. Note the malunion of the os pubis (*green*).

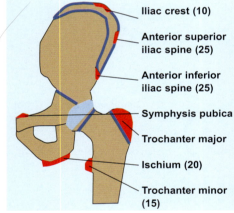
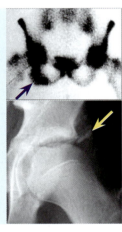

B Avulsion fractures of the pelvis Numbers represent percentage incidence. Scintigramme shows increased uptake at ischial apophyseal avulsion (*blue*) in a gymnast. Röntgenogramme shows avulsion of the anterior inferior iliac spine (*yellow*) in a soccer player.

Iliac crest (10)

Anterior superior iliac spine (25)

Anterior inferior iliac spine (25)

Symphysis pubica

Trochanter major

Ischium (20)

Trochanter minor (15)

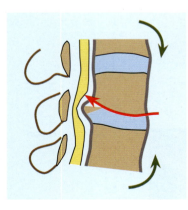

C Slipped vertebral epiphysis The lesion represents a Salter-Harris I or II fracture of the vertebral epiphysis. Under axial loading and flexion (*green*), the intervening physis gives way before the stronger fibers of the anulus. Rotation accounts for laterality. The epiphysis slips posteriorward into the vertebral canal, where it may encroach upon the theca and cauda equina. The lesion has been typed as cartilaginous or osteochondral, small or large, and central or lateral. Most frequent location is low lumbar.

PELVIS

Fractures of the pelvis are managed according to general principles, for example, identify associated visceral injury such as bladder disruption. Several factors distinguish the child from the adult:

- Incidence of pelvic fractures in children is <0.2% of all fractures, compared with 2% for adults.
- Energy for fracture is higher in children, while energy of hip dislocation is lower. In syndromes such as trisomy 21, hip dislocation does not have the same grave consequences of avascular necrosis and osteochondral fracture as in adults.
- The triradiate cartilage is at risk for growth disturbance [A].
- Apophyseal avulsion fractures are managed mostly by protected weight bearing [B]. These typically are acute, occurring during sports characterized by sudden acceleration, for example, running for a soccer ball. Tenderness localizes the injury and röntgenogrammes confirm the diagnosis. MRI allows accurate measurement of displacement. There is no consensus on unacceptable displacement: >2 cm may result in weakness of attached muscle, for example, of hamstrings in ischial avulsion, to which gymnasts are particularly vulnerable. Most heal with rest over a 3-month period. Use a screw if there is a sufficiently large osseous fragment. Union takes longer than closed primary healing. Otherwise, excise the fragment and repair the tendon to donor site *via* drill holes or anchors.

SPINE

Prevalence of spine fractures in children is 1% of adults. There are two injuries that are unique to children.

SCIWORA

The acronym stands for *Spinal Cord Injury Without Radiographic Abnormality*. This is seen principally in the first decade. There is a mismatch in elasticity between the pædiatric spine and spinal cord. The former stretches up to 5 cm but returns to the original position without residual displacement to appear radiographically normal. The latter does not tolerate stretch beyond 5 mm, resulting in traumatic myelopathy. Myelopathy may be acute or delayed (≤48 h) and transient or complete. Its severity correlates inversely with age: the younger the patient, the greater the mismatch in elasticity. While röntgenogrammes are negative, MRI will show the spinal cord injury.

Management is focused on the neural injury. Immobilize the spine and protect activity for 3 months. Reassess spinal stability with dynamic imaging. The spinal column heals but the spinal cord may not.

Slipped Vertebral Epiphysis

Each vertebral body is rimmed by an *epi*physis, which is articular at the intervertebral disc. The epiphysis is thickened along its circumference like a "ring" into which insert the fibers of the anulus similar to an "apophysis" [C].

Evaluation The patient presents with back pain, without or with radiculopathy, and a flexed posture with tilting opposite to any laterality of displacement in order to increase the capacity of canal and intervertebral foramen. The principal differential is herniated intervertebral disc. This, along with the circumpubertal age of presentation, accounts for the typical delay in diagnosis.

IMAGING Röntgenogrammes may show an osseous fragment off the posterior corner of the vertebral body, although CT is definitive. Myelography shows a sharp thecal indentation. MRI, which may miss the osseous fragment, delineates the associated protrusion of the intervertebral disc.

Management This is symptomatic unless pain is unacceptable in intensity or duration, there is neural compromise, or the osseous fragment encroaches upon >50% of the vertebral canal. Excision of the fragment may be more successful than discectomy for back pain because the intervertebral disc is relatively spared.

TRAUMATIC DISLOCATION

Traumatic joint dislocations in children are treated with a controlled reduction. Reduction may be closed with sedation in an emergency setting or in the operating room adding chemical paralysis as indicated. Operative reduction allows conversion to open reduction if closed method is unsuccessful, and fixation of associated fractures.

Elbow Dislocation

This may be associated with fracture of the medial epicondyle (*q.v.*). The dislocation may spontaneously reduce, giving a normal appearance on röntgenogramme, including no significant displacement of the medial epicondyle. Significant and diffuse elbow swelling with tenderness and variable ecchymosis over the medial epicondyle betray the gravity of the injury. Beware that the medial epicondyle may become incarcerated in the joint, which is an indication for open reduction.

Elbow instability occurs when fracture of the lateral condyle (*q.v.*) extends into the intercondylar groove (Milch type II), necessitating reduction of the elbow at the time of open reduction and internal fixation of the fracture.

Dislocation of the head of radius may be congenital or traumatic. Traumatic may be isolated or in conjunction with fracture, for example, of Monteggia (*q.v.*). Confirm anatomic reduction of the head of radius by demonstrating that it points at the capitulum in every radiographic view, including at all angles of elbow flexion in the lateral projection and on a radiocapitular view. Add an arthrogram or MRI when in doubt.

Ankle Dislocation

Physeal fractures, such as a triplane of the distal tibia (*q.v.*), may present as an ankle dislocation [A]. At the time of operation, raise an anterior flap over the fibula to evaluate the syndesmosis: if this is disrupted, reduce the fibula into the incisura of the tibia under direct vision before fixation. This manœuver avoids posterior displacement under indirect clamp reduction with image intensification, which may narrow the mortise and restrict talar movement.

Knee Dislocation

This may be atraumatic. Atraumatic knee dislocation may be isolated, referred to as congenital (*cf.* Lower Limb chapter), or associated with another condition, for example, in Larsen syndrome (*cf.* Syndromes chapter). The majority of traumatic knee dislocations in children are patellar (*q.v.*), which may or may not spontaneously reduce. Traumatic tibiofemoral knee dislocations in adolescents are managed according to adult principles.

Hip Dislocation

Most hip dislocations in children are posterior, presenting as an adducted, flexed, and medially rotated thigh [B]. As a general rule, hip dislocation requires less energy in children compared with adults, whereas it takes more energy to fracture the proximal femur of a child. The teenager represents a transitional stage. Reduce a hip dislocation within 6 hours, in case the retinacular vessels are stretched or kinked rather than torn. In the setting of an open proximal femoral physis, perform the manœuver in the operating room, where chemical paralysis will reduce the risk of physeal fracture [C]. The physis is the weakest site and will yield at the rim of the acetabulum if the pericoxal muscles are not relaxed. The resulting epiphysial separation may tear the retinacular vessels, resulting in osteonecrosis of the proximal epiphysis of femur. Opening the hip to clear an obstacle to reduction, such as entrapped labrum, is preferable to a forcible closed reduction.

An eccentric reduction, or a joint width relatively greater than the contralateral side or absolutely >3 mm, is an indication for imaging such as a CT or MRI to evaluate the hip for an intra-articular fragment. Such imaging also examines the pelvis for associated injury. In the operating room, an arthrogram may be performed to confirm concentric reduction. Scintigraphy to evaluate blood flow to the head of femur has been unreliable in predicting osteonecrosis. An intra-articular fragment may be extracted by arthroscopic or an open approach.

GENERAL

Harris HA. Line of arrested growth in the long bones in childhood: the correlation of histological and radiographic appearances in clinical and experimental conditions. *Br. J. Radiol.* 4(47):561–569, 1931.

Hübner U, Schlicht W, Outzen S, Barthel M, Halsband H. Ultrasound in the diagnosis of fractures in children. *J. Bone Joint Surg.* 82(8)-B:1170–1173, 2000.

Matsen FA III, Veith RG. Compartment syndromes in children. *J. Pediatr. Orthop.* 1(1):33–41, 1981.

Poland J. *Traumatic Separation of the Epiphysis.* London: Smith, Elder & Co.,; 1898.

Salter RB, Harris WR. Injuries involving the epiphyseal plate. *J. Bone Joint Surg.* 45(3):587–622, 1963.

Skaggs DL, Friend L, Alman B, Chambers HG, Schmitz M, Leake B, Kay RM, Flynn JM. The effect of surgical delay on acute infection following 554 open fractures in children. *J. Bone Joint Surg.* 87(1)-A:8–12, 2005.

PHYSEAL BRIDGE

Langenskiöld A. An operation for partial closure of an epiphysial plate in children, and its experimental basis. *J. Bone Joint Surg.* 57(3)-B:325–330, 1975.

NONACCIDENTAL TRAUMA

Akbarnia BA, Torg JS, Kirkpatrick J, Sussman S. Manifestations of the battered-child syndrome. *J. Bone Joint Surg. Am.* 56(6)-A:1159–1166, 1974.

Caffey JP. Multiple fractures in the long bones of infants suffering from chronic subdural hematoma. *Am. J. Radiol. Radium Ther.* 56:163–173, 1946.

Kempe CH, Silverman FN, Steele BF, Droegenmueller W, Silver HK. The battered child syndrome. *JAMA* 181:17–24, 1962.

Kleinman PK. *Diagnostic Imaging of Child Abuse.* Baltimore, MD: Williams & Wilkins; 1998.

FOOT

Buch BD, Myerson MS. Salter-Harris type IV epiphyseal fracture of the proximal phalanx of the great toe. A case report. *Foot Ankle Int.* 16(4):216–219, 1995.

Johnson G. Pediatric Lisfranc injury: "bunk bed" fracture. *Am. J. Roentgenol.* 137(5):1041–1044, 1981.

Smith JW, Arnoczky SP, Hersh A. The intraosseous blood supply of the fifth metatarsal: implications for proximal fracture healing. *Foot Ankle* 13(3):143–152, 1992.

ANKLE

Caterini R, Fursetti P, Ippolito E. Long-term follow-up of physeal injury to the ankle. *Foot Ankle* 11(6):372–383, 1991.

Lynn MD. The triplane distal epiphyseal fracture. *Clin. Orthop.* 86:187–190, 1972.

Ramsey Pl, Hamilton W. Changes in tibiotalar area of contact caused by lateral talar shift. *J. Bone Joint Surg.* 58(3)-A:356–357, 1976.

TIBIA

Cozen L. Fracture of the proximal portion of the tibia in children followed by valgus deformity. *Surg. Gynecol. Obstet.* 97(2):183–188, 1953.

McLennan JG. The role of arthroscopic surgery in the treatment of fractures of the intercondylar eminence of the tibia. *J. Bone Joint Surg.* 64(4)-B:477–480, 1982.

Meyers MH, McKeever FM. Fracture of the intercondylar eminence of the tibia. *J. Bone Joint Surg.* 41(2)-A:209–222, 1959.

Polakoff DR, Bucholz RW, Ogden JA. Tension band wiring of displaced tibial tuberosity fractures in adolescents. *Clin. Orthop.* 209:161–165, 1986.

PATELLA

Houghton GR, Ackroyd CE. Sleeve fractures of the patella in children: a report of three cases. *J. Bone Joint Surg.* 61(2)-B:165–168, 1979.

FEMUR

Bar-On E, Sagiv S, Porat S. External fixation or flexible intramedullary nailing for femoral shaft fractures in children. A prospective, randomised study. *J. Bone Joint Surg.* 79(6)-B:975–958, 1997.

Basener CJ, Mehlman CT, DiPasquale TG. Growth disturbance after distal femoral growth plate fractures in children: a meta-analysis. *J. Orthop. Trauma* 23:663–667, 2009.

Ender J, Simon-Weidner R. Die fixierung der trochanteren bruche mit runden, elastischen condylennageln. *Acta Chir. Austriaca* 1:40–42, 1970.

Gonzalez-Herranz P, Burgos-Flores J, Rapariz JM, Lopez-Mondejar JA, Ocete JG, Amaya S. Intramedullary nailing of the femur in children. Effects on its proximal end. *J. Bone Joint Surg.* 77(2)-B:262–266, 1995.

Kregor PJ, Song KM, Routt ML, Sangeorzan BJ, Liddell RM, Hansen ST. Plate fixation of femoral shaft fractures in multiply injured children. *J. Bone Joint Surg.* 75(12)-A:1774–1780, 1993.

Illgen R II, Rodgers WB, Hresko MT, Waters PM, Zurakowski D, Kasser JR. Femur fractures in children: treatment with early sitting spica casting. *J. Pediatr. Orthop.* 18(4):481–487, 1998.

Küntscher G. Die marknägelung von knochenbrüchen. *Arch. Clin. Chir.* 200:443–450, 1940.

Ligier JN, Metaizeau JP, Prevot J, Lascombes P. Elastic stable intramedullary nailing of femoral shaft fractures in children. *J. Bone Joint Surg.* 70(1)-B:74–77, 1988.

Moon ES, Mehlman CT. Risk factors for avascular necrosis after femoral neck fractures in children: 25 Cincinnati cases and meta-analysis of 360 cases. *J. Orthop. Trauma* 20:323–329, 2006.

Ratliff AH. Fractures of the neck of the femur in children. *J. Bone Joint Surg.* 44-B:528–542, 1962.

Rush LV. Dynamic intramedullary fracture-fixation of the femur. Reflections on the use of the round rod after 30 years. *Clin. Orthop.* 60:21–27, 1968.

Townsend DR, Hoffinger S. Intramedullary nailing of femoral shaft fractures in children via the trochanter tip. *Clin. Orthop.* 376:113–118, 2000.

CLAVICLE

McKee RC, Whelan DB, Schemitsch EH, McKee MD. Operative versus nonoperative care of displaced midshaft clavicular fractures: a meta-analysis of randomized clinical trials. *J. Bone Joint Surg.* 94(8)-A:675–684, 2012.

Robinson CM, Goudie EB, Murray IR, Jenkins PJ, Ahktar MA, Read EO, Foster CJ, Clark K, Brooksbank AJ, Arthur A, Crowther MA, Packham I, Chesser TJ. Open reduction and plate fixation versus nonoperative treatment for displaced midshaft clavicular fractures: a multicenter, randomized, controlled trial. *J. Bone Joint Surg.* 95(17)-A:1576–1584, 2013.

HUMERUS

Holstein A, Lewis G. Fractures of the humerus with radial-nerve paralysis. *J. Bone Joint Surg.* 45(7)-A:1382–1388, 1963.

Sarmiento A, Kinman PB, Galvin EG, Schmitt RH, Phillips JG. Functional bracing of fractures of the shaft of the humerus. *J. Bone Joint Surg.* 59(5)-A:596–601, 1977.

ELBOW

Babal JC, Mehlman CT, Klein G. Nerve injuries associated with pediatric supracondylar humeral fractures: a meta-analysis. *J. Pediatr. Orthop.* 30(3):253–263, 2010.

Culp RW, Osterman AL, Davidson RS, Skirven T, Bora FW Jr. Neural injuries associated with supracondylar fractures of the humerus in children. *J. Bone Joint Surg.* 72(8):1211–1215, 1990.

de Jager LT, Hoffman EB. Fracture separation of the distal humeral epiphysis. *J. Bone Joint Surg.* 73(1)-B:143–146, 1991.

el-Sharkawi AH, Fattah HA. Treatment of displaced supracondylar humerus fractures of the humerus in children in full extension and supination. *J. Bone Joint Surg.* 47-B:273–279, 1965.

Gartland JJ. Management of supracondylar fractures of the humerus in children. *Surg. Gynecol. Obstet.* 109(2):145–154, 1959.

Greenspan A, Norman A. The radial head, capitellum view: useful technique in elbow trauma. *Am. J. Roentgenol.* 138(6):1186–1188, 1982.

Haraldsson S. On osteochondrosis deformas juvenilis capituli humeri including investigation of intra-osseous vasculature in distal humerus. *Acta Orthop. Scand. Suppl.* 38:1–232, 1959.

Jakob R, Fowles JV, Rang M, Kassab MT. Observations concerning fractures of the lateral humeral condyle in children. *J. Bone Joint Surg.* 30(4)-B:430–436, 1975.

Mintzer CM, Waters PM, Brown DJ, Kasser JR. Percutaneous pinning in the treatment of displaced lateral condyle fractures. *J. Pediatr. Orthop.* 14(5):462–465, 1994.

Roberts NW. Displacement of the internal epicondyle into the elbow-joint: four cases successfully treated by manipulation. *Lancet* 227(2):78–79, 1934.

Smith RW. Observations on dysfunction of the lower epiphysis of the humerus. *Dublin Quart. J. Med. Sci.* 9:63–74, 1850.

Swenson AL. The treatment of supracondylar fractures of the humerus by Kirschner-wire transfixation. *J. Bone Joint Surg.* 30(4)-A:993–997, 1948.

White L, Mehlman CT, Crawford AH. Perfused, pulseless, and puzzling: a systematic review of vascular injuries in pediatric supracondylar humerus fractures and results of a POSNA questionnaire. *J. Pediatr. Orthop.* 30(4):328–335, 2010.

FOREARM

Bado JL. The Monteggia lesion. *Clin. Orthop.* 50:71–76, 1967.

Bell Tawse AJS. The treatment of malunited anterior Monteggia fractures in children. *J. Bone Joint Surg.* 47(4)-B:718–723, 1965.

Friberg KSI. Remodelling after distal forearm fractures. II. The final orientation of the proximal and distal epiphyseal plates of the radius. *Acta Orthop. Scand.* 50:731–739, 1979.

Lanfried MJ, Stenclik M, Susi JG. Variant of Galeazzi fracture-dislocation in children. *J. Pediatr. Orthop.* 11(3):332–335, 1991.

Rush LV. *Atlas of Rush Pin Technics.* Meridian, MS: Berivon; 1955.

Seel MJ, Peterson HA. Management of chronic posttraumatic radial head dislocation in children. *J. Pediatr. Orthop.* 19(3):306–312, 1999.

Tarr RR, Garfinkel AI, Sarmiento A. The effects of angular and rotational deformities of both bones of the forearm. An in vitro study. *J. Bone Joint Surg.* 66(1)-A:65–70, 1984.

Waters PM, Kolettis GJ, Schwend R. Acute median neuropathy following physeal fractures of the distal radius. *J. Pediatr. Orthop.* 14(2):173–177, 1994.

WRIST AND HAND

Dorsay TA, Major NM, Helms CA. Cost-effectiveness of immediate MR imaging versus traditional follow-up for revealing radiographically occult scaphoid fractures. *Am. J. Roentgenol.* 177:1257–1263, 2001.

Seymour N. Juxta-epiphyseal fracture of the terminal phalanx of the finger. *J. Bone Joint Surg.* 48(2)-B:347–349, 1966.

Vadivelu R, Dias JJ, Burke FD, Stanton J. Hand injuries in children: a prospective study. *J. Pediatr. Orthop.* 26(1):29–35, 2006.

AXIAL SKELETON

Bradford DS, Garcia A. Lumbar intervertebral disk herniations in children and adolescents. *Orthop. Clin. N. Am.* 2(2):583–592, 1971.

Pang D, Wilberger JE Jr. Spinal cord injury without radiographic abnormalities in children. *J. Neurosurg.* 57(1):114–129, 1982.

Rossi F, Dragoni S. Acute avulsion fractures of the pelvis in adolescent competitive athletes: prevalence, location and sports distribution of 203 cases collected. *Skel. Radiol.* 30(3):127–131, 2001.

SPORTS

BACKGROUND

Participation in sports is on an inexorable rise in Western culture. At play in this trend are the societal prioritization of physical fitness; a zeal for competition; the building of character, for example, confidence, self-image, discipline, and teamwork; a recognition that occupying a child's time with sports is diverting from other allurements of youth, for example, the "screen–refrigerator" complex; and the financial incentives for sports industry and participant, for example, the promise of remuneration in college and beyond. Fueling the frenzy is the presumption that enjoyment is not enough: excellence and success are the driving goals, which may be achieved only by means of early adoption and specialization, for example, preschool, and long hours.

This chapter focuses on the distinctive aspects of sports in the immature skeleton, in contrast with the late teenager, who blends with the adult.

Physis

This provides the single sharpest contrast between children and adults with regard to injury and treatment (*cf.* Trauma chapter).

Maturation

Age is a stricter defining criterion in children than in adults, for example, 1 year separates middle school from high school, yet an ocean separates them socially, psychologically, and physically. Children mature at different rates, whereas adults are mature by definition. Differences are amplified by the growth acceleration of puberty, which correlates with the peak of serious injuries presenting to an emergency facility. The principal stratifier in sports participation during childhood is chronologic age. These factors account for unanticipated psychic and physical risks to children finding their place in sports. A method of stratification based upon assessment of biologic maturity, including such factors as Tanner stage, is more appropriate and safer.

Numbers	Comment
3%	High-school participants in soccer, basketball and American football who go on to play in division I or II
1%	Obtain a college scholarship for athletics
$10,000	Average scholarship
1/5000	Play at the professional level

A **Success in youth sports** The average scholarship covers half the cost of a state school and <1/4 the cost of a private institution. This must be balanced against the costs of lessons, camps, and time raising the elite athlete.

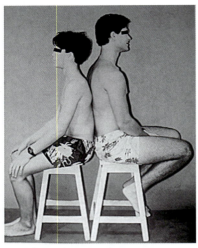

B Differential maturation Even though both are the same age, a boy sits next to a man. This has far-reaching implications on sports participation and performance [Blount].

Age	70's	00's
Preschool	5%	10%
Prepuberty	4%	15%
Adolescents	6%	15%

Food	Cost 1990 → 2007
Energy dense	Cola: ↓ 35% Fast food: ↓ 10%
Vegetables	↑ 10%

C Childhood obesity Childhood obesity was stable until the early 1970s. Its rise coincides with the crossing of child *per diem* consumption of milk (decline) and cola (increase). It has doubled or tripled in a generation. Reductions in the price of food account for 1/3 of the rise in body mass index in children and young adults. There is no evidence that family income impacts obesity. However, maternal employment does (e.g., less time, more prepared food), correlating with a 10% to 33% rise in obesity of children in upper socioeconomic strata.

Gender

Vigorous physical activity delays menarche. A practical outcome is elimination of this as a measure of maturity in the management of conditions affected by growth, for example, scoliosis. Beware of the triad of amenorrhœa, eating disorder, and osteoporosis, which puts the female athlete at increased risk of overuse injuries or stress fractures. Maturation has a narrower window in girls than in boys, in whom it has a long tail, for example, running performance plateaus after puberty in girls whereas it continues to increase in boys.

Thermoregulation

Children's capacity to regulate body temperature is less developed compared with that of adults. A greater surface area to body mass means greater heat absorption from the environment. A growing body produces more metabolic heat *per* mass unit during physical activity. Children sweat less, reducing heat dissipation by evaporation. They have a duller thirst response and so replenish fluid loss later than adults. These characteristics increase the risk of heat-related illness.

Obesity

Childhood obesity is multifactorial and in tumultuous evolution. Obesity may be defined as body mass index >95th percentile. Risk factors include urban residence, which highlights the effects of a sedentary lifestyle with greater access to food, uterine exposure to maternal diabetes and adiposity, and genetic factors in association with certain diseases, for example, Prader-Willi. Musculoskeletal complications include accelerated maturation, lower limb deformity such as Blount disease and slipped capital femoral epiphysis, and increased musculoskeletal complaints such as back pain, all of which may limit activity.

Even though input, for example, eating, and all the forces that influence it, including the economics of food, are ultimately more influential than is output, for example, exercise, sports are intimately intertwined and integral to abatement of the obesity epidemic.

Genetics

The type of sport in which a child participates is determined by interest (of child and parent), social environment, and continual competitive selection. The genetic basis for physical ability and psychological aptitude has remained veiled except for the most rudimentary characteristics such as height for basketball or weight for wrestling. An expanding body of research is uncovering gene polymorphisms that will allow a much more sophisticated understanding. For example, polymorphism in the gene encoding actin-binding protein α–actinin-3, a highly conserved component of fast-twitch skeletal muscle fibers, may separate power and speed athletes from endurance athletes. A recognition that genetics is an immutable component of the performance phenotype may decompress the family when the child does not meet expectations. Genetic testing to identify child aptitude, and the development of sports profiles, will enable more informed and rational decision making.

EPIDEMIOLOGY

Reporting (e.g., in sports that place a premium on toughness) and definitions (e.g., by a coach vs. trainer vs. physician) introduce imprecision in statistical analysis of sports injuries.

Two million children *per annum* are seen in an emergency setting for a sports-related injury. Another 2 million receive nonemergency medical care. Total cost of management of pædiatric sports injuries is $2 billion *per annum*. Most injuries are benign [A]. American football is most injurious [B] and most dangerous, having a 10 times greater rate of catastrophic event, such as permanent nerve deficit, than do other sports. Annual attrition from organized sports is 1/3, while total attrition by adolescence is 3/4. Boys sustain more injuries than do girls, whose rate is increasing more steeply due to more rapid increase in sports participation. Fractures and physeal overuse injuries predominate in preteens, whereas ligamentous injuries come to the forefront in teenagers.

Injury Prevention

Sports and play injuries are unique in that exposure is elective, recurrence is not unusual, and prevention is possible. There are several strategies that may be taken to make these activities safer for children [C]. Three-fourths of school playground fractures involve the upper limb, of which >1/2 are supracondylar humerus fractures (*cf.* Trauma chapter).

THE DISABLED CHILD

The International Wheelchair Games were hosted by Dr. Ludwig Guttmann (German-born refugee to England) on the opening day of the 1948 Summer Olympics in London, for World War II veterans with spinal cord injury. The first Paralympic (Greek παρα: "beside") Games took place in Rome in 1960. There are six categories of disability: limited mobility or wheelchair, amputation, blindness, cerebral palsy, intellectual impairment, and other. The disabled realize the same benefits of sports as able-bodied children. Because they are less active at baseline, sports and strength training are essential for the disabled, including to control obesity, reduce contractures, increase muscle strength, build bone mass, and integrate into the society around them.

In children with Down syndrome, a requirement for participation in Special Olympics is no evidence of instability on lateral flexion–extension röntgenogrammes of the cervical spine. Special considerations for patients with spina bifida relate to vulnerability of skin to breakdown, including from brace wear; fractures, which restrict them from high-contact sports; and wheelchair use. For cerebral palsy, seizure control is essential.

Wheelchair injuries are primarily soft tissue. This ranges from blisters on the hand to decubitus ulcer, due to the design that raises the knees above the pelvis. Overuse injuries are common, in particular of the shoulders.

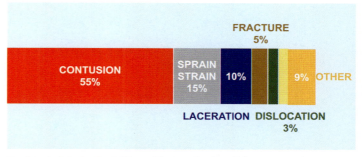

A Sports injuries in children Most are benign. *Yellow* represents concussion at 3%, which will command a larger proportion as focus is brought upon it.

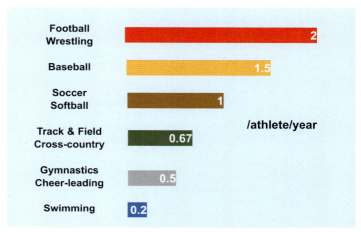

B Injuries brought to medical attention by sport American football leads, followed closely by wrestling. Categories are simplified: in each, the upper has a slightly greater rate. For bigender sports, there are no significant differences. Softball approximates soccer rather than baseball.

PLAYGROUND	
Surface	Soft: shredded rubber, sand, ? wood chips Hard: grass, soil, cement
Fall zone	9 ft between equipment
Height	1 ft/year age up to 6 ft
Entrapment	6" between bars to avoid entrapment of limb or head No open hooks that may catch clothing
PRACTICE & GAME	
Athlete	Fitness Strength training Rest Hydration Protective clothing
Coach	Use and maintenance of correct equipment Education, e.g., first aid, CPR, injury protocols Enforcement of safety rules Reporting of injury Multiple sports with no specialization
Community	Pre-participation assessment Funding, e.g., facilities, monitoring, medical care Evidence based rules and regulations Behavior modification

C Injury prevention in youth sports Recommendations in an evolving landscape. Some are straightforward, others nebulous. An example of the latter is behavior modification, yet 1/3 of athletes who quit include negative interactions with a coach or parent as a reason. Softness of wood chips is debated.

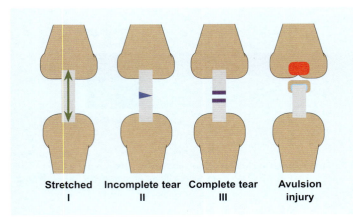

Stretched **I** Incomplete tear **II** Complete tear **III** Avulsion injury

A   Grading of ligamentous injury In type I, there is injury and pain but no instability. In type II, there is more motion but a clear endpoint on manual testing. Type III is characterized by instability, is associated with capsular injury, and lacks an endpoint. Avulsion is a reflection that ligament is stronger than bone in the immature child. The quintessential example is fracture of the intercondylar eminence of tibia.

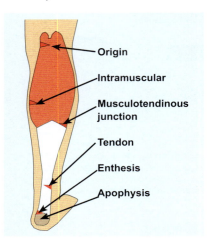

- Origin
- Intramuscular
- Musculotendinous junction
- Tendon
- Enthesis
- Apophysis

B   Triceps suræ injury Different levels of injury present a constellation: muscle strain; tendinitis, including in association with retrocalcaneal bursitis; enthesitis, for example, associated with ankylosing spondylitis; and apophysitis (Sever).

Common Sites	Sport
Medial epicondyle	Throwing, (e.g., baseball)
Iliac spine	Kicking, (e.g., soccer)
Ischial apophysis	Jumping and landing, (e.g., gymnastics)
Apex of patella	Jumping, (e.g., basketball)
Tibial tubercle	Jumping, (e.g., basketball)
Calcaneal apophysis	Running and jumping, (e.g., soccer)

C   Apophyseal injury These result from traction during activities exemplified by the most common sports with which they are associated. The knee dominates in frequency.

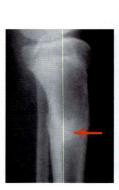
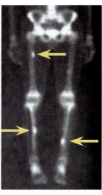

D   Stress fracture Multiple may occur, as in this cross-country runner. Röntgenogramme shows hyperostosis (*red*). Scintigramme reveals involvement of both tibia and femur (*yellow*).

TYPE OF INJURY

Sports injuries may be acute or chronic, which may be described as overuse. Overuse injury results from repetitive submaximal loading, leading to microtrauma that may be reversed by rest. In the absence of rest, cumulative microtrauma results in stress injury. It is a diagnosis of exclusion:

- Pain is intermittent, punctuated by periods of normal function. It does not awaken the child from sleep, even though it may delay falling asleep and require the comfort of a parent. It is not localized, for example, child cups the patella with the hand.
- There are no objective signs of macroinjury, such as joint effusion or other inflammatory sign, deformity, instability, or atrophy.

While initially more benign than acute injury, overuse may take longer to heal; requires active involvement of the child for recovery and future prevention, for example, stretching program and other behavior modifications; and may result in more time away from sports. Rest is simple and cheap and effective, yet may be the most vexing prescription to child and family.

Sports injuries may be divided anatomically into ligament, muscle, physis, fibrocartilage and bone.

Ligament

Ligaments fail suddenly in most cases, by contrast with physeal injuries, which tend to result from repetitive stress. Ligament injuries may be classified [A]. Ligament injuries are most common around the ankle and knee. They may coexist with bony injuries, as seen in tibial spine fractures.

Muscle

Injuries may be of muscle belly, tendon, or enthesis [B].

Physis

In addition to acute fracture (*cf.* Trauma chapter), children involved in sports may present with chronic repetitive stress injuries, for example, Little League shoulder (*q.v.*). Unlike acute fracture, the physis becomes widened, irregular, and tender, but not grossly unstable. One type of injury may usher in the other, for example, Osgood-Schlatter condition preceding fracture of the tibial apophysis. Certain synchondrosis disruptions are classified separately, for example, accessory navicular (*cf.* Foot chapter).

Fibrocartilage

This consists of meniscus and labrum. In the knee, the medial meniscus is more contrained (2-3 mm excursion) compared with the lateral meniscus (10 mm). The medial meniscus is more susceptible to trauma, leading to tear, while the lateral meniscus is more susceptible to reactive hypertrophy, as in the genesis of the discoid form. In the shoulder, the labrum is essential to stability, while in the hip the rôle of the labrum is less clear (cf. Hip chapter).

Bone

Acute fractures are discussed in Trauma. Chronic injuries may result from traction [C] or compression, for example, stress fracture and osteochondritis dissecans.

Stress fractures occur most frequently in the tibia (*cf.* Trauma chapter), metatarsal bones, and femur, for example, in runners [D], and the distal radius and at the pars interarticularis, producing spondylolysis, for example, in gymnasts (*cf.* Spine chapter).

Osteochondritis dissecans represents segmental avascular necrosis of subchondral bone with injury to overlying cartilage. Causes include repetitive microtrauma and a genetic predisposition to localized juxta-articular ischæmia. A subgroup of patients may have been given this diagnosis for disordered epiphysial maturation. It is classified based upon the geographic extent of injury, as determined by injury and at time of operation [E]. Cartilage and stability guide treatment.

- Stage I. Cartilage is intact and fragment is stable. Manage closed.
- Stage II. Cartilage is partially disrupted but fragment is stable. Manage closed or open.

- Stage III. Cartilage is completely disrupted. Fragment remains in place but is loose and at risk for displacement. Manage open, and include fixation.
- Stage IV. Osteochondral fragment has displaced. In the acute setting, it may be returned to the donor site and fixed, with the expectation that it will heal. In the chronic setting, the fragment becomes eroded such that it cannot be put back. Reconstruct the donor site.

CONCUSSION

This also may be referred to as mild traumatic brain injury. Rapid short-duration neural impairment results from biomechanical force applied or transmitted to the head. The pathophysiology includes force resulting in ion dysregulation and vasoconstriction that lead to an energy crisis in the brain. Grading is retrospective, with severity determinable only after recovery. By definition, brain imaging is negative. It is impossible to estimate the scope of the problem because definition, classification, and diagnosis are in flux; however, there is universal agreement that concussion has been underestimated and is increasing.

Preparticipation screening is essential to establish a child's baseline cognitive function. Concussion varies by sport [A]. Symptoms and signs may not appear until hours after the inciting event [B]. Loss of consciousness is rare, and if it lasts more than 30 seconds, should raise concern for a significant intracranial lesion. Assess an athlete away from the field in an environment that will be used for follow-up, such as a quiet room. Any evidence of a structural brain injury is an indication for brain imaging. Postconcussive symptoms and signs typically resolve after a week.

Remove a concussed athlete from the game, from physical exertion, and from school, for a period of "cognitive rest." Allow a return to sports after resolution of signs and symptoms, but not sooner than a week. Because most repeat concussions occur within the first 2 weeks after injury, this may be regarded as a window of vulnerability and a guide for return to sports [C]. Recurrence of symptoms after exertion indicates incomplete recovery. There is no consensus on retirement of an athlete from a sport. This may be considered for the athlete who sustains three concussions in the same season or in whom postconcussive symptoms and signs persist beyond 3 months.

STRENGTH TRAINING

This also is known as resistance or weight training. Strength training enhances muscle power (by resistance) and endurance (by repetition). Strength training differs from body building, which is occupied with æsthetics and stands on its own as a competitive sport. Goals of strength training include both improved performance and reduced injury.

Weights may be free, for example, dumbbell, or static, for example, machine. By requiring control of a limb in space, free weight improves coordination and balance as well as strength. Static weight, in a supported position, is safer. Closed chain exercises are performed with the hand or foot stabilized. A free hand or foot opens the chain. Isotonic exercise maintains a fixed resistance while muscle length varies. In isometric exercise, a muscle contracts without changing its length, for example, in an immobilized limb. Muscle contraction may be concentric, in which length decreases, or eccentric, characterized by lengthening of the muscle during resistance. The latter may accelerate power acquisition at the expense of an increase in injury rate. Alternating concentric and eccentric contraction in rapid succession forms the basis of plyometrics, or jump training, which may reduce the rate of anterior cruciate ligament tears in female athletes.

Strength training in prepubertal children is effective without muscle hypertrophy by recruitment of motor neurons for a given muscle mass.

Begin strength training after 7 years of age, by when a child has developed adult balance and posture control. A schedule of 2 to 3 times/week for 3 months will yield significant results safely. Start with large muscle groups and transition to small. Maintain high repetitions (10) and titrate resistance in 10% increments. Perform 1 to 3 sets with 1 to 3 minutes of

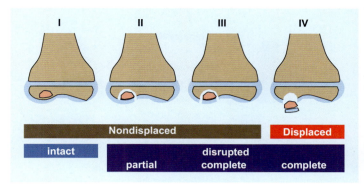

E Classification of osteochondritis dissecans I: Osteonecrosis. II: Dead bone has become separated from surrounding bone, as evidenced by a "halo." Cartilage (*blue*) is partially injured. III: Overlying cartilage is completely broken. Fragment remains in place but is loose and at risk for displacement. IV: Osteochondral fragment has separated or become "dissected" (König) to become a mobile body. There is no desiccation, or "drying."

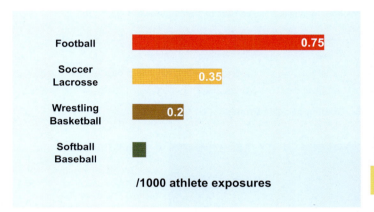

A Concussion by sport American football leads. Data for certain high-risk sports, for example, ice hockey, are limited.

Physical	Cognitive	Emotional	Sleep
Headache	'Foggy'	Irritable	Drowsy
Nausea	Difficult	Sad	Altered
Vomiting	concentration	Nervous	pattern
Balance	Amnesia		
Visual			
Fatigue			
Sensory hypersensitivity			

B Symptoms and signs of concussion Balance may be tested by three positions: standing on both feet with hands on iliac crests with open and shut eyes and standing on the nondominant foot.

Concussion rehabilitation
No physical activity + cognitive rest
Light aerobic exercise
Sports-specific exercise
Noncontact drills
Full-contact practice
Game

C Concussion rehabilitation Return to sports is gradual. Once symptoms and signs have resolved, the athlete may progress through each stage no faster than every 24 hours.

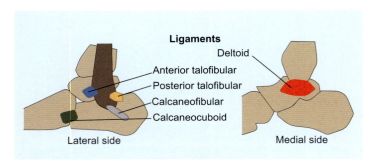

A   Ankle ligaments The anterior talofibular ligament, extending from anterior margin of the fibular malleolus to the talus distal to its lateral articular facet, is most frequently injured. The calcaneofibular ligament, the longest, is a rounded cord that courses from fibular malleolus to a tubercle on the lateral surface of the calcaneus, where the peronei longus and brevis run over it. The posterior talofibular ligament, the strongest of the lateral complex, runs from fibular malleolus to a tubercle on the posterior surface of the talus lateral to the groove for flexor hallucis longus. The deltoid drapes over the tibial malleolus and has two laminæ. Superficial consists of tibionavicular, calcaneotibial, and posterior talotibial. Deep consists of anterior talotibial fibers.

Attenuation	Mild swelling and tenderness
Partial tear	Moderate swelling, unable to bear weight
Complete tear	Marked swelling, bleeding, instability, and disability

B   Grading of ankle sprains.

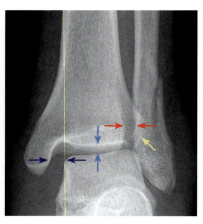

C   Deltoid disruption The ankle of this mature teenager was stepped on, resulting in an acceptably displaced distal fibula fracture. The force emerged through the deltoid ligament, widening the medial joint (*navy*) compared with the superior tibiotalar distance (*blue*). Normal clear space is <6 mm (*red*) and normal overlap of fibula and tibia is >1 mm (*yellow*) on mortise view.

rest between them. Book end each session with a 10-minute period of warm up, including stretching, and a 10-minute cool down. "Detraining," or loss of strength, occurs at 5% to 10%/week. There is no deleterious effect on growth. With proper technique and supervision at no lower than 1:10 instructor:student ratio, there is no increase in injury.

ANKLE

The ankle accounts for the largest number of orthopædic complaints in the child athlete. Sports as a stress test may awaken silent conditions, such as tarsal coalition, or turn normal into abnormal, such as irritation of the calcaneal apophysis.

Ankle Sprain

This represents tear of one or more ankle ligaments, which may be divided into medial and lateral [A]. The medial is termed deltoid, after its resemblance to an upside-down Greek letter delta, Δ. The lateral group consists of three independently named ligaments. Ankle sprains may be classified by severity [B]. With increasing severity, more of the ligamentous complex is torn, bearing with it more pain and instability. The peak incidence of ankle sprain is in latter teenage years. Basketball is the most abundant source (25%), followed by soccer (20%) and American football (15%).

Ankle sprains may be recurrent, due to excessive force in the coronal plane transmitted to the ankle by a tarsal coalition that limits subtalar motion. Also in the differential diagnosis are peroneal retinacular tear and traction on an accessory os subfibulare.

Most ankle sprains are produced by an inversion mechanism. Eversion (1%) produces the high ankle sprain, in which there is disruption of the tibiofibular syndesmosis. Direct force to the lateral leg results in a valgus moment on the knee and external rotation of the ankle.

Evaluation Ask about the mechanism of injury, such as "rolling" the ankle. Swelling may be focal, for example, anterolateral at the anterior talofibular ligament, or diffuse, suggesting a more complete injury that includes the entire lateral ligamentous complex. The deltoid ligament is injured rarely in children. Cutaneous change, for example, ecchymosis, may track beyond the ankle, marking the extent of soft tissue disruption. Look for foot deformity, and range the subtalar joint, to rule out tarsal coalition. Percussion, which will transmit force to bone while minimizing stretch to injured soft tissues, above the tip of fibula may reveal physeal injury; immediately beyond the tip, it may reveal os fibulare avulsion.

Examination of motion is not feasible in the acute setting. In the chronic setting, talar tilt or inversion of the ankle tests the anterior talofibular and calcaneofibular ligaments. The anterior drawer manœuvre also stresses the anterior talofibular ligament. External rotation with valgus tests the deltoid ligament. External rotation and maximal ankle flexion test the syndesmosis, which also may be stressed by manually compressing tibia and fibula.

For eversion testing, ask a patient to stand and rotate the pelvis away from the affected side, reproducing the mechanism of injury. A single limb calf raise will hurt.

IMAGING For a child who is unable to bear weight, or for clinical suspicion of an osseous injury, röntgenogrammes are indicated. Check the trochlea of talus for osteochondral fracture. MRI is the imaging modality of choice to evaluate ligamentous injury, although this rarely is necessary.

Management Ankle sprains are the most undertreated sports injury and have the highest rate of recurrence. Do not hesitate to place a child in a cast to immobilize the ankle enough for the torn ligament(s) to heal. Stiffness is not a concern. Most difficult to achieve is behavior modification: support and rest the ankle and stay out of sports until clinically healed. For a cooperative older child, a cam walker worn full-time for up to 6 weeks suffices. No walking until no pain; no jumping and no running. Healing is evidenced by no swelling, no tenderness, full motion, and unfettered ability to bear weight, which may be assessed by observing no limp, single limb calf raise, hopping, squatting, and "duck walking."

For a syndesmosis injury, as evidenced by widening of the medial joint or tibiofibular clear space, treat with a syndesmotic screw or suture button or both. Remove the screw in 3 months if you don't want it to break.

Osteochondral Lesion of Talus

Anterolateral lesions of the trochlea are more often associated with a recognized traumatic event than posteromedial lesions, which are the product of repeated microtrauma [A]. Mechanism for the former is compression in ankle flexion (dorsiflexion) and eversion, as when an athlete pivots on a planted foot. For the latter, the ankle is extended (plantar flexed) and inverted, as in push off during running. There is no gender predilection. Peak incidence is in the second decade.

Evaluation There may be a history of trauma. The patient complains of ankle pain, which is associated with effusion and stiffness. The patient may sense a mobile body. Chronic ankle pain or persistent ankle pain after there has been sufficient time for an acute injury to heal should raise suspicion for this diagnosis.

IMAGING Obtain röntgenogrammes in ankle flexion and extension to view the anterior and posterior margins of trochlea [B]. Röntgenogrammes may not identify stage I lesions, which will be detected on scintigramme. Cartilage is best seen on MRI, which permits classification and guides management.

Management Prognosis for healing of lesions when they present in the first decade is better than second decade. Acute lesions have a higher healing rate than chronic lesions, of which half heal by closed methods. Stable lesions may be managed closed. Unstable lesions require operative treatment.

STAGE I AND II Cast for 6 weeks with touchdown weight bearing. The lesion is stable, and the cartilage remains partially intact. If the lesion does not heal, operative treatment is indicated. The necrotic bone may be drilled retrograde through the lateral body of talus [C]. Use an image intensifier or an arthroscope to make sure the overlying cartilage is not disturbed. Harvest autogenous bone graft from calcaneus or distal tibia and pack through the drilled tunnel to support the cartilage surface. Alternatively, the lesion may be opened like a book arthroscopically, hinging on the intact cartilage. The bed is débrided of necrotic tissue and drilled or fractured with an awl to stimulate bleeding and healing of the bone. Because opening the lesion may destabilize it, add fixation.

Small lesions and those that are difficult to access may be excised, although there is no consensus on size or location.

STAGE III Treat as an unhealed stage II. Add fixation because the lesion is unstable.

STAGE IV If the fragment is viable and has a reasonable osseous component for union, treat as a stage III. Sculpt the donor site to match the fragment. Otherwise, remove the mobile body. If the defect is small, excise, débride, and drill. If large, reconstruct, which requires open access. Lateral lesions may be accessed by an oblique fibular osteotomy emerging distal to the syndesmosis or ligament and capsular release with subluxation of the talus anteriorward. Posteromedial lesions may require osteotomy of the tibial malleolus [D]. Reconstruction options include osteochondral allo- or autograft transfer and autogenous chondrocyte implantation. The latter has the disadvantage that it requires two stages. The first consists of harvest of full-thickness cartilage with superficial layer of subchondral bone from the knee or retrieval of the osteochondral lesion from the talus. The chondrocytes are isolated and grown in laboratory. In the second stage, the lesion is débrided and oversewn with a periosteal flap obtained from the distal tibial, after which the chondrocyte suspension is injected. Advantages of autogenous chondrocyte implantation include ability to treat large and rim lesions, obviating concerns about shape matching.

Outcomes Prognosis for healing of lesions when they present in the first decade is better than second decade. Acute lesions have a higher healing rate than chronic lesions, of which half heal by closed methods. Stable lesions heal more reliably and by closed methods. The fate of lesions requiring open reconstruction is unclear.

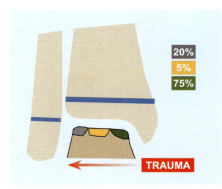

A   Location of osteochondritis dissecans of the talus Lateral lesions tend to be due to acute trauma.

20%
5%
75%

TRAUMA

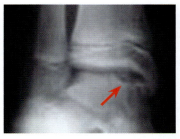

B   Röntgenographic appearance of osteochondritis dissecans There is sclerosis of the trochlea and a halo surrounding the lesion (*red*).

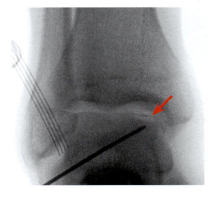

C   Retrograde drilling of osteochondritis dissecans A guidewire is passed through the lateral body of talus into the lesion (*red*). An image intensifier confirms that the wire is centered on the lesion in all planes. An arthroscope monitors the cartilage to make sure it is not disturbed. The guidewire is overdrilled to break up the necrotic bed. The drill tunnel is curetted and irrigated. Bone graft is tamped through the tunnel to support the overlying cartilage until the lucency is filled.

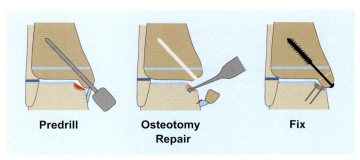

Predrill   Osteotomy Repair   Fix

D   Osteotomy for exposure This aids orthogonal approach to a posteromedial lesions.

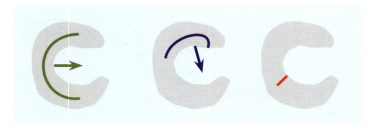

A   Patterns of meniscal tears Tears may occur in every direction and in every plane. Medial displacement of the longitudinal tear is likened to a bucket handle (*green*). Displacement may also produce a flap (*blue*). Radial tears start in the avascular zone (*red*). Complex tears combine fundamental patterns.

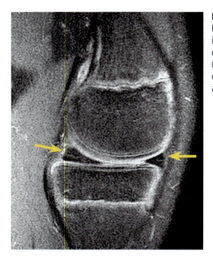

B   Meniscal vascularity Posterior horn shows vascular ingrowth from periphery into center of healthy meniscus (*yellow*). The articular surface of meniscus is intact, arguing against tear.

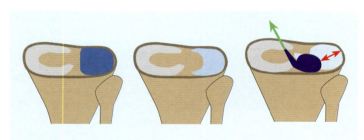

C   Classification of discoid meniscus tear Two-thirds are complete (*blue*), covering the entire lateral tibial articular surface, and 1/3 are incomplete (*light blue*), covering <80%. One-fourth of these demonstrate rim detachment and instability, 50% at the anterior horn, followed by 40% posterior horn and 10% in the middle third. A variant (*navy*) is degenerative and lacks meniscocapsular ligaments to anchor to the lateral capsule, detaching it from the tibia (*red*). Its only attachment (*green*) is the meniscofemoral ligament of Wrisberg, which travels posterior to posterior cruciate ligament to reach femur.

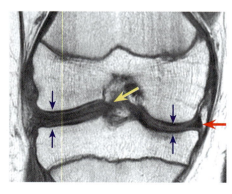

D   Discoid meniscus Lateral discoid meniscus appears rectangular on cross section (*yellow*) as opposed to the typical triangular shape (*red*). The complete fullness separates and flattens the lateral condyles, an increased distance and morphology that raises suspicion on röntgenogramme. The discoid meniscus extends into the intercondylar notch.

KNEE

The knee accounts for the greatest burden of surgical care in the pædiatric athlete.

Meniscus Tear

This is a second-decade injury. Mechanism is twisting and compression, without or with coronal plane deflection. They may be longitudinal or radial, described according to the surface of the meniscus, incomplete or complete, based upon the depth of tear. Longitudinal tears may be intra-substance, which may displace as a bucket handle. They may be break through one horn, where displacement creates a flap. There are other patterns, including horizontal cleavage and complex combinations.

The adolescent meniscus may be divided into outer third, described as red because it is well perfused by a blood supply that enters from synovial membrane into the outer margin, middle third, or red-white, and inner third, which is white and avascular. At birth, the entire meniscus has a vascular network, which retreats to the adult state by the second decade.

Evaluation There may be a history of sudden onset pain without or with hearing a noise from, or feeling a click in, the knee. Presentation includes knee pain, often around the joint line, mechanical signs such as locking and crepitus, and effusion, which is a sign of instability. Provocative testing, including twisting in and out in single limb stance on a partially flexed knee (Thessaly) and maximal flexion, elicits pain.

IMAGING Röntgenogrammes are negative except in a discoid meniscus (*q.v.*). MRI is the modality of choice, but exercise caution. Do not interpret blood vessels coursing through the meniscus, visible on MRI in particular in the prepubescent child, as a tear. A tear requires an interruption in the articular surface of the meniscus. On the other hand, MRI may underestimate lateral meniscal injuries.

Management Most meniscal tears in children are longitudinal in the peripheral red zone, which heal well with repair. Reserve débridement only for untidy or unstable tears or those in the central avascular region, repairing any extension into the red zone. Reduction in meniscal surface area will increase joint pressure, accelerating degeneration of the knee. Meniscal débridement in children has greater consequence than in adults, because they have longer to walk on the knee.

Discoid Meniscus

The term describes resemblance of the meniscus to a disc rather than a crescent (Greek μηνη "*moon*," Latin *luna*, hence the alternate term semi-lunar cartilage) due to preservation of its central portion. The majority are lateral. They are rarely bilateral. Cause is unknown. Incidence is 4%. A disorganized collagen fiber scaffold makes them vulnerable to tear, at twice the rate of normal menisci. Classification is based upon shape and stability [C].

Evaluation Most discoid menisci escape detection in childhood because they are stable and not torn. An unstable discoid meniscus may shift into the intercondylar fossa with extension, presenting as a snapping knee: there is audible crepitus, a palpable shift, and a visible bulge at the anterior lateral joint line. This is intermittent and activity related. Absent instability, the patient may present with pain due to a tear.

IMAGING Röntgenogrammes may show widening of the lateral joint width associated with squaring of the condyles, suggesting an interposed block of tissue. MRI is the modality of choice [D]. Three or more body segments will be visible on sequential images. Continuity between meniscal horns gives the appearance of a "bow tie."

Management Observe discoid menisci identified incidentally. Even though they are more prone to tear, there is no evidence that prophylactic treatment reduces this rate. Symptomatic discoid menisci are saucerized, in which the central portion is arthroscopically débrided leaving a 6- to 8-mm rim. Repair or débride associated tear. Repair rim detachment to the capsule. Counsel the patient and family that what you leave behind is not a normal but a better meniscus.

Patellar Instability

Habitual instability or dislocation differs from the congenital dislocation, which is irreducible (*cf.* Lower Limb chapter). Peak incidence is puberty. Redislocation rate is 20% after index event, which in more than half of cases occurs during sports. Girls are affected more than are boys. There are several predisposing factors.

*   Soft tissue. This includes generalized ligamentous laxity, contracture of lateral patellar retinaculum, and attenuation of the medial patellofemoral ligament, which is a static stabilizer of the patella. This courses from the superomedial margin of patella to the medial femoral epicondyle between adductor tubercle and attachment of tibial collateral ligament, adjacent physis.
*   Muscular weakness, in particular vastus medialis obliquus and core muscles, which act as dynamic stabilizers of the patella.
*   Osseous. A patella supera is displaced out of the trochlea. A dysplastic trochlea does not retain the patella. How much this is a primary factor, or one that develops due to erosion by an instable patella, is unknown. Genu valgum increases the lateral force vector, as does lateral torsion of tibia along with tibial tubercle, and medial torsion of femur.

In knee extension, the patella is not engaged in the trochlea, held in place by dynamic and static soft tissue stabilizers. By 30 degrees of flexion, the patella is fully seated in the trochlea, which takes over as the osseous restraint.

Evaluation Ask about the inciting event, to assess likelihood of an associated fracture in the event of significant trauma. Medial patellofemoral ligament injury occurs in 2/3 of traumatic dislocations, and fracture in 1/3 [E]. Ask about the number of recurrent events, which may include pain and giving way in routine activities such as changing direction. Pain is associated with swelling in the acute setting. Note the position of the patella in knee extension, and track it during flexion. Manipulate the patella for laxity. Check apprehension in extension and during knee flexion, which is more reliable. Measure intermalleolar distance for genu valgum. Determine the rotational profile of the lower limbs.

IMAGING Full-length standing anteroposterior view röntgenogrammes allow calculation of genu valgum and quadriceps angle. Lateral view may demonstrate patella supera, as well as the sclerotic line of a trochlea *en profil* crossing the condyles anterior to the anterior femoral cortex, which is a sign of trochlear dysplasia. Merchant view shows patellar tilt and translation and allows calculation of the sulcus angle [F]. The sulcus angle may be underestimated on a single view röntgenogramme. MRI in habitual dislocators may show that the trochlea is flattened by overlying articular cartilage despite an osseous groove. Calculate the tibial tubercle–trochlea distance, which is a measure of lateral torsion: abnormal is >20 mm. Trace the medial patellofemoral ligament, and look for an avulsion fracture or bone bruising.

Management Nonoperative management focuses on strengthening of vastus medialis obliquus, gluteal, and core muscles. This is successful in most first time dislocators but only half of second time dislocators, who are manifesting intrinsic patellofemoral disease. Similarly, family history is a risk factor for failure of nonoperative management. This highlights the importance of static restraints, both soft tissue and bony.

*   Correct genua valga by growth modulation (*cf.* Lower Limb chapter).
*   Correct medial torsion of femur by derotational osteotomy.
*   Lateral retinacular release is indicated for lateral patellar tilt without significant translation. This is not a stand-alone procedure but is combined with more complete reconstruction.
*   Proximal realignment includes advancement of vastus medialis obliquus and nonanatomic medial soft tissue imbrication.
*   Distal realignment is indicated for tibial tubercle–trochlea distance >20 mm. In the immature, consider medialization of the lateral half of ligamentum patellæ to periosteum or sartorius (Roux-Goldthwaite). This may be augmented by transfer of semitendinosus to patella (Galeazzi). For the mature adolescent, perform a tibial tubercle medial transfer.

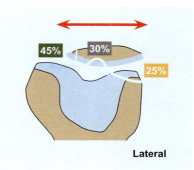

E Fracture after traumatic dislocation The lateral condyle or the articular surface of patella may be fractured as the patella dislocates. The medial margin may be fractured as the patella relocates or as an avulsion by the medial patellofemoral ligament.

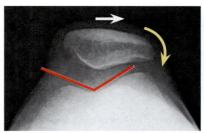

F Merchant view The sulcus angle (*red*) measures depth of trochlea: dysplasia is >145 degrees. The patella is tilted (*yellow*) and translated (*white*): abnormal is >10 mm. Note that Greek τροχιλεια means "pulley, groove, *trochlea*."

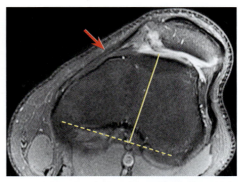

G Trochlear dysplasia The trochlea is flat and does not restrain patella from lateral displacement. The medial patellofemoral ligament (*red*) is attenuated. The position of trochlea is determined by a perpendicular (*yellow*) to the posterior condylar margin (*dashed*). This is compared with a perpendicular to the tibia tubercle by overlapping axial images to measure the tibial tubercle–trochlea distance.

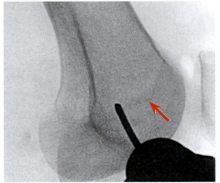

H Medial patellofemoral ligament The isometric femoral tunnel site is immediately proximal to the distal physis of femur (*red*) and anterior to the posterior cortex extension line.

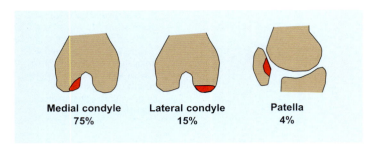

I **Distribution of osteochondritis dissecans of the knee** Other lesions that have been reported include of trochlea and tibial condyle.

CHARACTERISTIC	POOR PROGNOSIS
Stability	Halo or mobile body
Size	> 400 mm²
Age	2nd decade
Location	Atypical

J **Prognostic factors in osteochondritis dissecans of the knee.**

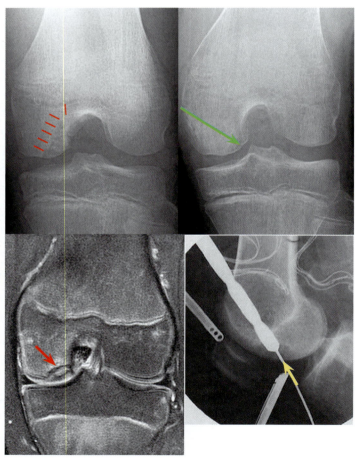

K **Drilling of osteochondritis dissecans of the knee** The lesion is seen on notch view röntgenogrammes and MRI (*red*). It was drilled antegrade (*green*) through epiphysis away from physis. Most of the lesion was healed by 6 months after operation. The technique may be facilitated by inserting the guidewire through the center of the lesion as viewed and probed at arthroscopy (*yellow*).

- For patella supera, a distal transfer of tibial tubercle is indicated in the mature adolescent.
- Just like muscle strengthening harnesses dynamic stabilizers to compensate for static stabilizers, medial patellofemoral ligament reconstruction relies on a static soft tissue restraint to compensate for loss of static osseous restraint. Tendon graft is more durable than primary repair or medial soft tissue imbrication for the repeat dislocator. A medial strip of quadriceps may be sewn to the femoral attachment site, or a strip of adductor may be sewn to the patellar attachment site. Tension the graft at 30 degrees of knee flexion such that it allows 25% of lateral patellar displacement. These techniques avoid the distal physis of femur [H]. For the mature child, autogenous gracilis tendon or allograft may be secured by drill holes in patella and tensioned through a tunnel in femur.
- Trochleoplasty may deepen the trochlea by elevating the lateral condylar surface or depressing the center. Concerns about alteration of the articular surface, and the consequences of patellofemoral arthritis, have slowed acceptance of this procedure.

Osteochondritis Dissecans

Incidence is 1%, peaking at puberty and affecting boys twice as often as girls. Most lesions occur on the lateral aspect of the medial condyle of femur [I]. Up to ¼ are bilateral.

Evaluation There may be a history of trauma. The patient complains of knee pain, which is associated with effusion and stiffness. The patient may sense a mobile body. Gait may be characterized by lateral rotation of tibia, to move the intercondylar eminence away from a medial condylar lesion. This may be tested by extending the knee while medially rotating the tibia, which elicits pain that is relieved by lateral rotation (Wilson test). In terminal knee flexion, a condylar lesion may be tender directly.

IMAGING A condylar lesion may be obscured on anteroposterior projection röntgenogramme. It may be exposed by a 45-degree "notch view," which brings the beam tangent to the lesion. A "halo" of sclerosis may surround the lesion. Scintigraphy may have value in predicting healing: "hot" lesions, like an acute fracture, may heal by nonoperative means, whereas "cold" lesions, like a nonunion, will not. Cartilage is best seen on MRI, which permits classification (*cf.* Type of Injury). Dissection of fluid on T2-weighted pulse sequence to form a "halo" indicates a breach of overlying cartilage and instability. The size of the lesion may be measured on MRI: >400 mm² have a poor prognosis [J].

Management Prognosis for healing of lesions when they present in the first decade is better than second decade. Nonoperative treatment focuses on symptoms. The benefits of activity modification, limited weight bearing, casting or bracing, and physiotherapy are unproven.

Indications for operation include presence of a "halo," which on röntgenogramme indicates that the lesion has been walled off by the rest of the bone and represents a nonunion, large lesions >400 mm² in size, and mobile body. For stable but large lesions, or lesions surrounded by sclerosis, drill the bone to break up the wall and stimulate ingrowth. Drilling may be arthroscopic through the articular surface with a pin. Alternatively, an antegrade approach through the epiphysis beyond the physis with a cannulated drill may be utilized, using an image intensified to center the pin tip in the lesion and an arthroscope to ensure that the articular surface is not violated [K]. Graft the lesion through the drill tunnel. Unstable lesions and mobile bodies are treated as for the talus (*q.v.*).

Ligament Tear

Ligaments are at once unyielding and pliant. Posttraumatic knee instability is discussed in the Hippocratic Corpus. Knee ligaments may be divided into intra- and extra-articular. The former were termed cruciate by Galen after the manner in which they "cross" the joint (Latin *crux*: "cross"). They are distinguished as anterior and posterior based upon their site of attachment on the tibia. The latter are termed collateral and are named according to their site of distal attachment as tibial and fibular or after their location medial and lateral.

Injured collateral ligaments heal with closed methods. A posterior cruciate ligament tear can heal primarily by closed or by surgical methods. An anterior cruciate ligament does not heal primarily and is treated by replacement. Potential reasons for higher anterior cruciate ligament injury rates in girls include a narrower intercondylar fossa, a smaller cross-sectional diameter, differences in strength, flexibility and neuromuscular control, and hormonal profile. The anterior cruciate ligament consists of anteromedial bundle, the predominant constraint against translation, and a more horizontal posterolateral bundle, which predominates against rotation (pivot shift).

Evaluation Ask about the mechanism, such as valgus blow to the knee with the foot planted. The child may remember a noise from the knee and giving way. Was there swelling? A traumatic hæmarthrosis is associated with an anterior cruciate ligament tear in half or more of cases [L]. Are there repeated episodes of instability and effusion? When the knee is not inflamed and the patient does not guard, perform varus/valgus tests in 30 degrees of flexion, a posterior drawer at 90 degrees of flexion, an anterior drawer at 30 degrees of flexion (Lachman), and a pivot shift test. Check for concomitant meniscal injury, including palpation of the joint line and maximum flexion. Estimate the maturity of the child clinically.

Imaging Röntgenogrammes screen the knee for fracture, such as of the intercondylar eminence (*cf.* Trauma chapter), or other lesion, and provide an assessment of the physes. MRI shows the ligaments [M], as well as associated articular lesions such as meniscus tear.

Management Partial anterior cruciate ligament tears may be treated nonoperatively if the physical examination shows no significant instability, in particular if the posterolateral bundle is preserved.

The natural history of a complete anterior cruciate ligament tear in a child is poor, because recurrent instability leads to articular injury, in particular irreparable medial meniscal tear and chondral injury.

Physeal Sparing In the extra- and intra-articular technique, the iliotibial tract is harvested leaving its distal attachment intact, wrapped around the lateral femoral condyle (where it is fixed), passed through the knee, under the intermeniscal ligament, and sewn to the periosteum over the anterior margin of the medial tibial condyle [N]. This may overconstrain the knee in rotation. Alternatively, the semitendinosus and gracilis may be harvested leaving their insertion intact, tunneled through the tibial epiphysis, secured to the femoral footprint by a staple, and looped back through the tibial tunnel.

The physes may be spared by staying intraepiphysial. Advocates reserve this for the "prepubescent." The femoral physis may be spared, or the tibial physis, or both [O].

Transphyseal This is indicated for any child. It is isometric and well established. Autogenous semitendinosus and gracilis grafts traverse, but are fixed remote from, the physes. Do not place bone (e.g., ligamentum patellæ) across the physis, where it will produce a bridge. Do not insert an implant across the physis, which eventually will stop growing. Remember that the treatment of a physeal bridge is resection with soft tissue interposition. Keep tunnels <7% of the cross-sectional area or <10 mm. Anatomic femoral tunnel placement increases the percentage of physeal removal, which argues for single bundle technique.

Posterior cruciate ligament injury is rare in children. Avulsion from the tibia is more likely than intrasubstance tear. This may be repaired arthroscopically, which allows evaluation of the knee for associated injury, or open, by a direct popliteal fossa approach.

HÆMARTHROSIS	Pre-puberty	Adolescent
ACL tear	45%	65%
Meniscal tear	45%	45%
Fracture	15%	5%

L Lesions associated with hæmarthrosis of the knee Prepubescent is defined as Tanner stage 1 or 2, <12 years for boys and <11 years for girls.

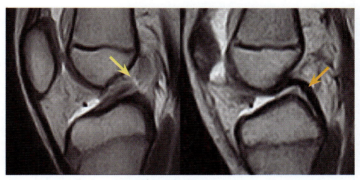

M MRI of the knee The anterior cruciate ligament is torn, as evidenced by discontinuity and fraying at the femur in contrast with the tibial stump that appears cord-like (*yellow*). The posterior cruciate ligament is dense and preserved (*orange*).

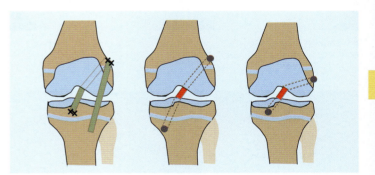

N Techniques for anterior cruciate ligament reconstruction The iliotibial tract (*green*) may be looped around the lateral femoral condyle, drawn through the knee under intermeniscal ligament, and sewn over the anterior tibial margin. Transphyseal (*middle*) hamstring graft reconstruction is isometric. Intraepiphysial (*right*) hamstring graft reconstruction seeks isometry while avoiding the physes.

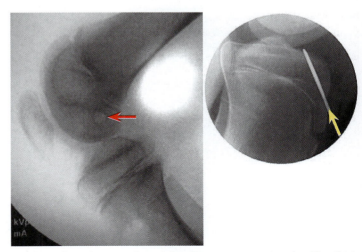

O Physeal-sparing anterior cruciate ligament reconstruction The distal physis of femur may be spared by drilling a transverse tunnel in the distal femoral epiphysis (*red*). The proximal tibial physis may be spared by staying within the proximal tibial epiphysis (*yellow*).

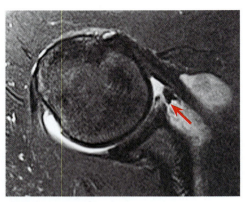

A Bankart lesion Labral avulsion from anterior glenoid cavity is seen on MRI (*red*).

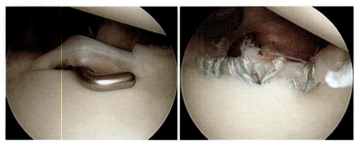

B Bankart lesion A tear in the glenoid labrum, through which the probe is advanced, is repaired arthroscopically.

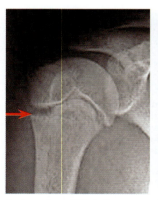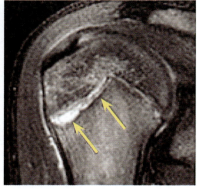

C Imaging of Little Leaguer's shoulder Anteroposterior view röntgenogramme, taken in external rotation, shows widening of the lateral proximal physis of humerus. This is confirmed on MRI.

SHOULDER

The proximal physis gives 80% of longitudinal growth to the humerus. Three secondary ossification centers, for head and tubercles, coalesce by 7 years. The proximal physis fuses in the late teens. Peri-omal muscles—rotator cuff, deltoid, biceps brachii, scapular—dynamically stabilize the glenohumeral joint by concavity compression during motion. The glenohumeral capsule and ligaments are recruited as static stabilizers at the extremes of motion. The other static stabilizer is the labrum, which deepens the glenoid cavity.

Traumatic Instability

A third of acute traumatic shoulder dislocations occur in children. One half will recur, the rate being inversely correlated with age. The majority are anterior. The mechanism is a direct blow or forced abduction, lateral rotation, and extension. Most chronic instability also is anterior. Laxity develops from repetitive microtrauma, sustained during overhead sports

Evaluation Ask about type of activity, for example, a contact sport such as ice hockey or overhead sport such a pitching. Determine the direction of instability. Is there anterior apprehension with shoulder abduction and external rotation? Is this improved with anterior pressure applied by the palm? Is there apprehension with posterior force applied through the humerus with the shoulder flexed, adducted, and internally rotated? Is there inferior instability, as evidenced by a sulcus sign with distraction? Can the head of the humerus be subluxated manually in the glenoid cavity?

IMAGING Röntgenogrammes, including axillary view, may show associated fracture, such as a Hill-Sachs lesion. MRI, without or with arthrography, determines the presence of a labral or glenoid rim avulsion (Bankart) as well as other soft tissue injury [A].

Management Most chronic instability is managed successfully by directed physiotherapy. If symptoms and signs persist beyond 6 months, consider surgical treatment, which may include imbrication of attenuated capsule and ligaments.

For anterior traumatic instability, in the absence of a Bankart lesion, immobilize for 3 weeks, after which begin dynamic shoulder stabilization under the guidance of a physiotherapist.

A Bankart lesion, as well as age at dislocation, are associated with recurrence in 3/4 of patients with nonoperative care. In addition, delayed has a higher recurrence than early operative repair. Less dissection is necessary by arthroscopy, in particular of subscapularis, which permits more rapid rehabilitation. Recurrence after operation is 10%.

Atraumatic Instability

This is multidirectional. Causes include ligamentous laxity and repetitive overhead activity.

Evaluation Patients complain of anterior shoulder pain with abduction and external rotation. Posterior pain may be elicited in the flexed and adducted position, such as when pushing in front of an object. Inferior instability may be felt when carrying a heavy load. Examine both shoulders, because the condition usually is bilateral. The sulcus sign is readily produced. The head of the humerus may be subluxated with ease. Look for other signs of ligamentous laxity, such as hyperextension of elbows, knees, metacarpophalangeal joints, and thumb on volar forearm.

IMAGING MRI may show capsular redundancy.

Management This resembles traumatic instability. Postoperative rehabilitation is slower, as this is a laxity and not a stiffness problem.

Little Leaguer's Shoulder

This is named after the inciting sport, namely, pitching a baseball. It represents an overuse proximal humeral physeolysis [C]. It may be exacerbated by rotator cuff weakness for the demands put upon it.

Evaluation The patient complains of diffuse upper arm and shoulder pain of insidious onset. Rule out shoulder instability. Ask about activity, including pitch count and rest periods between pitching.

IMAGING Röntgenogrammes show widening of the proximal physis of humerus. Contralateral images show no widening of the nondominant upper limb. MRI, obtained if presentation is atypical, confirms physeolysis [C].

Management This is nonoperative. Stop throwing. Strengthen the rotator cuff. Begin throwing in a monitored training program after 6 weeks. Return to a game after 3 months if pain has resolved. Do not exceed 600 pitches/season, which increases risk of this injury.

Impingement

This is the most common cause of posterior shoulder pain in adolescents who are involved in overhead sports, such as baseball pitchers, swimmers, and tennis players. In external rotation and abduction, supra- and infraspinatus abut against the posterosuperior labrum, leading to tear, partial articular supraspinatus tendon avulsions, and stretching of the anteroinferior capsuloligamentous complex. This is exacerbated by subtle instability.

Evaluation Provocative manœuvres for impingement are positive, such as internal rotation with the shoulder flexed to 90 degrees, which elicits pain when supraspinatus impinges upon coracoacromial ligament and anterior acromion (Hawkins). Resisted abduction by supraspinatus in the plane of the scapula is painful with internal rotation (empty can) as the greater tubercle approaches the acromion, where the tendon may be squeezed. There may be an associated glenohumeral internal rotation deficit.

IMAGING Röntgenogrammes are normal. MRI will show increased T2-weighted signal intensity in the rotator cuff and subacromial space. Rotator cuff tear is rare.

Management Physiotherapy to strengthen the rotator cuff, in order to decrease risk of tear, and scapular stabilizers, as well as posterior capsular stretching, are effective in most patients. Refractory pain may be addressed arthroscopically, with subacromial bursectomy, labral repair, posterior capsular release, and capsular plication for associated instability as indicated.

ELBOW

The elbow is more often injured than the shoulder, with fractures accounting for the lion's share (*cf.* Trauma chapter). Sports injuries combine poor mechanics and more enthusiasm than skill. The mechanisms are similar for both joints, including overhead activity such as pitching a baseball, and involvement of the dominant upper limb. The flexor-pronator mass provides dynamic valgus stability to the elbow, while the static stabilizers are the ulnar collateral ligament and the radiocapitular joint.

Medial Little Leaguer's Elbow

This represents a traction apophysitis of the medial epicondyle of humerus, from which originate the flexor–pronator muscles of the forearm. The mechanism is excessive valgus loading of the elbow at cocking and initiation of acceleration [E], which is exacerbated by flexor–pronator contraction to flex the wrist during ball release. This is the more common injury—half of baseball pitchers will complain of this at least once—and the one for which the appellation was conceived. Force travels through the weaker medial epicondylar physis in the child, protecting the ulnar collateral ligament, which would be injured in the late teenager or adult.

Evaluation The patient complains of medial elbow pain associated with the offending sports activity. There is tenderness and swelling of the medial epicondyle. Terminal extension may be lost.

IMAGING Röntgenogrammes may be normal or show epicondylar fragmentation or overgrowth (Hueter-Volkmann principle). It also may show separation of the epicondyle (*cf.* Trauma chapter).

Management Absent a fracture, treatment resembles that of Little League shoulder. It may be challenging to counsel patient and family, invested in playing, about nonoperative care for protracted symptoms.

Age (years)	Pitches per game	Games per week
8-10	52 ± 15	2 ± 0.6
11-12	68 ± 18	2 ± 0.6
13-14	76 ± 16	2 ± 0.4
15-16	91 ± 16	2 ± 0.6
17-18	106 ± 16	2 ± 0.6

D   Maximum pitches These guidelines were developed by the American Academy of Orthopædic Surgeons to protect the shoulder of the pædiatric athlete.

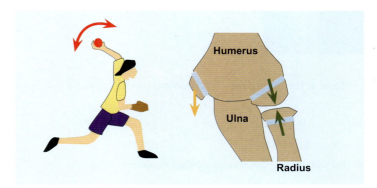

E   Overhead sports Overhead acceleration against resistance, for example, pitching a baseball or striking a tennis ball, produces a valgus load that distracts the medial side (*orange*) and compresses the lateral side (*green*) of the elbow.

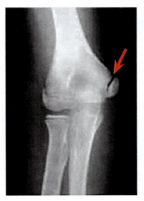

F   Little Leaguer's elbow Röntgenogrammes show physeolysis (*red*).

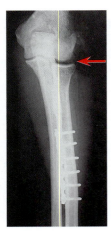

G Decompression of the radiocapitular joint In a cadaveric model, the radius was shortened the width of a saw blade (1 to 2 mm) and compression plated. The head of radius was thereby drawn away from capitulum (*red*), which reduces force and contact area across their articulation.

Time (after exercise)	Compartment Pressure
Rest	≥15 mm Hg
1 minute	≥30 mm Hg
5 minutes	≥20 mm Hg

A Pressure in exertional compartment syndrome These guidelines aid diagnosis.

Lateral Little Leaguer's Elbow

Excessive valgus loading of the elbow results in compression of the radiocapitular articulation. The capitulum is more vulnerable to osteochondritis dissecans than the head of radius. Osteochondritis dissecans, which affects pubertal and older adolescents, differs from Panner disease, which is an osteochondrosis in prepubescent children that involves the entire capitulum and resolves spontaneously without sequelae (akin to Köhler disease of the tarsal navicular).

Evaluation The patient complains of activity-related lateral elbow pain. There may be mechanical symptoms such as catching or locking. There often is an associated flexion contracture. Pain is exacerbated by extension and valgus stress.

    IMAGING The first röntgenographic sign is subchondral flattening. MRI allows measurement of size and classification and determines if there is a mobile body, all of which guide treatment.

Management This follows the general protocol for osteochondritis dissecans (*q.v.*). Stable lesions, characterized by open physis, flattening, and no contracture, heal with nonoperative treatment. Unstable lesions, in which physis is closed, capitulum is fragmented, and there is an associated contracture, benefit from operation. Surgical treatment includes anterior elbow capsulectomy for contracture >20 degrees.

A unique aspect is the role of decompression. This follows the experience of shortening osteotomy for Kienböck disease of the lunate. Shortening of the radius significantly reduces mean force, contact area, and pressure across the radiocapitular articulation. Alternatively, a lateral column shortening of the distal humerus may translate the capitulum proximalward and achieve the same effect; however, this may carry a higher risk, including osteonecrosis from injury to the posterior nonanastomotic blood supply of the capitulum.

OTHER

Exertional Compartment Syndrome

This first was described as march gangrene, after a mechanism and the ultimate outcome. It was named anterior tibial syndrome after the compartment most affected, although it also has been reported in lateral crural compartment, arm, forearm, hand, thigh, and gluteals. Adolescents are affected. While characterized by elevated muscular compartment pressures, the condition differs from its acute counterpart:

- Less pain.
- An intermittent course. It resolves with rest and is not progressive.
- Onset follows lower-energy trauma, for example, following running.
- Delayed presentation, typically 24 to 48 hours after inciting event.
- Chronic patients have increased intramuscular pressure at rest and a greater increase in this pressure with exercise.

Evaluation The patient complains of pain in the affected compartment that is brought on by exercise, which is stopped as a result. There may be associated neural findings such as paræsthesias. Pain resolves with rest without residuum. More than half have bilateral symptoms. Physical examination at rest is normal; after exercise, the compartment is tense.

    TESTING Compartment pressures after exercise have been characterized [A], although such measurements are invasive. Near-infrared spectroscopy measures reduced oxygen saturation of muscle. Increased T2-weighted signal intensity is seen on MRI after exercise. Thallium 201 single photon emission CT, which is superior to electrocardiogram in detection of ischæmic muscle from coronary artery disease, is effective and accurate for exertional compartment syndrome.

Management Many patients will accommodate to pain. Fasciotomy is indicated for patient in whom pain is unacceptable and prevents exercise. This may be open *via* a single incision according to compartment involved or endoscopically assisted *via* two smaller incisions. Proceed with caution, because the morbidity of surgical treatment is not insignificant, including scar, infection, neural injury, and chronic pain.

Plica

Plica synovialis represents a normal "fold" (Latin *plica*, whence "*plication*") of synovial membrane remnant from joint tricompartmentalization during fetal development. Locations are suprapatellar; medial parapatellar, which is most symptomatic; infrapatellar; and rarely lateral. Trauma incites inflammation, which hurts.

Evaluation There often is no history of a specific traumatic event. Presentation is in adolescence, including intermittent mechanical anterior knee pain, clicking with activity, catching or giving way, and palpable, tender crepitus with movement of the knee.

IMAGING This is a clinical diagnosis of exclusion. Röntgenogrammes are negative; MRI is variable.

Management Most patients respond to rest, activity modification, patellar taping, as well as quadriceps and core strengthening. Pain persistent for more than 6 months may be addressed arthroscopically. Surgical findings include hypertrophy, injection, cord or ledge morphology, bowstringing and snapping over, and erosion of femoral condyle or patella [B].

Reflex Neurovascular Dystrophy

This is the childhood equivalent of complex regional pain syndrome in adults. The concept has evolved since the original description from the American Civil War (Mitchell). The name described loss of descending pain inhibition at the spinal cord that sets up a vicious cycle of vascular constriction, hypo-oxygenation, and hyperacidosis, followed by more pain. Girls outnumber boys 3:1. The lower limb is affected twice as often as the upper limb.

Evaluation There is a history of trauma, for example, articular fracture of the knee. The child complains of amplified or disproportionate pain after healing has been demonstrated by objective measures. Pain does not follow an anatomic or dermatomal pattern. Associated findings include limp, stiffness, hyperæsthesia, atrophy of disuse, and cutaneous change in temperature and color.

IMAGING This confirms healed injury. Röntgenogrammes may show osteopenia. Scintigramme may show asymmetric uptake due to dysautonomia [C].

Management This is a diagnosis of exclusion, which requires at once confidence and sensitivity to establish and accept. Delay in diagnosis is typical. Take time to educate and assure patient and family. Vigorous physiotherapy is the cornerstone, even through pain: do not immobilize or otherwise support that the child is vulnerable. Do not operate, for example, arthroscopy to lyse adhesions: this is an additional trauma that exacerbates the problem. Enlist a psychologist to explore other stressors in the child's life, both at school and in the home. A 2- to 3-week hospitalization may be beneficial in fulminant cases. The objectives are to ensure compliance with physiotherapy, up to 5 hours daily, and to control the environment, including sequestration from parents. The role of vitamin C as prophylaxis, administered daily starting at the time of injury or in the emergency setting, is not well defined.

Most patients recover completely or are significantly improved. Five percent develop chronic pain. Up to 15% may relapse.

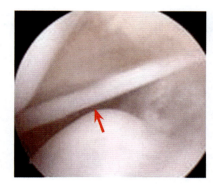

B Symptomatic plica synovialis This normal structure is bowstrung across the femoral condyle.

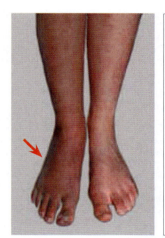 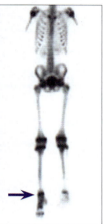

C Reflex neurovascular dystrophy after severe ankle sprain The leg and foot have diffuse soft swelling and discoloration (*red*), which corresponds with increased signal on scintigramme (*blue*).

GENERAL

Blount WP. *Fractures in Children*. Baltimore, MD: Williams & Wilkins Co.; 1954.

Cawley J. The economics of childhood obesity. *Health Aff.* 29(3):364–371, 2010.

Faigenbaum AD, Myer GD. Resistance training among young athletes: safety, efficacy and injury prevention effects. *Br. J. Sports. Med.* 44(1):56–63, 2010.

König F. Veber freie korper in der gehenken. *Dtsch. Z. Chir.* 27:90–109, 1888.

Halstead ME, Kevin D, Walter KD, Council on Sports Medicine and Fitness. Clinical report: sport-related concussion in children and adolescents. *Pediatrics* 126(3):597–615, 2010.

Lippi G, Longo UG, Maffulli N. Genetics and sports. *Br. Med. Bull.* 93(1):27–47, 2010.

Norton C, Nixon J, Sibert J. Playground injuries to children. *Arch. Dis. Child.* 89(2):103–108, 2004.

Wilt F, Yessis M. *Soviet Theory, Technique and Training for Running and Hurdling*. Ames, Iowa: Vol. 1. Championship Books, 1984.

ANKLE

Berndt AL, Harty M. Transchondral fractures (osteochondritis dissecans) of the talus. *J. Bone Joint Surg.* 41-A:988–1020, 1959.

Flick AB, Gould N. Osteochondritis dissecans of the talus (transchondral fractures of the talus): review of the literature and a new surgical approach for medial dome lesions. *Foot Ankle* 5(4):165–185, 1985.

Tol JL, Struijs PAA, Bossuyt PMM, Verhagen RAW, van Dijk CN. Treatment strategies in osteochondral defects of the talar dome: a systematic review. *Foot Ankle Int.* 21(2):119–126, 2000.

KNEE

Kennedy A, Coughlin DG, Metzger MF, Tang R, Pearle AD, Lotz JC, Feeley BT. Biomechanical evaluation of pediatric anterior cruciate ligament reconstruction techniques. *Am. J. Sports Med.* 39(5):964–971, 2011.

Hefti F, Beguiristain J, Krauspe R. Osteochondritis dissecans: a multicenter study of the European Pediatric Orthopedic Society. *J. Pediatr. Orthop.* 8(4)-B:231–245, 1999.

Hui C, Roe J, Ferguson D, Waller A, Salmon L, Pinczewski L. Outcome of anatomic transphyseal anterior cruciate ligament reconstruction in Tanner stage 1 and 2 patients with open physes. *Am. J. Sports Med.* 40(5):1093–2008, 2012.

Joo SY, Park KB, Kim BR, Park HW, Kim HW. The 'four-in-one' procedure for habitual dislocation of the patella in children: early results in patients with severe generalised ligamentous laxity and aplasia of the trochlear groove. *J. Bone Joint Surg.* 89(12)-B:1645–1649, 2007.

Kocher MS, DiCanzio J, Zurakowski D, Micheli LJ. Diagnostic performance of clinical examination and selective magnetic resonance imaging in the evaluation of intraarticular knee disorders in children and adolescents. *Am. J. Sports Med.* 29(3):292–296, 2001.

Lawrence JT, Argawal N, Ganley TJ. Degeneration of the knee joint in skeletally immature patients with a diagnosis of an anterior cruciate ligament tear: is there harm in delay of treatment? *Am. J. Sports Med.* 39(12):2582–2587, 2011.

MacIntosh DL, Darby TA. Lateral substitution reconstruction. *J. Bone Joint Surg.* 58-B:142–146, 1976.

MacNab I. Recurrent dislocation of the patella. *J. Bone Joint Surg.* 34(4)-A:957–967, 1952.

Nelitz M, Dornacher D, Dreyhaupt J, Reichel H, Lippacher S. The relation of the distal femoral physis and the medial patellofemoral ligament. *Knee Surg. Sports Traumatol. Arthrosc.* 19(12):2067–2071, 2011.

Rohren E, Kosarek FJ, Helms CA. Discoid lateral meniscus and the frequency of meniscal tears. *Skeletal Radiol.* 30(6):316–320, 2001.

Stanitski CL, Harvell JC, Fu F. Observations on acute knee hemarthrosis in children and adolescents. *J. Pediatr. Orthop.* 13(4):506–510, 1993.

Vavken P, Murray MM. Treating anterior cruciate ligament tears in skeletally immature patients. *Arthroscopy* 27(5):704–716, 2011.

Wilson JN. A diagnostic sign in osteochondritis dissecans of the knee. *J. Bone Joint Surg.* 49(3)-A:477–480, 1967.

Young R. The external semilunar cartilage as a complete disc. In: Cleland J, Mackey JY, Young RB, eds. *Memoirs and Memoranda in Anatomy*. London, UK: Williams and Norgate; 1987:179–187.

SHOULDER

Bottoni CR, Smith EL, Berkowitz MJ, Towle RB, Moore JH. Arthroscopic versus open shoulder stabilization for recurrent anterior instability. A prospective randomized clinical trial. *Am. J. Sports Med.* 34(11):1730–1737, 2006.

Dotter WE. Little leaguer's shoulder—fracture of the proximal humeral epiphyseal cartilage due to baseball pitching. *Guthrie Clin. Bull.* 23(1):68–72, 1953.

Hovelius L, Augustini BG, Fredin H, Johansson O, Norlin R, Thorling J. Primary anterior dislocation of the shoulder in young patients. A ten-year prospective study. *J. Bone Joint Surg.* 78(11)-A:1677–1684, 1996.

Pasque CB, McGinnis DW, Griffin LY. Shoulder. In: Sullivan JA, Anderson ST, eds. *Care of the Young Athlete*. Rosemont, IL: American Academy of Orthopaedic Surgeons, and Elk Grove Village, IL: American Academy of Pediatrics; 2000.

ELBOW

Bennett GE. Shoulder and elbow lesions distinctive of baseball players. *Ann. Surg.* 126(1):107–110, 1947.

Diab M, Poston JM, Huber P, Tencer AF. The biomechanical effect of radial shortening on the radiocapitellar articulation. *J. Bone Joint Surg.* 87(6)-B:879–883, 2005.

Takahara M, Mura N, Sasaki J, Harada M, Ogino T. Classification, treatment, and outcome of osteochondritis dissecans of the humeral capitellum. *J. Bone Joint Surg.* 89(6)-A:1205–1214, 2007.

OTHER

Goldschneider KR. Complex regional pain syndrome in children: asking the right questions. *Pain Res. Manag.* 17(6):386–390, 2012.

Johnson DP, Eastwood DM, Witherow PJ. Symptomatic synovial plicae of the knee. *J. Bone Joint Surg.* 75(10)-A:1485–1496, 1993.

Mavor GE. The anterior tibial syndrome. *J. Bone Joint Surg.* 38(2)-B:513–517, 1956.

Mitchell SW, Morehouse GR, Kean WW. *Gunshot Wounds and Other Injuries of Nerves*. New York: Lippincott, 1864.

Nallamothu N, Pancholy SB, Lee KR, Heo J, Iskandrian AS. Impact on exercise single-photon emission computed tomographic thallium imaging on patient management and outcome. *J. Nucl. Cardiol.* 2(4):334–338, 1995.

Pedowitz RA, Hargens AR, Mubarak SJ, Gershuni DH. Modified criteria for the objective diagnosis of chronic compartment syndrome of the leg. *Am. J. Sports Med.* 18(1):35–40, 1990.

INFECTION

Musculoskeletal infections risk life, deformity, and disability. Infections and their treatment are evolving. Pyarthritis due to *Hæmophilus influenzæ* has declined due to vaccination. Antibiotic resistance is rising, for example, methicillin-resistant *Staphylococcus aureus* (MRSA) is the causative pathogen in up to 1/3 of cases, is more invasive, and leads to more complications. Diagnosis is improving with new modalities, for example, polymerase chain reaction. Duration of intravenous administration of antibiotics and total duration of therapy have been shortened significantly.

Osteomyelitis is twice as frequent as pyarthritis. This increased rate may be due to MRI detection of bone infection before radiographic change. Musculoskeletal infections show no gender predilection. Presentation skews to the middle of the first decade (6.6 years).

PATHOPHYSIOLOGY

Most infections are hæmatogenous [A]. Joints may be seeded through the vascular network of the synovial membrane and by local extension from infection of intra-articular bone (neck of femur, neck of radius, distal fibula, proximal humerus). Direct inoculation is an occupational hazard of childhood (scrapes and falls) and has particular relevance to the surgical incision.

Bacteræmia occurs daily and, often, as does trauma in a child. The metaphysis of bone is vulnerable to infection because of normal vascular stasis in hairpin capillary loops turned back by an impervious physis [B]. Hæmatoma results in a similarly favorable environment. Bacteria may gain access to epiphysial bone and a joint from metaphyseal bone *via* transphyseal vessels, which remain patent in infancy and account for a high rate of hip pyarthritis [C].

Bacteria secrete a glycocalyx (Greek γλυκος: "sugar" and καλυξ: "coat"), a viscous polysaccharide slime that coats their surface. The glycocalyx protects against drying, traps nutrients, allows adherence to surfaces to aid colonization and resist flushing, and prevents engulfment by phagocytes. Bacteria gain advantage by formation of a community within an adhesive matrix known as a biofilm, which impedes diffusion of antibiotics and where the bacteria communicate by quorum sensing and adapt to their environment (e.g., reduce metabolism) as a population, akin to a multicellular organism, rather than as individuals.

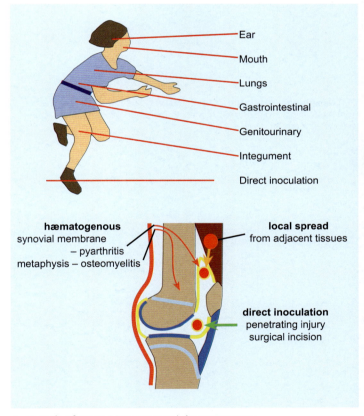

Ear
Mouth
Lungs
Gastrointestinal
Genitourinary
Integument
Direct inoculation

hæmatogenous
synovial membrane
– pyarthritis
metaphysis – osteomyelitis

local spread
from adjacent tissues

direct inoculation
penetrating injury
surgical incision

A   Portals of entry Most common is hæmatogenous.

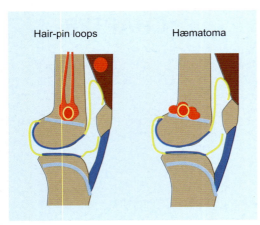

B   Vascular anatomy Stasis in hairpin loops or a hæmatoma provides a favorable environment for bacterial proliferation.

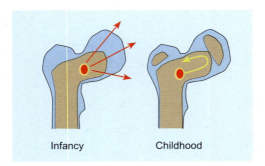

C   Transphyseal extension Transphyseal vessels allow spread of infection from metaphysis into joint (*red*) in infancy. The physis becomes impervious (*yellow*) with growth.

Most exposures do not amount to infection, because the immune system clears the infectious organisms [D]. When organism virulence overcomes host defense, an acute infection follows, which may escape local confines to threaten the child systemically, including life. A stalemate between organism and host results in chronic infection, including abscess, posing a local threat to the limb. This is defined as > 6 weeks but may last for years. Impaired hosts include the malnourished, those with chronic disease or tumor, those receiving immunosuppressive medication, and the premature. They may become infected even by low-virulence organisms, which can penetrate porous defenses.

SELECT ORGANISMS

Bacteria may be distinguished morphologically as coccus (Greek κοκκος: "grain, seed"), rod or bacillus (Latin *baculus* = Greek βακτηρία: "staff, cane"), vibrio (comma shaped), spirilla (spiral), and spirochete (tightly coiled). The organisms may occur in pairs (diplococcus), for example, *Neisseria*; in chains, for example, *Streptococcus*; in bunches, for example, *Staphylococcus* (Greek σταφυλη: "grape"); in filaments, for example, *Actinobacter*; and in complex structures resembling fungi, for example, *Nocardia*.

Gram-positive bacteria are characterized by a thick cell wall containing many layers of peptidoglycan and teichoic acids, which retain crystal violet in the Gram stain technique (Danish scientist Hans Christian Gram, 1853–1938). Gram-positive cocci are the most common pathogens in musculoskeletal infections. By contrast, Gram-negative bacteria have a relatively thin cell wall consisting of a peptidoglycan layer surrounded by a second lipid membrane containing lipopolysaccharides, the endotoxin responsible for much of their toxicity. Acid-fast bacteria, like *Mycobacterium*, are resistant to decolorization by acids during staining procedures (e.g., Gram stain), on account of the high lipid content of its wall (mycolic acid), which also contributes to virulence and resistance. L-form bacteria are strains of bacteria that lack cell walls. The main pathogenic bacteria in this class is Mycoplasma.

Certain genera of Gram-positive bacteria, such as *Clostridium tetani* (puncture wounds), form resistant endospores that may lie dormant for millions of years. Aerobic organisms use oxygen as the electron acceptor, while anaerobic organisms use other inorganic compounds (e.g., nitrate, sulfate, carbon dioxide) as electron acceptors, in a redox reaction that releases energy to synthesize ATP and drive metabolism.

Type of pathogen depends upon several factors:

- Age. While *Staphylococcus aureus* is most common overall, Gram-negative bacteria and in particular *Kingella kingæ* account for more than half of infections in children under 4.
- Vaccination history. Vaccination against *Hæmophilus influenzæ B* in the last decade of the 20th century has essentially eliminated pyarthritis due to this organism compared with a prevaccination rate of 1/3 of pyarthritis.
- Host environment. Because of its ability to rapidly develop a biofilm, *Staphylococcus epidermidis* is of particular concern to patients with implants.

- Socioeconomics. *Hæmophilus influenzæ* remains relevant in developing countries lacking vaccination programs.
- Geography. Tuberculous spondylitis, rare in North American children, remains a significant burden in Africa.

Staphylococcus Aureus

New strains of this Gram-positive bacterium may be methicillin (MRSA) or vancomycin resistant. MRSA secretion of the necrotizing toxin Panton-Valentine leukocidin results in more invasive infection, longer hospitalization, more surgery, and higher complication rates.

Staphylococcus Epidermidis

This Gram-positive bacterium is responsible for nosocomial infection. It is a threat to patients who are immune compromised. The ability to form biofilms on implants is a major virulence factor. It is a frequent contaminant in laboratory analysis.

Kingella Kingæ

Infections by this Gram-negative coccobacillus are rising, in particular in infants. Presentation is benign, including fever in less than 1/5 of children and a normal C-reactive protein (CRP) in more than 1/3.

Propionibacterium Acnes

This ærotolerant anaerobic Gram-positive bacterium is a commensal colonist of the sebaceous glands of the skin around puberty. The indolent nature of this organism explains the delayed presentation of postoperative infection (including revision), in particular in spine surgery, where it requires implant removal for eradication.

Pseudomonas æruginosa

Opportunistic Gram-negative rod that rarely causes disease in the healthy, except when a physical barrier is breached, such as after a puncture wound to the sole of the foot in a shoe. It also is found in the setting of immune compromise, such as in the gastrointestinal tract of a child with leukæmia and the lungs in cystic fibrosis.

Salmonella

This Gram-negative enterobacterium is of particular concern in children with sickle cell disease. Capillary occlusion secondary to sickling may infarct the gut, permitting *Salmonella* invasion. Reticuloendothelial dysfunction and expanded marrow with sluggish flow leads to osteonecrosis with *Salmonella* infection. The infection is distinguished by diaphyseal involvement [A], multiple sites, and a high rate of complications due to vasculopathy and immune compromise.

Borrelia Burgdorferi

This spirochete causes Lyme disease (Old Lyme, Connecticut, USA), a zoonosis transmitted from rodents by the *Ixodes* tick. Lyme disease is characterized by a delayed, warm though not itchy, target rash, termed erythema chronicum migrans, and pyarthritis. The disease also may affect the heart and central nervous system. Be alert to travel and exposure history: due to the relative indolence of pyarthritis, delay in diagnosis is typical.

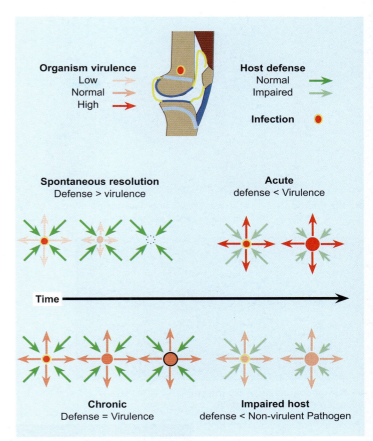

D   Organism *versus* host The balance of virulence *versus* defense influences outcome.

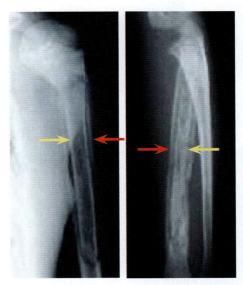

A   Salmonella osteomyelitis in sickle cell disease This polyostotic infection elicits extensive subperiosteal osteogenesis (*red*) that completely surrounds the native diaphysis (*yellow*).

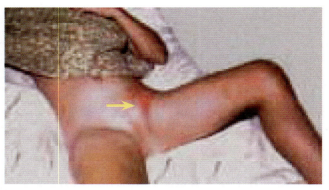

A   Hip infection Presentation was delayed until swelling, redness, and warmth appeared externally. The hip is held in flexion, lateral rotation, and abduction.

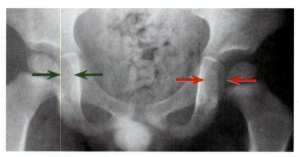

B   Röntgenogramme of hip infection The left hip has an effusion based upon increased medial joint width.

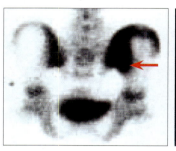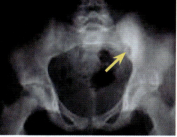

C   Scintigraphy for osteomyelitis Increased uptake in the left ilium (*red*) despite negative röntgenogrammes, which showed a lesion 3 weeks later (*yellow*).

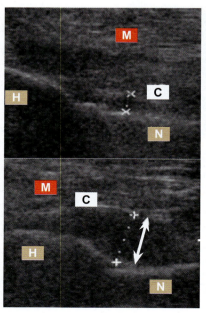

D   Ultrasonography for hip effusion The joint capsule is elevated (*white*) off the femur by fluid. H, head of femur; N, neck of femur; C, capsule; M, muscle.

EVALUATION

History

Determine if there is comorbidity. What is the vaccination status? Have there been any significant exposures or travel? Was the child injured? Duration of symptoms in pyarthritis is of prognostic value: while there is biochemical evidence of cartilage within several hours of exposure to pus, clinical outcomes, including postinfectious arthritis and growth disturbance, deteriorate after 3 days. Did the patient already receive antibiotics? If so, this will reduce culture yields from blood and other tissue specimens.

Physical Examination

Take the temperature. Perform a screening examination first. Is the child in distress? This suggests an overwhelmed host worthy of expeditious attention. It argues against more benign confounding conditions such as transient synovitis. Similarly, lack of movement of, or bearing weight on, a limb, known as "pseudoparalysis," is a sign of such extreme pain that the child will not use the affected part. Even if the examiner tries, the child will splint to present joint rigidity. In children, infected joints do not move; by contrast, only half of adjacent joints show reduction of motion in osteomyelitis. Look for inflammatory signs in the soft tissues, including swelling, redness, and warmth [A]. In order to relax these inflamed soft tissues, joints are flexed and at the hip rotated lateralward [A]. Percuss the bone to determine tenderness: this transmits force effectively to the bone while manipulating surrounding soft tissues less than palpation. Check the skin for stigmata that may predispose to infection, such as a pock or a laceration.

Imaging

Röntgenogrammes Signs of infection include the following:

- Soft tissue swelling. This includes alteration of cutaneous contour, distortion of intermuscular planes, and contrasting densities.
- Joint diastasis. At the hip, measure the distance between proximal femoral epiphysis and medial wall of acetabulum [B]. An effusion may be sufficiently large to dislocate a joint.
- Periosteal elevation. This represents repair of osseous destruction.
- Bone loss. A reduction of bone density of >30% is necessary before there are radiographic changes.

Röntgenogrammes are significant only if positive; negative images are inconclusive.

Scintigraphy This is indicated for clinical suspicion of osteomyelitis with normal röntgenogrammes. Technetium (99mTc) medronic acid is taken up preferentially by bone, concentrating (hot) where bone is inflamed. The immediate or flow phase (seconds after injection) assesses bone perfusion. The second or blood pool phase (minutes) is a measure of surrounding vascularity, as capillary dilatation slows the flow of blood. The third or delayed phase (hours) is a reflection of bone turnover. Reduced uptake ("cold" scan) is concerning for infarction and osteonecrosis, which limit antibiotic access. The scintigramme is unaffected by bone or joint aspiration.

Ultrasound This is indicated for evaluation of the joint (in particular axial), such as effusion [D], and soft tissue, such as abscess. It is noninvasive, nonradiating, dynamic, portable, versatile, and cheap. However, it is user dependent, both for technique and for interpretation. Both quantitative and qualitative assessment of joint effusion is possible. At the hip, >2 mm elevation of the capsule off the neck of femur at the anterior joint recess defines distension. Echogenicity of the fluid suggests pus. Synovial membrane hypertrophy distinguishes transient synovitis (absent) from infection or other inflammatory process (present). Joint aspiration may be facilitated by ultrasonogramme, which confirms articular location of the needle. False negatives may occur early in disease, before sufficient fluid has accumulated to be detectable.

MRI This shows soft tissue best [E]. It also shows bone and its reaction. The modality allows for early identification with high sensitivity, before röntgenogrammes change, and provides anatomic detail for surgical planning. Gadolinium enhancement enables identification of infection of nonossified cartilage, including the epiphysis. This is a tissue target for MRSA and *Kingella kingæ*. Thus, treatment may be instituted earlier to mitigate damage from these pathogens.

Exercise sobriety and correlate MRI findings with the entire evaluation of the child. Because it reveals everything in such detail, it may raise alarm and promote zealous intervention. Remember that it requires sedation for the young child who will not lie still.

CT/PET This may be superior to MRI in monitoring response to treatment for osteomyelitis and in distinguishing ongoing infection from repair. However, the radiation dose limits the use of this modality.

Laboratory Studies

Blood Only half of children will have an elevated white blood cell count (WBC) > 12,000/mm^3 at presentation. Most patients will have erythrocyte sedimentation rate (ESR) > 20 mm/h and C-reactive protein (CRP) > 20 mg/L; in combination, these markers approach 100% sensitivity for infection. Isolated musculoskeletal infection is characterized by a range of CRP 20 to 90 mg/L; CRP > 90 mg/L suggests disseminated infection. With successful treatment, ESR rises by 3 to 4 days and normalizes by 4 to 6 weeks, while CRP rises by 1 to 2 days and normalizes within 2 weeks [F]. ESR is useful for long-term follow-up and CRP for the acute treatment period.

Bone and joint This may be fluid from arthrocentesis or blood from bone or surgical specimen. The emergency setting, where the child may be sedated and before antibiotics are administered, is an opportunity to obtain fluid directly from the site of infection, rather than peripherally from a vein. If an appendicular joint is swollen, stick a needle in it. Decompression in this case may be therapeutic, by decreasing bacterial load, in addition to diagnostic. Infected metaphyseal bone is soft. Insert a needle while aspirating in the event that there is a periosteal abscess. Once bone is encountered, advance the needle while rotating through a small arc to burrow into the bone, from where a blood specimen may be aspirated. At operation, physical deep and superficial tissue is preferable to swabs.

Gram stain may show bacteria. WBC > 50,000/mm^3 with predominance of polymorphonuclear leukocytes in joint fluid is consistent with infection, although there may be overlap with juvenile idiopathic arthritis.

Culture Only half of blood, joint, and bone specimens will yield an organism. The rate is reduced by antibiotics, of which administration should be delayed in the stable child until all specimens are obtained. For *Kingella kingæ*, nasopharyngeal cultures (due to colonization) are significantly more positive than joint fluid.

Polymerase chain reaction Heat-stable polymerase selectively amplifies, using complementary primers, a specific region, or target of DNA after melting the double helix into independent strands. It provides results within 3 hours. It identifies fastidious organisms difficult to grow in culture, such as *Kingella kingæ*. It accelerates identification of virulent pathogens, such as MRSA, allowing earlier treatment to limit their morbidity. Early identification also promises more targeted antibiotic regimens, reducing iatrogenic bacterial resistance.

Due to diagnostic dilemma, burden of disease, and gravity of negative outcomes, diagnostic criteria have been developed for pyarthritis of the hip [G]. Added to this has been repeat presentation, suggesting deterioration during a period of observation. Remember that these are guidelines and not rules.

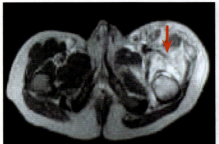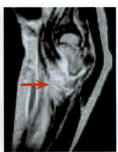

E   MRI showing a thigh abscess Osteomyelitis of the proximal femur was associated with an abscess of the upper thigh (*red*). This guided the approach to drainage.

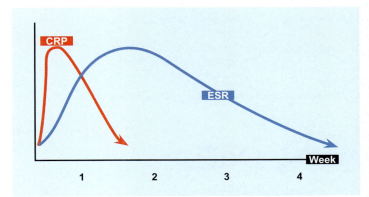

F   Temporal pattern of CRP and ESR CRP is a better acute measure, ESR better as a chronic measure.

Predictor	#: Likelihood of infection
	0: Not infection.
Refusal to bear weight	1: Unlikely.
Fever (> 38.5 degrees)	2: Unlikely, observe.
Leukocytosis (> 12,000/mm^3)	3: Likely, act.
Erythrocyte sedimentation rate (ESR)	4: Highly likely, act.
C-reactive protein (CRP)	Negative predictive value: > 80%
	Positive predictive value: 50%

G   Prediction of pyarthritis of the hip Do not rely on these guidelines at the expense of judgment. Normal value of ESR is <20 mm/h. Normal value of CRP is <10 mg/L.

Antibiotic	Comment
First generation cephalosporin (e.g., cephalexin)	Standard empirical therapy MSSA, *Kingella kingæ*
Clindamycin	For cephalosporin hypersensitivity *Kingella kingæ* resistant Covers Gram positive cocci + anaerobic Gram negative rods + some MRSA
Vancomycin	MRSA Concerns about iatrogenic resistance
Third generation cephalosporin (e.g., ceftriaxone)	Gram negative coverage in neonates

A   Initial antibiotic therapy Clinical assessment guides treatment.

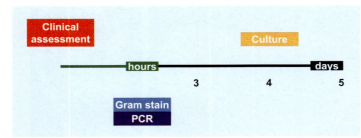

B Timing of antibiotic therapy Selection of antibiotics is influenced by sequence of evaluation.

Indication	Timing of treatment
Active infection	• Days *per venam* • Weeks *per orem*
Surgical prophylaxis	Single dose *per venam*: • prior to surgical incision • at emergency presentation

C Timing of antibiotic therapy This varies according to indication.

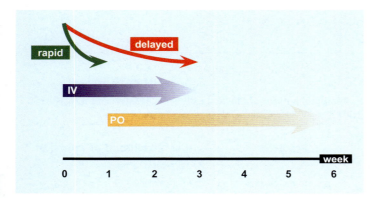

D Timing of antibiotic therapy Duration and route are determined in part by clinical response (rapid or delayed), and overall are contracting. IV, intravenous; PO, *per orem*.

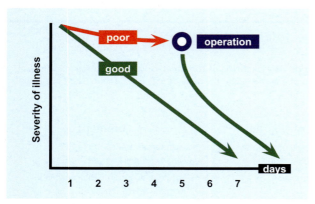

E Variability in the course of treatment Several factors impact treatment approach, such as operation for drainage and débridement when intravenous antibiotics alone do not elicit a good response.

MANAGEMENT

Established principles stand in a setting of changing practice that admits variability.

Antibiotics

The potential for healing pædiatric musculoskeletal infection is remarkable. For example, diskitis may resolve without antibiotics, of which the effect is limited to shortening the duration of symptoms. Balancing this is the vulnerability of children. For example, physeal involvement may disturb growth, leading to malangulation or arrest. Empirical therapy commences after specimens have been obtained. Clinical assessment [A], in particular age and history, Gram stain, PCR, and culture, guides treatment. Time is an essential factor:

- Selection and focusing of type of antibiotic [B].
- Active treatment *versus* prophylaxis [C]:

There is clear evidence to support a single dose of preoperative intravenous antibiotics within 6 hours of incision as surgical prophylaxis. Further administration is moot and if prolonged >48 hours may increase infection by selection for resistant organisms.

- Duration and route of antibiotic therapy [D]:

The advantage of the intravenous route is rapidity of delivery, due to 100% bioavailability. The oral route is affected by compliance and bioavailability, which in turn is determined by gastrointestinal disease (absorption) and metabolism. Initial hospital treatment allows close observation for response. The traditional 6 weeks of intravenous route and treatment has undergone fundamental revision. The following is an idealized approach.

- Begin intravenous antibiotics:

Ensure that the child does not develop cephalosporin-induced neutropenia. Calculate antibiotic blood levels and modify dosing as indicated.

- Observe for clinical and laboratory response:

The former includes fever, pain, swelling, warmth (Celsius), function, and surgical incision. Pain includes that to palpation and with joint motion. Function includes gait assessment, for example, will the child who refused to bear weight at presentation now attempt this? A good response to the operation is a dry wound for 24 hours after drain removal. The latter may be limited to CRP, due to the rapidity of its response to infection and treatment. Observe the trend: a steady decline to <20 mg/L is deemed a success.

- Convert to oral antibiotics:

This is done once a good response has been realized. Observe in hospital for 24 hours to ensure no relapse and to educate family on regimen and follow-up.

- Stop oral antibiotics when ESR normalizes to <20 mm/h:

This may be followed weekly in the ambulatory setting.

Most (>80%) primary infections can be treated successfully with antibiotics *per venam* < 1 week and *per orem* for 3 weeks. However, this idealized approach will be modified according to patient. Specimen analysis may reveal that initial antibiotic selection was ineffective, requiring a change that prolongs intravenous duration. Persistent or worsening clinical (e.g., fever, pain, wound drainage) and laboratory (e.g., elevated CRP) response should prompt further investigation, such as with imaging, a broadening of antibiotic spectrum for occult organism, and possible repeat operation [E]. The socioeconomic status of the patient and family has implication on compliance and follow-up.

Pyarthritis

Pus in a joint causes damage of hyaline and physeal cartilage by inflammatory mediators and of bone by ischæmia due to vascular thrombosis and pressure occlusion. Consequences include arthritis, growth disturbance, and osteonecrosis. Susceptibility to injury is determined principally by time: cartilage degradation is detectable microscopically after hours, though macroscopic, clinical injury becomes significant after 3 days. Anatomy also is a determinant. Swelling is more apparent in an appendicular joint, whereas for an axial joint, ultrasonogramme may be necessary to diagnose a joint effusion. Tenuity of blood supply limits tolerance to pressure and collateral compensation. The hip is the quintessential example of anatomic vulnerability. Thus, even though the knee represents the highest burden numerically, the hip is the greatest source of consternation [A].

While osteomyelitis may resolve without surgical intervention, or even with no treatment at all (e.g., diskitis), pyarthritis requires treatment, and invasion, at least with a needle.

Infected joints may be divided into axial (hip and shoulder) and appendicular [B]. Appendicular pyarthritis may be treated with aspiration and antibiotics. Aspiration may be combined with irrigation *via* two large-bore angiocatheters until clear. Confirm by physical examination that the joint has no more fluid, in case loculations prevent complete decompression. This approach decreases the bacterial load sufficiently in a child that antibiotics will be able to eradicate the rest of the infection. It is diagnostic and therapeutic. Despite a success rate > 80% with aspiration, many surgeons prefer arthroscopic or open lavage, influenced in large measure by the grave consequences of delayed evacuation of pus from the joint: the child may be able to tolerate serial aspirations but the cartilage will not. A hybrid approach consists of aspiration and lavage at presentation in the emergency setting, where a child may be adequately sedated, followed by a more open approach if there is repeat accumulation of fluid or other evidence of poor response.

Because axial joints are deep and fluid accumulation cannot be assessed as a response to treatment, open irrigation and drainage is the first choice:

- Approach the hip *via* a Smith-Petersen approach and the shoulder *via* a deltopectoral approach.
- Perform a 1-cm² capsulectomy to allow egress of fluid after operation.
- Place a drain of sufficient caliber not to occlude. Remove the drain once there has been a good response and output is "minimal," although there is no consensus on amount. The drain offers a path of lesser resistance to decompress the joint in order to allow healing of the wound, which must be observed to remain dry for 24 hours after drain removal before discharge is considered.
- Fenestration and curettage of intra-articular bone are indicated if röntgenogrammes show osseous change. Drilling of radionegative bone is controversial. If osteomyelitis has extended to infect the joint, it has achieved a spontaneous decompression. If the bone is uninvolved, drilling provides a direct and deep path for extension of infection into the bone.
- Repair the wound loosely and with interrupted monofilament suture.

Suppressing the immune response to infection by adding intravenous dexamethasone to intravenous antibiotic therapy may reduce fever, pain, and other inflammatory signs, lower acute-phase reactants, and thereby accelerate clinical response as well as shorten duration of intravenous treatment and hospitalization.

Osteomyelitis

Osteomyelitis is an infection of the bone. This is classified temporally as acute (<3 weeks), subacute (3 to 6 weeks), and chronic (>6 weeks). Acute is radionegative, subacute has röntgenographic change, and chronic is characterized by abscess formation with osteonecrosis [A]. The femur is most affected [B]. Infection typically begins in the metaphysis, from where it expands toward the diaphysis and through the cortex, where it may be contained by the periosteum or it may escape to form a soft tissue abscess [C]. Long bones are more susceptible, due to a thick and relatively hypovascular cortex, compared with flat bones, such as the pelvis, which have thin cortices and rich medullæ.

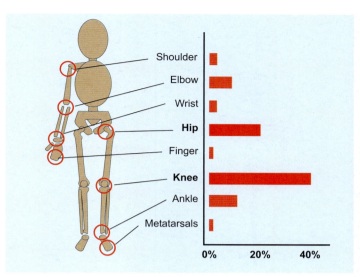

A Geographic distribution of pyarthritis.

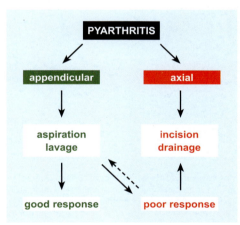

B Treatment of pyarthritis The approach differs according to type of joint and response to initial intervention.

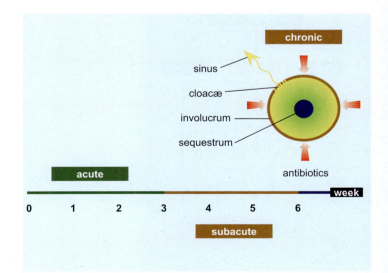

A Classification of osteomyelitis Chronicity is defined as >6 weeks. Chronic osteomyelitis is characterized classically by a sequestrum, dead piece of bone "isolated" from the surroundings in a pool of pus; an involucrum, "a wrapper" of sclerotic bone that forms as a barrier around the infection; and cloacæ, "drains" that eventually perforate the involucrum to allow flow of pus out toward the skin via a sinus, "tract." Antibiotics cannot penetrate the involucrum, hence the indication for operative drainage.

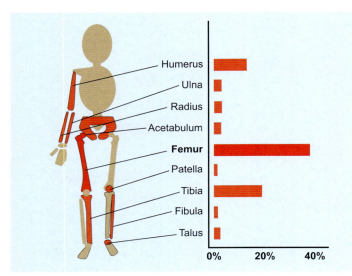

B Geographic distribution of osteomyelitis.

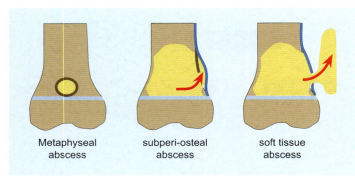

C Subacute progression of osteomyelitis Metaphyseal abscess (Brodie) may erode the cortex, where it may be contained as an abscess by a repeatedly reactive periosteum that gives an "onion-skin" appearance, or from where it escapes into surrounding soft tissues.

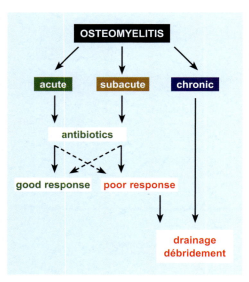

D   Treatment of osteomyelitis The approach differs according to type of joint and response to initial intervention.

The child presents with signs of inflammation, such as fever, tenderness, swelling, and erythema. There may be a history of trauma forming a hæmatoma that creates a favorable environment for bacterial growth. Percussion amplifies force in bone. While the patient may limit use of a limb, such as limp, individual joints will not be stiff as they are in pyarthritis.

If röntgenogrammes are negative, scintigramme may show a locus of increased uptake. It focuses the clinical examination in a child with a vague presentation, such as refusal to walk. It also casts a wide net to evaluate remote sites, such as the spine in diskitis, and multiple sites, as may be affected in a generalized process such as leukæmia. Ultrasonogramme rules out a joint effusion in when there is a diagnostic dilemma between pyarthritis and osteomyelitis. The imaging modality also evaluates soft tissues, including for periosteal abscess, which may be aspirated. MRI gives greater detail of extent of bone involvement and of soft tissue extension. MRI does not influence management in primary or otherwise uncomplicated cases, except to raise anxiety.

For radionegative osteomyelitis, which is typical of an acute presentation, antibiotics are the initial treatment of choice [D]. If there is a good response, a full recovery without sequelæ is expected. If there is a poor response, investigate further, including more detailed imaging such as MRI. Consider operative intervention to decrease bacterial load if there is a defined site of disease, such as a soft tissue abscess that was not visible on röntgenogrammes.

Subacute osteomyelitis may be managed initially with antibiotics. Unlike pyarthritis, where pus damages articular cartilage if not evacuated, bone will recover fully from injury even if surgical treatment is delayed, so long as the child is stable. If there is a poor response over 2 to 3 days, surgical drainage and débridement are indicated. There has been significant bone destruction, suggesting that the balance has tipped away from host toward organism.

In the chronic setting, antibiotic access may be blocked by an involucrum, which must be physically disrupted [E]:

- Preoperative imaging will aid in surgical planning, including incision and need for consultants.
- Explore and drain the soft tissues.
- Débride all tissue that is not viable.
- If there is cortical softening, excise this to make a wide window.
- If the cortex is robust, outline an ovoid window with a drill like a postage stamp and remove with an osteotome.
- Débride until bleeding bone, manually or with a motorized burr.
- Do not injure an adjacent physis.
- Preserve periosteum to promote bone healing.
- Lay adjacent healthy muscle into the osseous bed, a process known as "saucerization." The muscle will bring the blood supply that was absent in the abscess, thereby bringing antibiotics to the infected site.
- Extensive sinus may require plastic closure, including flap coverage, after complete excision.

Complications

Generalized Infection that escapes the confines of bone, joint, or soft tissue may threaten the child systemically. Accelerate evaluation and make management more aggressive if a child is in distress.

Localized Pyarthritis may result in the following:

- Postinfectious arthritis, due to irreversible articular cartilage injury. There is no good solution for this.
- Growth disturbance, malangulation, or arrest, due to physeal cartilage injury. Excise a discreet bridge once diagnosis is made and before deformity sets in. Add osteotomy for established deformity. Perform distraction osteogenesis for shortening, without or with correction as indicated.
- Osteonecrosis, due to vascular thrombosis and pressure occlusion [A]. Observe for recovery.

These complications are the result of delayed or incomplete treatment, virulence of pathogen, and host immunity, in particular the neonate.

Osteomyelitis may result in the following:

- Advance of acute to chronic infection, an evolution from simple infection to abscess, from radionegative to radiopositive, and from nonoperative to operative treatment.
- Morbid fracture. Deossification lags the activity of infection by 2 to 3 weeks. Fracture is a risk of operative débridement.
- Growth disturbance due to adjacent physeal injury. This may be infectious or iatrogenic.

OTHER INFECTION

Chronic Recurrent Multifocal Osteomyelitis

The name is descriptive, except that this is "inflammation" of the bone in a general sense: pathologic analysis shows bone that is reactive as if infected, yet no organism is isolatable. Because of this, and because solitary lesions are possible, the disorder also is known as chronic non-bacterial osteomyelitis (CNO).

The patient complains of pain without other systemic or local inflammatory symptoms or signs. The pain comes and goes in different sites of the body. Duration is months to years. Laboratory analysis is normal. Röntgenogrammes show a sclerotic heterogeneous lesion typically in metaphysis of a long bone abutting physis, although any bone may be affected. Scintigramme shows increased uptake in the lesion and identifies other skeletal sites. The unusual presentation often leads to MRI (T2-weighted and enhanced with gadolinium-diethylene triamine penta-acetic acid), which may be difficult to differentiate from a neoplastic process. Biopsy often is inconclusive, leading to more invasive and extensive surgical intervention. Lesions abutting a physis are at risk of iatrogenic growth disturbance.

Autoinflammation, immune dysregulation without autoantibodies, error of metabolism, and postinfectious reaction have been posited as causes. There may be overlap with enthesitis-related arthritis. CRMO has been associated with chronic inflammatory bowel disease and hypophosphatasia. CRMO is equivalent in the adult to SAPHO syndrome (synovitis, acne, pustulosis, hyperostosis, and osteitis), which is managed in a similar manner.

Based upon a high haplotype relative risk, a gene has been identified in the region of a rare allele of marker D18S60 that may contribute to the cause of CRMO. In an animal model, restriction fragment length polymorphism analysis indicates that a CRMO gene may reside on murine chromosome 18.

Recognize the entity and exercise restraint. Spend the time to educate patient and family, who often require considerable assurance given chronicity, appearance on imaging, and the inevitable previous opinion. The patient is not ill. Pain is frustrating but manageable symptomatically, including nonsteroidal anti-inflammatory drugs. Other agents, indicated for severe pain, include immunosuppressants (corticosteroids, methotrexate, and tumor necrosis factor blockers), immunomodulators (intravenous immunoglobulins, interferon, colchicine, and dapsone), calcitonins, and bisphosphonates. Observe clinically. Alter laboratory analysis, röntgenogrammes, and other imaging if presentation changes significantly. There is debate about whether a good prognosis with spontaneous resolution is universal.

Pelvis

The pelvis is complex [A]. Its cavitary nature makes evaluation indirect. The patient may complain of flank, back, hip, or groin pain. Examine the abdomen for rebound tenderness associated with appendicitis. Diskitis may present as refusal to walk or abdominal pain in the first decade; only in the second decade does a child reliably localize this to the back. Palpate and move the spine. The sacroiliac joint may be stressed by *flexion–abduction–external rotation* manœuvre (FABER, Patrick). A rectal examination may reveal a deep pelvic abscess. Prone hip extension stretches the iliopsoa.

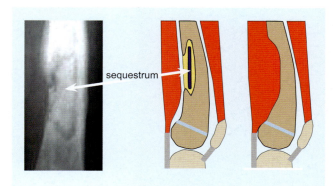

E Operative treatment of chronic osteomyelitis The approach differs according to type of joint and response to initial intervention.

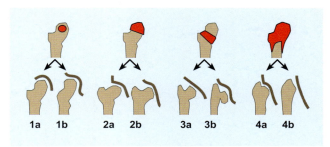

A Classification of sequelaæ of hip pyarthritis Initial necrosis (*red*) determines severity of final deformity.

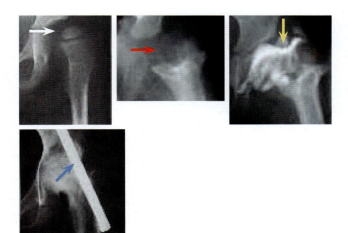

B Sequelæ of hip pyarthritis Unrecognized infection (*white*) resulted in delayed treatment, which was complicated by osteonecrosis (*red*). Arthrogram shows hinged deformity of the proximal femoral epiphysis (*yellow*). Because of unacceptable pain and stiffness, the patient underwent hip arthrodesis with an anterior plate at age 14 years (*blue*).

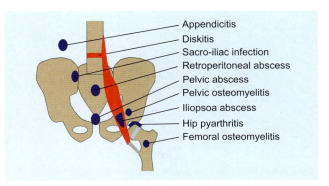

A Sites of infections about the pelvis.

Due to the overlap between multiple organ systems, imaging for pelvic infection prioritizes soft tissue. While screening with ultrasonogramme or scintigramme may focus the evaluation, CT and MRI are the modalities of choice.

Management of infections of the pelvis (and spine) is exceptional. Because of the morbidity of access, and because of rich vascularity, principles of treatment are skewed toward antibiotics without and with image-guided aspiration and drainage and away from operation initially, because most will resolve without the latter.

Pyomyositis

This represents a hæmatogenous bacterial infection of skeletal muscle. It is seen in healthy children in tropical regions; by contrast, in temperate zones, it most often involves immunocompromised children, including with diabetes mellitus, viral infection (e.g., HIV), and poor nutrition. Most affected are quadriceps femoris, gluteal, and iliopsoa muscles. In the majority of cases (>75%), the pathogen is *Staphylococcus aureus*. Three clinical stages are distinguished:

- Stage 1 (first week) is characterized by localized muscle ache, pain, and low-grade fever. Physical examination reveals induration of muscle with mild pain but without cutaneous manifestation. This accounts for delay in diagnosis. T2-weighted MRI shows nongeographic hyperintense signal and muscle enlargement. Have a high index of suspicion and obtain this test early. Treatment is intravenous antibiotics and close observation.
- Stage 2 (2 to 3 weeks). Suppuration makes the child appear ill and the muscle exquisitely tender. Abscess presents rim enhancement on MRI. Perform urgent drainage and débridement.
- In stage 3, the child has become septic. Supplement drainage and débridement with supportive measures as indicated.

Necrotizing Fasciitis

The condition is described in the Corpus Hippocraticum in association with erysipelas. The name emphasizes disproportionate destruction of superficial fascia with relative sparing of subjacent muscles (Wilson). Spread is rapid along deep fascial planes. Two types are distinguished, based upon pathogens:

- Type I is polymicrobial, including ærobes *Streptococcus pyogenes, MSSA, and MRSA* and anærobes *Clostridium perfringens, Bacteroides fragilis, and Aeromonas hydrophila.* This represents the majority of cases.
- Type II is monomicrobial.

It also may be classified based upon fulminance. Immune compromise is a risk factor. Skin is the richest source of pathogens, where infection reflects anatomic distribution, for example, perineal infection (Fournier gangrene) by anærobes. One source of MRSA is nosocomial. Bacterial exotoxins and superantigens set up a vicious cycle of thrombosis followed by necrosis followed by bacterial growth and invasion. The limbs are more affected than the trunk, which is associated with a higher mortality rate due to proximity of vital viscera and lack of amputation as an option.

The condition resembles an infected compartment syndrome. The inciting event is a breach of skin, including a surgical incision. Appearance is one of acute distress, often panic. Pain is the first sign and is out of proportion with the remainder of the early presentation. Within hours, other inflammatory signs manifest: fever, swelling, compartment tension, cutaneous crepitus, violaceous discoloration, and bullæ, which leak gray "dishwater" pus [A]. Systemic signs develop, such as tachycardia, hypotension, diarrhœa, and vomiting. No matter the external manifestation, the internal ones are much worse. Tissues are devitalized, black, œdematous, indurated yet friable, unstable due to loss of normal anchoring architecture, liquefied, and foul. Inflammatory markers are very elevated, for example, CRP > 100 mg/L and WBC > 20,000/mm^3, whereas hæmoglobin is reduced <10 g/dL.

A Necrotizing fasciitis There are severe changes in the lower limbs (*red*) in a child who requires ventilatory support (*yellow*).

Do not let laboratory analysis distract from the fact that this is a clinical diagnosis. And it is a surgical emergency. Administer broad spectrum and multiple intravenous antibiotics. Imaging such as MRI may be too much of a delay, as are fine needle aspiration or biopsy. Operation requires courage, both on the side of the patient and family—who must be counseled on how much will be removed and that there will be many stages and risks including death—as well as the side of the surgeon. Make a big incision and débride widely: leaving dead tissue will threaten life for the misplaced concern about saving function. Explore everywhere and follow every tract. Amputation may be necessary. Reserve the ICU, plan for a return to the operating room, and assemble an interdisciplinary team (e.g., soft tissue reconstructive surgeons).

Hyperbaric oxygen therapy is not readily available and controversial. Intravenous immunoglobulins show efficacy as an adjunctive treatment.

Mortality rate increases with time to diagnosis and with age.

Tuberculosis

The disease is caused by *Mycobacterium tuberculosis*. It is highly aerobic (lung) and very slow growing, replicating over several hours compared with minutes for most bacteria. The German scientist Robert Koch (1843 to 1910) presented four postulates that proved this bacillus as the cause of consumption.

Less than 10% of tuberculosis is extrapulmonary, and skeletal involvement accounts for 2% of the total burden of the disease. Half of skeletal cases are spinal [A]. The disease is heavily weighted toward the developing world: 1/3 cases are in Asia and 1/3 in Africa. After socioeconomic status, immune compromise is the most frequent causative factor. The portal of entry is the lung, with hæmatogenous spread to the skeleton. Less than 10% of healthy children will contract tuberculosis after infection with *Mycobacterium tuberculosis*.

Evaluation Rarity in the developed world results in lack of clinical suspicion. This, together with slow progression of disease, results in delayed diagnosis (months). Inflammatory markers are only mildly elevated, including ESR, but often, CRP is normal. Ask about travel and exposure, as well as BCG (Bacille Calmette-Guérin) vaccination. Obtain a chest röntgenogramme. Place a tuberculin skin test. Because the disease is globally erosive of both sides of a joint and elicits a robust osseous reaction, tumor may be suspected on röntgenogrammes. MRI aids visualization of soft tissue abscess.

Management Despite or because of the slowness of progression, the disease is destructive. This results in significant postinfectious arthritis and deformity. It also necessitates a prolonged (12 months) and multiple (four drug: isoniazid, rifampin, ethambutol, pyrazinamide) antibiotic regimen. Drug resistance is a worldwide concern. Surgical débridement may require bone grafting of subchondral erosions. Osteotomy corrects malangulation. Arthrodesis may be necessary for end-stage arthritis.

Tuberculous spondylitis (Pott disease) starts in the metaphysis of the vertebral body (adjacent to intervertebral disk), where it produces a short sharp kyphosis [B]. Ten percent of cases are cervical, with thoracic slightly more frequent than lumbar. Cervical involvement may lead to atlantoaxial instability. Lumbar infection may extend along the psoa to the groin. Pott disease is the most dangerous manifestation of skeletal tuberculosis. Pain is universal. Neural involvement occurs in half of cases. Röntgenogrammes measure deformity. MRI shows the abscess and neural elements. CT is useful for operative planning.

In addition to antibiotic treatment, surgical reconstruction is indicated for the following:

- Neural compromise. This may be due to abscess or to severe deformity.
- Progression of deformity.

Operation is circumferential, because abscess compromises the integrity of the anterior column of the spine [C] and rigidity requires vertebral column resection for correction. Hence the high surgical risk.

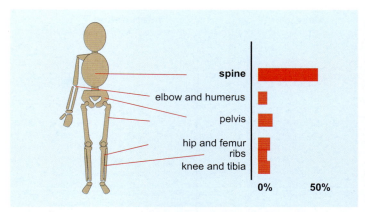

A   Geographic distribution of musculoskeletal tuberculosis.

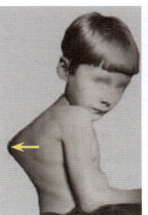

B   Tuberculosis of the spine This may produce a short sharp kyphosis (*yellow*).

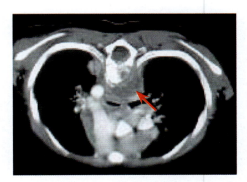

C   Tuberculous paravertebral abscess The abscess (*red*) infiltrates all columns of the spine, eroding the vertebral body leading to anterior collapse into kyphosis.

Measure		Intervention
Host		Maximize health, e.g., improve nutrition Minimize risk, e.g., treat pre-existing infection such as urinary tract
Skin		Clean: chlorhexidine, bleach Remove hair with depilatory agent (not razor)
Nose		Topical mupirocin
Antibiotics		Intravenous administration within 1 hr. before operation Redose during operation Antibiotic powder in wound Stop within 24 h after operation
Operating room		Heat to maintain patient normothermia Limit traffic to essential personnel Dedicated attire Close doors
Skin		Chlorhexidine preparation Do not use adhesive drapes
Instruments		Wipe and keep dry
Suction		Clamp when not in use Change the tip
Gloves		Change regularly
Dressing		Impervious Careful technique for postoperative change
Drain		Remove within 24 h
Dental prophylaxis		No consensus

A **Measures influencing surgical site infection** These may be divided into before (*gray*), at (*blue*), and after (*green*) operation.

Surgical Site Infection

Surgical site infection (SSI) represents nearly 1/5 of all hospital-acquired infections, second to urinary tract infection. It increases morbidity and mortality: national data show a 3% increase in death due to SSI. It deteriorates outcomes: for example, nonunion hurts and impedes function, threatens implant stability, and ultimately requires revision and reconstruction. It increases cost, including further testing, antibiotics, repeat operation, and prolonged length of stay in hospital (mean 1 week).

Sources of SSI include the physical environment, such as personnel, operating room, and equipment. The host brings normal cutaneous flora (nearly half of cases are due to *Staphylococcus aureus*) and may be compromised and colonized, such as in neuromuscular disease.

Several measures may be taken to reduce SSI [A]. Neuromuscular patients undergo preoperative assessment for health status and risk of infection, including laboratory analysis such as serum transferrin and urinalysis. They are managed accordingly, such as referral to a general surgeon for gastrostomy tube placement, before undergoing major operation. A bleach bath (1/2 cup, 20 minutes) is an effective chemical decontaminant, in particular to reduce MRSA, and does not risk iatrogenic resistance.

Antibiotics are most effective around the time of operation: practices that prolong postoperative use, for example, for the duration of wound drainage, may increase infection by selecting for resistant organisms. Consider earlier administration of antibiotics when a tourniquet is planned. Readminister in operation according to the half-life of the antibiotic.

The room where an operation takes place no longer can be regarded as a "theater," but as a place with strict and consistent controls. Wear clothing dedicated to the operating room: change scrubs between cases, and keep civilian clothes, bags, and other paraphernalia out. Warm the operating room: patient hypothermia is associated with increased infection. The most effective skin preparation is chlorhexidine: it has the same bactericidal properties as alcohol (both better than iodine) but lasts longer. Adhesive drapes may trap blood and other contaminants as they inevitably lift off the skin during long procedures, thereby increasing SSI. The instrument bath is a culture broth: dilute in a chemical bacteriocidal agent such as hydrogen peroxide or bleach, or wipe and keep instruments dry. Do not suck continually: minimize how much of the room air is circulated into the wound. Consider simple measures such as regularly changing sucker tip and outer pair of gloves, which are breached more frequently than realized. Irrigate the wound multiple times during long procedures, and use irrigant that is opened only when needed for this indication.

Apply an impervious dressing. Change it after 48 hours methodically: wear a gown and sterile gloves, replace soiled gauze and adhesive strips, clean the skin with an antiseptic solution, do not touch the wound edges. Avoid prolonged wound drainage: colonization provides a route for exogenous bacteria to access the wound. Administration of prophylactic antibiotics for dental care or other invasive procedures lacks consensus or consistent national treatment recommendations.

Abernethy LJ, Lee YC, Cole WG. Ultrasound localization of subperiosteal abscesses in children with late-acute osteomyelitis. *J. Pediatr. Orthop.* 13(6):766–768, 1993.

Appel M, Pauleto AC, Cunha LA. Osteochondral sequelae of meningococcemia: radiographic aspects. *J. Pediatr. Orthop.* 22(4):511–516, 2002.

Aroojis AJ, Johari AN. Epiphyseal separations after neonatal osteomyelitis and septic arthritis. *J. Pediatr. Orthop.* 20(4):544–549, 2000.

Belthur MV, Birchansky SB, Verdugo AA, Mason EO Jr, Hulten KG, Kaplan SL, Smith EO, Phillips WA, Weinberg J. Pathologic fractures in children with acute *Staphylococcus aureus* osteomyelitis. *J. Bone Joint Surg.* 94(1)-A:34–42, 2012.

Berger E, Saunders N, Wang L, Friedman JN. Sickle cell disease in children: differentiating osteomyelitis from vaso-occlusive crisis. *Arch. Pediatr. Adolesc. Med.* 163(3):251–255, 2009.

Bickels J, Ben-Sira L, Kessler A, Weintroub S. Primary pyomyositis. *J. Bone Joint Surg.* 84(12)-A:2277–2286, 2002.

Bos CF, Mol LJ, Obermann WR, Tjin a Ton ER. Late sequelae of neonatal septic arthritis of the shoulder. *J. Bone Joint Surg.* 80(4)-B:645–650, 1998.

Brodie BC. An account of some cases of chronic abscess of the tibia. *Med. Chir. Trans.* 17:239–249, 1832.

Brook I. Microbiology and management of infectious gangrene in children. *J. Pediatr. Orthop.* 24(5):587–592, 2004.

Canavese F, Krajbich JI, LaFleur BJ. Orthopaedic sequelae of childhood meningococcemia: management considerations and outcome. *J. Bone Joint Surg.* 92(12)-A:2196–2203, 2010.

Cavalier R, Herman MJ, Pizzutillo PD, Geller E. Ultrasound-guided aspiration of the hip in children: a new technique. *Clin. Orthop.* 415:244–247, 2003.

Ceroni D, Cherkaoui A, Combescure C, François P, Kaelin A, Schrenzel J. Differentiating osteoarticular infections caused by Kingella kingae from those due to typical pathogens in young children. *Pediatr. Infect. Dis. J.* 30:906–909, 2011.

Chambers JB, Forsythe DA, Bertrand SL, Iwinski HJ, Steflik DE. Retrospective review of osteoarticular infections in a pediatric sickle cell age group. *J. Pediatr. Orthop.* 20(5):682–685, 2000.

Choi IH, Pizzutillo PD, Bowen JR, Dragann R, Malhis T. Sequelae and reconstruction after septic arthritis of the hip in infants. *J. Bone Joint Surg.* 72(8)-A:1150–1165, 1990.

Dartnell J, Ramachandran M, Katchburian M. Haematogenous acute and subacute paediatric osteomyelitis: a systematic review of the literature. *J. Bone Joint Surg.* 94(5)-B:584–595, 2012.

Duffy CM, Lam PY, Ditchfield M, Allen R, Graham HK. Chronic recurrent multifocal osteomyelitis: review of orthopaedic complications at maturity. *J. Pediatr. Orthop.* 22(4):501–505, 2002.

Ezra E, Cohen N, Segev E, Hayek S, Lokiec F, Keret D, Wientroub S. Primary subacute epiphyseal osteomyelitis: role of conservative treatment. *J. Pediatr. Orthop.* 22(3):333–337, 2002.

Garron E, Viehweger E, Launay F, Guillaume JM, Jouve JL, Bollini G. Nontuberculous spondylodiscitis in children. *J. Pediatr. Orthop.* 22(3):321–328, 2002.

Giedion A, Holthusen W, Masel LF, Vischer D. Subacute and chronic 'symmetrical' osteomyelitis. *Ann. Radiol.* 15(3):329–342, 1972.

Girschick HJ, Zimmer C, Klaus G, Darge K, Dick A, Morbach H. Chronic recurrent multifocal osteomyelitis: what is it and how should it be treated? *Nat. Clin. Pract. Rheum.* 3(12):733–738, 2007.

Gram HC. Über die isolierte Färbung der Schizomyceten in Schnitt- und Trockenpräparaten. *Fortschr Med.* 2: 185–189, 1884.

Grimes J, Carpenter C, Reinker K. Toxic shock syndrome as a complication of orthopedic surgery. *J. Pediatr. Orthop.* 15(5):666–671, 1995.

Gristina AG, Shibata Y, Giridhar G, Kreger A, Myrvik QN. The glycocalyx, biofilm, microbes, and resistant infection. *Semin. Arthroplasty* 5(4):160–170, 1994.

Grogan DP, Love SM, Ogden JA, Millar EA, Johnson LO. Chondro-osseous growth abnormalities after meningococcemia. A clinical and histopathological study. *J. Bone Joint Surg.* 71(6)-A:920–928, 1989.

Hammond PJ, Macnicol MF. Osteomyelitis of the pelvis and proximal femur: diagnostic difficulties. *J. Pediatr. Orthop.* 10(2)-B:113–119, 2001.

Harris NH, Kirkaldy-Willis WH. Primary subacute pyogenic osteomyelitis. *J. Bone Joint Surg.* 47-B:526–532, 1965.

Hodgson AR, Stock FE, Fang HS, Ong GB. Anterior spinal fusion. The operative approach and pathological findings in 412 patients with Pott's disease of the spine. *Br. J. Surg.* 48:172–178, 1960.

Jaberi FM, Shahcheraghi GH, Ahadzadeh M. Short-term intravenous antibiotic treatment of acute hematogenous bone and joint infection in children: a prospective randomized trial. *J. Pediatr. Orthop.* 22(3):317–320, 2002.

Jaramillo D. Infection: musculoskeletal. *Pediatr. Radiol.* 41(Suppl 1):S127–134, 2011.

Jones HW, Beckles VL, Akinola B, Stevenson AJ, Harrison WJ. Chronic haematogenous osteomyelitis in children: an unsolved problem. *J. Bone Joint Surg.* 93(8)-B: 1005–1010, 2011.

Jung ST, Rowe SM, Moon ES, Song EK, Yoon TR, Seo HY. Significance of laboratory and radiologic findings for differentiating between septic arthritis and transient synovitis of the hip. *J. Pediatr. Orthop.* 23(3):368–372, 2003.

Khachatourians AG, Patzakis MJ, Roidis N, Holtom PD. Laboratory monitoring in pediatric acute osteomyelitis and septic arthritis. *Clin. Orthop.* 409:186–194, 2003.

Kim HK, Alman B, Cole WG. A shortened course of parenteral antibiotic therapy in the management of acute septic arthritis of the hip. *J. Pediatr. Orthop.* 20(1):44–47, 2000.

Kocher MS, Mandiga R, Zurakowski D, Barnewolt C, Kasser JR. Validation of a clinical prediction rule for the differentiation between septic arthritis and transient synovitis of the hip in children. *J. Bone Joint Surg.* 86(8)-A:1629–1635, 2004.

Konyves A, Deo SD, Murray JR, Mandalia VI, Von Arx OA, Troughton AH. Septic arthritis of the elbow after chickenpox. *J. Pediatr. Orthop.* 13(2):114–117, 2004.

Kucukkaya M, Kabukcuoglu Y, Tezer M, Kuzgun U. Management of childhood chronic tibial osteomyelitis with the Ilizarov method. *J. Pediatr. Orthop.* 22(5):632–637, 2002.

Lowden CM, Walsh SJ. Acute staphylococcal osteomyelitis of the clavicle. *J. Pediatr. Orthop.* 17(4):467–469, 1997.

Luhmann SJ, Jones A, Schootman M, Gordon JE, Schoenecker PL, Luhmann JD. Differentiation between septic arthritis and transient synovitis of the hip in children with clinical prediction algorithms. *J. Bone Joint Surg.* 86(5)-A:956–962, 2004.

Lundy DW, Kehl DK. Increasing prevalence of *Kingella kingae* in osteoarticular infections in young children. *J. Pediatr. Orthrop.* 18(2):262–267, 1998.

Mantadakis E, Plessa E, Vouloumanou EK, Michailidis L, Chatzimichael A, Falagas ME. Deep venous thrombosis in children with musculoskeletal infections: the clinical evidence. *Int. J. Infect. Dis.* 16(4):e236–243, 2012.

Maraqa NF, Gomez MM, Rathore MH. Outpatient parenteral antimicrobial therapy in osteoarticular infections in children. *J. Pediatr. Orthop.* 22(4):506–510, 2002.

Morrison MJ, Herman MJ. Hip septic arthritis and other pediatric musculoskeletal infections in the era of methicillin-resistant *Staphylococcus aureus*. *Instr. Course Lect.* 62:405–414, 2013.

Odio CM, Ramirez T, Arias G, AbdelNour A, Hidalgo I, Herrera ML, Bolan W, Alpizar J, Alvarez P. Double blind, randomized, placebo-controlled study of dexamethasone therapy for hematogenous septic arthritis in children. *Pediatr. Infect. Dis. J.* 22(10):883–888, 2003.

Orlicek SL, Abramson JS, Woods CR, Givner LB. Obturator internus muscle abscess in children. *J. Pediatr. Orthop.* 21(6):744–748, 2001.

Peltola H, Unkila-Kallio L, Kallio MJ. Simplified treatment of acute staphylococcal osteomyelitis of childhood. The Finnish Study Group. *Pediatrics* 99(6):846–850, 1997.

Perlman MH, Patzakis MJ, Kumar PJ, Holtom P. The incidence of joint involvement with adjacent osteomyelitis in pediatric patients. *J. Pediatr. Orthop.* 20(1):40–43, 2000.

Piehl FC, Davis RJ, Prugh SI. Osteomyelitis in sickle cell disease. *J. Pediatr. Orthop.* 13(2):225–227, 1993.

Pott P. The chirurgical works of Percivall Pott, F.R.S., surgeon to St. Bartholomew's Hospital, a new edition, with his last corrections. 1808. *Clin. Orthop.* 4–10, 2002.

Rasool MN. Osseous manifestations of tuberculosis in children. *J. Pediatr. Orthop.* 21(6):749–755, 2001.

Riise ØR, Kirkhus E, Handeland KS, Flatø B, Reiseter T, Cvancarova M, Nakstad B, Wathne KO. Childhood osteomyelitis-incidence and differentiation from other acute onset musculoskeletal features in a population-based study. *BMC Pediatr.* 8(45):2431–2438, 2008.

Roderick MR, Ramanan AV. Chronic recurrent multifocal osteomyelitis. *Adv. Exp. Med. Biol.* 764:99–107, 2013.

Rose CD, Fawcett PT, Eppes SC, Klein JD, Gibney K, Doughty RA. Pediatric Lyme arthritis: clinical spectrum and outcome. *J. Pediatr. Orthop.* 14(2):238–241, 1994.

Segev E, Hayek S, Lokiec F, Ezra E, Issakov J, Wientroub S. Primary chronic sclerosing (Garre's) osteomyelitis in children. *J. Pediatr. Orthop.* 10(4)-B:360–364, 2001.

Shallcross LJ, Fragaszy E, Johnson AM, Hayward AC. The role of the Panton-Valentine leucocidin toxin in staphylococcal disease: a systematic review and meta-analysis. *Lancet Infect Dis.* 13(1):43–54, 2013.

Song J, Letts M, Monson R. Differentiation of psoas muscle abscess from septic arthritis of the hip in children. *Clin. Orthop.* 391:258–265, 2001.

Spiegel DA, Meyer JS, Dormans JP, Flynn JM, Drummond DS. Pyomyositis in children and adolescents: report of 12 cases and review of the literature. *J. Pediatr. Orthop.* 19(2):143–150, 1999.

Stumpe KD, Strobel K. Osteomyelitis and arthritis. *Semin. Nucl. Med.* 39(1):27–35, 2009.

Tong CW, Griffith JF, Lam TP, Cheng JC. The conservative management of acute pyogenic iliopsoas abscess in children. *J. Bone Joint Surg.* 80(1)-B:83–85, 1998.

Tudisco C, Farsetti P, Gatti S, Ippolito E. Influence of chronic osteomyelitis on skeletal growth: analysis at maturity of 26 cases affected during childhood. *J. Pediatr. Orthop.* 11:358–363, 1991.

Unkila-Kallio L, Kallio MJ, Peltola H. The usefulness of C-reactive protein levels in the identification of concurrent septic arthritis in children who have acute hematogenous osteomyelitis. A comparison with the usefulness of the erythrocyte sedimentation rate and the white blood-cell count. *J. Bone Joint Surg.* 76(6)-A:848–853, 1994.

Willis AA, Widmann RF, Flynn JM, Green DW, Onel KB. Lyme arthritis presenting as acute septic arthritis in children. *J. Pediatr. Orthop.* 23(1):114–118, 2003.

Wilson B. Necrotising fasciitis. *Am. Surg.* 18(4): 416–431, 1952.

Yokoe DS, Mermel LA, Anderson DJ, Arias KM, Burstin H, Calfee DP, Coffin SE, Dubberke ER, Fraser V, Gerding DN, Griffin FA, Gross P, Kaye KS, Klompas M, Lo E, Marschall J, Nicolle L, Pegues DA, Perl TM, Podgorny K, Saint S, Salgado CD, Weinstein RA, Wise R, Classen D. A compendium of strategies to prevent healthcare-associated infections in acute care hospital. *Infect. Control Hosp. Epidemiol.* 29:S12–S21, 2008.

TUMORS

Malignant tumors of the musculoskeletal system constitute 10% of new cancers in children, numbering approximately 1,000 cases in the United States *per annum*. Benign tumors are 10 times the rate. We are presently on an exponential curve for advancement in oncology, for example, overall 5-year survival has risen from 10% to 20% in 1970 to better than 70% today. The most common pædiatric tumor is the benign fibrous cortical defect. The most common malignant tumor is osteosarcoma of bone and rhabdomyosarcoma of soft tissue; Ewing sarcoma traverses tissue types. This chapter focuses on common diagnoses.

EVALUATION

Because the word "tumor" may have sinister connotations, consider classifying tumors in simple terms for patients [A]. Most tumors are not life threatening. They may threaten local tissues, for example, risk of morbid fracture, and thus require surgical management. They may be stable, amenable to conservative measures, or incidental findings, which are left alone.

History

Duration may be difficult to determine. The tumor requires time to grow sufficiently to disturb function or to be physically apparent or visible. Hence the poorer prognosis for axial tumors compared with appendicular lesions. Age is the universal discriminator of disease, for example, 2/3 of rhabdomyosarcomas occur in the first decade, while osteosarcoma peaks at puberty [B]. Refine the presentation of pain [C]. Abrupt pain may indicate morbid fracture. Beware of being distracted by a sporting or other benign injury. Not all malignant or aggressive tumors elicit pain: rhabdomyosarcoma typically does not hurt. Race may be helpful, for example, Ewing sarcoma is less common in blacks than whites.

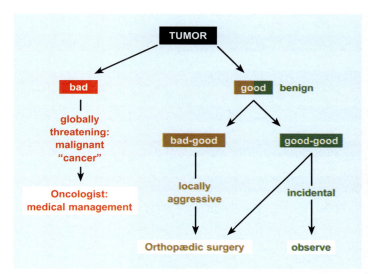

A Classification of tumors This simple approach provides clarity and perspective for patients.

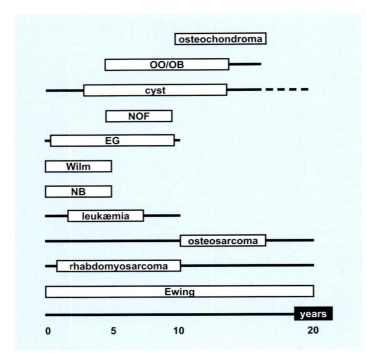

B **Age distribution of some tumors** NB, neuroblastoma; EG, eosinophilic granuloma; NOF, nonossifying fibroma; OO, osteoid osteoma; OB, osteoblastoma.

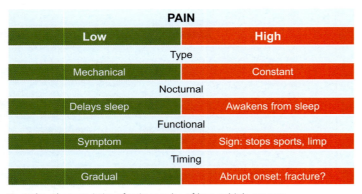

C **Pain** Characteristics of pain may be of low or high concern.

Physical Examination

Take the temperature. Ewing sarcoma may be mistaken for osteomyelitis at first. Observe gait for alteration due to pain or other interference with function. Does the child look ill, as if overcome by pain or a generalized process? Are the complaints focal or diffuse? Are there "hard" objective signs? Are the soft tissues reactive, as evidenced by swelling, redness, induration, and adhesion? Is there articular stiffness to suggest guarding? Is there atrophy of disuse or other asymmetry? If a mass is detectable, is it tender? Is it soft, firm, or hard? How large is it? Greater than 5 cm is ominous for soft tissue sarcoma.

Imaging

Develop a method that is clear, standard, efficient, and reproducible.

Röntgenogrammes The acronym ALLMDS facilitates communication [D]:

- A: Age.
- L: "Looks like." This admits descriptives such as "sunburst," "moth eaten," scalloped," and "expansile" [E].
- L: Location. Where within the bone, for example, metaphysis, diaphysis, or epiphysis [F], or what bone, for example, long bone such as the femur, irregular bone such as the spine, or flat bone such as the pelvis [G].
- M: Margins. These are divided into distinct, called "geographic," or nondistinct, called "nongeographic." The latter is more ominous, as it is a sign of rapid tumor growth and failure of bone to react and delimit this growth.
- D: Density. Lesions may be lytic, which are radiolucent; blastic, which are radiodense; or mixed, which are heterogeneous. This aids local assessment of bone but is not prognostic. Lytic lesions erode the integrity of bone and risk morbid fracture, influencing decision on internal fixation. On the other hand, while blastic lesions may be more stable, they may represent a high-grade osteosarcoma.
- S: Soft tissue. This may be reactive, such as elevation of periosteum, or a mass, for example, Ewing sarcoma.

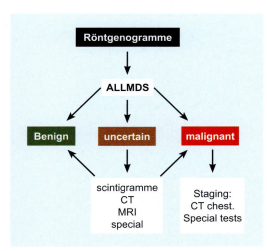

D Imaging for bone tumor Simple algorithm.

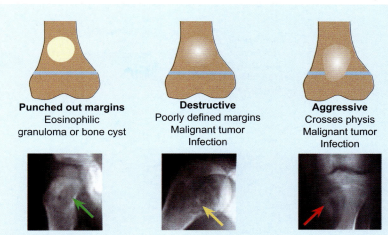

Effect of lesion on bone
Lytic eosinophilic granuloma (green), heterogeneous osteogenic sarcoma (yellow), and aggressive osteogenic sarcoma traversing the physis (red).

Effect of lesion on normal adjacent tissue
Scalloping in nonossifying fibroma (green), expanded cortex in aneurysmal bone cyst (yellow), and vigorous osseous reaction in osteoid osteoma (red).

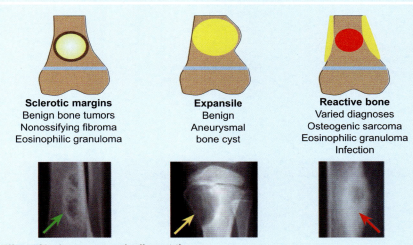

Special diagnostic features.
Ground glass appearance of fibrous dysplasia (green), speckled calcification in a cartilage tumor (yellow), and osteoblastic features of an osteogenic sarcoma (red).

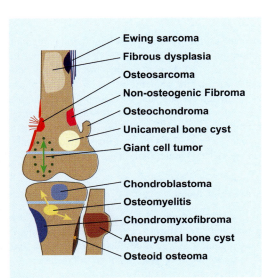

Ewing sarcoma
Fibrous dysplasia
Osteosarcoma
Non-osteogenic Fibroma
Osteochondroma
Unicameral bone cyst
Giant cell tumor
Chondroblastoma
Osteomyelitis
Chondromyxofibroma
Aneurysmal bone cyst
Osteoid osteoma

F Location of tumors within a long bone.

E Some diagnostic features by röntgenogramme.

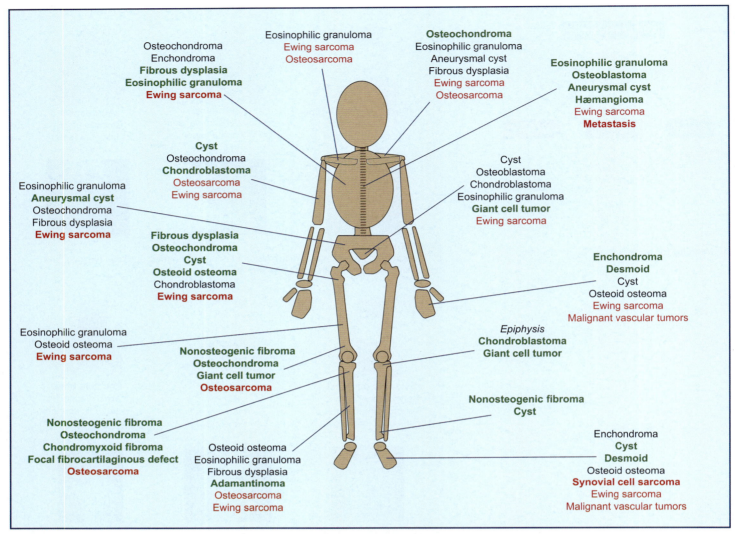

Osteochondroma
Enchondroma
Fibrous dysplasia
Eosinophilic granuloma
Ewing sarcoma

Eosinophilic granuloma
Ewing sarcoma
Osteosarcoma

Osteochondroma
Eosinophilic granuloma
Aneurysmal cyst
Fibrous dysplasia
Ewing sarcoma
Osteosarcoma

Eosinophilic granuloma
Osteoblastoma
Aneurysmal cyst
Hæmangioma
Ewing sarcoma
Metastasis

Cyst
Osteochondroma
Chondroblastoma
Osteosarcoma
Ewing sarcoma

Cyst
Osteoblastoma
Chondroblastoma
Eosinophilic granuloma
Giant cell tumor
Ewing sarcoma

Eosinophilic granuloma
Aneurysmal cyst
Osteochondroma
Fibrous dysplasia
Ewing sarcoma

Fibrous dysplasia
Osteochondroma
Cyst
Osteoid osteoma
Chondroblastoma
Ewing sarcoma

Enchondroma
Desmoid
Cyst
Osteoid osteoma
Ewing sarcoma
Malignant vascular tumors

Eosinophilic granuloma
Osteoid osteoma
Ewing sarcoma

Epiphysis
Chondroblastoma
Giant cell tumor

Nonosteogenic fibroma
Osteochondroma
Giant cell tumor
Osteosarcoma

Nonosteogenic fibroma
Cyst

Nonosteogenic fibroma
Osteochondroma
Chondromyxoid fibroma
Focal fibrocartilaginous defect
Osteosarcoma

Osteoid osteoma
Eosinophilic granuloma
Fibrous dysplasia
Adamantinoma
Osteosarcoma
Ewing sarcoma

Enchondroma
Cyst
Desmoid
Osteoid osteoma
Synovial cell sarcoma
Ewing sarcoma
Malignant vascular tumors

G **Tumor types by skeletal site** Common location of benign tumors in *green*. Malignant tumors in *red*, and common sites indicated in *bold*.

Ultrasonography This is indicated for a soft tissue mass when there is a low index of suspicion for malignancy. It may be used as a guide to aspiration or needle biopsy. It is simple to perform in an awake child without a special facility or medication.

Scintigraphy This is a measure of bone turnover and activity of a lesion. It may discern between a benign lesion that is incidental and not the explanation for regional pain and one that has a microfracture, thereby guiding treatment. It surveys the skeleton for other sites of disease. It has a high negative predictive value for malignant disease. Overlap between benign and malignant disease reduces the positive predictive value.

CT This is essential to staging as a survey of the chest and abdomen. Its fine bone detail aids operative decision making.

MRI Like CT, MRI is essential to staging. It is indicated for soft tissue tumors and bone tumors with a significant soft tissue component. It is supplanting CT for bone, for example, osteoid osteoma of a long bone. It has high sensitivity but specificity declines in differentiation of tumor from infection. The principal disadvantage is the requirement for sedation in the young child.

PET Detects gamma rays from the positron-emitting radioactive isotope fluorine-18 substituted for a hydroxyl group on glucose (fluorodeoxyglucose). The glucose analogue is taken up by actively dividing cells, where it is trapped but not metabolized, resulting in concentration of radioactive signal in tissue with high glucose uptake. This modality may enhance CT and surveys for metastases and is useful to follow response to treatment.

Laboratory Analysis

A peripheral blood smear is useful in leukæmia. White blood cell count may be difficult to interpret, for example, it may be reduced due to chronic disease. Inflammatory markers may be increased in tumor, for example, Ewing sarcoma, or in infection. Elevation of alkaline phosphatase may be sensitive though nonspecific, for example, in the active phase of fibrous dysplasia. It may serve as a marker of response to medical treatment, such as with bisphosphonates. Blood cultures distinguish infection. Special tests may be indicated, such as urinary catecholamines and metabolites, which are elevated in neuroblastoma.

Staging

There are three stages of benign tumor.

- Latent. These may be asymptomatic and incidentally found. They show little or no growth and do not disturb or escape the compartment.
- Active. There is growth of tumor, as well as destruction, remodeling, and possible fracture of bone, limited to the confines of the compartment.
- Aggressive. Tumor grows rapidly; destroys, distorts, and fractures bone; and escapes the compartment into surrounding soft tissue, including rare metastasis (e.g., giant cell tumor).

Staging of malignant tumors is complex and disease specific. It is essential to management and prognosis of malignant tumors. Several factors contribute to stage [H]. Surgical staging (Enneking) emphasizes pathologic grade and the compartmental nature of a lesion: fascia, joint, and bone define a compartment [I]. Broadly, stage 0 may be considered precancerous. For stage I, surgical treatment is sufficient. Surgery for stage IV is prophylactic or palliative, for example, for impending or actual morbid fracture. Stages II and III combine medical and surgical management.

Biopsy

This may be percutaneous or open. Percutaneous may be of bone marrow from the iliac crest, for example, in leukæmia or Ewing sarcoma, or with image guidance when open access is morbid, for example, in the spine, or when there remains uncertainty about the diagnosis of tumor. Plan a large and wide enough specimen from multiple locations to be definitive. Biopsy may be incisional for diagnosis, excisional when geographic and localized, or compartmental when margins are indistinct but there is no regional or distant spread [J]. The principles of open biopsy are well established, founded on the spirit that this must be undertaken with the same level of preparation as the definitive procedure.

- Plan for future reconstruction when selecting incision, which should be as small as possible and extensile.
- Perform a transmuscular approach to limit contamination within that compartment.
- Avoid major neurovascular structures. Unlike muscle, these are not expendable in the event of future resection.
- Include the margin of a lesion, where growth and atypia tend to be greatest.
- Strict hæmostasis reduces contamination.
- Intraoperative frozen section confirms that enough tissue has been obtained to establish diagnosis or that a lesion is benign before proceeding with definitive care.
- Consider referral before biopsy if the surgeon, pathologist, and institution are not equipped to manage the case regardless of diagnosis.

Differential Diagnosis

The adage "culture tumor, biopsy infection" was conceived in the diagnostic dilemma each can pose the other. Consider fever, systemic signs, age, location, and elevation of inflammatory markers. Presence or absence of a mass and appearance on imaging sharpen the diagnosis [K]. Biopsy may be necessary for certainty.

Distinguish osteosarcoma from myositis ossificans by zone reversal. The latter is characterized by central proliferating cells surrounded by a margin of ossification. In osteosarcoma, the rapidly growing periphery has not yet ossified.

Differentiate fractures by history, for example, trauma or repetitive stress, and empirically by treating with rest and immobilization. Distinguish anxiety time from biologic time: 4 to 6 weeks will not alter tumor prognosis. Laboratory analysis is normal. Advanced imaging may be necessary, such as MRI showing no soft tissue extension or mass. Resist biopsy.

Factor	Comment
Tumor	1: confined to site of origin 2: outside the site of origin
Nodal involvement	0: none 1: local 2: regional 3: distant
Metastasis	0: absent 1: present
Grade	1: low 4: high
Serum markers	Elevation
Resection	Measure of free or contaminated margins
Vascular	Invasion of vasculature
Lymphatic	Invasion of lymphatic system
Response	To chemotherapy, based upon % necrosis in surgical specimen
Imaging	e.g., MRI

H   Some factors considered for staging of tumors These may vary according to disease type.

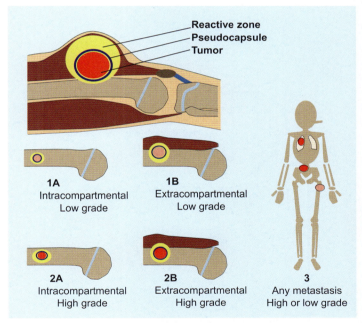

I   Staging of musculoskeletal tumors Surgical staging is determined by grade and physical extent of lesion.

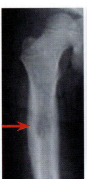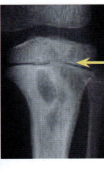

K   Infection, not tumor Atypical features of infection include periosteal reaction and diaphyseal location (*red*) and extension from metaphysis transphysis to epiphysis (*yellow*).

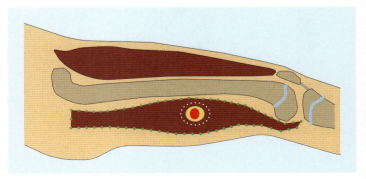

J   Biopsy of tumor This may be incisional, within the tumor (*red*), excisional (*white dots*), or compartmental (*green dots*).

	1	**2**	**3**
Pain	Mild	Moderate	Functional
Location	Upper limb	Lower limb	Proximal femur
Size	< 1/3	1/3-2/3	> 2/3
Density	Blastic	Mixed	Lytic

A   Assessing risk for morbid fracture of hole in bone 3 points are given for pain that is sufficiently severe to disturb function. A critical value is 9, which represents the beginning of the exponential part of the fracture curve (>1/3 will fracture). This system is a guide: it was developed for bone metastases in adults (Mirels).

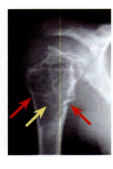

B   Active unicameral bone cyst There is a fracture fragment floating inside the cyst like a "fallen leaf" (yellow). The fracture takes up the entire width of the bone and has eroded the cortex to the point of fracture (red).

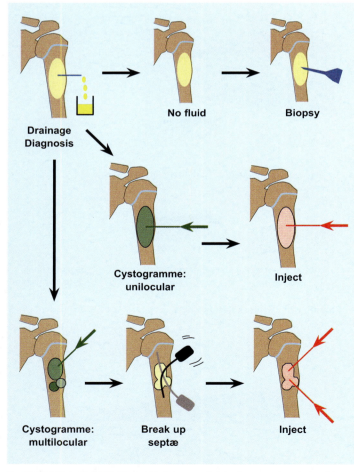

C   Aspiration and injection of a bone cyst Injection may be of steroid, bone marrow aspirate, or other adjuvant.

BONE CYST

Unicameral Bone Cyst

The name implies a "single chamber" (Latin *camera* = Greek καμαρα: "vaulted chamber") without loculation, although some have septæ. This most commonly occurs in the humerus and femur. Cause is unknown. The cysts are filled with yellow fluid and lined with a fibrous capsule.

Evaluation These may be incidental or may present with pain. They are metaphyseal and travel toward the diaphysis with growth. Incidental findings are assessed for fracture risk [A]. Pain indicates bending under load or fracture and may be severe enough to interfere with function. Lesions in the proximal femur are high risk because of concentration of the force of weight bearing and the grave anatomic consequences of fracture in this region.

RÖNTGENOGRAMME The lesion is central, nonexpansile, geographic with a sclerotic margin, and lytic. It may have septæ and an osseous fragment may float in its midst, known as "fallen leaf sign."

Management The natural history is spontaneous resolution of cysts by maturity in most cases. Latent cysts may be observed. Active cysts, which abut the physis, grow inexorably, and may fracture, tend to be treated surgically. Age, location, and fracture risk and consequences guide treatment.

LOW RISK EXCEPT FEMUR Observe. A humeral cyst that is small, asymptomatic, or acceptably painful may be managed conservatively, such as activity modification and nonnarcotic analgesics, and may resolve with maturity.

LOW RISK PROXIMAL FEMUR Observe or treat surgically because of concerns regarding load at, and fracture of, the hip.

HIGH RISK Observe if patient is very young and humerus is involved, or treat surgically. The proximal femur trumps age: consider fixation even in the very young.

FRACTURE EXCEPT FEMUR Treat by closed methods as long as alignment is acceptable. Healing of the fracture may partially heal cyst, potentially converting a cyst that is high risk by size into one that is low risk due to filling in with new bone.

FRACTURE FEMUR Treat surgically. Immobilization, for example, in hip spica cast, is associated with residual deformity, in particular coxa vara, due to intrinsic instability of the fracture and incomplete healing. For the proximal femur, improved alignment with surgical fixation may reduce complications of fracture such as malunion and osteonecrosis.

Surgical treatment may be divided into cases.

PERCUTANEOUS WITHOUT FIXATION This began as injection of steroid (Scaglietti), for its angiostatic and fibroblastic inhibitory effects. The method has evolved in multiple directions such that there is no consensus on best practice. It is preferred for the upper limb and lower risk lower limb lesions.

- The cyst is drained. If it is solid, reconsider diagnosis and perform an incisional biopsy.
- A cystogramme determines whether the cyst is uni- or multilocular. If the former, inject with steroid or other adjuvant. Bone marrow aspirate may bring mesenchymal stem cells that will promote bone ingrowth and healing. Calcitonin inhibits osteoclasts. Calcium sulfate cement is osteoconductive. Proprietary fibrosing agents have been promoted.
- If the latter, break up septæ to form a unilocular cyst. In the process, perforate the cyst to create channels of communication with the medulla, based upon the rationale that altered hæmodynamics with venous obstruction may be a causative factor, and to allow access to the cyst by bone stem cells.
- Repeat for recurrence.

OPEN WITH FIXATION This is indicated for high-risk lesions, such as proximal femur [D], or where open access is simple, for example, calcaneus.

- Create an ovoid window to avoid stress concentration at an angle. The cyst may dictate location of this at the eroded cortex.
- Débride the wall to remove all cells, manually or with power.
- Consider adjuvant intralesional therapy to kill residual cells, for example, liquid nitrogen (freezing), phenol (chemical), argon laser (coagulation), or hydrogen peroxide. For liquid nitrogen, leave in cavity until it evaporates; for other chemicals, let sit for 2 to 3 minutes. Cycle thrice. Reduce application hazard by controlling the agent within the osseous cavity in order to minimize injury to surrounding soft tissue. These augment but do not substitute for complete débridement.
- Pack the cyst with graft, allogenous or autogenous, or with a substitute. There are no robust data suggesting anything is better than bone, and allogenous bone avoids the morbidity of harvesting bone, in particular because much may be needed to fully fill a large cyst.
- If the bone is stable, apply a cast. If internal fixation is indicated, for example, proximal femur, medullary implants will load share and thereby be more durable in the event of recurrence. In the immature child, elastic medullary nails may be inserted antegradely or retrogradely. They provide stability even in proximal lesions because they may be anchored in the unaffected and hard proximal epiphysis: no physeal arrest will occur given their smooth surface and small fractional cross-sectional area [E].

Complications While bone cyst is a benign or "good" tumor, it is a "bad–good" tumor because outcomes can be vexing.

- Recurrence. Some factors cannot be controlled, such as abutment against a physis. The principal factor that is controllable is débridement; hence the recommendation to use a burr, to be methodical, to proceed until healthy bleeding bone, and to leave only periosteum in places (so long as the bone is not unreasonably destabilized or resected).
- Growth disturbance. This may be iatrogenic or related to activity of cyst. The former may be minimized by avoiding physis during operation. The latter is a reflection of duration and aggressiveness of cyst.
- Malunion. This is most common in the proximal femur. Likelihood increases with closed management.

Aneurysmal Bone Cyst

As the name implies, this is vascular and expansile. Cause is unknown, although vascular malformation is most subject to speculation. Evaluation and management principles overlap with unicameral cyst, with key distinctions. Aneurysmal cyst is more aggressive:

- Location. 1/4 arise in the axial skeleton, including posterior elements of the spine and the periacetabular region of the pelvis [F]. Consequences are greater morbidity of disease, for example, neural compromise, and of treatment, including more invasive dissection and more complex reconstruction.
- Recurrence. Correct surgical technique has reduced a formerly universal rate. Recurrence occurs within 2 years of operation, although children must be followed until maturity.
- Association with other tumors, including giant cell and osteosarcoma, in which it may represent the cystic component of a primary tumor.

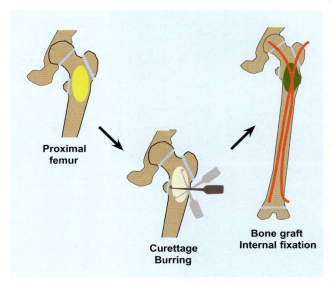

D Open treatment of bone cyst The cyst is débrided and bone grafted (*green*), after which the femur is stabilized with elastic medullary nails (*red*).

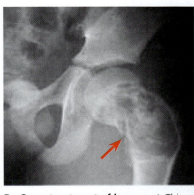 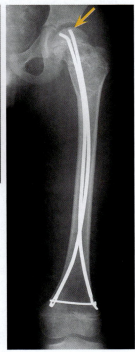

E Open treatment of bone cyst This cyst fractured (*red*). Retrograde elastic nailing was stable by purchase in the hard, unaffected proximal epiphysis (*orange*).

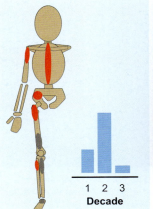 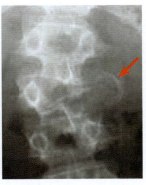

F Distribution of aneurysmal cyst The axial skeleton, including the spine (*red*) and the pelvis (*white*), makes advanced imaging and open treatment more typical.

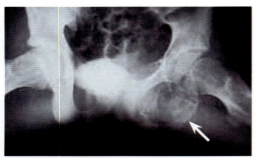

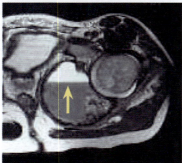

G Aneurysmal cyst of the pelvis The expansile and otherwise aggressive appearance on röntgenogramme led to MRI, which shows a characteristic blood–fluid level (*yellow*).

Evaluation On röntgenogramme, it is eccentrically expansile, lytic, and multiloculated, giving a "soap-bubble" appearance. The thin margin has been likened to an "eggshell." The radiographic appearance may raise concern and prompt further imaging. Scintigramme may show a "halo" of increased uptake surrounding a central cold region. MRI will show blood–fluid levels [G] and define soft tissue extension.

Management This tends to be open and has the additional considerations:

- Preoperative angiography and selective embolization before surgical treatment of large lesions, in particular in the pelvis, will decrease hæmorrhage and may shrink the lesion to decrease recurrence where complete resection is unrealistic.
- Entry into a cyst will return blood. Include soft tissue within, or the lining of, the cyst for biopsy, which will show proliferative fibroblasts, spindle cells, osteoid, and multinucleated giant cells.
- Break up all septæ to define the entire cyst wall, which may be interrupted.
- Consider an *en bloc* resection with reconstruction where feasible to reduce recurrence.
- In the spine, excision may result in instability necessitating reconstruction, including bone grafting, fusion, and internal fixation.

BENIGN FIBROUS TUMORS

Nonosteogenic Fibroma

Originally reported as a cyst of bone (Phemister), this was named separately as nonosteogenic (Jaffe) and nonossifying fibroma. The appellation fibrous cortical defect is reserved for small lesions confined to the cortex without medullary extension.

This is the most common benign lesion of bone in children, peaking in adolescence [A]. Cause in unknown, although it has been related to physis and traction by tendon or ligament, for example, at origin of the gastrocnemius from the distal femur.

Evaluation Most are incidental findings on röntgenogrammes obtained for injury followed by pain.

RÖNTGENOGRAMME The lesion is metaphyseal, eccentric, geographic with a "scalloped" margin, and lytic with one or more loculations [A]. A large lesion may show a cortical breach.

SCINTIGRAMME This is indicated when there is uncertainty whether the lesion is a source of pain, suggesting structural failure, or when the lesion risks morbid fracture, such as in the proximal femur or >50% diameter of the bone. Fracture will demonstrate increased signal.

Management The natural history is spontaneous resolution by maturity. Observe incidental findings and follow clinically based upon symptoms. For fracture through a lesion, immobilize and observe for (partial) healing. If the fracture cannot be immobilized effectively, or for lesions with significant risk of morbid fracture, treat like a unicameral cyst (*q.v.*).

Fibrous Dysplasia

Neoplastic fibrosis replaces and weakens bone, causing microfractures that hurt and lead to progressive deformity. It may arise in any bone, though the ribs and the proximal femur [B], as well as maxilla, are distinctive sites. Two types are distinguished: monostotic (80%) or polyostotic. The latter subtype is more severe and occurs in conjunction with café au lait spots and precocious puberty as part of McCune-Albright syndrome (*cf.* Syndromes chapter) and in conjunction with soft tissue myxomata in Mazabraud syndrome. Polyostotic fibrous dysplasia is caused by an activating gain of function mutation in the GNAS1 gene located on chromosome 20q13.2. This results in abnormal synthesis of both organic and inorganic components of the extracellular matrix, thereby compromising the structural integrity of bone.

Evaluation Pain is the most common presentation. Other signs include deformity and limb length discrepancy.

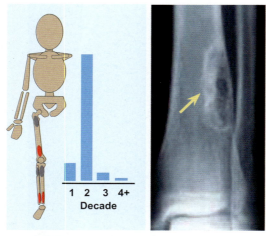

A Nonosteogenic fibroma It peaks in adolescence and commonly affects the tibia. It is eccentric, loculated with a scalloped margin (*yellow*).

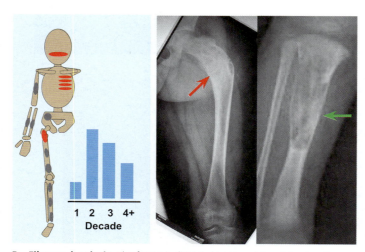

B Fibrous dysplasia The femur is distorted to resemble a "shepherd's crook" (*red*). Note the thick periosteal healing response. Appearance may be so varied, including provoking concern (*green*), that further imaging often is necessary.

IMAGING This tumor is one of the grand mimics. The classic appearance on röntgenogramme is the "shepherd's crook" deformity of the femur, which is slowly eroded and deformed progressively by subclinical microfractures. At the other extreme is the simple geographic lucent lesion, surrounded by a "rind" of sclerotic bone and producing no deformity. Opacity, resembling "ground glass," correlates with woven bone, with fibrous tissue being the principal tissue in lucent lesions.

The radiographic range is so broad that it often prompts further imaging. Scintigramme surveys the skeleton and may expose a fracture. CT is useful for complex lesions, in particular in the spine and craniofacial skeleton. MRI distinguishes this from malignancy and defines the extent of disease in bone and soft tissue.

Management

MEDICAL Bisphosphonates alleviate pain in polyostotic disease.

SURGICAL At biopsy, there is yellow-gray, gritty fibrous tissue with occasional cartilage foci forming a circumscribed mass that readily falls away from surrounding bone. Microscopically, a fibrous stroma is punctuated by "Chinese characters" or an "alphabet soup" of immature woven bone populated by some osteoblasts but many osteoclasts.

Indications for operation follow general principles, including pain, which is evidence of bone instability from microfracture, deformity interfering with function, or clinical fracture. Educate parents that operation may be the first stage before definitive management at maturity, when lesions stabilize. Medullary fixation is preferable because lesions progress during childhood and because recurrence is high. Follow meticulous technique for the cavity remaining after removal of the mass (*cf.* Cyst). Allograft bone will be resorbed partially by the neoplastic process.

Desmoid Tumor

Greek δεσμος = Latin *fibra*, which describes a tumor of fibrous tissue. It also is known as fibromatosis, reflecting an infiltrative and locally aggressive nature. This is a broad spectrum that encompasses Dupuytren contracture of the hand and Ledderhose disease of the foot.

Evaluation Firm smooth mass anchored to deep fascia but sparing overlying skin. In the limbs, 1/4 of cases are bilateral. An extraintestinal abdominal form of the disease affects 10% of patients with familial adenomatous polyposis (Gardner syndrome): both disorders are caused by mutation in the adenomatous polyposis coli gene on 5q22.2. Desmoid tumor may represent an error in response to injury, including a surgical incision. MRI demonstrates the nongeographic nature of the tumor and aids determination of extent of soft tissue infiltration. Biopsy shows a dense collagen matrix populated by myofibroblasts expressing platelet-derived growth factor-β proto-oncogene, which encodes the mitogenic β-chain of PDGF-B.

Management Because it is infiltrative and recurrence is high, nonoperative management is preferable. Because the injury of surgery may aggravate the tumor, plan to perform a wide excisional biopsy and confirm clear margins by intraoperative frozen section. Recurrence is high, and secondary operation is difficult in the setting of iatrogenic scarring. Collagenase, cryotherapy, and steroid injection may be helpful adjuncts. Radiation therapy for a benign condition raises concerns of physeal arrest and tumorigenesis in a child.

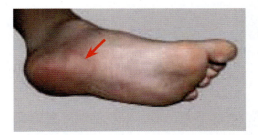

C Plantar fibromatosis Firm smooth mass associated with plantar aponeurosis.

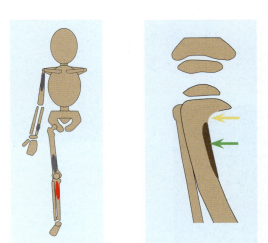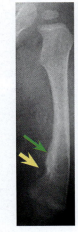

D Focal fibrocartilagenous dysplasia A lucent corticometaphyseal lesion (*yellow*) adjacent to the insertion of pes anserinus or hip adductors is interposed between proximal physis and a region of sclerotic reactive bone (*green*).

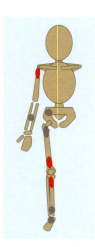

A Distribution of solitary osteochondroma The knee and proximal arm are most commonly affected. Multiple hereditary exostosis, which is more akin to a skeletal dysplasia, may affect the entire skeleton, except for relative sparing of the spine.

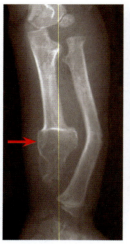
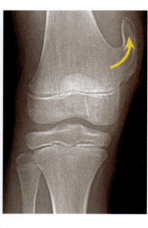

B Röntgenogramme of osteochondroma In multiple hereditary exostosis, the lesions deform affected bones and do not stand out alone (*red*). The presentation of solitary osteochondromata is classic, either sessile or pedunculated (*yellow*).

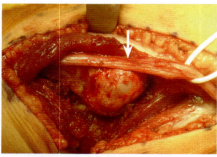
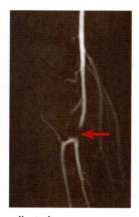
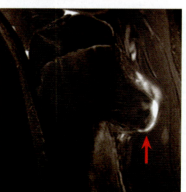

C Complicated osteochondroma Proximal fibula lesion may impinge upon the common fibular nerve, held by a silastic loop (*white*). A lesion arising from the posterior proximal tibia may obstruct the popliteal artery, before it bifurcates (*red*).

Focal Fibrocartilaginous Dysplasia

The name (Bell) reflects the tissue of which the tumor is composed. Cause is unknown. Trauma, including abnormal periosteal traction, for example, by pes anserinus at the proximal tibia or hip adductors at the distal femur, has been proposed.

Evaluation Onset is infancy in the lower limb and later in childhood for upper limb lesions. The most affected is the tibia [D]. It may be mistaken for pseudarthrosis of the tibia, which is bowed with a region of lucency, representing the lesion, adjacent to sclerosis produced by the osseous reaction [D].

Management Spontaneous resolution is possible, representing perhaps rupture of the periosteal tether. The rarity of the condition makes nonoperative guidelines, for example, bracing, impossible. Tibial lesions correct most predictably, in particular if deformity is <25 degrees. Persistent significant deformity, for example, genu varum, is treated with osteotomy and lengthening as indicated.

In the forearm, deformity and growth retardation may have deleterious effects on the uninvolved bone, such as ulnar tethering of the radius with radiocapitular instability. Early excision may allow restoration of growth and mitigate dysfunction.

BENIGN CARTILAGE TUMORS

Osteochondroma

The name describes a stem of "bone" capped by "cartilage." This also is known as exostosis, after the appearance of bone growing "away" from the main body. It is distinguished as such under the nail (*cf.* Foot chapter). It may arise from any bone [A]. Like fibrous dysplasia, osteochondroma may be solitary or multiple. The latter is a skeletal dysplasia having a genetic basis that is deforming [B] and associated with considerable morbidity, including malignant potential (*cf.* Syndromes chapter). Injury to the peripheral physis, followed by slow growth away with retention of physeal cartilage as a cap, may explain the pathogenesis.

Evaluation Pain and a mass are typical of the presentation. Prominence may take the mass vulnerable to physical trauma. The mass may hurt or limit motion if it interferes with muscle movement. In a critical location, or if sufficiently large, an osteochondroma may produce neurovascular compromise [C].

IMAGING Röntgenogrammes usually suffice. Solitary osteochondroma may be sessile, characterized by a smooth rounded lesion with a wide "base," or pedunculated, which is narrow and elongated like a "stalk" or finger [B]. It arises juxtaphyseal out of the metaphysis, from which it is directed and grows away. Medullary and cortical continuity between the main bone and osteochondroma gives rise to the description "aclasis" (Greek κλαω: "to break, interrupt"). For complex lesions in complex locations, MRI will show the structure of the lesion and the surrounding structures impacted by it to aid operative planning. Integrated PET/CT aids in identifying conversion of osteochondroma to chondrosarcoma in the multiple form of the disease.

Management Observe osteochondromata unless they significantly disturb a patient: there is no rôle for prophylactic removal. The natural history is unpredictable growth during childhood and stabilization after maturity. Follow clinically for unacceptable symptoms or signs. Indications for operation are pain; significant prominence, for example, at the medial condyle of the tibia, which is exposed during sports and where there is thin soft tissue coverage; dysfunction such as of joint or muscle; and neurovascular compromise.

Enchondroma

The name suggests a tumor of cartilage "inside" a long bone (medulla). However, it may occur in or on the cortex. It shows a predilection for the appendicular skeleton, where half occur in the hands and feet [D]. The tumor may be solitary or multiple (*cf.* Syndromes chapter), without (Ollier) or with hæmangiomata (Maffucci). Pathogenesis is an ectopic remnant of physeal cartilage. Macroscopically, lobules give the blue-gray hue of cartilage punctuated by yellow-white mineralized foci. Immunohistochemistry shows S100-positive chondrocytes.

Evaluation Solitary lesions typically are incidental findings. Pain may be a presenting sign of fracture. Lower limb length discrepancy may result, in particular for lesions about the knee.

Röntgenogramme Lytic, lobulated lesion with scalloped margins and speckled mineralization is a manifestation of endochondral ossification that accompanies these tumors.

Management For intractable pain, débride the cavity and bone graft. Add fixation as indicated. Lengthen a short limb, with deformity correction as indicated. Recurrence is rare (<5%).

Chondromyxoid Fibroma

The tumor is composed of lobular myxoid and chondroid tissue with occasional multinucleated giant cells and foci of calcification. It has been linked to mutation on 6q, in the region that includes the gene encoding the α-1 chain of collagen type XII.

Evaluation The majority (>80%) occur in long bones in the lower limb, most commonly about the knee. The tumor is associated with secondary aneurysmal bone cyst.

Röntgenogramme The eccentric, geographic, lytic, ovoid metaphyseal lesion looks like a "bite" out of the cortex [E]. It may extend to, but never is solely in, the epiphysis.

Management Manage according to general principles for hole in bone. *En bloc* resection, feasible for an eccentric lesion, reduces recurrence (25%). Reports of malignant transformation probably represent misdiagnosis of chondrosarcoma.

Chondroblastoma

This tumor is distinguished by the epiphysis or apophysis as the primary site [F]. It also is known as Codman tumor, after the original report of "chondromatous giant cell tumors" in the proximal humerus.

Evaluation Pain may be associated with joint swelling for epiphysial lesions. Absence of systemic involvement excludes other disease. Microscopically, chondroblastoma resembles giant cell tumor of the tendon sheath and pigmented villonodular synovitis. Chondroblastoma is S100 and vimentin positive. Metastasis has been reported, calling into question the appellation "benign" or the initial diagnosis.

Röntgenogramme The lesion is geographic, lytic, solely epiphysial, or apophyseal, with erosion into metaphysis.

Management Percutaneous radiofrequency ablation may be effective for small lesions and avoids articular dissection. Large lesions are at risk for articular collapse, which is an indication for open débridement and bone grafting. For the epiphysis, intralesional adjuvant risks injury to the physis and articular surface, which additionally limits surgical access on either side of the tumor. Epiphysial lesions have poorer outcomes due to incomplete excision, which leads to a high recurrence rate (30%), as well as to physeal and articular injury, which may be due to disease or iatrogenicity.

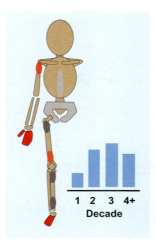
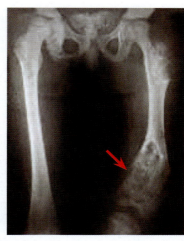

D Enchondroma The hands and feet are most affected. In the distal femur, growth disturbance may result in shortening and deformity (*red*).

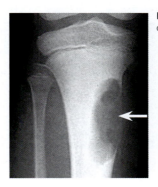

E Chondromyxoid fibroma A "bite" out of the cortex (*white*).

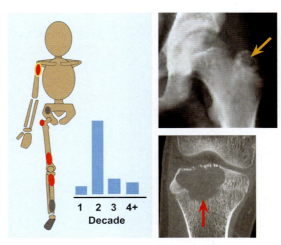

F Chondroblastoma The original report was in the proximal humerus. The lesion may be apophyseal, for example, trochanter major (*orange*), in addition to being epiphysial (*red*). Epiphysial lesions undermine the articular surface and may erode through the physis into the metaphysis.

	Osteoid Osteoma	Osteoblastoma
Size	≤ 2 cm	
Location	90% long bone	1/3 spine: 1/3 cervical 1/3 thoracic 1/3 lumbar
Symptoms	Intense, night pain	Less pain Less responsive to NSAIA
Sign	Swelling	Deformity

A Differences between osteoid osteoma and osteoblastoma NSAIA: nonsteroidal anti-inflammatory agent.

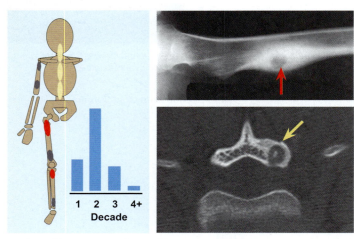

B Osteoid osteoma and osteoblastoma Osteoid osteoma most frequently occurs in the femur (*red*). The posterior elements of the vertebrae are the exclusive domain of osteoblastoma (*yellow*).

Letterer-Siwe	Hand–Schüller–Christian	Eosinophilic granuloma
Multifocal multisystem	Multifocal unisystem	Unifocal
Infant Diffuse disease Low survival	1st decade Triad: Exophthalmos Diabetes insipidus Osteolysis (skull)	Skeletal only Monostotic Polyostotic

C Forms of Langerhans cell histiocytosis.

BENIGN BONE TUMORS

Osteoid Osteoma and Osteoblastoma

Osteoid osteoma is a benign, bone-producing, highly vascular tumor that induces an intense reaction and a characteristic pain pattern. Several features distinguish this from osteoblastoma [A].

Evaluation The clinical course of osteoid osteoma consists of an acute phase lasting 1 to 3 years followed by a recovery phase characterized by healing of the lesion with maturity. Pain is intense, focal, and worst at night. Pain results from secretion by the central nidus (Latin "nest") of prostaglandins (in particular E2 and I2 or prostacyclin), inflammatory mediators that elicit a hypervascular response similar to that of injury. Pain is relieved by nonsteroidal anti-inflammatory agents, which block prostaglandin synthesis and are used as diagnostic and therapeutic tools. Osteoblastoma in the thoracolumbar spine presents with pain often associated with scoliosis (75%). In the cervical spine, it is one cause of torticollis.

IMAGING Röntgenogrammes show dense eccentric sclerosis without or with a radiolucent center. There may be surrounding osteopenia as a sign of disuse. Scintigramme shows focal increased uptake with 100% sensitivity, including early in cases when röntgenogrammes are negative, thereby accelerating diagnosis. CT reveals that the sclerosis forms an envelope surrounding a central nidus, likened to a "target." In the spine, osteoblastoma affects the posterior elements, with sparing of the vertebral bodies. CT is essential to operative treatment, localizing lesions for complete resection and demonstrating extent of disease for planning of reconstruction. MRI tracks CT, but the inflammatory nature of the tumor reduces accuracy.

DIFFERENTIAL DIAGNOSIS Signs such as swelling in a subcutaneous bone, for example, tibia, as well as the nidus surrounded by a sclerotic rim, raise the specter of infection. The periosteal reaction may be mistaken for stress fracture. Increased uptake in posterior elements of the spine on scintigramme raises the question of spondylolysis. The two may be distinguished by the fact that osteoblastoma will show uptake in the immediate or flow phase (seconds) when increased signal in spondylolysis is delayed until the second or blood pool phase (minutes). A herniated intervertebral disc may be suspected in an adolescent with sudden-onset back pain and deformity. The length and breadth of the differential list account for a characteristic delay in diagnosis (1 to 3 years).

Management The natural history is resolution with maturity in most children.

MEDICAL Nonsteroidal anti-inflammatory agents help but rarely are sufficient due to the intensity and duration of pain.

PERCUTANEOUS The rationale is limitation of morbidity, including dissection and bone compromise, which ease convalescence and reduce complications such as fracture. CT guides localization. Options include radiofrequency or laser coagulative (50°C to 90°C) necrosis. Repeat cycles for lesions >1 cm. The principal disadvantage is lack of immediate confirmation of tumor removal. A hybrid approach is percutaneous cannulated drilling with CT guidance until complete resection. The disadvantages are drill control and fracture risk.

OPEN EXCISION This may be intralesional débridement, with identification of the nidus, without or with bone grafting, or *en bloc* excision for noncritical bone to reduce recurrence. The nidus appears deep red, reflecting a microscopic architecture of osteoid within a highly vascular stroma. Intraoperative CT with navigation aids localization and resection and confirms completeness. Add fixation as indicated for stability. Advantages of open treatment are direct visualization to ensure sufficient resection, no size limitation, and ability to stabilize a critical site. Recurrence correlates inversely with aggressiveness of resection.

Spontaneous resolution of spine deformity after excision is more likely in younger patients with short duration of disease (<1 year).

Overall recurrence or persistence of pain regardless of percutaneous or open method is 10%.

Eosinophilic Granuloma

This is the most benign form of Langerhans cell histiocytosis [A], limited to the skeleton, most often as a solitary lesion. Langerhans cells are antigen-presenting immune cells, distinguished by Birbeck granules and populating skin and mucosa. Like fibrous dysplasia, eosinophilic granuloma imitates other disease. The two tumors also share a predilection for the craniofacial skeleton and ribs [B].

Evaluation Onset peaks in infancy. Pain may be associated with low-grade fever, which, together with elevated inflammatory markers and the radiographic appearance, makes differentiation from infection difficult. Skull lesions may resemble disorders of the central nervous system, such as arachnoid granulation (Pacchioni).

One-sixth of cases involve the spine, of which 1/2 have multilevel disease, 1/3 affect the cervical spine, and 1/6 will be deforming. Back pain is a universal finding. Deformity and soft tissue mass may encroach upon vertebral canal and intervertebral foramina to compromise the neural elements.

RÖNTGENOGRAMME Expansile, lytic lesions without or with periosteal reaction suggest aggressive destruction and simulate malignancy. Skull lesions may show "hole in hole" due to asymmetric erosion of the inner and outer tables. *Vertebra plana* (Calvé disease) describes "flattening" of the body, which collapses from a rectangle to a wedge or a line in anteroposterior and lateral projections. Image the entire spine.

OTHER IMAGING Scintigramme, which surveys the skeleton for polyostotic disease, may be cold in 1/3 of cases. CT provides best osseous detail, which is of particular importance for skull and spine lesions. MRI, enhanced with gadolinium, shows an associated soft tissue component.

Management While skull involvement and *vertebra plana* focus the differential, biopsy often is necessary for confidence in the diagnosis. Long bone lesions are treated according to principles of hole in bone (*cf.* Cyst). Operative indications for spine lesions are neural compromise and evidence of instability, including progressive deformity. Otherwise, support with a spinal orthotic primarily to control pain, with the secondary goal to protect alignment. The majority of cases (>90%) reconstitute without significant residual deformity. There is no consensus on chemotherapy. Do not irradiate children for this condition.

Giant Cell Tumors

While it peaks around the age of 30, 10% occur in children. 50% occur in the knee; it also has a predilection for the sacrum [F]. Measures of the aggressiveness of this benign tumor include the following:

- It traverses the physis between metaphysis and epiphysis, eroding to the articular surface.
- 3% metastasize to the lungs.
- 25% fracture.
- 25% recur.

It is more often solitary than polyostotic, which behaves more aggressively. It is characterized by giant cells with multiple central nuclei as opposed to the peripheral nuclei of Langerhans cells.

Evaluation Patients present with pain and swelling.

RÖNTGENOGRAMME Expansile and lytic lesion, erosive of bone yet eliciting little reaction, with soft tissue component. MRI aids determination of the extent of bone involvement and soft tissue extension.

Management Treat according to principles of hole in bone (*cf.* Cyst). Complications relate to involvement of the physis and erosion of subchondral bone, which lead to growth disturbance and arthritis. As for aneurysmal cyst and other high recurrence benign tumors, *en bloc* resection is preferable; however, this may not be feasible given proximity to joint. Like chondroblastoma, intralesional adjuvant risks iatrogenic injury to the physis and articular surface.

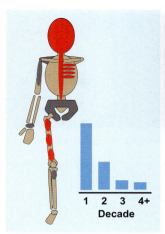

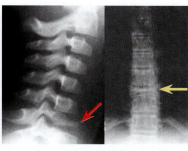

D Eosinophilic granuloma Vertebra plana may be seen on lateral projection in the cervical spine (*red*) and anteroposterior projection in the thoracic spine (*yellow*). Despite collapse, there is neither kyphosis nor scoliosis.

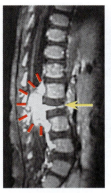

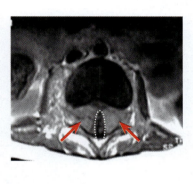

E Eosinophilic granuloma of the spine This lesion has eroded the vertebral body (*yellow*) and is associated with a large soft tissue mass (*red*), which occupies most of the spinal canal (*red*). The neural elements are outlined in white dots.

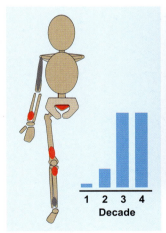

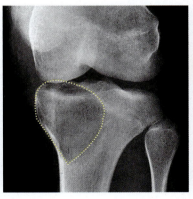

F Giant cell tumor It may extend between metaphysis and epiphysis, eroding the physis and subchondral bone (*yellow*).

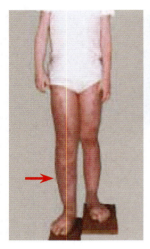

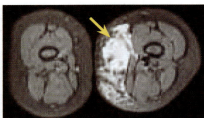

A   Hæmangioma This may represent an isolated tumor (*yellow*) or a vascular anomaly, such as in Klippel-Trénaunay-Weber syndrome (*red*).

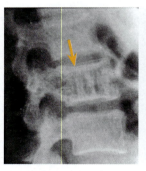

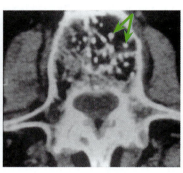

B   Hæmangioma of bone Radiodense longitudinal stripes reflecting osseous deposition along vascular channels give the appearance of a "jailhouse" or "corduroy" (*orange*) and appear as "polka dots" in transverse plane on CT (*green*). These findings contrast with thicker transverse striations parallel to end plates, as seen in the rachitic spine, which are likened to a "rugger jersey."

OTHER BENIGN TUMORS

Hæmangioma

Hæmangioma may be isolated, when it is regarded as a tumor, or part of a systemic condition, where it is an anomaly [A]. The tumors may be capillary, involving small vessels, or cavernous, involving large vessels. They may be distinguished according to tissue distribution.

Muscular   Most tumors occur in the lower limb, the majority in the thigh. Unlike vascular anomaly syndromes, skin is unaffected. Presentation includes pain without or with swelling, which may increase with dependent position of the limb or with activity. Röntgenogrammes show soft tissue swelling. MRI with gadolinium enhancement shows serpentine infiltration of muscle in early disease.

The natural history is spontaneous involution. Indications for surgical removal are unacceptable pain or dysfunction. Preoperative embolization may reduce hæmorrhage. Recurrence is associated with lesions having less defined margins and those that are in critical locations, for example, forearm, where wide margins may impair function.

Synovial   This may affect joint (mostly knee) or tendon sheath. Articular involvement is characterized by pain, hæmarthrosis, stiffness, and mechanical symptoms. Effusion should serve as an alert for further workup. Mechanical symptoms have been attributed to more innocent causes of internal derangement, thereby delaying diagnosis.

Treat arthroscopically for central lesions, or open for a peripheral lesion, where any capsule may be identified for a complete extralesional excision.

Osseous   Two-thirds occur in the craniofacial skeleton and spine [B], where the tumor affects the anterior column. Hæmangioma is the most common benign tumor of the vertebrae (10% of autopsies). Tumor may involve a single bone, adjacent bones, or separate sites. Osseous hæmangioma also includes massive osteolytic hæmangiomatosis (Gorham), where increased blood supply is stimulatory of osteoclasts more than osteoblasts, tipping the normal state toward resorption.

Most are asymptomatic. Consider embolization for pain that is not alleviated by conservative methods. Vertebroplasty alleviates pain and stabilizes deformity. Spinal canal decompression and reconstruction are indicated for neural compromise.

Pigmented Villonodular Synovitis

This disorder affects synovial joints, most frequently the knee, and tendon sheaths, most frequently in the hand, where it is known as giant cell tumor of the tendon sheath. Fusion transcripts of the gene encoding α-1 chain of collagen type VI and colony-stimulating factor-1 have been found, although causation has not been established.

Evaluation   Patients present with pain, swelling, and stiffness. There are two types: diffuse and focal. Röntgenogrammes show shadow of soft tissue swelling and may show saucerized erosions on both sides of the joint in advanced disease. MRI with gadolinium enhancement reveals hyperplastic and hypervascular synovial membrane, hæmosiderin deposition, and hæmorrhagic effusion. Histologic analysis shows synovial cell proliferation and multinucleated giant cells.

Management   Definitive treatment consists of complete synovectomy, arthroscopically or open, and with radiation if necessary. The articular location and infiltrative nature of this tumor raises recurrence.

MALIGNANT SOFT TISSUE TUMORS

These tumors account for about 7% of malignant tumors of childhood. They may be divided into five general categories [A].

Rhabdomyosarcoma

This is a sarcoma of the skeletal muscle and constitutes more than half of malignant soft tissue tumors in children. It is the most common pædiatric soft tissue sarcoma [B].

Evaluation Two-thirds occur in the first decade. Blacks and Asians are affected less commonly than Whites. Rhabdomyosarcoma may occur anywhere, and presentation varies accordingly [C]. One-quarter occur in the head and neck and 1/4 in the limbs. In a limb, it typically manifests as a firm, painless mass, without or with nodal involvement. Nodal extension is predictive of metastasis. By contrast with muscle, osseous lesions are painful. In the orbit, it produces proptosis. In the bladder or prostate, it produces urinary tract obstruction or hæmaturia, which may be gross or detected by urinalysis. In the chest, abdomen, or pelvis, it may grow large before manifestation.

There are 2 principal histologic types of rhabdomyosarcoma: embryonal (80%) and alveolar (20%), which have 2/3 the survival rate. Tumors arising in sites other than the limbs typically are embryonal, whereas limb tumors are alveolar, hence the poorer prognosis.

Embryonal rhabdomyosarcoma may be caused by somatic mutation in the SLC22A18 gene on chromosome 11p15.5, resulting in loss of heterozygosity of a tumor suppressor gene. Alveolar rhabdomyosarcoma results from fusion of the PAX3 gene on chromosome 2 with the FKHR gene on chromosome 13 as a result of a translocation t(2;13), or from fusion of the PAX7 gene on chromosome 1 with the FKHR gene as a result of a translocation t(1;13). Such translocations produce hybrid molecules that serve as potent transcription activators, deinhibiting myoblast proliferation. These mutations may be detected by fluorescent *in situ* hybridization (FISH) and reverse transcriptase–polymerase chain reaction (RT-PCR) testing of a biopsy specimen.

Management Survival for solitary lesions is >70%, which declines to the historical level <30% for metastatic disease. Operative treatment includes resection with a wide margin (>2 cm) and sampling of local lymph nodes.

Synovial Sarcoma

This occurs most frequently in the lower limbs, around the knee. It is the most common malignant soft tissue tumor of the foot. It is caused by the chromosomal translocation t(X;18)(p11;q11), leading to fusion of the SYT gene (18) with the SSX gene (X). The fusion proteins may function as aberrant transcriptional regulators to activate proto-oncogenes or inhibit tumor suppressor genes.

Evaluation Delay in diagnosis is characteristic, often >12 months. This is due to varied presentation, including latency, which gives the impression of benignity but which may be followed by rapid growth. The tumor is associated with deep fascia, manifesting as a deep, tender mass. Intralesional calcification ("snowstorm") on röntgenogramme is pathognomonic though infrequent. MRI is the imaging modality of choice for diagnosis and surgical staging. Cytogenic analysis (FISH, RT-PCR) confirms diagnosis.

Several factors influence survival [C].

Management Adjuvant monoclonal antibody against a cell surface receptor (FZD10) unique to synovial cell sarcoma cells may improve outcomes, including need for amputation and survival.

Wide resection (2-cm margin) limits recurrence. Location in the knee may involve popliteal artery and tibial nerve, which may preclude limb salvage.

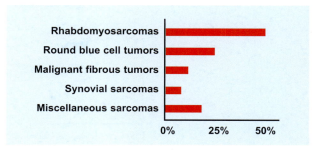

A Types of soft tissue sarcomas.

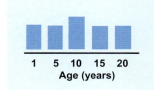

B Rhabdomyosarcoma age distribution 2/3 occur in the first decade.

Size	Histology		Location
< 5cm	Biphasic:	synovial cells in glandular architecture	Distal limb
5-10 cm	Monophasic:	spindle + round cells	Proximal limb
> 10 cm	Poorly differentiated		Central

C Prognosis for synovial cell sarcoma For good prognostic factors (*green*), survival rate is >80%. This declines to <20% for poor prognostic factors. Distal limb signifies hand and foot. Central location is the trunk, head, and neck.

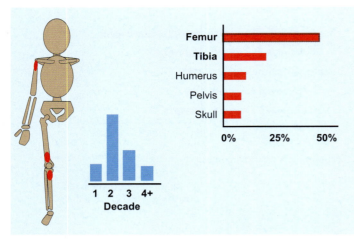

A   Geographic and age distributions of osteosarcoma Growth influences distribution, both geographic (knee) and temporal (adolescence).

Factor	Prognosis
Grade	Low: favorable
Location	Distal limb (best) - proximal limb - axial skeleton (worst)
Metastasis	Absence better than presence
Response to neo-adjuvant chemotherapy	Increasing tumor cell kill improves prognosis
Resectability	Complete primary resection improves prognosis
Alkaline phosphatase Lactate dehydrogenase	Elevation unfavorable
Clinical subtype	Parosteal and peri-osteal favorable
Relapse	Poor prognosis

B   Prognostic factors.

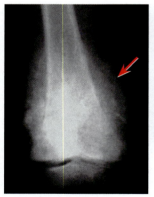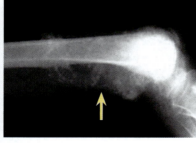

C   Radiographic appearance of osteosarcoma Osteogenesis look like a "sunburst" (red) or resemble "cotton wool" (yellow).

Estimated lower limb length discrepancy >8 cm in immature child
Poor response to neo-adjuvant chemotherapy
Tumor contamination beyond compartment, e.g., after biopsy or due to hæmatoma after morbid fracture
Major infection
Unresectable lesion, e.g., due to extensive soft tissue involvement, such as penetration of neurovascular structures.

D   Contraindications to limb salvage.

MALIGNANT BONE TUMORS

Osteosarcoma

Osteosarcoma is third in frequency to blood and brain cancers in childhood. It is the most common malignant tumor of bone. It is related to rapid growth, as evidenced by geographic distribution in the knee (more than half of cases) and the proximal humerus, as well as peak incidence during adolescence [A].

Loss of heterozygosity and tumor suppressor allelic inactivation at chromosome 3q13.31 have been found in osteosarcoma. A genetic predisposition is suggested by association of osteosarcoma with retinoblastoma (mutation in the RB1 gene on 13q14), Paget disease of bone (mutation in the TNFRSF11A gene on 18q22), Li-Fraumeni syndrome-1 (mutation in the TP53 gene on 17p13), Li-Fraumeni syndrome-2 (mutation in the CHEK2 gene on 22q12), and Rothmund-Thomson syndrome.

Evaluation Pain, limp, stiffness, inflammatory swelling, and focal mass are characteristic. Systemic presentation is uncharacteristic, except in metastasis. There is no gender or race predilection. Several factors are critical to prognosis [B].

LABORATORY Alkaline phosphatase elevation correlates with risk of metastasis. Elevation of lactate dehydrogenase bears a worse prognosis. Histologic analysis shows osteoid and cells that may be distinguished as osteoblastic, fibroblastic, chondroblastic, and telangiectatic, which contain loculi of blood. The tissue distinctions do not correlate with prognosis. Two clinical subtypes, parosteal, which is intracortical, and periosteal, which is low grade and encircles (Greek περι: "around") the bone, have a favorable prognosis.

RÖNTGENOGRAMME One-half of cases are blastic, including osteogenesis in a radiating "sunburst" or "cotton wool" pattern [C], 1/3 are lytic, and others are mixed. Repeated periosteal elevation and reaction results in lamellar bone deposition likened to "onion skin." The telangiectatic type may resemble aneurysmal bone cyst.

SCINTIGRAMME Survey the skeleton for metastasis, within both the same osseous compartment and extracompartmental.

CT CT of the chest is essential to staging. Of the site, it is essential to operative planning.

MRI This best visualizes medullary disease and soft tissue involvement.

PET This may detect disease missed by other modalities, predict response to chemotherapy, and aid in determination of response after treatment.

Management Neoadjuvant chemotherapy aids prognostication and improves surgical outcomes, including limb salvage, by shrinking the tumor. Osteosarcoma is radioresistant, leaving surgical as the only treatment for local control.

Operation for cure may include wide margins (> 5 cm); radical margins, defined as the entire osseous compartment from joint to joint; or amputation. Limb salvage is the first goal in a child, but is not always feasible [D]. For every patient, balance the functional benefits, including appearance, and the morbidity, physical and psychic, of limb salvage and reconstruction against early amputation and prosthetic fitting: there is no universal approach.

Ewing Sarcoma

Ewing sarcoma is part of a family of small, round, blue cell tumors that includes peripheral primitive neuroectodermal tumor and neuroepithelioma. The family shares the same reciprocal translocation of the EWS gene on chromosome 22q12 with various members of the ETS family of transcription factors on 11q24. The fusion protein is a target of current molecular treatment modalities (e.g., YK-4-279). Ewing sarcoma is the second most common malignant bone tumor of childhood. It may be osseous, medullary, or soft tissue.

Evaluation It peaks in the second decade [E]. In contrast with osteosarcoma, Ewing sarcoma occurs with equal frequency in flat bones, such as the pelvis, and long bones, where it may arise in the diaphysis. It also may arise in soft tissues. Whites are affected onefold more than blacks. Focal osseous symptoms and signs include pain, limp, stiffness, inflammatory swelling, and mass, while petechiae and other signs of blood dyscrasia are medullary manifestations and fever is systemic. Back pain may be spinal, retroperitoneal, or pelvic in origin. Most important determinants of prognosis are metastasis [F], followed by location (*cf.* Osteosarcoma).

LABORATORY Findings include abnormal blood cell count such as thrombocytopenia, and elevated inflammatory markers, including CRP and ESR. Histology shows characteristic small, round cells of which the glycogen-rich cytoplasm stains blue with hematoxylin and eosin. Immunohistochemical marker MIC2 antigen (CD99) stains the cell membrane. Cytogenetic studies of tissue specimen confirm the t(11;22) translocation.

RÖNTGENOGRAMME This is one of the diaphyseal lesions. It is permeative (wide zone of transition between disease and normal), destructive of bone, and eliciting a periosteal reaction.

MRI This tumor is characterized by a soft tissue mass, which is best visualized by MRI. MRI also reveals medullary extent.

PET This is sensitive for metastasis, though scintigramme and whole-body MRI may substitute.

Management Principles resemble those for osteosarcoma. A difference is the use of radiation therapy to augment surgery for local control of disease. A cost is radiation-induced sarcoma, in particular leukæmia.

Leukæmia

This is the most common cancer of childhood. The most common subtype is acute lymphoblastic.

Evaluation This peaks early in the first decade. Patients with chromosomal anomalies (e.g., trisomy 21) are at increased risk for leukæmia. 20% of children with leukæmia present with bone pain, of which the characteristic is a migratory pattern, and 10% present with a limp. An orthopædic surgeon or rheumatologist may be the first medical consultant. Keys to the diagnosis include physical evidence of systemic disease, such as fever, malaise, lymphadenopathy, hepatosplenomegaly, and signs of myelophthisis, such easy bruising and bleeding, infection, and pallor of mucous membranes.

LABORATORY Abnormal blood counts and peripheral smear, for example, leukocytosis (hence the name of the disease by Virchow), are diagnostic.

RÖNTGENOGRAMME "Leukæmic lines," transverse radiolucent metaphyseal bands, are rare though pathognomonic. More common is periosteal new bone formation in a background of disuse osteopenia and, in severe cases, geographic osteolysis.

Management The essential component for the surgeon is recognition. Bone marrow aspiration establishes the diagnosis.

Metastasis

The spine is third in frequency after the lung and liver as a destination for metastasis [G]. Most patients are symptomatic and half have multiple level involvement, hence the importance of survey imaging such as scintigramme or PET. Greater than 90% of lesions are vertebral or epidural, with <10% intradural. Most metastasis represents vascular seeding, including *via* Batson plexus, a network of valveless veins that drain the body cavities to the vertebral veins.

The tumor that most frequently metastasizes to bone is neuroblastoma [H]. This small, round, blue cell tumor has onset in infancy, is of sympathetic neural origin, may spontaneously regress to benign ganglioneuroma, and in more than half of cases presents with metastasis. 2/3 originate in the abdomen and pelvis; in the spine, 10% reach into the vertebral canal to encroach upon the neural elements.

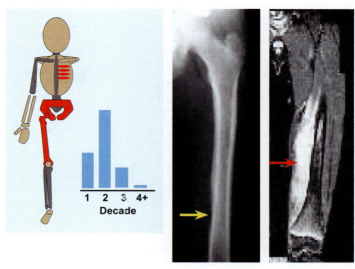

E Ewing sarcoma Half are axial and half are appendicular. Subtle radiographic change (*yellow*) despite a large soft tissue component (*red*).

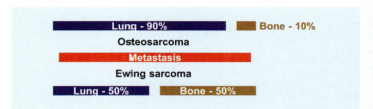

F Metastasis of osteosarcoma and Ewing sarcoma Metastasis at diagnosis halves the 5-year relapse-free survival.

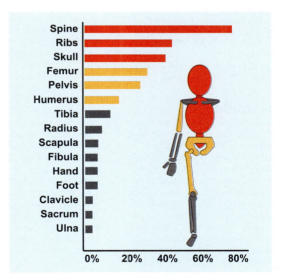

G Distribution of skeletal metastasis.

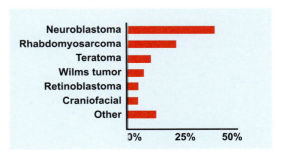

H Tumors metastasizing to bone.

BENIGN BONE TUMORS

Bergstrand H. Uber eine eigenartige, warscheinlich bisher nicht beschreibene osteoblastische Krankheit in den langen Knochen in der Hand und des Fusses. *Acta Radiol.* 11:596–613, 1930.

Campanacci M, Ruggieri P, Gasbarrini A, Ferraro A, Campanacci L. Osteoid osteoma. Direct visual identification and intralesional excision of the nidus with minimal removal of bone. *J. Bone Joint Surg. Br.* 81(5):814–820, 1999.

Canavese F, Soo BC, Chia SK, Krajbich JI. Surgical outcome in patients treated for hemangioma during infancy, childhood, and adolescence: a retrospective review of 44 consecutive patients. *J. Pediatr. Orthop.* 28(3):381–386, 2008.

Garg S, Mehta S, Dormans JP. Langerhans cell histiocytosis of the spine in children: long-term follow-up. *J. Bone Joint Surg. Am.* 86(8):1740–1750, 2004.

Geschickter CF, Keasbey LE. Tumors of blood vessels. *Am. J. Cancer* 23:568–591, 1935.

Green JA, Bellemore MC, Marsden FW. Embolization in the treatment of aneurysmal bone cysts. *J. Pediatr. Orthop.* 17(4):440–443, 1997.

Jaffe HL, Lichtenstein L. Solitary unicameral bone cyst with emphasis on the roentgen picture, the pathologic appearance and the pathogenesis. *Arch. Surg.* 44:1004–1025, 1942.

Kolodny A. Bone sarcoma: the primary malignant tumors of bone and the giant cell tumor. *Surg. Gynec. Obstet.* 44(1):214–241, 1927.

Mammano S, Candiotto S, Balsano M. Cast and brace treatment of eosinophilic granuloma of the spine: long-term follow-up. *J. Pediatr. Orthop.* 17(6):821–827, 1997.

Möller E, Mandahl N, Mertens F, Panagopoulos I. Molecular identification of COL6A3-CSF1 fusion transcripts in tenosynovial giant cell tumors. *Genes Chromosomes Cancer* 47(1):21–25, 2008.

Ramirez AR, Stanton RP. Aneurysmal bone cyst in 29 children. *J. Pediatr. Orthop.* 22(4):533–539, 2002.

Scaglietti O, Marchetti PG, Bartolozzi P. The effects of methylprednisolone acetate in the treatment of bone cysts. Results of three years follow-up. *J. Bone Joint Surg. Br.* 61(2):200–204, 1979.

Stanton RP, Abdel-Mota'al MM. Growth arrest resulting from unicameral bone cyst. *J. Pediatr. Orthop.* 18(2):198–201, 1998.

BENIGN FIBROUS TUMOR

Bell SN, Campbell PE, Cole WG, Menelaus MB. Tibia vara caused by focal fibrocartilaginous dysplasia: three case reports. *J. Bone Joint Surg. Br.* 67(5):780–784, 1985.

Bianco P, Riminucci M, Majolagbe A, Kuznetsov SA, Collins MT, Mankani MH, Corsi A, Bone HG, Wientroub S, Spiegel AM, Fisher LW, Robey PG. Mutations of the GNAS1 gene, stromal cell dysfunction, and osteomalacic changes in non-McCune-Albright fibrous dysplasia of bone. *J. Bone Miner. Res.* 15(1):120–128, 2000.

Couture J, Mitri A, Lagace R, Smits R, Berk T, Bouchard H-L, Fodde R, Alman B, Bapat B. A germline mutation at the extreme 3-prime end of the APC gene results in a severe desmoid phenotype and is associated with overexpression of beta-catenin in the desmoid tumor. *Clin. Genet.* 57(3):205–212, 2000.

Godette GA, O'Sullivan M, Menelaus MB. Plantar fibromatosis of the heel in children: a report of 14 cases. *J. Pediatr. Orthop.* 17(1):16–17, 1997.

Guille JT, Kumar SJ, MacEwen GD. Fibrous dysplasia of the proximal part of the femur. Long-term results of

curettage and bone-grafting and mechanical realignment. *J. Bone Joint Surg. Am.* 80(5):648–652, 1998.

Jaffe H, Liechtenstein L. Non-osteogenic fibroma of the bone. *Am. J. Pathol.* 18:205–221, 1942.

BENIGN CARTILAGE TUMORS

Chew DK, Menelaus MB, Richardson MD. Ollier's disease: varus angulation at the lower femur and its management. *J. Pediatr. Orthop.* 18(2):202–208, 1998.

Codman EA. Epiphyseal chondromatous giant cell tumors of the upper end of the humerus. *Surg. Gynecol. Obstet.* 52:543, 1931.

Dadfarnia T, Velagaleti GV, Carmichael KD, Eyzaguirre E, Eltorky MA, Qiu S. A t(1;9)(q10;q10) translocation with additional 6q23 and 9q22 rearrangements in a case of chondromyxoid fibroma. *Cancer Genet.* 204(12):666–670, 2011.

Jaffe HL, Lichtenstein L. Chondromyxoid fibroma of bone: a distinctive benign tumor likely to be mistaken especially for chondrosarcoma. *Arch. Path.* 19:541–551, 1943.

Konishi E, Nakashima Y, Iwasa Y, Nakao R, Yanagisawa A. Immunohistochemical analysis for Sox9 reveals the cartilaginous character of chondroblastoma and chondromyxoid fibroma of the bone. *Hum. Pathol.* 41(2):208–213, 2010.

Purandare NC, Rangarajan V, Agarwal M, Sharma AR, Shah S, Arora A, Paradar DS. Integrated PET/CT in evaluating sarcomatous transformation in osteochondromas. *Clin. Nucl. Med.* 34(6):350–354, 2009.

Yasuda T, Nishio J, Sumegi J, Kapels KM, Althof PA, Sawyer JR, Reith JD, Bridge JA. Aberrations of 6q13 mapped to the COL12A1 locus in chondromyxoid fibroma. *Mod. Pathol.* 22(11):1499–1506, 2009.

MALIGNANT SOFT TISSUE TUMORS

Barr FG, Galili N, Holick J, Biegel JA, Rovera G, Emanuel BS. Rearrangement of the PAX3 paired box gene in the paediatric solid tumour alveolar rhabdomyosarcoma. *Nat. Genet.* 3(2):113–117, 1993.

Deshmukh R, Mankin HJ, Singer S. Synovial sarcoma: the importance of size and location for survival. *Clin. Orthop.* 419:155–161, 2004.

Galili N, Davis RJ, Fredericks WJ, Mukhopadhyay1 S, Rauscher FJ III, Emanuel BS, Rovera G, Barr FG. Fusion of a fork head domain gene to PAX3 in the solid tumour alveolar rhabdomyosarcoma. *Nat. Genet.* 5(3):230–235, 1993.

Kawai A, Woodruff J, Healey JH. Brennan MF, Antonescu CR, Ladanyi M. SYT-SSX gene fusion as a determinant of morphology and prognosis in synovial sarcoma. *N. Engl. J. Med.* 338(3):153–160, 1998.

Shapiro DN, Sublett JE, Li B, Downing JR, Naeve CW. Fusion of PAX3 to a member of the forkhead family of transcription factors in human alveolar rhabdomyosarcoma. *Cancer Res.* 53(21):5108–5112, 1993.

Sharp R, Recio JA, Jhappan C, Otsuka T, Liu S, Yu Y, Liu W, Anver M, Navid F, Helman LJ, DePinho RA, Merlino G. Synergism between INK4a/ARF inactivation and aberrant HGF/SF signaling in rhabdomyosarcomagenesis. *Nat. Med.* 8(11):1276–1280, 2002.

Stout AP. Rhabdomyosarcoma of the skeletal muscles. *Ann. Surg.* 123(3):447–472, 1946.

MALIGNANT BONE TUMORS

Batson OV. The function of the vertebral veins and their role in the spread of metastasis. *Ann. Surg.* 112(1):138–149, 1940.

Delattre O, Zucman J, Melot T, Garau XS, Zucker J-M, Lenoir GM, Ambros PF, Sheer D, Turc-Carel C, Triche

TJ, Aurias A, Thomas G. The Ewing family of tumors—a subgroup of small-round-cell tumors defined by specific chimeric transcripts. *N. Engl. J. Med.* 331(5):294–249, 1994.

Ewing J. Diffuse endothelioma of bone. *Proc. New York Pathol. Soc.* 21:17–24, 1921.

Honoki K, Stojanovski E, McEvoy M, Fujii H, Tsujiuchi T, Kido A, Takakura Y, Attia J. Prognostic significance of p16(INK4a) alteration for Ewing sarcoma: a meta-analysis. *Cancer* 110(6):1351–1360, 2007.

Link MP, Goorin AM, Miser AW. Green AA, Pratt CB, Belasco JB, Pritchard J, Malpas JS, Baker AR, Kirkpatrick JA, Ayala AG, Shuster JJ, Abelson HT, Simone JV, Vietti TJ. The effect of adjuvant chemotherapy on relapse-free survival in patients with osteosarcoma of the extremity. *N. Engl. J. Med.* 314(25):1600–1606, 1986.

Miller CW, Aslo A, Won A, Tan M, Lampkin B, Koeffler HP. Alterations of the p53, Rb, and MDM2 genes in osteosarcoma. *J. Cancer Res. Clin. Oncol.* 122(9):559–565, 1996.

Ottaviani G, Jaffe N. The etiology of osteosarcoma. *Cancer Treat. Res.* 152:15–32, 2009.

Pasic I, Shlien A, Durbin AD. Recurrent focal copy-number changes and loss of heterozygosity implicate two noncoding RNAs and one tumor suppressor gene at chromosome 3q13.31 in osteosarcoma. *Cancer Res.* 70(1):160–171, 2010.

Riccio I, Marcarelli M, Del Regno N, Fusco C, Di Martino M, Savarese R, Gualdiero G, Oreste M, Indolfi C, Porpora G, Esposito M, Casale F, Riccardi G. Musculoskeletal problems in pediatric acute leukemia. *J. Pediatr. Orthop. B.* 22(3):264–269, 2013.

Schimke RN, Lowman JT, Cowan AB. Retinoblastoma and osteogenic sarcoma in siblings. *Cancer* 34(6):2077–2079, 1974.

OTHER TUMOR

Abe T, Tomatsu T, Tazaki K. Synovial hemangioma of the knee in young children. *J. Pediatr. Orthop. B.* 11(4):293–297, 2002.

Müller H, Horwitz A, Kuhl J. Acute lymphoblastic leukemia with severe skeletal involvement: a subset of childhood leukemia with a good prognosis. *Pediatr. Hematol. Oncol.* 15(2):121–133, 1998.

OTHER

Adler C-P, Kozlowski K. *Primary Bone Tumors and Tumorous Conditions in Children: Pathologic and Radiologic Diagnosis.* Berlin, Germany: Springer-Verlag; 1993.

Cheng EY, Thompson RC. New developments in the staging and imaging of soft-tissue sarcomas. *J. Bone Joint Surg. Am.* 81(6):882–891, 1999.

Enneking WF, Spanier SS, Goodman MA. A system for the surgical staging of musculoskeletal sarcoma. *Clin. Orthop.* 153:106–120, 1980.

Lowry PA, Carstens MC. Occult trauma mimicking metastases on bone scans in pediatric oncology patients. *Pediatr. Radiol.* 27(2):114–118, 1997.

Malkin D, Li FP, Strong LC, Fraumeni JF, Nelson CE, Kim DH, Kassel J, Gryka MA, Bischoff FZ, Tainsky MA. Germ line p53 mutations in a familial syndrome of breast cancer, sarcomas, and other neoplasms. *Science* 250(4985):1233–1238, 1990.

Mankin HG, Lange TA, Spanier SS. The hazards of biopsy in patients with malignant primary bone and soft-tissue tumors. *J. Bone Joint Surg. Am.* 64(8):1121–1127, 1982.

Mirels H. Metastatic disease in long bones. A proposed scoring system for diagnosing impending pathologic fractures. *Clin. Orthop.* 249:256–264, 1989.

NEUROMUSCULAR DISORDERS

Neuromuscular disorders account for the greatest burden of chronic disability in children. Because motor dysfunction is often an early manifestation, the orthopædic surgeon may be the first to evaluate the child.

Injury to the central nervous system may include several outcomes [A]. The prevalence of neuromuscular disease is evolving [B]. Poliomyelitis has declined due to immunization, and spina bifida has declined due to dietary supplementation with folic acid during pregnancy. Cerebral palsy remains unchanged, in part because advances in obstetrical knowledge and practice are balanced by increased survival of premature infants.

Neuromuscular disorders may be distinguished based upon level of disease [C]. Such a simplified system serves as a basis upon which to organize the approach to complex patients.

EVALUATION

History

Inquire about pregnancy and birth. Were fetal movements reduced or delayed? Was there perinatal distress? What were the Apgar scores? Was the child premature? What about hospitalizations and procedures? Is the child sufficiently interactive that desires and pain are known? The family is essential to determination of how much a deformity impairs care and hurts the child. Inquire about milestones. Delay in motor development is least variable among patients and most reliable from parents [D]. Early hand dominance is not a sign of advanced development but suggests unilateral loss of function. Initiate a neurologic assessment for walking delayed beyond the 2nd year. In older children with severe delay, absence of independent sitting by 4 years or independent walking by 7 years is prognostic of never walking. Do not underestimate a parent's intuition, which may identify correctly a problem that escapes quantification. For most patients with neuromuscular disease, the diagnosis will be established before orthopædic consultation.

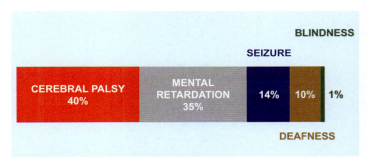

A Outcomes of central nervous injury Most result in cerebral palsy or mental retardation.

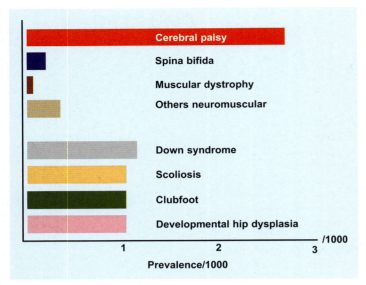

B   Prevalence of neuromuscular disorders Cerebral palsy is dominant.

		Brain	Spinal cord	Peripheral nerves	Muscle
Congenital		Cerebral palsy Spina bifida Mental retardation Aneurysm	Diastematomyelia	Insensitivity pain	Congential myopathy Arthrogryposis Absent muscles
Degenerative-Inherited		←	Friedreich ataxia ———————→ Syringomyelia Spinal muscle atrophy	Hereditary Motor Sensory Neuropathy Herniated disc	Muscular dystrophy Myotonia
Infectious, inflammatory		Meningitis Encephalitis	Poliomyelitis Transverse myelitis Guillain-Barre syndrome ———————→		Myositis Collagen disorders Dermatomyositis
Tumor		For example, medulloblastoma	For example astrocytoma	Neurofibromatosis	
Traumatic		Shaken baby Near drowning	Paraplegia	Obstetric palsy	Torticollis
Presentation		Spastic paralysis Hyper-tonicity Hyper-reflexia Sensation: abnormal Primitive reflexes MRI: abnormal	Flaccid paralysis Hypotonicity Hyporeflexia Sensation: abnormal EMG: variable Nerve conduction: normal	Distal weakness Hypotonicity Hyporeflexia Sensation: abnormal Family history +/– Nerve conduction: abnormal	Proximal weakness Hypotonicity Sensation: normal Family history + EMG: abnormal Creatine kinase high

C   Neuromuscular disease according to level of disease.

Physical Examination

The neural examination includes:

- Cognition. Cognitive function is essential to evaluation, management, and outcomes. For example, it may be difficult to determine pain in a cognitively impaired child with cerebral palsy.
- Motor function. Assess strength manually and against body weight. In addition to individual muscle groups, a functional assessment is based upon standing and walking ability: standing for demonstration, standing to assist transfer, walking at home, and walking in the community. For walkers, determine total distance as a general measure of function. Assistive devices are not limiting but liberating.
- Sensory function. Altered sensation may be direct, due to neural loss, for example, spina bifida, or indirect, due to cognitive loss.
- Special signs, for example, a child using the hands to "walk up" the anterior legs and thighs in order to rise from a seated position in the setting of muscle weakness. Divide tone into normal, reduced (hypotone), or increased (hypertone).

Gait Evaluate by observation (*cf.* Lower Limb chapter). Gait is divided into stance and swing phases, which overlap for 20% of the normal cycle. Stability during single-limb stance can be limited by cognition, balance, proprioception, coordination, standing posture, bony deformity, contractures, and weakness. Without stability in stance, it is impossible to develop an effective gait pattern. Each swing phase requires clearance of the off-loaded foot to preposition that foot in terminal swing. Ankle equinus, weakness in dorsiflexors, and cospasticity are examples that will prevent clearance and prepositioning and lead to an ineffective gait, one with inadequate stride length, poor cadence, or otherwise biomechanically impaired and energy inefficient. Gait also may be assessed in a laboratory, including instrumented motion analysis, dynamic electromyography, pedobarography, and energy consumption test. Include walking and running, which as a stress test will amplify deficit, for example, asymmetry of the limbs in hemiplegia.

There are several morbid gaits [E].

HIP ABDUCTOR WEAKNESS This produces a Trendelenburg gait, which is characterized by shifting of the center of mass over the affected joint in stance to eliminate the moment arm. Because the patient has the tendency to fall away from the weak limb in stance, a compensatory mechanism is to raise the walking velocity, thereby reducing time for the effect of gravity, for example, advanced hip deformity.

HIP EXTENSION WEAKNESS Walking slows to reduce forward momentum. Lumbar lordosis increases to move center of mass posteriorward. Knee flexion decreases to limit hip flexion, for example, muscular dystrophy.

SCISSORING Adductor spasticity slows walking velocity and narrows the base of stability, for example, diplegic cerebral palsy.

QUADRICEPS WEAKNESS This reduces knee control and is the principal determinant of walking. Body weight flexes the knee, which is counteracted by hip extension, plantar flexion, and locking of the knee in extension. Additionally, the limb may be rotated lateralward to move the force vector medialward away from the sagittal plane, for example, spina bifida.

CIRCUMDUCTION GAIT Hamstring weakness, or quadriceps contracture or spasticity, reduces knee flexion, which is a major hindrance during swing. The limb is functionally lengthened, necessitating that it be swung outward for the foot to clear the ground.

CROUCHED GAIT This may be compensatory to reduced hip extension, due to knee flexion contracture, or a result of triceps suræ weakness. The gait cycle is shortened, there is forward trunk lean to reduce demand on quadriceps, and energy consumption increases, for example, overlengthening of tendo Achillis.

STEPPAGE GAIT Anterior crural muscle weakness is compensated for by increasing hip and knee flexion for swing phase toe clearance.

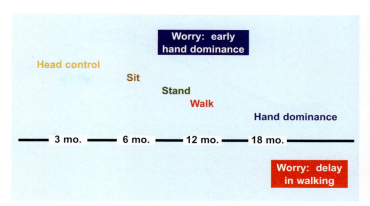

D   Select milestones.

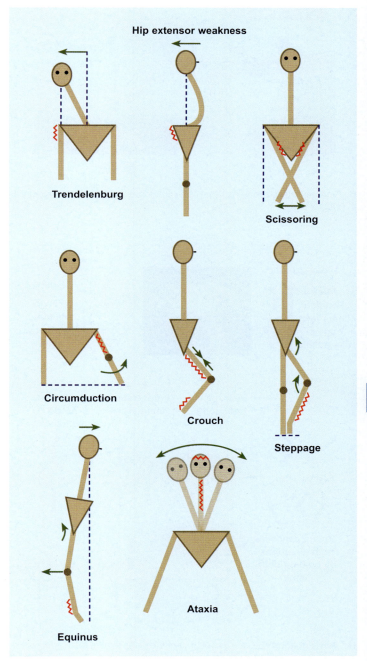

E   Abnormal gait Site of disease in *red* and motion, compensatory and morbid, in *green*.

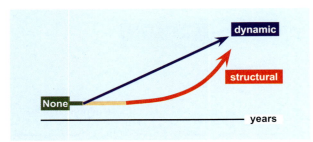

F Effect of time on contracture formation The orange part of the curve may be lengthened by early intervention such as stretching and bracing.

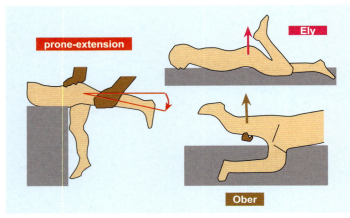

G Some contracture tests These are common tests to assess contractures in cerebral palsy.

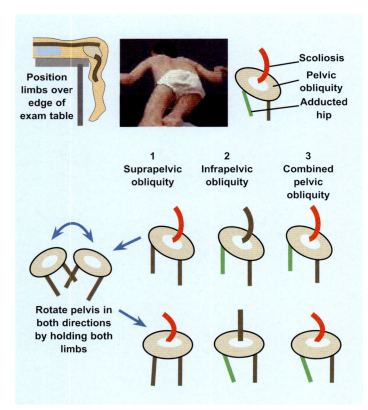

H Pelvic obliquity Rotate and neutralize the pelvis to unmask a primary spine deformity (*red*) that persists despite neutral alignment of pelvis and hips or a primary hip deformity (*green*) that remains despite pelvic and spine position. Combined deformities are present when pelvis rotation has no influence.

EQUINUS GAIT Reduced ankle flexion leads to a toe–toe gait, concentrating force at the forefoot during stance. There is reduced flexion or extreme hyperextension of the knee. In the neuromuscular patient, with compromised proximal muscle strength and control, forward translation of the center of mass reduces the effective base of support, thereby reducing stride length, for example, muscular dystrophy.

HINDFOOT VARUS This concentrates force over the lateral border of the foot during stance, for example, Charcot-Marie-Tooth disease.

ATAXIC GAIT Greek (α-: "not," ταξις: "precise arrangement"). This is a sign of central nervous disease, for example, in the cerebellum. It is characterized by a broad base, short stride, and titubation due to impaired balance.

The neuromuscular patient must balance benefits against energy consumption of walking. Speed declines first, to maintain energy cost *per* time. However, energy cost *per* distance increases: most patients will select a wheelchair for mobility once this exceeds thrice the normal.

Deformity Deformity may be dynamic or static.

DYNAMIC This reflects errant neural signaling. It may vary by position, for example, upright posture increases tone that accentuates dynamic deformity. Surgical correction is compensatory and less predictable.

STRUCTURAL Dynamic deformity may become fixed or structural with time [F], such as due to spasticity or positioning in wheelchair. Manual interventions before structural deformity sets in, such as stretching and bracing, may delay onset. Sites of contracture include the skin, muscle, and joint capsule or ligaments. Surgical correction is direct, but may be limited by concomitant contracture of neurovascular structures, which would be intolerant of stretch, for example, popliteal artery and tibial nerve behind a flexed knee. With more time, fixed contractures lead to joint deformity and instability, for example, flattening of the head of the femur subluxated against the rim of acetabulum in cerebral palsy.

Deformity may develop even in the setting of hypotonia, for example, scoliosis. Contracture matters when compensatory mechanisms are overwhelmed, thereby interfering with function. Titrate expectations and interventions according to function. For example, a child in a wheelchair has less demand than does an ambulatory child; by contrast, a plantigrade foot is a universal goal.

HIP FLEXION This tips the trunk forward, which is compensated for by lumbar hyperlordosis or knee flexion into a crouched gait. Assess this by the prone extension test [G] or by extending the affected hip in the supine position with the opposite hip maximally flexed to eliminate compensatory lumbar lordosis (Thomas). 30 degrees is a guide to release.

HIP ABDUCTION Hip abduction is important for perineal access and care. While limitation of abduction <45 degrees is a guide to release, let function be the ultimate guide.

ILIOTIBIAL TRACT The patient lies decubitus with affected limb up and with opposite hip and knee flexed. Flex, abduct, and extend the affected hip to bring tract over the trochanter major, where it will be tensioned to prevent the ipsilateral knee from adducting beyond midline under gravity (Ober).

GRACILIS In the prone position, abduct the hip with the knee flexed: tensioning the biarticular gracilis by extending the knee causes hip adduction (Phelps).

RECTUS FEMORIS This biarticular muscle flexes the hip and extends the knee. In the prone position, flexion of the knee tensions the muscle: contracture is revealed by the elevation of the buttock as the hip is obligatorily flexed (Duncan-Ely). Rectus femoris contracture also may limit knee extension and draw the patella proximalward (alta).

KNEE FLEXION Measure this by the popliteal angle. Hip flexion to 90 degrees tensions the hamstrings, thereby exposing contracture as the knee is extended.

KNEE EXTENSION Genu recurvatum is abnormal. It may be a direct result or a compensatory mechanism for weakness at the knee.

EQUINUS Invert the hindfoot to lock the subtalar joint. Flex and extend the ankle in knee flexion (gastrocnemius relaxed) and knee extension (gastrocnemius tensioned). 10 degrees of flexion allows heel–toe gait.

0 degree allows a plantigrade foot in the nonambulatory. >30 degrees risks crouch gait in the setting of weakness.

ROTATIONAL PROFILE This often is abnormal in neuromuscular patients. Medial femoral torsion is a characteristic of cerebral palsy. Lateral tibial torsion is a characteristic of spina bifida.

PELVIC OBLIQUITY This may be suprapelvic, originating in the spine, or pelvic, due to hip deformity [H].

SPINE Deformity is common in neuromuscular disease. Assess this in the unweighted prone position, upright, and with traction. Pay attention to the skin for signs of decompensation, such as sore, due to limited movement, and for surgical incisions, for example, spina bifida repair.

Reflexes Knowledge of reflexes, reactions, and signs is essential to understanding normal and delayed development [I].

MORO A startled baby, for example, simulated fall or clapping, abducts and extends all limbs and spine, which may be followed by opposite movement into an embrace [J]. The reflex is lost by 6 months. This aids differentiation of neonatal paralysis, for example, brachial plexopathy, from pseudoparalysis, for example, due to clavicle fracture.

PLACING REACTION In the vertical suspension position, the anterior leg is brought into contact with an edge: the normal infant flexes hip, knee, and ankle to surmount the edge and spontaneously extends the lower limb when the sole is planted. The reflex also may be elicited in the upper limb with the dorsal forearm as initial point of contact. This is normal up to 12 months.

ASYMMETRIC TONIC NECK Supine and neutral neck. Turn head in one direction then the other: the limbs toward which the head is turned extend while the opposite flex, assuming a "fencer position." This is lost by 6 months.

PARACHUTE Suspend the baby prone by holding the waist. Simulated fall elicits extension of the upper limbs toward and to protect the head. This appears at 6 months and remains.

EXTENSOR THRUST In the vertical suspension position, pressing the soles down against a flat surface elicits hip and knee extension for support. This reflex is lost by 6 months. Persistence will interfere with normal reciprocal hip and knee flexion during swing phase.

VERTICAL SUSPENSION A baby suspended vertically by the axillæ with examiner's thumbs supporting the neck flexes the hips and knees until 6 months. Extension and scissoring are signs of spasticity.

PALMAR GRASP The digits contract to receive an object inserted into the palm, and tone in the entire limb increases as the object is withdrawn. This reflex is lost by 6 months.

BABINSKI Plantar stimulation results in extension of the hallux and fanning out of the lesser toes. This reflex is lost by 2 years.

TONIC LABYRINTHINE In the supine position, tilting the head backward produces opisthotonos. This reflex is lost by 6 months.

DEEP TENDON Corticospinal reflex to acute muscle stretch. Hyperreflexia, including clonus >5 beats, indicates upper motor neuron disease.

While primitive reflexes aid diagnosis of developmental delay, they also are prognostic: loss of these reflexes by 2 years is predictive of independent walking.

Imaging

MRI This is the modality of choice for evaluation of the brain. It shows congenital malformations, such as polymicrogyria, heterotopia, and schizencephaly. Other findings in developmental delay include intracranial hæmorrhage or ischæmia, periventricular leukomalacia, cystic encephalomalacia and ventriculomegaly. It also allows determination of whether myelination is appropriate for age.

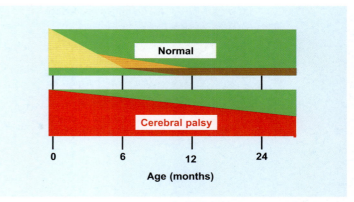

I **Natural history of reactions, patterns, and reflexes.** Most reflexes are lost by 6 months (*yellow*) and others by 12 months (*orange*). Persistent primitive reflexes and pathologic patterns represent a delay in development, such as in cerebral palsy (*red*). Appearance of the parachute reflex (*brown*) at 6 months and its persistence are normal.

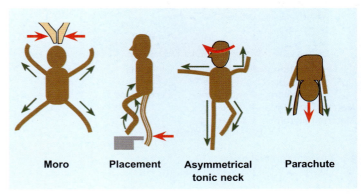

J **Common reflexes.** Provocation in red and response in *green*.

Study	Value
Total lymphocyte count	> 1500/mm³
Albumen	> 3.5 g/dL
Transferrin	> 175 mg/dL

K **Laboratory analysis before operation.** These values are associated with reduced infection rate.

Laboratory analysis The diagnosis of neuromuscular disease is typically not dependent upon laboratory analysis.

CYTOGENETICS Chromosomal analysis for a genetic disorder.

INFECTION Because of the high prevalence in this patient population, tests such as urinalysis often are indicated. Infectious workup also screens the mother for *in utero* exposure.

NUTRITION Preoperative assessment may reduce infection rate after major operation, for example, spine fusion for cerebral palsy [K].

PULMONARY FUNCTION Preoperative testing estimates risk of prolonged ventilator dependence after spine fusion in muscular dystrophy.

ELECTROENCEPHALOGRAPHY Diagnosis and evaluation of seizure.

ELECTROMYOGRAPHY AND NERVE CONDUCTION Diagnosis of muscular dystrophy and neuropathy.

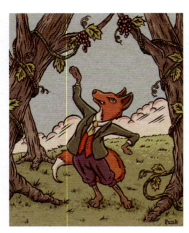

A Cognitive dissonance In Æsop's fable, the fox decides that the grapes he cannot reach are not ripe yet but sour, thereby reconciling his desire with his inability to fulfill it. In surgery, this may set into motion a cycle in which family perceives benefit despite equivocal outcomes, which confirms both their and the surgeon's choice of treatment, perpetuating the process.

		GENETIC		
PRENATAL 18%	PERINATAL 33%	POST-NATAL 16%	10%	UNKNOWN 23%
Infection Toxic Vascular Maternal seizure Maternal thyroid	Traumatic delivery Hypoxia Bradycardia Preterm Apgar < 4 Weight < 2,000 g	Infection Trauma Kernicterus		

A Causes of cerebral palsy.

Tone		Comment
Pyramidal	Spasticity	Velocity-dependent hypertonicity 80%
Extra-pyramidal	Athetosis	Greek αθετος: "unable to position" Slow, writhing, convoluted
	Choreiform	Greek χορεια: "dance" Sequential, rhythmic, ballistic
	Ataxia	Imbalance, incoordination, tremor
Mixed		Heterogeneity of disease

B Tonal classification of cerebral palsy Spasticity is caused by loss of inhibition of the reflex arc. Velocity dependence is manifested by tone that is dependent on the rate of stretch. Spastic patients have hyperreflexia, clonus, and myostatic contracture. Many patients will defy distinct classification. Response to surgical intervention is most predictable in spasticity.

Site	Features
Hemiplegia	Affects half the body in sagittal plane (Greek 'εμι: "half") Focal intracranial hæmorrhage or infarct
Diplegia	Affects "both" lower limbs (Latin bis: "both") Periventricular leukomalacia due to vascular insufficiency 3/4 are premature
Tetraplegia	Affects "four" limbs (Greek τεττταρες: "four") Variable cognitive dysfunction, including total involvement characterized by diffuse brain disease.
Monoplegia	Rare
Mixed	For example, asymmetric diplegia, double hemiplegia

C Geographic classification of cerebral palsy.

MANAGEMENT PRINCIPLES

Balance the burden of disease with the morbidity of intervention. Orthopædic care addresses the downstream effects of a primary disease that it cannot cure. Prioritize function over deformity: "normal" is unrealistic and unattainable. Prioritize communication, independence, and mobility over walking.

Appreciate the significance of sensation and perceptive disabilities. Terms such as "spasticity" and "plegia" do not acknowledge sensory impairment in cerebral palsy.

Account for all costs: pecuniary, social, and familial. Think of the family as a computer: running too many and incompatible programs may crash it.

Beware of cognitive dissonance. This describes the tension that results from attempting to reconcile two contradictory beliefs or realities, a tension that may be relieved by changing one of the two to be consistent with the other. To parents and caregivers with high expectations before operation, a poor or even fair outcome may be dissonant whereas a good outcome will be harmonious. This may explain how a positive subjective outcome is not contradicted by a negative objective outcome. An understanding of cognitive dissonance may bridge the divide between family expectations and surgeon restraint.

Recognize that natural history may be harnessed when favorable, such as in nonprogressive conditions or those with spontaneous improvement, yet it can be an obdurate force against influence, hence the failure to preserve walking despite the best intentions and surgical interventions.

Adhere to the proof razor: the burden of proof lies with one who makes a claim and not with one challenged by it. Exhaustive and exhausting remedies, foisted upon vulnerable families, may be rejected absent evidence. Do not be dogmatic: absence of proof is not proof of absence. Alternative remedies are acceptable when they do not harm the child or family; when they do not delay, interrupt, or otherwise interfere with proven treatments; and when there are no other effective options. Recognize the ethical limitations of caregivers consenting to high-risk procedures on behalf of a cognitively impaired patient. Be mindful of the ethical imperative *primum non nocere*: "first do no harm."

CEREBRAL PALSY

The name describes motor dysfunction caused by a disease of the brain. The suffix -plegia is derived from Greek πληγη: "a blow, stroke," used by Hippocrates to describe "paralysis" resulting from being struck by disease. While it is referred to as static encephalopathy, in recognition of a defined insult resulting in a stable brain disorder, the musculoskeletal consequences are progressive. It also is known as Little disease, after the English physician W. J. Little (1810–1894), who championed tenotomy (having undergone the procedure himself) and who attributed the disease to difficult pregnancy, premature birth, and neonatal asphyxia.

The appellation encompasses a group of disorders resulting from pre- and perinatal brain insult as well as postnatal causes such as near drowning and traumatic brain injury [A]. 1/4 walk independently, 1/2 have capacity with walking aids, and 1/4 do not walk.

Classification

The disorder is classified according to tone [B] and geographically [C]. Pyramidal pathways (in particular corticospinal) directly continue to the motor neurons of the spinal cord. The extrapyramidal system, including the basal ganglia and cerebellum, indirectly modulates motor function. A lesion in this system results in "dyskinetic" movements, characterized by abnormalities in control, posture, and timing. The geographic classification correlates with timing and mechanism of brain injury [D]. For example, the basis for prematurity as a risk factor is incomplete development of the cerebrum. Vasculature, resulting in hypoperfusion to the periventricular white matter, the region most susceptible to injury because it is a watershed zone between striate and thalamic arterial systems. These areas carry fibers responsible for lower limb motor function, manifesting as spastic diplegia. Geographic subtypes have several characteristics [E]. A final component of classification is the Gross Motor Function Classification System [F].

Medical Considerations

Multiple comorbidities beyond the musculoskeletal system impact decision making and outcomes.

Cognition Half of patients with cerebral palsy have cognitive impairment. This correlates with severity. It is exacerbated by dysarthria, which impedes expression of intellectual capacity.

Skin Hygiene is difficult, impeded by contracture, and dependent on caregivers. Skeletal distortion without the ability to accommodate due to movement restriction may lead to decompensation such as decubitus ulcer.

Gastrointestinal Poor oromotor control has several consequences:

- Failure to thrive due to feeding and swallowing difficulty. Patients may require gastrostomy or jejunostomy to augment nutrition. Low weight is the greater concern, by contrast with spina bifida, where overweight challenges function.
- Gastrœsophageal reflux and associated aspiration pneumonia.
- Constipation.

Teeth Dental caries, enamel dysgenesis, and malocclusion.

Respiratory Aspiration pneumonia due to oromotor dysfunction and seizure. Motor dysfunction impairs cough. Reduced mobility reduces mechanical factors that aid lung inflation. Prolonged recumbency after operation adds risk.

Seizure 1/3 of patients have epilepsy, a direct result of brain insult. This correlates with extent of involvement, increasing with cognitive impairment and tetraplegia.

Visual Visual field defects due to cortical injury. Premature infants may develop retinopathy.

Hearing Loss is seen in patients with history of kernicterus.

Diagnosis

Presentation demonstrates a temporal evolution:

- At birth, if risk factors are recognized in mother, such as toxic or infectious exposure, or in child, such as asphyxia or prematurity.
- In the first few months for tone abnormality, hypotonia precedes hypertonia. Failure to thrive also may manifest in this period.
- In the first couple of years for abnormal developmental milestones, such as delayed walking and premature hand dominance. Milestones are delayed but not lost: regression suggests a hereditary neurodegenerative disease rather than cerebral palsy.

Movement Management

This may be focal, to address local or segmental spasticity, or it may be generalized.

Botulinum toxin This neurotoxin, produced by the Gram-positive anaerobic rod *Clostridium botulinum* (Latin botulus: "sausage," after poisoning from contamination), binds to motor nerve terminals where it cleaves SNARE proteins to inhibit release of acetylcholine. It first was used to treat strabismus. It is injected into the skeletal muscle to produce a dose-dependent reversible paresis to overcome spasticity and potentiate manual lengthening. Needle placement may be determined anatomically or aided by ultrasonogramme or electromyography.

Botulinum toxin may be administered therapeutically or diagnostically. It is most effective in the lower limb, in particular triceps suræ in combination with casting for equinus. Other applications include the hip adductors for scissoring, to reduce subluxation of femoral head, and to facilitate perineal care, the rectus femoris to alleviate stiff knee gait, and the upper limb for flexion deformities of elbow and wrist. It may serve as

	Tetraplegia	Diplegia	Hemiplegia
	Global brain injury	Periventricular leukomalacia	Discrete lesion

week — 20 ... 25 ... 35

D   Timing of brain insult Although correlations are imprecise, the earlier the event during gestation, the greater the injury.

Features	Hemiplegia	Diplegia	Tetraplegia
Disability	Mild	Moderate	Severe
Feet	Equinovarus, equinovalgus		
Knees	Mild	Moderate	Severe
Hips	OK	Subluxation	Dislocation
Spine	OK	OK	Scoliosis
Upper Limbs	Variable	Little	Major
Seizure	Common	Rare	Common
Walking	Yes	Variable	No

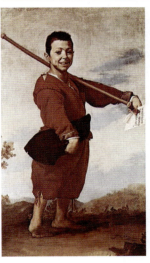

E   Characteristics of geographic subtypes *Boy with a clubfoot* by Jusepe de Ribera (1591–1652) is a vivid depiction of hemiplegia. The boy stands in equinus, with the forearm pronated and the wrist and fingers flexed.

Level	Function
I	Walking: without limitation. Running and jumping. Decreased speed, balance, coordination
II	Walking: with limitation For example, railing for stairs. Difficulty on uneven surface or interactive environment
III	Walking: at home with hand-held mobility device Community: wheel-chair.
IV	Does not walk. Stands to transfer. Supported sitting. Wheel-chair for mobility.
V	Global impairment. Unable to independently walk, stand or sit: requires transportation

F   Gross Motor Function Classification System Because it measures self-initiated movement and ability, this is a functional assessment, as opposed to systems that describe type of movement or part of body affected. It consists of 66 measures of sitting (truncal control) and walking ability, subdivided according to age.

an adjunct to preoperative assessment of tendon lengthening, providing a reversible preview of the operative effect. Because it blocks dynamic muscle activation, it is not effective for fixed contracture.

Maximum dose of botulinum toxin is 20 U/kg, distributed as 2 U/kg in small muscles and 6 U/kg in large muscles, and 600 U total. Maximal effect is seen in 1 to 2 weeks. Duration of effect is 3 to 6 months; redosing should be no more frequent, in order to avoid immunity.

Phenol This also is known as carbolic acid, after its discovery from coal tar. It was the agent used by the Scottish surgeon Sir Joseph Lister (1827–1912) to clean wounds and soak bandages in his development of antisepsis. It targets a major motor nerve directly (rather than diffusing over muscle endings), which is identified with a nerve stimulator under general anæsthesia. It is most effective for musculocutaneous nerve to improve extension of the elbow and obturator nerve to improve hip abduction.

Baclofen This activates GABAB receptor, opening potassium channels and closing sodium and calcium channels, thereby blocking neurotransmitter release and muscular contraction. It is indicated for generalized movement disorder. It may be administered *per orem* or *via* a pump placed in the anterior abdominal wall connected by a catheter with the subarachnoid space at a level in the spine determined by how much upper limb effect is desired [G]. The intrathecal route allows better control of dose and limits side effects. The pump is refilled every month and replaced once batteries are spent.

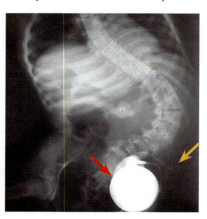

G Intrathecal baclofen Pump is implanted in the anterior abdominal wall (*red*), and catheter leads to subarachnoid space in lumbar spine (*orange*).

Rhizotomy This refers to "cutting" (Greek τομη) of dorsal nerve "roots" (Greek ριζα). The rationale is section of afferents to counteract loss of descending central nervous system inhibition of spinal cord stretch reflex [H]. The procedure consists of:

- L1–S2 laminoplasty. This gives access to the cauda equina while potentially reducing the development of postoperative spinal deformity, including hyperlordosis, spondylolisthesis, and scoliosis.
- Dorsal nerves are divided into rootlets that are stimulated to threshold using intraoperative electromyography, including external anal sphincter. Rootlets selected for section are those demonstrating abnormal response (≥2 muscles having a titanic or crescendo pattern), which typically represents 1/3 of the total.

Vigorous postoperative physical therapy is necessary to overcome associated weakness. Controversy surrounding this procedure is due in large measure to lack of strict criteria for patient selection. The ideal candidate is a 4- to 8-year diplegic who is cognitively spared and ambulatory. The child is intelligent and old enough to succeed with postoperative therapy, but young enough to have few if any permanent contractures. Furthermore, in patients who harness spasticity to stand or walk, underlying weakness may be exposed by rhizotomy. Even though the procedure improves range of motion and function in the lower limbs, orthopædic procedures are required in more than half of cases. Postoperative spinal deformity typically is self-limited, rarely requiring active management.

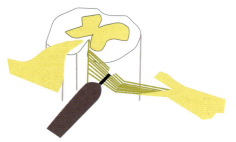

H Dorsal rhizotomy Afferent fibers in dorsal roots are sectioned to decrease spasticity.

Spine

Development of scoliosis correlates disease severity: 2/3 of tetraplegics are affected, hemiplegics rarely [I].

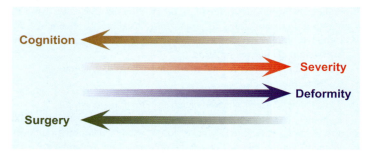

I Deformity correlates with disease severity Consider doing more for less: exercise restraint in the totally involved child, where risk may outweigh benefits in the setting of severe deformity and reduced demands.

These curves differ from idiopathic scoliosis:

- Onset is earlier, typically first decade.
- Increased likelihood and magnitude of progression.
- Bracing does not alter natural history.

Thoracic scoliosis may impact pulmonary function. Lumbar lordosis influences posture, including the need for assistive device to sit and engagement of the upper limbs for truncal support. It also may aggravate gastrointestinal dysfunction, such as constipation and swallowing. Deformity, including pelvic obliquity, with limited compensatory mechanisms risks overlying skin and soft tissues and may hurt.

Evaluation Disability may be difficult to determine in the cognitively impaired. Ask family and third parties about burden of care, such as ability to sit and feed. Assess flexibility of curve by comparing magnitude upright, supine, and with traction. Check the skin for any lesion that might increase infection risk. Refer to a nutritionist or abdominal surgeon for failure to thrive.

IMAGING Follow general principles (*cf.* Spine chapter), including traction views for flexibility since many patients may not be able to cooperate fully when asked to bend in the sagittal plane. Specialized modalities may be necessary in severe deformity.

LABORATORY EVALUATION This includes measures of infection and nutrition. There is no consensus on pulmonary function testing for cerebral palsy.

Management Outcomes are based more upon caregivers than upon the patient. They tend to be subjective, for example, sitting in a wheelchair is facilitated, more than objective. Objective measures, which might include such postoperative hospitalization, treatment of pneumonia, use of analgesics, rate or size of decubitus ulcer, have eluded demonstrated improvement.

Observe the relaxed, unweighted spine: this will buy time for the early-onset patient. Modify a wheelchair and consider an orthotic.

For postural support. Indications for surgical treatment follow general rules: >10 years of age with progressive curve >50 degrees. There are several special considerations:

- Infection rate approaches 10%. Contributing factors include the burden of chronic disease, malnourishment, multiple procedures and hospitalizations that result in polymicrobial colonization and may disturb the soft tissue envelope on the trunk, complex procedures with prolonged wound exposure, and impaired cognition and global involvement that interferes with aftercare. Addition of antibiotic powder directly to the wound after final irrigation may reduce the infection rate in such high-risk patients.
- Pelvis. Establish whether an oblique pelvis is part of the structural curve, acting like a spinal segment in continuity with the scoliosis, or is independent, based upon orientation and flexibility testing on physical examination and röntgenogramme [J]. To include the pelvis in a spine fusion may be debated [K]. If flexible, sparing it reduces operative time, blood loss, and risk of pseudarthrosis (highest at the lumbosacral junction) and preserves flexibility that may be of value for positioning. That such flexibility improves walking ability is unproven. Including it avoids a subsequent operation to extend the fusion in a curve type known for progression and a patient population that is fragile. Differentiate pelvic obliquity due to hip disease. There is no rule for whether spine deformity or hip deformity takes precedence for correction.
- Fusions tend to be long. Follow-up operations after the index may not be feasible. Spared curves are unpredictable. The benefits of preserving mobility are outweighed by the morbidity of a secondary operation.
- Blood loss. This is high in an ill patient who presents with anæmia of chronic disease and who has depleted reserves upon which to draw. This may be reduced by the use of antifibrinolytic agents such as tranexamic acid.
- Anterior procedure. Avoid this in a patient who has baseline pulmonary decline and a high-risk profile. Have realistic and reasonable goals: a stable spine with head balanced on pelvis does not need to be straight. Do not add to the morbidity of the procedure.
- Tissue quality. Patients may have a thin soft tissue envelope to cover prominent implants, increasing the risk of breakdown. Be mindful of the axiom: "the soft tissue is hard and the bone is soft." Osteopenia reduces implant stability, while contractures can be unyielding. Exercise restraint during spinal reduction.
- Complications are many [L]. Synchronize incentives and expectations, and educate and keep the family actively involved from the outset.
- Resource utilization. Spine fusion for neuromuscular patients taxes facility, such as intensive care unit, and health care providers, including other consultant physicians and therapists.

Hip

Like the spine, acquired deformity of the hip correlates with severity of disease, affecting more than half of tetraplegics. It is a manifestation of asymmetric neuromuscular control that does allow the hip to remain centered and is exacerbated by medial femoral torsion that twists the head of femur out the front of the acetabulum.

Evaluation Monitor the hip with serial röntgenogrammes, because subtle changes may not be perceptible manually and because the earlier dysplasia is detected the simpler the treatment. Limited hip abduction (<45 degrees) due to hypertonia of adductors is an at-risk sign. Ask the family if there is pain or other difficulty with perineal care. This may not be evaluable during a limited consultation.

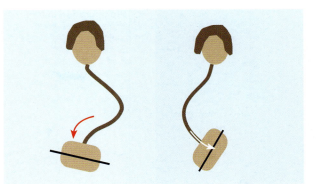

J Pelvic obliquity in neuromuscular scoliosis Both pelves are oblique. One (*red*) is not part of the structural C-shaped curve, as evidenced by opposite deflection, even though there is not enough spine remaining for the pelvis to return to horizontal. The other (*white*) is part of the curve, which continues into a pelvis that acts like a scoliotic spinal segment.

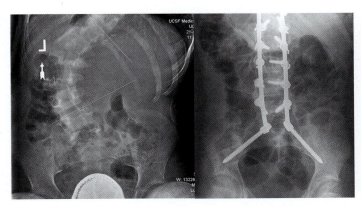

K Spine fusion for cerebral palsy The pelvis was included in a nonambulatory patient to reduce risk of secondary operation. Because the lumbosacral junction is at greatest risk of pseudarthrosis, the pelvis was rigidly fixed with S1 and S2 iliac screws. Simple AO screws in pedicles attached to a unit rod *via* wires looped through washers provide stability, allow gradual correction by creep, stay out of the canal to reduce hæmorrhage and permit unrestricted laminar decortication and are cost-effective.

Complication	Factors
Pain and regression	Proportional to extent of operation Cause unknown Minimize duration by upright positioning, early and active therapy, reduced immobilization Partial loss may be permanent for example, marginal walker before operation does not walk after operation
Infection	Multifactorial, including chronic disease Malnutrition Complex disease requiring prolonged procedures Impaired movement and cognition
Decubitus ulcer	Impaired movement and cognition Unclear communication Sensory disturbance Use of casts and braces
Aspiration pneumonia	Oromotor dysfunction Reduced movement Prolonged recumbency

L Select complications after spine surgery for cerebral palsy These are common to all big surgery.

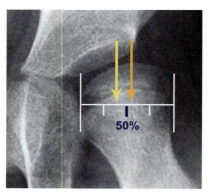

M Hip migration index
Measurement error results from determination of where articular surface ends (*yellow*) *versus* edge of ilium on a two-dimensional image (*orange*). Note valgus orientation of the neck of femur, exaggerated by medial torsion.

50%

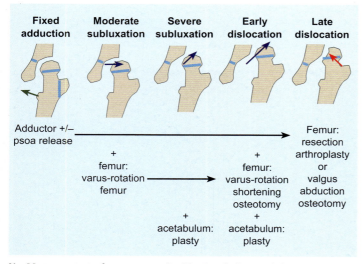

Fixed adduction	Moderate subluxation	Severe subluxation	Early dislocation	Late dislocation

Adductor +/– psoa release

Femur: resection arthroplasty or valgus abduction osteotomy

+
femur: varus-rotation femur → femur: varus-rotation shortening osteotomy

+
acetabulum: plasty

+
acetabulum: plasty

N Management of neuromuscular hip dysplasia Hip deformity in cerebral palsy tends to be progressive, as is reconstruction. Begin with contracture release (*green*), follow by reconstruction osteotomy (*blue*), and end with ablation (*red*).

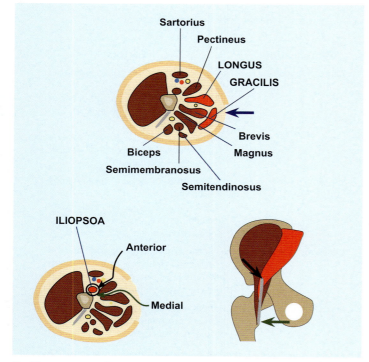

Sartorius
Pectineus
LONGUS
GRACILIS
Brevis
Magnus
Biceps
Semimembranosus
Semitendinosus

ILIOPSOA
Anterior
Medial

O Management of neuromuscular hip dysplasia Adductor release is performed through a medial incision (*blue*). Iliopsoa may be released through a medial (*green*) or anterior (*black*) incision.

Management Several factors influence management. The natural history is variable. There may be progression of subluxation to dislocation and of deformity from femur, for example, conoid epiphysis, to acetabulum, that is, obliquity, to degenerative joint disease. Risk of progression is related to the severity of involvement and walking ability. The gross motor function classification system is most predictive of progression. Progression often is silent, hence the importance of surveillance röntgenogrammes of at-risk hips. If pain arises, it is worst for subluxation: half of dislocated hips are asymptomatic. Intervention in the young child depends upon function, of which the ultimate level often is unknown, and later in childhood pain, of which again the level may be unclear. A proactive rather than reactive strategy is predicated on the recognition that outcomes of reconstruction of a good hip are better than salvage of a bad hip.

In contrast with developmental dysplasia, the hip in cerebral palsy is normal at birth and later becomes deformed by a combination of delayed walking and neuromuscular imbalance. There is a frameshift delay in the temporal schedule of operative treatment compared with developmental dysplasia of the hip (*cf.* Hip chapter). In addition, more deformity is tolerated at younger age, in part because function is delayed and functional demands are less predictable. Consider intervention for hip migration index (Reimers) >1/3 on röntgenogramme [M].

0 to 4 years Hip abduction brace. Augment abduction by adductor release as indicated.

Greater than 4 years Osteotomy without or with open reduction [N]. Because torsion is a significant feature of neuromuscular hip dysplasia, varus and derotation osteotomy of the femur is a central component of correction. Fix rigidly (e.g., blade plate) to avoid postoperative immobilization and associated morbidities, such as pressure phenomena and pulmonary compromise. Add innominate osteotomy based upon acetabular dysplasia. The neuromuscular acetabulum often is patulous due to constant microinstability; plasty (Pemberton) corrects this as it wraps the acetabulum around the head of the femur to contain it.

In the older child, take into consideration function, pain, and appearance on röntgenogrammes, which may show femoral head deformity as well as (sub)luxation and acetabular deformity. If the child stands to transfer and walks, perform a complex reconstruction to maximize hip function. Add open reduction, which may uncover significant degenerative change in the femoral articular surface where it has been rubbing against the edge of the acetabulum. In this setting, pain may persist due to osteoarthritis despite deformity correction. If the child does not walk, let pain guide treatment. If the deformity is painful, perform a proximal femoral resection arthroplasty (Castle-Schneider) or a proximal femoral valgus–abduction osteotomy (Schanz). Both procedures remove the head of the femur from acetabular contact, the source of pain. The former markedly improves hip motion and obviates the need for contracture release, but is plagued by proximal migration and reossification. The latter leaves the head of the femur in the buttock, which may break down over the prominence.

Contracture release This may be a part of hip reconstruction, or it may be an independent procedure [O]. For passive hip abduction <45 degrees, the adductors are approached *via* a direct medial approach (Ludloff). Cut gracilis and adductor longus. Neurectomy of obturator, of which the branches are defined as anterior and posterior relative to their position relative to the adductor brevis, is the ultimate release; however, it may be complicated by abduction contracture.

For hip flexion contracture >30 degrees, iliopsoa may be sectioned *via* same medial incision at its insertion into the trochanter minor, in the very young or the older patient who does not walk, or *via* the anterior approach (Smith-Petersen) for innominate osteotomy, where it is fractionally lengthened at the pelvic brim. For the latter approach, recognize that femoral nerve lies on the superficial surface of the iliopsoa, while its tendinous portion begins to form deep and medial in the muscle.

For popliteal angle >45 degrees, hamstrings may be released *via* the medial approach by traveling deep to the adductor magnus to reach ischial tubercle. Differentiate tendons that originate from the bone and may be tensioned more by knee extension from the sciatic nerve, which may be apposed to the posterior surface of ischium. Consider a nerve stimulator. Alternatively, hamstrings may be lengthened at the knee by a direct approach: cut gracilis, cut or Z-lengthen semitendinosus, fractionally lengthen semimembranosus by cutting surrounding aponeurosis, and resist the biceps femoris for fear of weakening and extension contracture of the knee.

Tailor amount of release to achieve symmetry. Consider performing releases in the lower limbs simultaneously (including with other lower limb reconstruction), to limit number of independent surgical and anæsthetic exposures and to not weaken disproportionately one level, thereby amplifying the deformity at other levels.

Lower Limb

Leg Lateral torsion of the ankle axis reduces push-off power by shortening the lever arm of the foot. This may be addressed by supramalleolar rotational osteotomy and fixed with percutaneous wires or with plate to obviate the need for a postoperative cast.

Sagittal deformity Patterns emerge from a sea of variations that elude comprehensive classification and universal rules of care [P].

EQUINUS The child may compensate by knee flexion or the knee may be driven into recurvatum by the ankle equinus. At early stage, botulinum toxin may allow fitting of an ankle foot orthotic. Later, operative lengthening of triceps suræ may be necessary. While equinus in cerebral palsy is tenacious, gastrocnemius recession is preferable if Silfverskiold sign is present. Based upon concern that this may be insufficient or not durable, lengthen tendo Achillis: err on less ankle flexion at operation in order to avoid weakening an already weak and contracted patient who thereby will be driven into a crouch gait. Add tibialis posterior fractional lengthening above the tibial malleolus for associated varus.

STIFF KNEE Spasticity of the rectus femoris, which is abnormally active during swing, leads to decreased knee flexion during swing, foot clearance problems, and reduced gait velocity and stride length. It may be defined as decreased knee excursion throughout the whole gait cycle of <30 degrees. Distal transfer to sartorius fascia or medial hamstrings improves peak, timing of, and range of knee flexion in swing. Advocates of release of distal rectus femoris cite simplicity and failure of transfer (20%).

"JUMP KNEE" The term describes the appearance of bouncing up and down during walking. The knee and possibly the hip are flexed throughout stance, with equinus occurring in late stance. Diplegic patients with this presentation may be candidates for selective dorsal rhizotomy (*v.s.*) or multilevel single-event surgical release.

CROUCH GAIT This may result from weakness due to disease or that is iatrogenic, that is, tendo Achillis overlengthening. Release hip and knee, and support the ankle in an orthotic.

Foot Evaluation and management in the ambulatory child follow general principles (*cf.* Foot chapter).

For the nonambulatory child, the goal is a plantigrade foot that can be stabilized in an ankle foot orthosis. Procedures for arthrodesis, stiffening, or limiting motion of the subtalar joint are attractive due to the limited demands of such a child and are indicated when rigid deformity precludes joint-preserving procedures such as lateral column lengthening [Q]. Procedures may be categorized as arthrodesis (e.g., Dennyson-Fulford), extra-articular fusion (e.g., Grice-Green), and extra-articular stabilizing or blocking procedures that limit eversion by an implant adjacent to the subtalar joint (e.g., Smith). The simplicity of these procedures has spilled them over into the flexible foot. Long-term outcomes remain pain and degenerative osteoarthritis, even if they may be less clearly or more slowly perceived in an involved child.

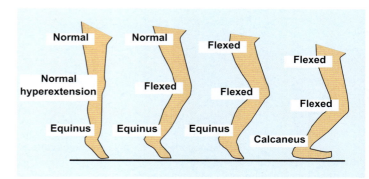

P Sagittal deformity in the lower limb Hemiplegia is characterized by greater distal involvement with relative proximal sparing and limb shortening that is advantageous to clear the floor in the setting of limited movement altering swing phase of gait.

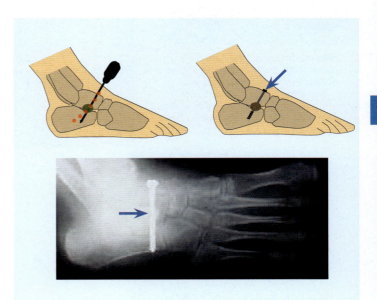

Q Subtalar arthrodesis for rigid flat foot in a nonambulatory An Ollier incision is used to approach the sinus tarsi (*red*). Decorticate the talus and calcaneus or use a dowel cutter to excise a part of the subtalar joint; bone is grafted (*green*). The foot is placed in a neutral position and fixed with a screw (*blue*). This is combined with soft tissue releases, such as triceps suræ lengthening.

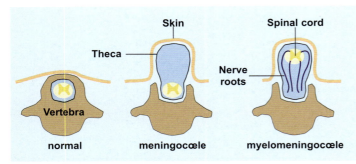

A Pathology of meningocœle and myelomeningocœle Meningocœle (<10%) may have no neural deficit, whereas in myelomeningocœle, by definition, the neural elements are stretched, exposed, and thereby injured.

Complication	Factors
Folate deficiency	1/2 cases 0.4 mg *per diem* preconception
Metabolic	Gestational diabetes
Toxic	Gestational exposure to drugs (e.g., neuroleptics)
Genetic	Chromosome anomaly (e.g., trisomy 13, 18)
Race	Whites = 3 X Blacks

B Causes of spina bifida Folic acid consumption and supplementation must be instituted when pregnancy is planned, because the lesion occurs before pregnancy is determined. Folic acid enrichment of cereal grain began in 1992 upon the recommendation of the U.S. Public Health Service, as a disease prevention measure.

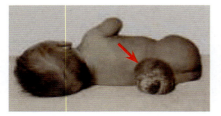
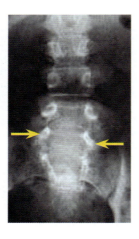

C Spina bifida Spina bifida (*red*) may be repaired *in utero* or in the neonatal period. Patients will walk with anatomic lesion L4 or below (*yellow*), which is seen on röntgenogramme as pedicular dysplasia, absent spinous process contour and interpedicular widening.

SPINA BIFIDA

Spina bifida (Latin *bifidus*: "cloven in two") may be closed, designated occulta (Latin: "occult"), or aperta (Latin: "open"), also termed cystica (Greek κυστις: "bladder, sac of fluid"). Occulta affects >20% of the Caucasian population at the lumbosacral junction and is an incidental finding on röntgenogrammes that has relevance to the surgeon operating on the spine in this region in order to avoid inadvertent entry into the vertebral canal. Cystica may be divided into two structural types [A]. The meninges (Greek μηνιγξ: "membrane"), dura mater and arachnoid, protrude to present a "sac" (Greek θηκη: "sheath" = Latin *theca*) filled with fluid without or with spinal cord (Greek μυελος: "marrow" of the vertebral column) and nerves. A variation is lipomyelomeningocœle, in which a fibrofatty mass traverses the lumbodorsal fascia through a neural arch and theca to infiltrate and tether the spinal cord. While the clinical spectrum of disease is broad, the principal morbidities are cognitive, genitourinary, and musculoskeletal.

Pathophysiology

Spina bifida results from failure of closure of the neural tube during 3rd and 4th weeks following conception. Because the neural tube folds and fuses from its middle toward each end, there are associated cranial defects. These include Chiari II malformation, which consists of caudal displacement through foramen magnum and squeezing of the brainstem that retards flow of cerebrospinal fluid to produce hydrocephalus. This and other brain anomalies account for varying degrees of mental impairment, which is worse the more craniad the lesion.

Many factors have been implicated in causation [B].

Natural History

Untreated, mortality is 80%, within the first year, from infection and hydrocephalus. With surgical repair, the two factors most important to long-term functional outcomes are hydrocephalus and anatomic level. Cognitive function correlates with early and unobstructed shunting of hydrocephalus (>80% of cases). Walking ability peaks toward the end of the first decade and declines with the onset of the pubertal growth spurt, due to increasing body weight, worsening contractures and deformities, and complications of comorbidities and multiple medical and surgical treatments. Renal failure is the leading cause of death in adults.

Presentation

Diagnosis may be made *in utero* based upon elevated a-fetoprotein and acetylcholinesterase due to an open neural tube detected by amniocentesis performed at the end of the first trimester of pregnancy. This may be confirmed by fetal ultrasonogramme, which shows ventriculomegaly and Chiari II malformation.

Myelomeningocœle is evident at birth [C]. Lipomyelomeningocœle may be more subtle, including soft tissue mass and stigmata of dysrrhaphism such as hypertrichosis or sinus. Clinical presentation may be divided according to the locus of the disease.

- Central nervous system disease. Signs of encephalopathy due to hydrocephalus and anomalies include cognitive impairment and seizures. Brainstem and upper cervical compression due to Chiari II malformation may lead to upper limb weakness, spasticity, and incoordination. In addition, swallowing difficulty, gastrœsophageal reflux, and aspiration pneumonia result in failure to thrive and are life threatening in the infant.
- Spinal cord disease. This includes myeloschisis, tethering, and syrinx as an extension of hydrocephalus. The zone of neural injury may be imprecise: functional level often does not correspond with anatomic level. Sensory level may not match motor level, and flexors are more proximally affected than extensors. Patients with upper thoracic lesions have poor trunk control. Those with lower thoracic and upper lumbar lesions do not walk. L4 or below walk, due principally to preserved quadriceps function.

Fetal repair for myelomeningocœle reduces the need for shunting and improves motor, at the expense of preterm delivery and uterine dehiscence at delivery. Neural function may change longitudinally due to several factors, such as hydrocephalus and spinal cord tethering. By contrast with spasticity and dyskinesia in cerebral palsy, most patients with spina bifida present with flaccid paralysis.

- Musculoskeletal deformities, which reflect functional level. Upper thoracic level is characterized by scoliosis, thoracolumbar kyphosis, and lumbar hyperlordosis. Asymmetry of pericoxal muscle function in low thoracic/upper lumbar level leads to hip dislocation. Knee, ankle, and foot contractures and deformities are the principal features of more distal levels.
- Cutaneous breakdown. This is related to abnormal sensation; immobility that does not allow pressure relief; deformity concentrating pressure, such as over a gibbus or due to posture asymmetry; and lower limb distal vasculopathy. It is exacerbated by orthotics and casting and by maceration due to bowel and bladder dysfunction.
- Neurogenic bowel and bladder, accounting for routine urinalysis and preoperative coverage for urinary tract infection.

Spine

Because of the pathogenesis, spinal deformity in spina bifida has two components. Like cerebral palsy, it may be acquired as a result of neuromuscular imbalance to produce scoliosis. It may be congenital, such as hemivertebral failure of formation, to produce kyphosis. With progressive deformity, the erector spinæ dislocate anterioward to the vertebral bodies to become flexors, thereby worsening the deformity.

An orthotic provides stability to a child with poor truncal control. Surgical indications include the following:

- For kyphosis, intractable soft tissue breakdown over gibbus. This is facilitated by cordectomy if there is no useful function in the lower limbs or bowel and bladder.
- For scoliosis, recruitment of the upper limbs to correct posture. Liberation of the upper limbs is critical for the child to interact with the environment.

The benefits of surgical treatment of spine deformity have evaded demonstration. Accordingly, there is no clear role for prophylactic intervention to arrest progression or in anticipation of pulmonary or other visceral compromise.

There are several special considerations relevant to spine surgery in spina bifida.

- Infection. Multiple hospitalizations and operations, as well as neurogenic bowel and bladder requiring catheterizations and manipulations, result in polymicrobial colonization. The soft tissue envelope, stretched and bruised by deformity, and repeatedly incised, for example, starting with the spina bifida repair, is fragile and attenuated. Exposure of the theca risks dural tear, which may require synthetic reconstruction to prevent chronic leak. Sensory loss may remove protective mechanisms to decompress the wound.
- Pseudarthrosis. The posterior elements, and therefore the surface for fusion, are absent. This requires combination with anterior fusion, performed *via* separate approach, posterior interbody access, or vertebral column resection.
- Tethered spinal cord. 1/3 of patients will undergo detethering procedure. Evaluate level of conus medullaris (below L2) and filum terminale (thickened, fatty) by MRI, and solicit a neurologic surgeon for release before correction, lest the spinal cord be stretched by correction and there be a loss of neural function. Orthopædic procedures are not reduced by detethering, and retethering is not uncommon.
- Latex allergy. This is not exclusive to spina bifida [F]. Anaphylaxis may be life threatening. Best practice is primary prophylaxis in a latex-minimized environment.

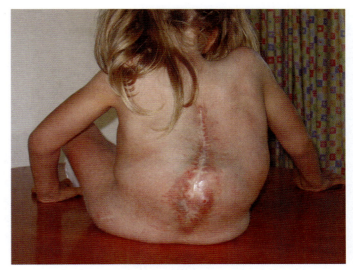

D   Cutaneous breakdown Despite decompression of the gibbus by a gel support with cut out, the soft tissue is eroded by a progressive and rigid deformity.

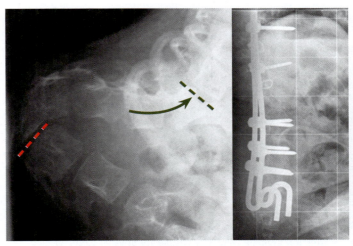

E   Kyphectomy for spina bifida Perform a circumferential dissection from a posterior approach: the great vessels are safely anterior to the vertebral column. The resection includes the anomalous apical vertebra (*red*) and proximal lordotic segment (*green*), of which the total length is determined by what is necessary to reconnect a straightened spine. If a cordectomy is performed, then the junctional vertebrae may be removed one by one as necessary, instrumented, and returned to shape the reconstruction akin to the Sofield-Millar technique for osteogenesis imperfecta. In a young or thin child, S rods placed over the iliac alæ provide pelvic fixation that is stable against sagittal displacement and not prominent. Monitor the hallux to make sure the great vessels are not stretched by correction. Excise the area of breakdown widely to close healthy wound edges, feasible by posterior soft tissues, including relocated paraspinous muscles, that will be relaxed by the kyphectomy.

Fraction	Disease
1/2	Spina bifida
1/4	Cerebral palsy
1/4	Other, e.g., ventriculoperitoneal shunt, muscular dystrophy, exstrophy of bladder,

F   Latex allergy in neuromuscular disease This represents a type I IgE-mediated immune response to the highly elastic rubber polymer manufactured from the sap of the tropical tree *Hevea brasiliensis*. The allergy has as common factors multiple hospitalizations and procedures, including urinary catheterization and as early as ventriculoperitoneal shunt placement for hydrocephalus in the neonate.

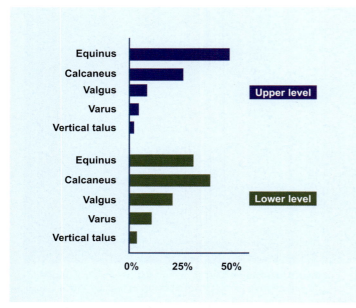

G   Foot deformity in spina bifida Most (>80%) upper level children present with significant foot deformity. The foot represents the greatest burden of deformity in lower level ambulatory child.

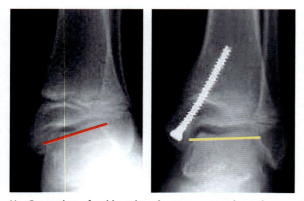

H   Correction of ankle valgus by temporary physeal screw Valgus inclination of talar trochlea (*red*) improves (*yellow*) with growth modulation of the distal tibia by a percutaneous screw, which is bent by the effect.

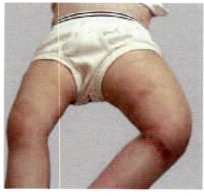
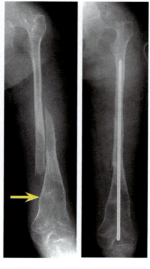

I   Fracture in spina bifida The left thigh is swollen and red. Röntgenogramme shows osteopenia and evidence of previous fracture based upon cortical irregularity (*yellow*). Fracture was fixed with medullary device that shares the load with and stabilizes the femur against further injury.

Hip

In an infant with demonstrated quadriceps function, and in a child who walks, hip dysplasia is evaluated and managed according to general principles (*cf.* Hip chapter). Hip dislocation may be seen in upper lumbar or higher levels, in whom it does not affect walking ability. This is managed according to general neuromuscular principles (*v.s.* cerebral palsy). Pain is mitigated by sensory loss, which may remove pain *per se* as an indication for surgical treatment. Asymmetric hip contracture and dislocation may lead to proximal femoral or pelvic prominence and sitting imbalance. These risk pressure concentration and soft tissue ischæmic necrosis, which may be exacerbated by sensory loss and reduced mobility. Despite such theoretical considerations, there is no consensus on operative indications: follow patients regularly, and intervene if a problem is imminent or arises rather than as prophylaxis in anticipation of one.

Lower Limb

Knee The child who does not walk is more tolerant of a flexion contracture. Be prepared to combine tendon lengthening and release with posterior capsulotomy. Extension without or with shortening osteotomy of the distal femur may be necessary in the older child.

Foot and ankle Every deformity is possible in spina bifida [G]. Treat the foot and ankle of the walking child according to general principles (*cf.* Foot chapter). For the nonambulatory, the goal is a supple plantigrade foot.

- Deformity tends to be severe, stiff, and recurrent.
- Be careful when casting a foot in the setting of incomplete or absent sensation.
- Preserve motion: a flexible foot that bears weight on the sole will be most stable, easiest to maintain in brace, and least at risk for soft tissue breakdown.
- Tenodesis is useful and effective in the setting of absent voluntary control.
- Consider tendon exsection for release, to reduce recurrence of deformity.
- As with the knee, add capsulotomy of the ankle and subtalar joints as necessary.
- Supplement releases with osseous procedures, including decancellation and talectomy.

Distinguish hindfoot valgus from ankle valgus, which may be treated simply and effectively by distal medial tibial temporary physeodesis with percutaneous screw [H].

Fracture 30% of children will sustain a fracture, peaking at puberty, when the child is adapting to an increase in size and weight. Thoracic and nonambulatory patients are at highest risk: disuse osteopenia from motor loss and sensory neuropathy conspire to raise the risk with the level of disease. Correspondingly, most fractures involve the femur and tibia. In an ambulatory child, consider medullary fixation for repeated fracture or to prevent malunion, which may impair walking or increase risk for subsequent fracture [I]. Physeal fractures heal more slowly and have a higher rate of growth disturbance. Balance prolonged immobilization against exacerbating osteopenia. Growth disturbance and deformity may require correction, or tip a patient with marginal ambulatory status toward the wheelchair.

Fractures in spina bifida may be confused with infection and occasionally neoplasm due to a vigorous inflammatory response characterized by swelling and redness, an exuberant callus on röntgenogramme, and the fact that many fractures occur after imperceptible trauma. Fever and inflammatory markers may be elevated, but in reduced proportion to the physical examination to be consistent with infection. Immobilization confirms fracture empirically as inflammatory signs subside.

MUSCULAR DYSTROPHY

The term describes a group of hereditary, primary, progressive diseases of the muscle [A]. The pathogenesis is muscle cell death leading to weakness (fatty degeneration) followed by contracture (fibrosis).

Duchenne Muscular Dystrophy

This is the most common type of muscular dystrophy and has the distinction of being the most lethal genetic disease of childhood. It is caused by a mutation in the gene encoding dystrophin on Xp21.1-2. Dystrophin is a sarcolemma protein that connects cytoskeleton with extracellular matrix. 1/3 are new mutations. The tissue distribution of dystrophin in cardiac and smooth muscle, as well as brain, in addition to skeletal muscle explains the pleiotropy of the gene defect.

Evaluation The French neurologist and electrophysiologist G-B-A Duchenne de Boulogne (1806–1875) recognized in his appellation "pseudohypertrophic muscular paralysis" that the most striking sign is weakness in the setting of apparently potent, overgrown calves. The first consultation may be for a general complaint that the child is unable to keep up physically with his peers. In addition to calf hypertrophy, discrepant with the early age, Gower sign may reveal proximal muscle weakness [B]. Characteristics of gait include an abductor lurch (Trendelenburg), hyperlordosis of the lumbar spine (to compensate for hip extensor weakness) [C], posterior thrust of the knee (to compensate for quadriceps weakness), and toe walking. Cardiac disease must be addressed and function optimized before operation. Gastrointestinal and urinary dysfunction reflect smooth muscle disease. Mean intelligence quotient is 20 below normal (105).

The natural history is predictable [D].

LABORATORY ANALYSIS Abnormal dystrophin allows leakage of intracellular components such as creatine phosphokinase, which is >100 times normal level (<200 IU/L). Polymerase chain reaction confirms the mutation. Pulmonary function testing is part of preoperative evaluation.

IMAGING Ultrasonogramme reveals altered signal due to fibrofatty infiltration of muscle.

Medical management Steroids suppress immune-mediated cell destruction, temporarily improving muscle strength and delaying progression of scoliosis. Deflazacort is bone and carbohydrate sparing, limiting osteoporosis and weight gain. Creatine monohydrate, which improves muscle performance in healthy athletes, has been shown to increase muscle strength and functional performance. It remains early to determine efficacy of other avenues of investigation, such as gene therapy and disease-modifying drugs that act at a genetic level, for example, codon read-through and exon skipping. For example, eteplirsen and drisapersen are morpholinos (knockdown tools that block RNA and thereby modify gene expression) that results in skipping of exon 51 of the dystrophin gene. For a subset of patients with Duchenne muscular dystrophy due to a frame-shift mutation, such drugs may restore the reading frame to produce a functional protein.

Spine Steroids and improvements in cardiopulmonary care have reduced surgical treatment of scoliosis. Bracing is contraindicated due to potential of thoracic constriction negatively impacting pulmonary function. Scoliosis is a marker of advanced disease, which also is marked by pulmonary decline. Recommendations for surgical treatment beginning at 20 degrees are indications that curve progression is inevitable and that the window for intervention is narrowed by pulmonary function. Preoperative cardiac evaluation and pulmonary function tests are essential. Operative ventilatory risk, including permanent postoperative dependence, rises sharply after forced vital capacity drops below 30%. Spine fusion rectifies and stabilizes the back, which is critical to a child with weak upper limbs. It slows the decline of pulmonary function, which is primarily affected by respiratory muscle weakness. Perform a long fusion that includes the pelvis, in order to reduce the risk of a second procedure and insult to the patient's lungs. Operative risks include increased hæmorrhage because of reduced constriction of the vascular muscle wall

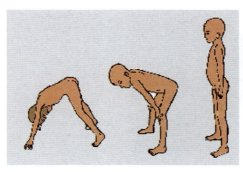

X-linked
• Duchenne
• Becker
• Emery-Dreifuss
Autosomal dominant
• Myotonic
• Facioscapulohumeral
• Emery-Dreifuss
• Oculopharyngeal
• Distal
Autosomal recessive
• Limb-girdle muscular dystrophy
• Emery-Dreifuss

A Muscular dystrophies They may be classified according to inheritance pattern. There are many subtypes, for example, the limb–girdle phenotypic series includes 20 forms with unique mutations affecting >20 protein products. There are other forms of muscular dystrophy.

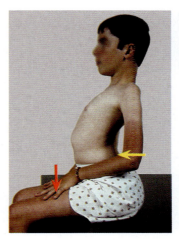

B Gower sign The child walks up the front of the legs and thighs when asked to stand from a seated position. Muscle weakness advances from proximal to distal in Duchenne muscular dystrophy.

C Lumbar hyperlordosis Hip flexion contracture and hip extensor weakness drive the lumbar spine into increasing lordosis to balance head over pelvis. Note the use of the hands for stability.

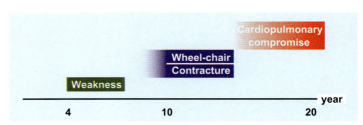

D Natural history of Duchenne muscular dystrophy Contracture, such as scoliosis and equinovarus, coincides with confinement to the wheelchair. Cardiopulmonary compromise accounts for death in the third to fourth decades. Walking after 13 years is Becker muscular dystrophy, which has a later onset and milder course, with survival into the fifth decade.

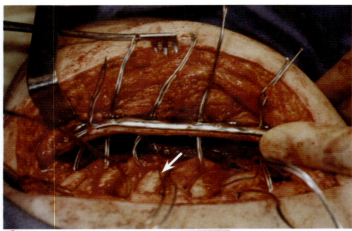

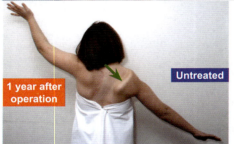

E Scapulothoracic fusion for FSHMD By a vertebral border of scapula approach, ribs are exposed for circumferential wiring (*white*), which is secured to a contoured LCDC plate to the dorsal scapular surface. Scapula and ribs are compressed with intervening bone iliac crest bone graft.

and malignant hyperthermia. The latter results from uncontrolled skeletal muscle oxidative metabolism, leading to a rise in end-tidal CO_2 concentration as the first anæsthetic sign and cyanosis as the first sign in the operative field. Increased body temperature occurs late. Avoid volatile anæsthetics, and treat with nondepolarizing muscle relaxants.

Foot and ankle While the patients walk, deformity typically remains flexible. Support and maintain neutral position with orthotics, without or with casting. Gastrocnemius recession for toe walking is safe in a weakening condition. Equinovarus may be addressed effectively by the Rancho Los Amigos procedure:

- Split transfer of tibialis anterior to cuboid bone.
- Tibialis posterior fractional lengthening proximal to tibial malleolus.
- Open tendon of Achilles Z-lengthening.

In the nonambulatory child with profound weakness, in whom a plantigrade foot is the goal, tendo Achillis lengthening may be combined with transfer of tibialis posterior through the interosseous membrane to the dorsum, where tenodesis may suspend the foot in a neutral position.

Myotonic Dystrophy

Myotonia refers to delayed muscle relaxation after contraction. This is the most common muscular dystrophy in adults, with onset in the second decade. Heterogeneity manifests by type 1 caused by a heterozygous mutation in the dystrophia myotonica protein kinase gene on 19q13.32 and type 2 caused by mutation in the zinc finger protein 9 gene on 3q21.3. It is distinguished by weakness that proceeds from distal to proximal, facies myopathica giving a haggard appearance, cataracts, insulin-resistant diabetes mellitus, encephalopathy, and male hypogonadism.

Facioscapulohumeral Muscular Dystrophy

FSHMD is the third most common muscular dystrophy. It is associated with contraction of the D4Z4 macrosatellite repeat on 4q35. The disease is characterized by facial weakness, for example, inability to whistle, as well as weakness of the shoulder and proximal arm muscles, including serratus anterior, trapezius, and rhomboid major and minor, which results in the winging of the scapula and diminished shoulder abduction and flexion. Penetrance of this autosomal dominant disorder is 95% by 20 years age. An infantile form is characterized by hip flexion contracture and extensor weakness, lumbar hyperlordosis, foot drop, sensorineural hearing defects, and retinal vasculopathy.

The origin of deltoid, which is relatively spared, is reversed. Activation will anchor deltoid in the heavier upper limb to move a lighter scapula when not stabilized against the thorax. Patients complain of shoulder ache, inability to perform overhead activities such as combing the hair, and unsightly winging of the scapula. Surgical stabilization of the scapula against the posterior thorax [E] alleviates discomfort, advantages the deltoid to abduct and flex the shoulder, and improves shoulder appearance.

Emery-Dreifuss Muscular Dystrophy

The phenotypic series includes X-linked subtypes (emerin gene on Xq28, FHL1 gene on Xq26.3), autosomal dominant forms (lamin A/C gene on 1q22, TMEM43 gene on 3p25.1, SYNE1 gene on 6q25.1-2, SYNE2 gene on 14q23.2), and an autosomal recessive form (1q22). The common feature is mutation of proteins associated with the nuclear membrane. The original appellation humeroperoneal dystrophy emphasizes triceps weakness leading to flexion contracture of the elbow and loss of hindfoot eversion and ankle flexion, leading to equinovarus. Other features are paraspinous muscle contracture limiting neck motion and cardiac disease, such as conduction defects that risk sudden death and are indications for insertion of a pacemaker. Onset peaks in the second decade. Creatine kinase is elevated 10 times normal, which contrasts with Duchenne muscular dystrophy.

OTHER NEUROMUSCULAR DISEASES

Charcot-Marie-Tooth disease

This is named after Jean-Martin Charcot (1825–1893) and his student Pierre Marie (1853–1940) of France and Howard Henry Tooth (1856–1926) of England, whose contribution was to recognize that this represents neuropathy and not myelopathy. While Charcot is regarded as the "Father of Neurology," he acknowledged Duchenne as "My Master in Neurology."

CMT is the most common hereditary neural disease. It represents a heterogeneous group of hereditary motor and sensory neuropathies, of which there are 7 phenotypic types, based upon the clinical presentation (e.g., age of onset), and >50 genetic subtypes, based upon identified mutation. CMT may be divided into demyelinating and axonal forms. Autosomal dominant and recessive as well as X-linked patterns of inheritance occur.

Pathophysiology Most types, including CMT types 1, 3, and 4, are demyelinating. Degradation of abnormal myelin results in dysfunction of motor and sensory axons, which thicken like an "onion bulb" due to attempts at repair and remyelination. Pain and temperature are preserved because they are carried by unmyelinated nerve fibers. In axonal forms of disease, such as CMT type 2, there is primary neuron death followed by wallerian degeneration. X-linked types include both forms of the disease.

Evaluation Family history varies according to type, whether this represents a new spontaneous mutation, and penetrance, which may be so low that affected relatives may not perceive the disease. Peripheral neuropathy manifests as weakness, muscle wasting, and loss of sensation, progressing from distal to proximal, involving the lower limbs before the upper limbs. Onset typically is in childhood. The earliest complaints are motor, such as clumsiness and frequent falls. As the disease advances, signs emerge such as steppage gait, deformity of the foot, and calf and interosseous muscle atrophy. Deep tendon reflexes, vibratory sensation, and proprioception are diminished, with normal pain and temperature sensation. In the foot, weakness begins in the interossei, producing clawing, followed by tibialis anterior weakness, producing cavus due to unopposed peroneus longus, and peroneus brevis weakness, allowing unopposed tibialis posterior to drive the hindfoot into the varus. 1/3 of children develop spine deformity. 5% to 10% develop hip dysplasia, which is acquired due to neuromuscular imbalance, silent in the first decade and progressive, and which is an indication for screening röntgenogramme of the pelvis. Enlarged peripheral nerves may be palpable.

Peripheral nerve thickening, for example, median, may be imaged with ultrasound. Nerve conduction is slowed in demyelinating forms of the disease. Sensory nerve action potentials and compound muscle action potentials are reduced in axonal forms, while nerve conduction is normal. Cytogenetic testing, such as for mutation in the gene encoding peripheral myelin protein-22 on 17p12 (CMT types 1A and 1E, Dejerine-Sottas disease, Roussy-Levy syndrome), confirms the diagnosis, although it is not available for all types.

Management Manage cavovarus and clawing of the foot according to general principle (*cf.* Foot chapter). Intervene surgically before the subtalar joint becomes stiff, in order to preserve motion. Spine and hip deformities also are managed according to general principles (*cf.* Spine, Hip chapters).

Type	Traditional Classification	
I	Werdnig-Hoffman, acute	onset < 6 mo.
II	Werdnig-Hoffman, chronic	onset 6–24 mo.
III	Wolfhart-Kugelberg-Welander	onset > 24 mo.
IV	no eponym	adult onset
International Spinal Muscular Atrophy Consortium		
I	Infantile	Onset <6 mo. Unable to sit, death in infancy
II	Intermediate	Onset 6–24 mo. Unable to walk, death by third decade
III	Juvenile	Onset >2 years Marginal walking, lost by second decade
IV	Adult	Mean onset fourth decade.

A   Classification of spinal muscular atrophy Severity correlates inversely with age of onset.

Spinal Muscular Atrophy

This represents a group of disorders characterized by anterior horn cell degeneration and progressive weakness and muscle atrophy [A]. It is the second most common autosomal recessive inherited disorders after cystic fibrosis. Sensation and cognition are unaffected. Spinal muscular atrophy is caused by mutation of the survival of motor neuron 1 gene on 5q13.2.

Evaluation A history of fetal hypokinesia may be elicited. Boys are affected more than girls, lower limbs more than upper limbs, and proximal more than distal weakness. Facial muscles are spared, except tongue fasciculation. There is absent tendon reflexes but no central neural signs. Type I presents as a floppy baby. Type II typically is diagnosed based upon hypotonia and delayed or missed motor milestones, in particular independent sitting and walking. Most common cause of death in spinal muscular atrophy is pulmonary infection.

Compound muscle action potentials are reduced, with neurogenic patterns on electromyography. Sensory nerve conduction is normal. Cytogenetic testing confirms diagnosis.

Management The spine and hip are most deformed and most treated. Follow general principles for the patient with muscle weakness and spine deformity (*cf.* Duchenne Muscular Dystrophy) and for the neuromuscular patient with acquired hip dysplasia based upon pain and walking ability (*cf.* Cerebral Palsy).

Friedreich Ataxia

This is the most common hereditary ataxia. It is an autosomal recessive disorder caused by trinucleotide repeat mutation in the frataxin gene on 9q13.21. Disease severity is related to the number of repeats. It is characterized by degenerative changes in spinocerebellar tracts, dorsal columns, pyramidal tracts, cerebellum, and medulla.

Evaluation As the name implies, ataxia is the first and defining sign, with titubation and a tabetocerebellar gait, to which contribute both loss of position and vibratory sense in dorsal columns of spinal cord and degeneration of cerebellum. Additional features include dysarthria, dysphagia, absent tendon reflexes, preserved Babinski reflex, variable cognitive impairment, and rare chorea. Upper limbs and face are affected less and later than lower limbs and trunk. Typical course is onset toward the end of the first decade with loss of ambulation following in the second decade. Like spinal muscular atrophy, morbidity correlates inversely with onset. Contractures develop, resulting in kyphoscoliosis and cavovarus foot deformity in half of patients. Insulin receptor abnormality leads to diabetes mellitus in 10%. 25% have optic atrophy, and 10% have sensorineural hearing loss. Most patients succumb to hypertrophic cardiomyopathy in midadult life.

Nerve conduction is mildly slowed. Sensory nerve action potentials are reduced or absent. Somatosensory evoked potentials are abnormal. Echocardiography is an essential part of preoperative workup. Cytogenetic testing confirms the diagnosis.

Management This mirrors management of other neuromuscular disorders (*cf.* Cerebral Palsy).

Poliomyelitis

This infection is caused by neurotropic enteroviruses of the *Picornaviridæ* family. It is transmitted *via* an orofæcal route from contaminated water. In 1% of cases, from the gut, there is viræmia followed by lodgment and destruction of anterior horn cells and brain stem motor nuclei, causing paralysis over a 1- to 2-week period. Muscles with motor nuclei extending over several segments are particularly vulnerable. There may be partial or complete recovery. Neural imbalance leads to contractures, which are amplified by growth, which is stunted.

The disease peaked in the mid-20th century, since which it has declined by 99% due to immunization. Eradication is near.

GENERAL

Babinsky JFF. Sur le spasme du peaucier du cou. *Rev. Neurol.* 9:693–696, 1901.

Duncan WR. Release of the rectus femoris in spastic paralysis. *J. Bone Joint Surg. Am.* 37(1):634–636, 1955.

Moro E. Das erste tremenon. *München Med. Wochenschr.* 65:1147–1151, 1918.

Ober FR. The relation of fascia lata to conditions in the lower part of the back. *JAMA.* 109:554–558, 1937.

CEREBRAL PALSY

Arens L, Peacock W, Peter J. Selective posterior rhizotomy: A long-term follow-up study. *Childs Nerv. Syst.* 5(3):148–152, 1989.

Bell KJ, Ounpuu S, De Luca PA, Romness MJ. Natural progression of gait in children with cerebral palsy. *J. Pediatr. Orthop.* 22(5):677–682, 2002.

Bleck EE. Locomotor prognosis in cerebral palsy. *Dev. Med. Child. Neurol.* 17(1):18–25, 1975.

Castle ME, Schneider C. Proximal femoral resection-interposition arthroplasty. *J. Bone Joint Surg. Am.* 60(8):1051–1054, 1978.

Dreher T, Wolf SI, Maier M, Hagmann S, Vegvari D, Gantz S, Heitzmann D, Wenz W, Braatz F. Long-term results after distal rectus femoris transfer as a part of multilevel surgery for the correction of stiff-knee gait in spastic diplegic cerebral palsy. *J. Bone Joint Surg. Am.* 94(19):1–10, 2012.

Jevsevar DS, Karlin LI. The relationship between preoperative nutritional status and complications after an operation for scoliosis in patients who have cerebral palsy. *J. Bone Joint Surg. Am.* 75(6):880–884, 1993.

Kay RM, Rethlefsen SA, Fern-Buneo A, Wren TA, Skaggs DL. Botulinum toxin as an adjunct to serial casting treatment in children with cerebral palsy. *J. Bone Joint Surg. Am.* 86(11):2377–2384, 2004.

Little WJ. On the influence of abnormal parturition, difficult labours, premature birth, and asphyxia neonatorum, on the mental and physical condition of the child, especially in relation to deformities. *Trans. Obstet. Soc.* 3:293, 1862.

Nordmark E, Josenby AL, Lagergren J, Andersson G, Strömblad LG, Westbom L. Long-term outcomes five years after selective dorsal rhizotomy. *BMC Pediatr.* 8:54, 2008.

Noonan KJ, Halliday S, Browne R, O'Brien S, Kayes K, Feinberg J. Interobserver variability of gait analysis in patients with cerebral palsy. *J. Pediatr. Orthop.* 23(3):279–287, 2003.

Palisano R, Rosenbaum P, Walter S, Russell D, Wood E, Galuppi B. Development and reliability of a system to classify gross motor function in children with cerebral palsy. *Dev. Med. Child Neurol.* 39(4):214–223, 1997.

Phelps WM. Description and differentiation of types of cerebral palsy. *Nerv. Child.* 8(2):107–127, 1949.

Reynell JK. Post-operative disturbances observed in children with cerebral palsy. *Dev. Med. Child Neurol.* 7(4):360–376, 1965.

Rodda JM, Graham HK, Carson L, Galea MP, Wolfe R. Sagittal gait patterns in spastic diplegia. *J. Bone Joint Surg. Br.* 86(2):251–258, 2004.

Schanz A. Zur Behandlung der veralteten angeborenen Hüftverrenkung. *Z. Orthop.* 42:442–444, 1921.

Soo B, Howard JJ, Boyd RN, Reid SM, Lanigan A, Wolfe R, Reddihough D, Graham HK. Hip displacement in cerebral palsy. *J. Bone Joint Surg. Am.* 88(1):121–129, 2006.

Sutherland DH, Larsen LJ, Mann R. Rectus femoris release in selected patients with cerebral palsy: a preliminary report. *Dev. Med. Child Neurol.* 17(1):26–34, 1975.

Tachdjian MO, Minear WL. Hip dislocation in cerebral palsy. *J. Bone Joint Surg. Am.* 38(6):1358–1364, 1956.

SPINA BIFIDA

Alman BA, Bhandari M, Wright JG. Function of dislocated hips in children with lower level spina bifida. *J. Bone Joint Surg. Br.* 78(2):294–298, 1996.

Adzick NS, Thom EA, Spong CY, Brock JW III, Burrows PK, Johnson MP, Howell LJ, Farrell JA, Dabrowiak ME, Sutton LN, Gupta N, Tulipan NB, D'Alton ME, Farmer DL. A randomized trial of prenatal versus postnatal repair of myelomeningocele. *N. Engl. J. Med.* 364(11):993–1004, 2011.

Centers for Disease Control and Prevention. Spina bifida and anencephaly before and after folic acid mandate-United States, 1995-1996 and 1999-2000. *MMWR Morb. Mortal. Weekly Rep.* 53(17):362–365, 2004.

Drennan JC, Freehaffer AA. Fractures of the lower extremities in paraplegic children. *Clin. Orthop.* 77:211–217, 1971.

Mercado E, Alman B, Wright JG. Does spinal fusion influence quality of life in neuromuscular scoliosis? *Spine* 32(19):S120–S125, 2007.

Nutter AF. Contact urticaria to rubber. *Br. J. Dermatol.* 101(5):597–598, 1979.

Sharrard WJW, Drennan JC. Osteotomy-excision of the spine for lumbar kyphosis in older children with myelomeningocele. *J. Bone Joint Surg. Br.* 54(1):50–60, 1972.

MUSCULAR DYSTROPHY

Alman BA, Raza SN, Biggar WD. Steroid treatment and the development of scoliosis in males with duchenne muscular dystrophy. *J Bone Joint Surg. Am.* 86(3):519–524, 2004.

Conte G, Gioja L. Scrofola del sistema muscolare. *Annali Clinici dell'Ospedale degli Incurabili di Napoli* 2:66–79, 1836.

Diab M, Darras B, Shapiro FL. Scapulothoracic fusion for adolescent and infantile facioscapulohumeral muscular dystrophy. *J. Bone Joint Surg. Am.* 87(10):2267–2275, 2005.

Duchenne GBA. Recherches sur la paralysie musculaire pseudo-hypertrophique ou paralysie myo-sclerosique. *Arch. Gen. Med.* 11:5–25, 1868.

Drachman DB, Toyka KV, Myer E. Prednisone in Duchenne muscular dystrophy. *Lancet* 2(7894):1409–1412, 1974.

Hoffman EP, Brown RH, Kunkel LM. Dystrophin: the protein product of the Duchenne muscular dystrophy locus. *Cell* 51(6):919–928, 1987.

Kley RA, Tarnopolsky MA, Vorgerd M. Creatine for treating muscle disorders. *Cochrane Database Syst. Rev.* 2:CD004760, 2011.

Landouzy L, Dejerine J. De la myopathie atrophique progressive (myopathie hereditaire debutant dans l'enfance, par la face, sans alteration du systeme nerveux). *Compt. Rend. Hebomadaires Acad. Sci.* 98:53–55, 1884.

Shapiro FL, Specht L. The diagnosis and orthopaedic treatment of inherited muscular diseases of childhood. *J. Bone Joint Surg. Am.* 75(3):439–454, 1993.

Weimann RL, Gibson DA, Moseley CF. Surgical stabilization of the spine in Duchenne muscular dystrophy. *Spine* 8(7):776–80, 1983.

OTHER NEUROMUSCULAR DISEASES

Brzustowicz LM, Lehner T, Castilla LH, Penchaszadeh GK, Wilhelmsen KC, Daniels R, Davies KE, Leppert M, Ziter F, Wood D. Genetic mapping of chronic childhood-onset spinal muscular atrophy to chromosome 5q11.2-13.3. *Nature* 344(6266):540–541, 1990.

Chamberlain S, Shaw J, Rowland A, Wallis J, South S, Nakamura Y, von Gabain A, Farrall M, Williamson R. Mapping of mutation causing Friedreich's ataxia to human chromosome 9. *Nature* 334(6179):248–250, 1988.

Charcot JM. *Clinical Lectures on Diseases of the Nervous System [Leçons sur les maladies du système nerveux]* 1889. Thomas Savill, translator ed., London: The New Sydenham Society; 2010.

Friedreich N. Über degenerative atrophie der spinalen, hinterstränge. *Arch. Anat. Physiol.* 26:391, 1863.

Holmes JR, Hansen ST Jr. Foot and ankle manifestations of Charcot-Marie-Tooth disease. *Foot Ankle* 14(8):476–486, 1993.

Kugelberg E, Welander L. Heredofamilial juvenile muscular atrophy simulating muscular dystrophy. *Arch. Neurol. Psychiat.* 75(5):500–509, 1956.

Kumar SJ, Marks HG, Bowen JR, MacEwen GD. Hip dysplasia associated with Charcot-Marie-Tooth disease in the older child and adolescent. *J. Pediatr. Orthop.* 5(5):511–514, 1985.

Milbrandt TA, Kunes JR, Karol LA. Friedreich's ataxia and scoliosis: the experience at two institutions. *J. Pediatr. Orthop.* 28(2):234–238, 2008.

Ward CM, Dolan LA, Bennett DL, Morcuende JA, Cooper RR. Long-term results of reconstruction for treatment of a flexible cavovarus foot in Charcot-Marie-Tooth disease. *J. Bone Joint Surg. Am.* 90(12):2631–2642, 2008.

Wetmore RS, Drennan JC. Long-term results of triple arthrodesis in Charcot-Marie-Tooth disease. *J. Bone Joint Surg. Am.* 71(3):417–422, 1989.

CHAPTER 12

SYNDROMES

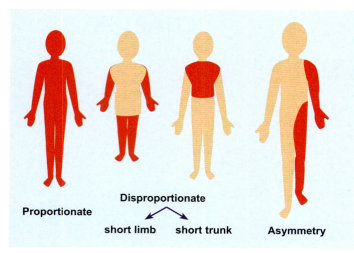

A   Short stature This may proportionate or disproportionate, or it may affect a region of the body asymmetrically.

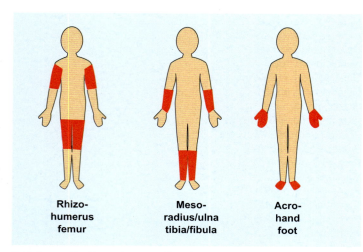

B   Micromelia Shortening may affect the "root" or proximal segment, the "middle" segment, or the "tip" of the limb.

Syndrome	Facies
Achondroplasia	Frontal bossing, depressed nasal bridge
Apert	Proptosis, downsloping palpebral fissures
Camptodactyly	Flat face
Cantu syndrome	Full lips, long philtrum
Cornelia de Lange	Synophrys, "carp" mouth
de Barsy	Progeroid
Down	Mongoloid
Emanuel	Low-hanging columella
Freeman-Sheldon	Whistling face
Hurler	Gargoyle
Larsen	Dish face
Pseudoachondroplasia	Normal face
Proteus	Elephant man
Rubinstein-Taybi	Squinting smile
Silver-Russell	Triangular face

C   Facies Many syndromes may be distinguished by appearance of the face.

GENERAL CONSIDERATIONS

The title *syndromes* is used for lack of a more inclusive term. Syndromes are arranged in alphabetical order for simplicity. There is no comprehensive system of classification that is complete, because of diverse causes, heterogeneity of presentation, evolution of expression with growth, as well as rapid and continual medical discovery. These are diseases first and orthopedic problems second: most important is evaluation, because orthopedic management will not solve the primary problem and may deliver a fair outcome at best. This contrasts with disorders of the musculoskeletal system that occur in an otherwise normal child, where orthopedic management is the focus. All tissues of the skeleton may be affected, from bone to cartilage to surrounding soft tissues. The clinical presentation is broad, from premature osteoporotic fracture in the adult to perinatal lethal. While individually the disorders may be rare, collectively, their incidence may be as high as 1/5,000 births. It is important to realize that many diagnoses do not represent a single disease but rather a heterogeneous group of disorders of which only some subtypes are well characterized while others originate in single case reports.

Language

Syndrome, used by Galen as a compound of Greek συν: "with, together" and δρομοσ: "a course, race, running," signifies "a concurrence" of signs in, or the clinical presentation of, a disease.

Short stature may be defined as <2 standard deviations below mean height or below 2.5 percentile. An alternative guideline is height <5 ft. (150 cm). Short stature may be divided into proportionate, affecting the entire body equally, or disproportionate. Terms such as midget for the former and dwarf for the latter are not universally accepted. Little person is neutral and is aligned with the Little People of America.

Disproportion of short stature may arise from the limbs, referred to as micromelia (Greek μικρος: "small" and μελος: "limb"). Disproportionate shortening of the "trunk" is known as microcormia (Greek κορμος) [A]. Limb shortening may be asymmetric. Alternatively, limbs may be short at the "root," known as rhizomicromelia (Greek ριζα); at the "middle" segment, known as mesomicromelia (Greek μεσος); or at the "tip," known as acromicromelia (Greek ακρος) [B]]. This terminology comes from radiographic classification based upon the region of bone principally affected, such as epiphysis *versus* metaphysis versus diaphysis. The convenience of this system has led to its wide adoption; however, it is simplistic, bears no relationship to morbidity, and frequently suggests a connection between entities where there is none.

Of the skeleton, dysplasia (Greek δυς: "bad" and πλασσω: "I form") represents a generalized affection of the skeleton. Dysostosis (Greek οστεον: "bone") refers to involvement of a single bone or a group of physically or functionally related bones. Dysmorphism (Greek Morpheus, God of Sleep who may take any human "form" in dreams) is applied to a "bad form" of body part, often the *facies* (Latin) or "face" that can distinguish a specific disorder [C].

Classification

These disorders have been given descriptive names according to clinical presentation, pathogenesis, or radiographic appearance. Achondroplasia emphasizes cartilage as locus of disease, while osteogenesis imperfecta distinguishes bone as the abnormal tissue. Other skeletal dysplasia may be grouped according to whether they affect the metaphysis or the epiphysis of a long bone. Identification of genetic mutations has allowed molecular typing. For example, the type II collagenopathies span a spectrum from the severe Kniest dysplasia to spondyloepiphysial dysplasia and Stickler disease to the relatively mild precocious osteoarthritis. Challenges of molecular classification include:

- The molecular defects are numerous and evolving.
- Clinically unrelated disorders may have the same molecular defect. Achondroplasia is caused by mutation of one type (3) of fibroblast

growth factor receptor, while other types produce the craniosynostosis syndromes of Pfeiffer (1) and Crouzon (2).

- Clinically related disorders may have different molecular defects. Mutations in the gene encoding type IX collagen and the gene encoding cartilage oligomeric matrix protein both have been found in multiple epiphysial dysplasia.
- The molecular defects are heterogeneous, obscuring the biologic pathways to disease. The highest expression of fibroblast growth factor receptor 3 is in the brain, yet it is the expression in cartilage during endochondral ossification that is responsible for the clinical manifestations of achondroplasia.

Despite these limitations, knowledge of molecular biology may aid understanding of the tissue distribution of disease. Type I collagen is the principal structural protein of bone, dentin, and sclera, hence the association (and clinical subclassification) of osteogenesis imperfecta with dentinogenesis imperfecta and blue sclerae. Type II collagen occurs in cartilage and vitreous humor. As a result, Stickler arthroophthalmopathy may include osteoarthritis and retinal detachment.

Evaluation

Assess clinical features, support with imaging, and verify with histologic analysis and laboratory studies if available.

Stature After facial appearance, stature is most distinguishing. Stature may be short, normal, or tall. Short stature may be proportionate, such as in endocrinopathy, or disproportionate, such as skeletal dysplasias. Few syndromes feature tall stature, such as Marfan. Neuromuscular disorders do not affect stature significantly.

Family history Many syndromes are inheritable. They may be autosomal or X-linked and dominant or recessive. Others represent new spontaneous mutations. Neurofibromatosis type 1 is transmitted as an autosomal dominant to half affected children, while in the other half, the disorder arises spontaneously.

Development Some syndromes are characterized by global delay, such as Prader-Willi syndrome. Others affect cognitive or motor function separately, such as muscular dystrophy. Developmental delay may be temporal or permanent; for example, in achondroplasia, motor development may be delayed in the first 2 years, due to macrocephaly and ligamentous laxity.

System Divide conditions into those that affect the musculoskeletal system and those that affect other systems and viscera [D]. Within the musculoskeletal system, conditions may be categorized geographically according to the part affected.

Pathognomonic features From Greek παθος: "disease" and γιγνωσκω: "I know," these may form the nidus around which other findings may be assembled. This approach represents a primary focus on the disease, in contrast with the system approach, which focuses on the manifestation [E].

Imaging

RÖNTGENOGRAMMES These form the basis of evaluation. They may describe a disease geographically.

- Part of the skeleton, for example, spondylo- for spine
- Part of a long bone, for example, epiphysial, metaphyseal, and diaphyseal

Röntgenogrammes may describe the skeleton qualitatively.

- Increased density, for example, osteopetrosis
- Reduced density, for example, osteogenesis imperfecta
- Mixed, for example, stippling of epiphyses in chondrodysplasia punctata

Röntgenogrammes may reveal features that, while not always present in every patient, are pathognomonic [E].

Radiographic features vary according to age. Many features that may aid diagnosis in childhood disappear by adulthood, such as epiphysial stippling. These features are considered dynamic, a manifestation of abnormal bone development.

Part	Abnormality	Syndrome
Spine	Kyphosis— thoracolumbar	Achondroplasia; metatropic dysplasia; mucopolysaccharidoses
	Kyphosis— cervical	Diastrophic dysplasia; Larsen
	Atlantoaxial instability	Down; Dyggve—Melchior—Causen; Kniest; mucopolysaccharidoses; spondyloepiphysial dysplasia
	Sacrococcygeal	Carpenter; caudal regression
Hip	Coxa vara	Type II collagenopathy
Foot	Club	Arthrogryposis; Bruck; camptomelic dysplasia; caudal regression; diastrophic dysplasia; Escobar; Freeman—Sheldon; Larsen; Melnick—Needles; Möbius; nail—patella
	Polydactyly	Carpenter; chondrodysplasia punctata; chondro—ectodermal dysplasia; Grebe; Rubinstein—Taybi
	Syndactyly	Apert
Long bone	Bowing	Neurofibromatosis (tibia); multiple exostosis (forearm); mesomelic dysplasia
Knee	Patella	Meier—Gorlin; nail—patella; Rubinstein—Taybi; small patella
Elbow	Radial head dislocation	Beals; Cornelia de Lange; nail—patella; mesomelic dysplasia; otopalatodigital
Forearm	Radial anomaly	Goldenhar; Holt—Oram; TAR; VACTERL
Wrist	Supernumerary fusion	Apert; chondro—ectodermal dysplasia; multiple synostosis; otopalatodigital
Hand	Polydactyly	chondro—ectodermal dysplasia
	Syndactyly	Apert
Skin	structure	Bruck; chondrodysplasia punctata; Ehlers—Danlos; melorheostosis; multiple synostosis; pterygium; oculodentodigital dysplasia; proteus; pterygium
	pigmentation	McCune—Albright; neurofibromatosis; oculodentodigital
Joint		Arthrogryposis; epiphysial dysplasia
Muscle		Amyoplasia; Poland
Nerve		cerebral palsy; Friedreich ataxia; Lesch—Nyhan; oculodentodigital dysplasia; Sanfilippo
Blood		Ehelers—Danlos; Klippel—Trénaunay—Weber; Marfan; melorheostosis
Nail		Apert; chondro—ectodermal dysplasia; multiple synostosis; nail—patella; oculodentodigital; otopalatodigital; pycnodysostosis
Hair		Metaphyseal chondrodysplasia of McKusick; oculodentodigital dysplasia; trichorhinophalangeal

D Geographical distribution Syndromes may be distinguished and grouped by anatomic part affected.

Pathognomonic feature	Syndrome
Caudal reduction in interpedicular distance	Achondroplasia
Champagne pelvis	
Elephant ilia	
Cloverleaf skull	Antley-Bixler
Mitten hand and foot	Apert
Macroglossia	Beckwith-Wiedemann
Accordion femora	Osteogenesis imperfecta
Saber tibiae	
Wormian bones	
Blue sclerae	Marshall-Smith, osteogenesis imperfecta
Cauliflower ears—calcification of pinnae	Diastrophic dysplasia
Hitch-hiker thumb—bracchydactyly of first metacarpal	
Cervical kyphosis	
Iliac horns	Nail-patella
Patella: a-/hypo-plasia	Meier-Gorlin; nail-patella
Absent or bifid clavicles	Cleidocranial dysostosis
Hot-cross bun skull	
Double hump vertebrae	Dygvve-Melchior-Clausen
Exostoses directed away from physis	hereditary multiple exostosis
Exostoses directed toward physis	metachondromatosis
Accessory calcaneal apophysis	Larsen syndrome
Lace-border iliac crests	Dyggve-Melchior-Clausen
Monophalangic hallux	Fibrodysplasia ossificans progressiva
Whistling face	Freeman-Sheldon
Ashkenazim	Familial dysautonomia; Gaucher; Tay-Sachs
Erlenmeyer flask femur	Craniometaphyseal dysplasia; Gaucher
Swiss cheese epiphysial degeneration	Kniest dysplasia
Café-au-lait patches	'Coast of Maine': McCune-Albright
	'Cost of California': neurofibromatosis
Lisch nodule	Neurofibromatosis
Coccyx prolongation like a tail	Metatropic dysplasia
Synostosis	Antley-Bixler; Apert; femoral-facial syndrome; mesomelic dysplasia; multiple synostosis
Madelung deformity	Leri-Weill dyschondrosteosis
Sandwich vertebrae, rugger jersey spine, endobones.	Osteopetrosis (of Albers-Schönberg)
Tree frog feet.	
Secondary ossification center at base of second metacarpal and metatarsal	otopalatodigital
Second metacarpal pseudo-epiphysis	Silver-Russell

E Pathognomonic features These may offer direction in a sea of complexity.

ULTRASONOGRAPHY This modality may establish a prenatal diagnosis. The fundamental finding is short limbs for gestational age. A small thorax (including reduced thoracic:abdominal ratio) is a feature of lethal skeletal dysplasias. There may be clinical expression of osseous disease, for example, fractures in osteogenesis imperfecta. There may be delayed or absent ossification, for example, of the clavicles in cleidocranial dysplasia. There may be regional abnormalities, for example, clubfoot in diastrophic dysplasia.

OTHER IMAGING MODALITIES These are employed according to specific relevance to disease. In achondroplasia, foramen magnum stenosis may be measured on computed axial tomography. Published disease-specific standards are available based upon such measurements. Critical stenosis of the vertebral canal due to spine deformity may be evaluated by magnetic resonance imaging.

Laboratory analysis This most commonly is performed of blood, urine, and skin. Chromosome number, size, position, and staining pattern may be determined by karyotyping blood. Hormone serum levels, for example, growth hormone, thyroxine, and thyroid stimulating hormone, identify endocrinopathy. The mucopolysaccharidoses are characterized by enzyme deficiency leading to reduction of product and accumulation of precursor that is detected by urine assay. The clinical diagnosis of Marfan syndrome may be confirmed by immunohistochemical staining or pulse-chase analysis of fibrillin-1 protein in cultured skin cells obtained from skin biopsy. Biochemical and molecular analysis of skin and blood for type I collagen mutation aids the diagnosis and typing of osteogenesis imperfecta. Ehlers-Danlos VI may be confirmed by insufficiency of hydroxylysine on analysis of hydrolyzed dermis, reduced lysyl hydroxylase activity in cultured skin fibroblasts, and altered ratio of lysyl pyridinoline to hydroxylysyl pyridinoline in urine.

Algorithm

The following is a singular and simplified approach to turn the key and open the door to this multidisciplinary area into which may be drawn the orthopedic surgeon at times insecure and intimidated [F].

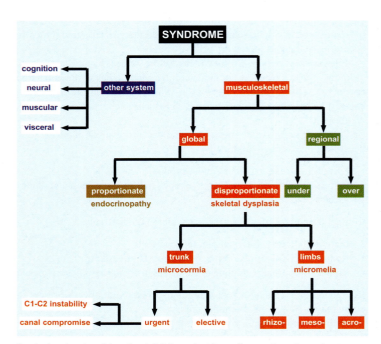

F A simple algorithm for initial navigation of a syndromic patient.

ACHONDROPLASIA

Most common skeletal dysplasia, with incidence ~ 1:25,000 live births.

Gain-of-function fibroblast growth factor receptor 3 (FGFR3) mutation on chromosome 4p16.3 codon 380 glycine. Chondrocyte activation of FGFR3 increases bone formation and accelerates fusion of ossification centers with premature synchondrosis closure, limiting endochondral bone growth.

This may be transmitted as autosomal dominant with complete penetrance; however, most are new spontaneous mutations. A family of FGFR3 mutations is recognized ranging from mild (hypochondroplasia) to moderate (achondroplasia) to severe (thanatophoric dysplasia).

Features do not become apparent on ultrasonogram until after 16 weeks.

Abnormal endochondral with spared membranous ossification produces a large head with narrow foramen magnum, "champagne pelvis" with constricted triradiate cartilage [A], long clavicles with broad shoulders, long fibulae with varus ankles and knees [B], and short pedicles with lumbar spinal stenosis [C]. Hypotonia in infancy, rhizomicromelia [D], frontal bossing with midface hypoplasia, trident hand [E], thoracolumbar kyphosis, joint contractures (including at the hips exaggerating lumbar lordosis), and "chevron" metaphyses.

Decompression of brainstem for foramen magnum stenosis, based upon MRI compared with normative data, somatosensory evoked potentials, and polysomnography. Spine osteotomy and fusion for thoracolumbar kyphosis. Due to pedicle hypoplasia, decompression for lumbar spinal stenosis must include articular process excision, requiring fusion and instrumentation. Osteotomy for genua vara. Physeodesis of distal fibula for ankle varus.

Nonsurgical treatment includes weight control, management of frequent middle ear infections and dental crowding, adenotonsillectomy and nasal mask continuous positive airway pressure for obstructive sleep apnea.

Pharmacotherapy includes growth hormone (although there is no consensus), and BMN-111, a stabilized version of C-type natriuretic peptide that inhibits the FGFR3 pathway.

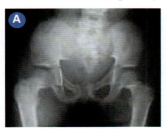

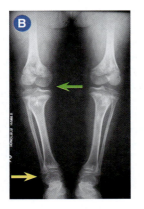

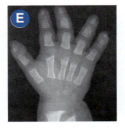

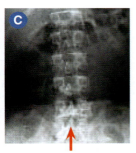

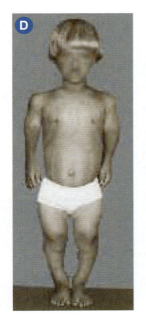

Future strategies for treatment include the following:

- Chemical inhibitors of FGFR3 tyrosine kinase
- Antibodies to interfere with binding of FGF ligands to FGFR3
- C-type natriuretic peptide antagonism of FGFR3 downstream signaling by inhibition of mitogen-activated protein kinase pathway in growth plate chondrocytes, thereby recovering bone growth

ACRODYSOSTOSIS

Type 1 caused by heterozygous mutation in PRKAR1A gene on chromosome 17q24, and type 2 by mutation in PDE4D gene on chromosome 5q12.

Peripheral dysostosis (short tubular bones) of hands and feet. Reduced interpedicular distance producing spinal stenosis. Stippling of cone-shaped epiphyses resolves spontaneously in the first few years of age.

AMNIOTIC BAND SYNDROME

Also known as Streeter anomaly.

Herniation of members through ruptured amnion results in constriction, vascular occlusion, and necrosis. ADAM (amniotic deformity, adhesions, mutilations) complex includes associated terminal transverse defects and cleft lip and palate. LBWD (limb body wall defect) includes associated body wall and visceral defects explained by pressure on the embryo during the first 4 weeks.

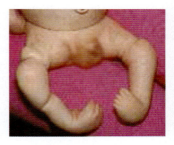

AMYOPLASIA

See arthrogryposis.

ANTLEY-BIXLER SYNDROME

Mutation of cytochrome P450 oxidoreductase on 7q11.23.

Trapezoidocephaly secondary to lambdoid and coronal synostosis, radiohumeral and radioulnar synostosis, and camptodactyly.

Abnormal steroidogenesis and genitourinary and cardiac anomalies.

Airway obstruction may lead to demise in the neonatal period.

APERT SYNDROME

Mutation in fibroblast growth factor receptor 2 gene (FGFR2). By contrast with dominant mutations in the FGFR3 gene, which affect endochondral ossification resulting in achondroplasia, dominant mutations of FGFR1 and FGFR2 cause the craniosynostosis syndromes of Apert, Crouzon, and Pfeiffer, which involve bones arising by membranous ossification.

Autosomal dominant; however, most *de novo* mutations.

Wheaton first reported two cases of what Apert called acrocephalosyndactyly. Acrocephaly is due to coronal synostosis [A]: early decompressive craniectomy may limit mental deficiency. Syndactyly and synonychia produce "mitten" hand [B] and "sock" foot [C]: the former is an indication for release, and the latter for osteotomy or ostectomy to relieve pressure. Failure of cervical segmentation, broad thumbs and halluces, and carpal and tarsal coalition. Cardiac, respiratory, nervous, abdominal, and genitourinary anomalies.

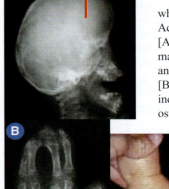

ARTHROGRYPOSIS

Originally termed arthrogryposis multiplex congenita. Arthrogryposis refers to a heterogeneous group of disorders of which the common feature is multiple congenital joint contractures. Fetal akinesia due to maternal disease, intrauterine constraint, or vascular compromise retards development of nerves, muscles, or connective tissues. The earlier and longer the loss of movement, the more severe the deformities. Muscle is replaced by fibrofatty tissue. Arthrogryposis without other system disease is subclassified as amyoplasia. Distal arthrogryposis, affecting hands and feet, is autosomal dominant. Intelligence is normal. Limited joint motion, medial rotation of shoulders, extension of elbows, flexion and ulnar deviation of wrists, camptodactyly, thumb in palm, hip dislocation, knee

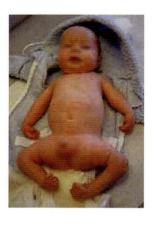

contracture, clubfoot, and scoliosis. Loss of cutaneous creases with joint dimpling. Operative reduction of dislocated hips is controversial. Femoral shortening facilitates treatment of flexion contracture. Center the arc of motion at 15 degrees: walking is easier on straight knees. Talectomy may be necessary for clubfoot. Stiffness limits correction of scoliosis.

BEALS SYNDROME

Type	Features
I	Known as auriculo–osteodysplasia. Autosomal dominant. Short stature, auricular anomalies including elongation of lobe with secondary posterior lobule, radiocapitular dysplasia with head of radius dislocation, hip dysplasia.
II	Known as congenital contractural arachnodactyly. Mutation in fibrillin-2 gene at 5q23-q31. Marfan syndrome without visceral involvement and with crumpled ear helices as the hallmark, due to expression of fibrillin-2 in auricular cartilage.

BECKWITH-WIEDEMANN SYNDROME

Mutations in several imprinted genes within 11p15.5 region, as well as mutation of 5q35. The former also is affected in Silver-Russell syndrome, while the latter in Sotos syndrome.

Autosomal dominant with variable expressivity, as well as *de novo* mutation.

Overgrowth, including macroglossia, exophthalmos, limb hypertrophy, and visceromegaly. Tumor diathesis, including Wilms tumor, hepatoblastoma, neuroblastoma, and adrenal carcinoma. Posterior helical ear pits, abdominal wall defects including umbilical hernia, and renal anomalies. Neonatal hypoglycemia and history of hydramnios and prematurity.

BRACHYDACTYLY

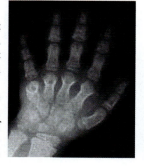

Multiple mutations identified for different types and subtypes. Classified into groups A to E, each of which are subclassified. First syndrome in humans in which Mendelian inheritance was described.

Premature physeal closure; variable short stature; short metacarpals, metatarsals, and phalanges; and variable shortening of humerus, radius, and ulna. Hypersegmentation with an extra ossicle producing phalangeal deviation distinguishes type C.

BRACHYOLMIA (BRACHYRHACHIA)

Named from Greek βραχυς: "short" and ολμος: "trunk," whence the synonym brachyrhachia, from Greek ραχις: "spine".

Type	Features
1	Hobaek, Toledo. Autosomal recessive. Scoliosis, endplate irregularity, intervertebral narrowing, corneal opacities (Toledo), precocious calcification of costal cartilage.
2	Maroteaux. Autosomal recessive. Affects the spine less, and is associated with precocious calcification of the falx cerebri.
3	Autosomal dominant, caused by a gain of function mutation in the gene for transient receptor potential cation channel subfamily V member 4, a Ca^{2+} channel. Allelic with Charcot-Marie-Tooth and spinal muscular atrophy, distal subtype. Kyphoscoliosis and flattened, irregular cervical vertebrae.
4	Autosomal recessive, caused by mutation in gene encoding enzyme bifunctional 3'-phosphoadenosine 5'-phosphosulfate synthetase 2. The enzyme synthesizes 3'-phosphoadenosine 5'-phosphosulfate from ATP and inorganic sulfate, providing the source for cellular sulfation.

BRUCK SYNDROME

Type	Mutation
1	Mutation of FKBP10 gene on 17q21.
2	Mutation of PLOD2 gene on 3q23-q24.

Deficiency of bone-specific telopeptide lysyl hydroxylase, resulting in aberrant cross-linking of type I collagen. Lysine residues in the triple helix are normally hydroxylated. Enzyme normal in cartilage and ligament.

Fractures and Wormian bones resemble osteogenesis imperfecta. Normal sclerae and teeth. Contractures resemble arthrogryposis, hence the appellation "osteogenesis imperfecta with joint contractures." Pterygia, scoliosis, and clubfoot.

CAFFEY DISEASE (INFANTILE CORTICAL HYPEROSTOSIS)

Mutation of 17q21.31-q22, which encodes the α-1 chain of type 1 collagen; however, no features of osteogenesis imperfecta.

Autosomal dominant as well as *de novo* mutation.

Onset in the first few months of life with spontaneous resolution by 2 years with minimal sequelae. Despite its name, it has been detected by ultrasonogram *in utero* (prenatal form) and in adulthood.

Inflammatory presentation, including fever and hot, tender long bones [A] and mandibles [B], which show diaphyseal periosteal deposition.

This is distinct among hereditary disorders in being transient and leaving no residue.

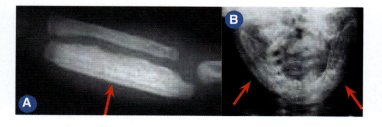

CAMP(T)OMELIC DYSPLASIA

Greek καμπη: "bending, flexion, and twisting" and μελοσ: "limb," to describe the characteristic feature of long bone bowing, especially of the tibiae, clubfoot, and hip dislocation.

17q24 mutation with haploinsufficiency of SOX 9.

Cutaneous dimpling at apex of bowing. Cleft palate, micrognathia, flat face, and pterygium colli. Thoracic dysplasia, including tracheobronchial hypoplasia, bladeless scapulae, slender or absent ribs, reduced cage volume, and sternal mineralization. Congenital heart and kidney disease. Death is frequent in infancy due to respiratory insufficiency.

Gonadal dysgenesis may culminate in sex reversal of affected XY cases.

CARPENTER SYNDROME

Autosomal recessive mutation in Ras-associated protein RAB23 gene on 6p11.

Also called acrocephalopolysyndactyly. Craniosynostosis produces a "pointed head." Brachysyndactyly of the hands and preaxial polysyndactyly of the feet. Correction of genu valgum to stabilize patellae. Pilonidal dimple with absent coccyx.

Variable mental retardation, short stature, obesity, and eye, ear, cardiovascular, and genitourinary anomalies.

CHONDRODYSPLASIA PUNCTATA (CONRADI-HÜNERMANN)

Dominant mutation in the gene encoding delta(8)-delta(7) sterol isomerase emopamil-binding protein on Xp11.23-p11.22, an enzyme essential to cholesterol biosynthesis. Rhizomicromelic dwarfism characterized by asymmetry of involvement and by calcific stippling of trachea, thorax, spine, pelvis, coracoid process, and glenoidal cavity. The latter typically resolves after first year of life. Kyphoscoliosis and clubfoot. Cutaneous disease, including striated ichthyosiform hyperkeratosis, whorled pigmentation, cicatricial alopecia, and "orange-peel" skin. Ocular anomalies, including cataracts, nystagmus, and glaucoma. Warfarin teratogenicity, by inhibition of synthesis of gamma-carboxyglutamic acid, which is involved in both clotting and calcification, may lead to chondrodysplasia punctata.

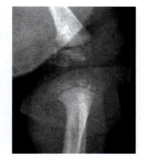

CHONDROECTODERMAL DYSPLASIA (ELLIS-VAN CREVELD)

Mutation in Ellis-van Creveld gene on 4p16. Micromelic dwarfism characterized by postaxial polydactyly, capitate–hamate fusion, genua valga, clubfoot, nail dystrophy, and rib hypoplasia with narrow chest. Upper lip anomaly described as "lip-tie" [A] and tooth eruption at birth described as "natal teeth." Cardiac and male genitourinary anomalies and variable mental retardation. Largest pedigree in the Old Order Amish of Lancaster County, Pennsylvania, whose members were described as having "six-fingered dwarfism." On the way to a pædiatric conference in England (1938), the Scott Ellis met the Dutchman van Creveld while sitting in the same compartment of a train, where they discussed a case they each had seen independently.

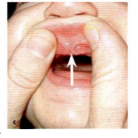

CLEIDOCRANIAL DYSPLASIA

Autosomal dominant loss-of-function mutation in runt-related transcription factor 2 gene (RUNX2) on 6p21.1.

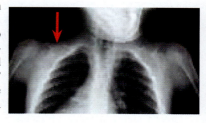

Head has been likened to a "hot cross bun" due to persistent open sutures. The head also is known as "Arnold" head, after a Muslim Chinese progenitor from South Africa with >1,000 descendants.

Midline defects, including hypoplastic or aplastic clavicles with hypermobile shoulders, short middle phalanges, coxa vara, symphysis pubis diastasis, scoliosis, and spondylolisthesis. Dental anomalies.

Formerly called "dysostosis" to emphasize the regional nature of anomalies of the head and shoulder.

CORNELIA DE LANGE SYNDROME

Autosomal dominant as well as *de novo* mutation in Nipped B-like (NIPBL) gene on 5p13.1, which encodes a component of cohesin, a protein complex that coheres sister chromatids during cell division. Characteristic facies, including synophrys, crescentic, or "carp" mouth, long philtrum, anteverted nares, and ptosis.

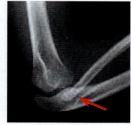

Mental and growth retardation, "growling" cry, hirsutism, and ocular, cardiac, genitourinary, gastrointestinal, and pulmonary anomalies. Self-injurious and autistic behavior. Micromelia disproportionately affecting the upper limb, including ulnar dysgenesis, radial head dislocation, oligodactyly, proximally placed thumb, clinodactyly of smallest finger, and single palmar flexion crease.

de Lange was Professor of Pædiatrics at the University of Amsterdam, where she was followed by van Creveld. The disorder was described 17 years earlier (1916) by Brachmann, whose studies were interrupted by a call to the German Army.

CRANIODIAPHYSEAL DYSPLASIA

Mutation in the SOST gene on 17q12-q21.

Hyperostosis of skull encroaches on foramina and osseous canals leading to cranial nerve palsy and hearing loss, of face results in "leonine facies," and of the skeleton bones produces diaphyseal sclerosis and medullary stenosis, in particular of ribs, clavicles, and sternum.

CRANIOMETAPHYSEAL DYSPLASIA

Autosomal dominant form caused by mutation in the human homolog of mouse progressive ankylosis gene on 5p15.2-p14.1. Additional autosomal recessive form mapped to chromosome 6q21-22.

Skull and facial manifestations similar though less severe than above. Metaphyseal rather than diaphyseal involvement is distinguished by "Erlenmeyer flask" deformity in long bones.

de BARSY SYNDROME

This is one of the progeroid syndromes, which are distinguished by cutis laxa with subcutaneous paucity of fat and prominence of veins, together with "pseudohydrocephalic" head, producing an "old appearance," from Greek γερων: "old man."

This type most affects the skeleton: multiple joint dislocations and subluxations, in particular of the hip, scoliosis, and vertical talus.

Other features include corneal clouding, short stature, and mental retardation.

DIASTROPHIC DYSPLASIA

Mutation in the solute carrier family 26 (sulfate transporter), member 2, gene (SLC26A2) on 5q32-q33.1. Allelic to epiphysial dysplasia, multiple. Greek δια-, an emphatic prefix, and στρεφω, "I twist," describe the "severely twisted" clubfeet and spine. The latter includes thoracolumbar kyphoscoliosis and cervical kyphosis [A]. Short first metacarpal producing "hitchhiker thumb" [B] and calcification of pinnae producing "cauliflower ear." The former permits diagnosis on ultrasonogram at 16 months *in utero*. Multiple joint contractures and malformations, in particular of the hips, which show flattening and a "double-hump" deformation.

Other features include cleft palate, collapse of the tracheobronchial tree, and restrictive pulmonary disease.

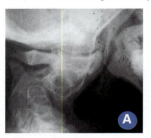 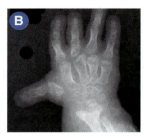

DOWN SYNDROME (TRISOMY 21)

Genomic dosage imbalance at 21q22.3 producing phenotypic variability. Diagnosis by Quad test (serum α-fetoprotein, estriol, β-HCG, and inhibin A) in second trimester of pregnancy: a positive test is followed by amniocentesis.

Risk increases with maternal age: 9-fold from 30 years to 40 years. Incidence is 1:1,000.

"Mongoloid" facies; simian (Latin *simia*: "ape") crease (single transverse palmar); hypotonia; ligamentous laxity; instability of C1-C2 [A], hips [B], and patella; flat feet; and scoliosis.

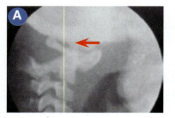 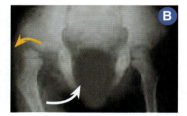

Screen for C1-C2 instability in symptomatic patient, including local signs, such as torticollis and neck stiffness, and global signs, such as myelopathy. Asymptomatic or general screening is contraindicated:

- Symptoms and signs precede neural injury.
- Radiographic instability may alternate with stability without clinical correlation.
- Atlantoaxial fusion has a high complication rate.

Cognitive impairment; hearing loss, usually conductive; hypothyroidism; and congenital malformation of heart, in particular atrioventricular septal defect; gut, such as duodenal atresia; blood, in particular leukemia; and brain, including senile plaques and neurofibrillary tangles leading to premature Alzheimer disease.

The disorder was first described by John Langdon Haydon Down of London, whose *Observations on an Ethnic Classification of Idiots* (1866) included a description of the "Mongoloid" type. While this study has been condemned as racist, the final sentence suggests no such intention, as Down regarded the "degeneracy" across racial barriers "to furnish some arguments in favour of the unity of the human species."

Down also first described a mentally delayed obese girl whose hands and feet remained small as a hypogonadal adult, seven decades before the report of Prader, Labhart, and Willi.

DYGGVE-MELCHIOR-CLAUSEN SYNDROME

Mutation in dymeclin gene at 18q21.1.

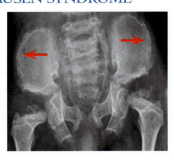

Dymeclin is necessary for correct organization of Golgi apparatus. Allelic with Smith-McCort dysplasia. Psychomotor retardation, hip instability with waddling gait, odontoid hypoplasia with C1-C2 instability, platyspondyly, vertebral anterior beaking and kyphoscoliosis, hypoplasia of scapula and glenoid cavity, epiphysial/apophyseal irregularity manifesting as "lace-border" iliac crests, widening of sacroiliac joints and symphysis pubis, and camptodactyly.

DYSPLASIA EPIPHYSIALIS HEMIMELICA

Also known as Trevor disease. Non-Mendelian and nonfamilial. Boys more than thrice girls. Osteocartilaginous tumors arising from epiphyses, often lower limb, multilevel, and ipsilateral. Lesions cause pain, swelling, and deformity, starting during infancy or early childhood. Radiolucency of lesions delays diagnosis. Manage by excision and osteotomy for deformity correction. Recurrence is common, necessitating repeat operation(s).

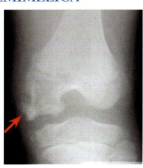

EHLERS-DANLOS SYNDROMES

A group of hereditable disorders characterized by:

- Skin hyperextensibility. Acrogeria. Collagen fibers seen on electron microscopy of skin have been likened to hieroglyphics.
- Articular hypermobility. Instability of hip, patella, elbow, and shoulder.
- Tissue fragility. Prematurity in 50% due to premature rupture of fetal membranes. Vascular and visceral rupture. Bruisable skin that heals with "cigarette paper" scars. Hernia and pneumothorax.
- Skeletal deformity. Kyphoscoliosis, spondylolisthesis, atlantoaxial rotatory displacement, flatfoot, and pectus deformity. Tendency to recurrent deformity after correction.

The disorder may be classified into 10 subtypes, but V, VIII, and X may not be distinct entities. The subtypes have distinguishing features, with variable overlap. Most have autosomal dominant transmission.

Type	Mutation
I	Type V collagen α-1 chain on 9q34.3. Type V collagen α-2 chain on 2q32.2. Type I collagen α-1 chain on 17q21.33.
II	Type V collagen α-1 chain on 9q34.3.
III	Tenascin-XB on 6p21.3. Type III collagen α-1 chain on 2q32.2.
IV	Type III collagen α-1 chain on 2q32.2.
V	Abnormal collagen cross-linking due to deficiency of lysyl hydroxylase.
VI	Lysyl hydroxylase on 1p36.22.
VII	Type I procollagen N-proteinase on 5q35.3.
VIII	12p13.
IX	Cu(2+)-transporting ATPase, alpha polypeptide on Xq21.1. Allelic to Menkes syndrome.
X	Fibronectin.

Type	Features
I	Classic gravis: "severe".
II	Classic mitis: "mild". Mildness may delay or preclude diagnosis.
III	Hypermobility without skeletal deformity.
IV	Vascular. Autosomal dominant or recessive. Spontaneous rupture of major vessels and viscera. Aneurysm, fistula.
V	X-linked.
VI	Ocular-scoliotic. Kyphoscoliosis from infancy. Retinal detachment, scleral fragility, rupture of ocular globe.
VII	Dermatosparaxis ("skin tearing") due to abnormal type I collagen in skin. Autosomal recessive.
VIII	Peri-odontitis: gingival recession, premature loss of teeth, resorption of alveolar bone.
IX	Skull. Occipital horns adjacent foramen magnum directed caudad. Wormian bones. Coarse hair.
X	Striae distensae. Petechiae due to defect in platelet aggregation.

EMANUEL SYNDROME

Malsegregation of the t(11;22)(q23;q11.2) translocation, a rare example in humans of reciprocal (non-Robertsonian) exchange of genetic material between chromosomes.

Kyphosis and scoliosis and hip dislocation.

Ear: preauricular tag and sinus, low set, hearing loss, and otitis media.

Eyes: hooded eyelids, strabismus, and myopia.

Psychomotor delay; seizures; cardiovascular anomalies, including aortic and pulmonary stenosis and septal defects; and genitourinary anomalies, including absent kidney and cryptorchidism.

EPIPHYSIAL DYSPLASIA, MULTIPLE

Genetic heterogeneity manifested by six types, designated EDM1-6.

Type	Features
1	Mutation in the gene for cartilage oligomeric matrix protein on 19p13.11. Includes milder form (Ribbing) and more severe form (Fairbank). Allelic to pseudoachondroplasia. Diagnosis aided by reduced serum levels of cartilage oligomeric matrix protein
2	Mutation in gene encoding type 9 collagen α-2 chain on 1p33-p32.2, which also has been implicated in susceptibility to intervertebral disc disease with sciatica.
3	Mutation in gene encoding type 9 collagen α-3 chain on 20q13.33. Myopathy may distinguish this type.
4	Mutation in the solute carrier family 26 (sulfate transporter), member 2 gene (SLC26A2) on 5q32-q33.1. Allelic to diastrophic dysplasia, atelosteogenesis II, achondrogenesis IB. Distinguished by clubfoot and double-layered patella (red arrows).
5	Mutation in matrilin-3 gene on 2p24.1. Allelic to one form of spondylo-epimetaphyseal dysplasia.
6	Mutation in gene encoding type 9 collagen α-1 chain on 6q13.

Normal to moderate short stature. Delayed and irregular epiphysial formation leads to long bone deformity, in particular coxa vara, genua vara or valga, and brachydactyly as well as premature osteoarthritis.

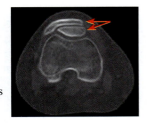

Multiple epiphysial involvement distinguishes this disorder from Legg-Calvé-Perthes disease. Sparing of the spine distinguishes it from spondyloepiphysial dysplasia.

ESCOBAR SYNDROME

See pterygium syndrome.

FAMILIAL DYSAUTONOMIA

Also known as Riley-Day syndrome, congenital insensitivity to pain, and hereditary sensory and autonomic neuropathy type III.

Mutations in the inhibitor of kappa light polypeptide gene enhancer in B cells, kinase complex-associated protein (IKBKAP) gene on 9q31.3.

Diminished pain and temperature perception leads to self-inflicted injuries. Vasomotor instability often triggered by stress, hyperhidrosis, alacrima, cutaneous blotching, and absence of fungiform papillae on tongue. Lack of axon flare after intradermal injection of histamine. Gastrointestinal and renal dysfunction. Increased prevalence in Ashkenazi Jewish descent.

Orthopedic problems include fracture, autoamputation, osteomyelitis, septic arthritis, neuropathic arthropathy, vibratory loss, areflexia, and scoliosis.

Emotional lability and absence of pain dictate conservative management.

FANCONI ANÆMIA

Genetically heterogeneous with 15 complementation groups. Common feature is abnormal DNA breakage, cross-linking, and repair.

Myelophthisis with pancytopenia requires bone marrow transplant.

Short stature. Radial defects, including hypoplastic/absent/bifid thumb as well as absent radius, require reconstruction.

Genitourinary anomalies, including hypoplastic/absent/horseshoe/ectopic kidney, hypogonadism, cardiac septal defects, hyperpigmentation with *café au lait* spots, and malignant diathesis.

FEMORAL–FACIAL SYNDROME

Facies characterized by long philtrum, thin upper lip, hypoplastic alae nasi, and microretrognathia.

Femoral hypoplasia/aplasia with acetabular dysplasia. Radioulnar and radiohumeral synostosis. Congenital scoliosis. Sacral dysplasia may resemble caudal regression syndrome. Feet with preaxial polysyndactyly and clubfoot. Sprengel anomaly.

Cardiac and genitourinary anomalies.

One-third of patients have a prenatal history of maternal diabetes.

FIBRODYSPLASIA OSSIFICANS PROGRESSIVA

Distinguish *myositis ossificans*, a general term for heterotopic ossification that may be subclassified as *traumatica* when it follows injury and is not hereditable.

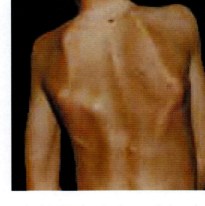

Mutation in activin A receptor type I gene on 2q24.1 results in abnormal signal transduction in response to bone morphogenetic protein type I.

Episodic and unpredictable heterotopic ossification of striated muscle, in craniocaudad, axial to appendicular, and proximal to distal directions.

Only signs at birth are halluceal deformation and monophalangism. Clinodactyly, digital reduction defects, vertebral fusion, hearing loss, and alopecia.

Pain and ankylosis, which may be exacerbated by trauma (both accidental and iatrogenic).

Mean age of onset 5 years; confinement to wheelchair by third decade.

Restrictive pulmonary disease may lead to respiratory failure.

Eighty percent of patients receive an incorrect initial diagnosis. Diagnosis is clinical: while lesions may be confused with malignancy, avoid biopsy as it exacerbates condition.

FREEMAN-SHELDON SYNDROME

Also known as whistling face–windmill vane hand syndrome and cranio-carpotarsal dystrophy.

Mutation in embryonic skeletal muscle myosin heavy chain 3 gene on 17p13.1.

A type of distal arthrogryposis.

Small mouth with pursed lips resembles whistling. Camptodactyly with ulnar deviation has been likened to a windmill vanes. Kyphoscoliosis. Contractures of hips (without or with dislocation), knees, and shoulders. Clubfoot and vertical talus.

Myopathy and seizure. Malignant hyperthermia may impact operation.

FRIEDREICH ATAXIA

Mutation in frataxin gene on 9q21.11. Second locus on 9p reflects genetic heterogeneity. Frataxin is involved in mitochondrial iron homeostasis.

Autosomal recessive. Most common inherited ataxia.

Ataxia, absent deep tendon reflexes, impaired proprioception and vibratory sense, dysarthria, extensor plantar response (Babinski), and nystagmus.

Pes cavus and scoliosis.

Preadolescent onset; confinement to wheelchair by fourth decade.

Hypertrophic cardiomyopathy: death most frequently from heart failure.

GAUCHER DISEASE

Mutation in gene encoding acid β-glucosidase on 1q22.

Autosomal recessive lysosomal storage disease cerebroside lipidosis.

Cells of mononuclear phagocyte origin (such as macrophages) laden with glucosylceramide (glucosylcerebroside), known as Gaucher cells, accumulate in bone marrow, spleen, liver, lung, ocular limbus, and skin, leading to pancytopenia, hepatosplenomegaly, interstitial restrictive lung disease, pingueculae, and cutaneous pigmentation.

Continuum and wide spectrum of severity: perinatal lethal to asymptomatic adult.

Osteolysis, bone crises, and pathologic fractures. Widening of distal

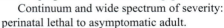

Type	Features
1	Non-neuropathic.
2	Neuropathic—acute. Perinatal or infantile lethal.
3	Neuropathic—chronic. Later onset, slower progression.

metaphysis of femur likened to "Erlenmeyer flask" (orange). Osteonecrosis of head of femur managed by hip arthroplasty.

Partial splenectomy for thrombocytopenia, to balance risk of sepsis.

Multifaceted treatment includes enzyme replacement, chemical chaperone, substrate reduction, and bone marrow transplantation.

Increased prevalence in Ashkenazi Jewish descent.

GOLDENHAR SYNDROME

Linked to 14q32.

Also known as oculoauriculovertebral dysplasia and hemifacial microsomia.

Anomalies of first and second branchial arch derivatives.

Facial reconstruction for asymmetric eye and ear anomalies.

Spine fusion for congenital scoliosis. Reconstruction for radial ray anomalies, which are ipsilateral to facial anomalies.

Congenital heart disease, including tetralogy of Fallot and coarctation of aorta. Central nervous system lesions, including hydrocephalus and cerebellar hypoplasia. Genitourinary anomalies, including multicystic or ectopic kidney.

GUILLAIN-BARRÉ SYNDROME

Familial type caused by mutation in the peripheral myelin protein 22 gene on 17p12. Allelic with Charcot-Marie-Tooth disease type 1.

Acute demyelinating polyneuropathy resulting from aberrant immune mechanism suggested by preceding upper respiratory infection or *Campylobacter jejuni* enteritis.

Ascending symmetric flaccid paralysis, proximal muscles more affected, ophthalmoplegia, and dysphagia. Variable sensory involvement, including loss of proprioception, and autonomic dysfunction, such as arrhythmia.

Involvement of respiratory muscles may necessitate ventilator support.

Cerebrospinal fluid analysis shows albuminocytologic dissociation: elevated protein without elevated cell count, in contrast with infection.

Treat with plasmapheresis or immunoglobulin *per venam*.

HAND–FOOT–GENITAL SYNDROME

Mutation in the homeobox A13 gene on 7p15.2.

Genitourinary anomalies, including double uterus and bifid scrotum.

Short first metacarpal and metatarsal result in proximal location of hypoplastic thumbs and halluces. Smallest finger clinodactyly–brachydactyly. Carpal and tarsal fusions.

HÆMOPHILIA

Type	Features
A	Mutation in gene encoding coagulation factor VIII on Xq28. Recessive affects boys. Mild (40% of cases): 6–30% factor level, hæmorrhage after trauma. Moderate (10%): 1–5%. Severe (50%): <1%, at least monthly spontaneous hæmorrhage. 1:10000
B Christmas disease	Mutation in gene encoding coagulation factor XI on Xq27.1. Recessive. 1:30,000 Named after patient Stephen Christmas (1947–1993). B(M): inhibition of factor VII by abnormal factor IX prolongs PT. B Leyden: factor IX increases after puberty to eliminate hæmorrhagic diathesis.

Laboratory tests show normal platelet count and prothrombin time (PT), but a prolonged activated partial thromboplastin time (aPTT).

Hemorrhage into joints and muscles, in contrast with bleeding disorders due to platelet defects or von Willebrand disease, in which mucosal bleeding predominates.

Hemarthrosis begins after walking and is characterized by swelling, pain, stiffness, and inflammatory arthritis. Muscle hemorrhage causes necrosis, contractures, and neuropathy by entrapment.

Chronic synovitis unresponsive to factor replacement is associated with HLA-B27 allele, which prevents downregulation of inflammatory mediators after hemarthrosis.

Orthopedic management includes synovectomy, arthroplasty, and radial head resection.

Medical treatment consists of factor VIII infusion. Add gamma globulin and cyclophosphamide to induce tolerance in 10% of patients who develop antibodies to factor VIII.

Heterozygous female carriers have 50% factor levels, reducing coagulability without clinical signs. Mortality is reduced 20% due to reduction in ischemic heart disease.

Hæmophilia affected the Romanov imperial dynasty of Russia and Queen Victoria of England, who was a carrier.

HOLT-ORAM SYNDROME

Autosomal dominant mutation in T-box 5 gene on chromosome 12q24.21. T-box 5 is a transcription factor involved in heart development and limb identity.

Also known by the descriptive appellations heart–hand syndrome and atriodigital dysplasia.

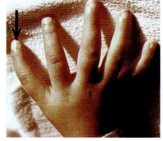

Congenital cardiac defects, including atrial septal defect and hypoplastic left heart.

Preaxial upper limb anomalies, including absent, bifid, or triphalangeal fingerlike thumb (arrow), proximal and distal thumb metacarpal epiphyses, radial club hand and hypoplasia, radioulnar synostosis, and carpal abnormality.

Anomalies of shoulder girdle and thorax. Asymmetric involvement of upper limbs, left greater than right, consistent with cardiac link.

HOMOCYSTINURIA

Autosomal recessive mutation in gene encoding cystathionine β-synthase on chromosome 21q22.3. Cystathionine β-synthase converts homocystine to cystathionine. Elevated homocystine and by-product methionine, diagnosed in urine.

Developmental delay, seizures, and ocular anomalies in particular ectopia lentis within the first decade, which requires operative treatment.

Thromboembolism is the major cause of morbidity and early death. Prophylactic anticoagulation for high-risk periods such as pregnancy.

Osteoporosis by second decade manifested by "codfish" vertebrae on lumbar röntgenogramme. Kyphoscoliosis and dolichostenomelia, but limited joint mobility, which distinguishes this disorder from Marfan syndrome.

Treat with dietary restriction of protein, betaine therapy, and pyridoxine (B6). Responsiveness to pyridoxine distinguishes a milder phenotype from the more severe nonresponsive phenotype.

KLIPPEL-FEIL SYNDROME

See Spine chapter.

KLIPPEL-TRÉNAUNAY-WEBER SYNDROME

Mutation of 8q22.3, or gain-of-function translocation of 8q22;14q13, possibly involving gain of function of the gene encoding the angiogenic factor VG5Q.

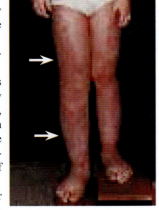

Also known as angioosteohypertrophy syndrome.

Klippel-Trénaunay syndrome refers to cutaneous hæmangiomata, slow-flow venous and lymphatic malformations, and limb hypertrophy (white). When arteriovenous fistulae are present, the cutaneous manifestations are more diffuse and more pink, and the name of Weber is appended.

Visceral dysfunction due to vascular malformations, such as thrombocytopenia, pulmonary embolus, high-output cardiac insufficiency, and seizure.

Length equalization by physeodesis of affected limb may be necessary. Synovial vascular hypertrophy may elicit pain and benefit from arthroscopic débridement. Surgical debulking is controversial.

Compression stockings reduce blood and lymph pooling and thereby pain, swelling, and ulceration. Sclerotherapy thickens and ultimately blocks abnormal vascular channels.

KNIEST DYSPLASIA

Mutation of a-1 chain of type II collagen on 12q13.11.

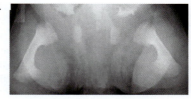

Severe type II collagenopathy.

Phenotype reflects distribution of type II collagen in cartilage and vitreous humor.

Disproportionate short stature, kyphoscoliosis, hypoplasia/aplasia of dens axis producing atlantoaxial instability, "dumbbell" long bones with splayed metaphyses/epiphyses, "Swiss cheese" epiphysial degeneration, coxa vara, joint narrowing, and contractures.

Myopia, retinal detachment, cataracts, and lens dislocation.

LARSEN SYNDROME

Autosomal dominant mutation of filamin B gene on 3p14.3. Filamin B cross-links protein actin to regulate communication between cell membrane and cytoskeletal network. This is allelic with atelosteogenesis type I.

Autosomal recessive mutation in β-1,3-glucuronyltransferase 3 gene on 11q12.3. The enzyme catalyzes glycosaminoglycan–protein linkage in proteoglycans.

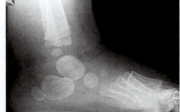

Cluster island of La Reunion (Indian Ocean off east coast of Africa).

1:1,500 compared with 1:100,000 in Western countries.

Dislocations of large joints, in particular hip, knee, and elbow.

Accessory calcaneal (green) and carpal ossification centers, equinovarus and equinovalgus, "spatula" fingers, brachydactyly, congenital scoliosis, and cervical kyphosis.

"Dish" facies due to prominent forehead with flat midportion.

Stabilize spine, reconstruct dislocations, and correct foot deformity.

LÉRI-WEILL DYSCHONDROSTEOSIS

Pseudo–autosomal dominant mutation in the short stature homeobox gene on Xp22.33 and Yp11.32, or deletion of the SHOX downstream regulator. Allelic with Langer mesomelic dysplasia, of which the phenotype is more severe.

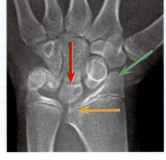

Mesomicromelia with bowing and Madelung deformity. Madelung deformity represents a growth disturbance of the volar ulnar part of the distal physis of radius, which results in volar translation of wrist and hand and dorsal displacement of the normally growing distal ulna. It is characterized by lucency (orange) at the locus of growth disturbance, triangular distortion of the distal epiphysis (green), and pyramidalization (red) of the wrist as it falls into the defect.

Girls more severely affected than boys.

LESCH-NYHAN SYNDROME

X-linked recessive mutation in hypoxanthine guanine phosphoribosyltransferase gene on Xq26.2-q26.3. The enzyme salvages purines from degraded DNA to reintroduce into purine synthetic pathways. While complete or severe (<1% activity) deficiency is the feature of Lesch-Nyhan syndrome, mild deficiency causes hyperuricemia and gout.

Hyperuricemia and hyperuricosuria causing nephrolithiasis.

Neural signs predominate: psychomotor delay, choreiform movements, athetosis and spasticity, dysarthria, and dysphagia.

Short stature, hip dysplasia, scoliosis, fractures, self-mutilation and digital autoamputations, and infections.

MAFUCCI SYNDROME

See Ollier disease.

MARFAN SYNDROME

Mutation of fibrillin-1 gene on 15q21.1.

Fibrillin-1 is the major constitutive element of extracellular microfibrils, distributed in elastic and nonelastic connective tissue. The microfibrils store in an inactivated form transforming growth factor-β (TGF-β); abnormal microfibrillar architecture results in increased release and thereby activation of TGF-β for cellular proliferation, differentiation, motility, and apoptosis. Thus, the effect of fibrillin-1 mutation is both primarily structural and secondary to hyperactivity of TGF-β.

Fibrillin-1 provides force-bearing structural support, its synthesis correlating with late morphogenesis and appearance of well-defined organ structures. Synthesis of fibrillin-2, of which mutation causes congenital contractural arachnodactyly (of Beals *q.v.*), coincides with early morphogenesis and the beginning of elastogenesis, during which it regulates elastic fiber assembly. Fibrillin is distributed in the periosteum, aortic media, and suspensory ligament of the lens, hence the three principal systems affected.

Tissue	Features
Skeletal	disproportionate tall stature • upper:lower segment < 0.85 • arm span:height > 1.05 • mean adult male height 190 cm • mean adult female height 175 cm dolichocephaly micro-/retro-gnathia pectus: carinatum, excavatum, asymmetry dural ectasia scoliosis + kyphosis spondylolisthesis protrusio acetabuli dolichostenomelia arachnodactyly articular hypermobility or contracture pes planus
Cardiac	aortic root dilatation: regurgitation + dissection aortic aneurysm pulmonary artery dilatation
Ocular	ectopia lentis myopia retinal detachment cataract
Other	high arched palate dental crowding pneumothorax striae distensae abdominal hernia

Puberty onset 2 years premature.

Trisomy 8, of which most cases are mosaic hence mildness of presentation, resembles skeletal features of Marfan syndrome.

Cardiovascular disease accounts for mortality. Treatment is pharmacologic, including β-adrenergic blockade and angiotensin II receptor antagonists, and surgical, such as aortic valve and root graft.

Orthopedic care is focused upon deformity of the spine (*q.v.*). Triradiate physeodesis has been advocated for protrusio acetabuli.

The condition first was described by Giovanni Morgagni (1682–1771), at autopsy of a prostitute distinguished by her tall stature and long, gracile limbs (in particular the fingers), who died *in coitu* of aortic dissection.

Antoine Marfan (1858–1942) described the condition in a 5-year-girl as dolichostenomelia, from Greek δολιχος: "long," στενοσ: "thin," and μελοσ: "limb." Niccolò Paganini (1782–1840), whose death was attributed to internal hemorrhage, is believed to have been affected by Marfan syndrome, including the arachnodactyly and articular hypermobility that aided his virtuosity at violin. Abraham Lincoln (1809–1865) probably had multiple endocrine neoplasia type 2B, which mimics the skeletal features of Marfan syndrome.

Diagnosis is based upon family history and a systemic score.

Family history	No family history
Aortic root dilatation Ectopia lentis systemic score ≥ 7	Aortic root dilatation AND • fibrillin-1 mutation • ectopia lentis • systemic score ≥ 7

Systemic score	
Wrist and thumb sign	3
Dural ectasia	2
Protrusio acetabuli	2
Pes planus	2
Pectus carinatum	2
Pectus excavatum, asymmetry	1
Scoliosis or kyphosis	1
Elbow contracture	1
Craniofacial dysmorphia	1
Myopia	1
Mitral valve prolapse	1
Striae distensae	1

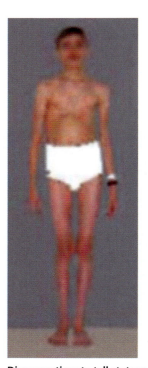

Disproportionate tall stature.

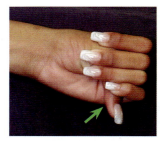

Arachnodactyly Thumb sign is defined as thumb interphalangeal joint reaching ulnar border of hand (*green*). Wrist sign is defined as ringing of the wrist by thumb reaching distal interphalangeal joint of smallest finger.

MARSHALL-SMITH SYNDROME

Mutation in nuclear factor 1 X–type gene on 19p13.3.

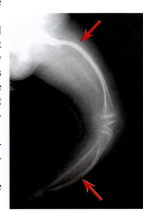

Accelerated or disharmonic skeletal maturation. Osseous fragility may result in "nontraumatic" fractures and secondary deformity. Absence of osteopenia suggests a qualitative rather than a quantitative defect in bone. Orthopedic management includes bisphosphonates and fracture stabilization.

Characteristic facies includes prominent forehead, micrognathia, exophthalmos, and blue sclerae.

Osseous fragility and blue sclerae resemble osteogenesis imperfecta.

Psychomotor delay and failure to thrive.

Respiratory compromise accounts for the majority of mortality.

MᶜCUNE-ALBRIGHT SYNDROME

Gain-of-function or constitutively activating postzygotic somatic cell mutation of guanine nucleotide–binding protein α-stimulating activity polypeptide 1 gene (GNAS1) on 20q13.32.

Clinical triad:

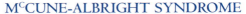

- Polyostotic fibrous dysplasia of long and craniofacial bones
- *Café au lait* cutaneous patches with irregular or "coast of Maine" borders
- Precocious puberty

Deformity, such as Shepherd crook femur, and morbid fracture produced by fibrous dysplasia require orthopedic intervention, including bisphosphonate and operation.

Craniofacial hyperostosis may produce deafness and blindness due to neural foraminal compression.

Cutaneous patches are asymmetric and often end abruptly at the body midline. They may be distinguished from those of neurofibromatosis, which have smooth or "coast of California" borders, are smaller, and include axillary freckling.

Signs of puberty, such as vaginal bleeding and spermatogenesis, may be seen in the first half of the first decade.

Endocrinopathy is variable in type and extent, including in addition to hyperthyroidism, pituitary gigantism, and Cushing syndrome due to hyperadrenocorticism.

MEIER-GORLIN SYNDROME

Five types caused by mutations in ORC1 gene on 1p32.3 (1), ORC4 gene on 2q22.3 (2), ORC6 gene on 16q11.2 (3), CDT1 gene on 16q24.3 (4), and CDC6 gene on 17q21.2 (5).

Also known as ear–patella–short stature syndrome.

Microtia, auditory canal atresia, hearing loss, micrognathia, and cleft palate.

Thoracic dysplasia with pulmonary compromise and genital anomalies.

Aplastic/hypoplastic patellae, congenital spine deformity, articular laxity, clubfoot, and camptodactyly–clinodactyly.

MELNICK-NEEDLES SYNDROME

See otopalatodigital syndromes.

MELORHEOSTOSIS

Mutation in the LEMD3 gene on 12q14.3. LEMD3 is a protein integral to the inner nuclear membrane that is involved in gene expression.

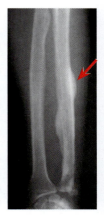

The term is derived from Greek μελος: "limb," ρεω: "I flow," and οστεον: "bone" to describe longitudinal flowing hyperostosis along the cortex of long bones resembling wax dripping along a candlestick. Bones are affected asymmetrically and may correspond with a sclerotome.

Involvement of surrounding soft tissues leads to painful and deforming contractures, muscle atrophy, and scleroderma. Associated vascular anomalies such as hæmangiomata, lymphangiectasis, vascular nevi, glomus tumors, stenosis, and aneurysms.

MESOMELIC DYSPLASIA

Mesomicromelia and synostosis are the cardinal features. Radioulnar, carpal, tarsal, and metatarsal synostosis, radial capital subluxation, and bowing of long bones, including "rhomboid" tibiae and fibulae.

Four types may be distinguished.

Type	Features
Kantapura	Mutation on 2q24-q32.
Langer	Mutation in short stature homeo box gene. Allelic with Léri-Weill dyschondrosteosis. Distinguished by mandibular hypoplasia.
Nievergelt	Autosomal dominant mutation of α–1 chain of type 10 collagen on 6q22.1. Mild short stature.
Savarirayan	Mutation of LAF4 gene on 2q11.2.

METACHONDROMATOSIS

Autosomal dominant mutation in protein tyrosine phosphatase nonreceptor type 11 gene on 12q24. The protein tyrosine phosphatase family are signaling proteins.

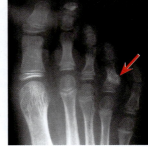

The disorder is allelic with Noonan syndrome (*q.v.*).

Combines features of enchondromatosis (of Ollier *q.v.*) and hereditary multiple exostoses (*q.v.*). Distinguished by:

- Direction of exostoses toward adjacent joints
- Predominance in hands and feet
- Potential for spontaneous regression
- Lack of malignant potential

Involvement of the hip may resemble.

Legg-Calvé-Perthes disease.

METAPHYSEAL CHONDRODYSPLASIA

Metaphyseal involvement contrasts with epiphysial sparing and results in contractures rather than primary osteoarthritis.

Bowing of long bones produces varus deformity in lower limbs.

Stature varies from mild (Schmid) to moderate (MᶜKusick) to severe (Jensen).

Type	Features
Jansen	Mutation in parathyroid hormone receptor 1 gene on 3p21.31. Ligand-independent activation disrupts endochondral ossification. Cranial sclerosis leading to deafness, choanal stenosis or atresia. Skeletal manifestations resemble hyperparathyroidism, including osteopenic fractures. Hypercalcæmia and hypercalcuria with nephrocalcinosis. Hypophosphatæmia, hyperphosphaturia, elevated 1,25 dihydroxy vitamin D and alkaline phosphatase.
McKusick	Autosomal recessive mutation of RNA component of mitochondrial RNA processing endoribonuclease on 9p13.3. Appellation 'cartilage-hair hypoplasia' reflects distinguishing feature of sparse, small caliber hair. Immune deficiency manifested as susceptibility to infection and increased risk of malignancy. Hæmocytopenia. Clustered in Old Order Amish and in Finland.
Schmid	Autosomal dominant mutation of a-1 chain of type 10 collagen on 6q22.1.

METATROPIC DYSPLASIA

Mutation in the transient receptor potential cation channel subfamily V member 4 gene on 12q24.11. TRPV4 is a Ca^{2+} channel.

Allelic with brachyolmia type 3, spondyloepiphysial dysplasia (Maroteaux), spondylometaphyseal dysplasia (Kozlowski), and Charcot-Marie-Tooth type 2C.

The term describes a "change" (Greek τροπη) in clinical presentation of severity of deformity from limbs (resembling achondroplasia) to trunk (resembling Morquio syndrome) with growth. At birth, the limbs are markedly affected with relative sparing of the trunk; with advancing age, progressive and severe kyphoscoliosis becomes the predominant feature.

Prolongation of the coccyx or the presence of a cutaneous fold over the posterior aspect of the pelvis gives the appearance of a tail.

Deformity of the iliac alae results in a "halberd" pelvis. The ends of femora and humeri are said to be "trumpeted," rather than "dumbbell" in Kniest dysplasia. Microcalcification of epiphyses, hyoid, and cricoid cartilages.

MÖBIUS SYNDROME

Gene locus on 13q12.2-q13.

Congenital cranial neuropathy, most frequently facial and abducens, leading to facial paralysis and impaired ocular abduction.

Arthrogryposis, digital anomalies, clubfoot, scoliosis with increased sagittal plane spine deformity.

Absence of pectoralis muscles reflects association with Poland syndrome.

MUCOPOLYSACCHARIDOSES

Characterized by intracellular accumulation and urinary excretion of mucopolysaccharides [A] due to deficiency in degradative lysosomal enzymes. Mucopolysaccharide is the historical term for glycosaminoglycan (GAG). Proteoglycans, formerly known as protein polysaccharides or mucoproteins, refers to a molecule of "protein and sugar." It has three components:

- Glycosaminoglycan (GAG). This represents an unbranched chain of repeating disaccharide units of which one is an amino sugar. With the exception of hyaluronic acid, the GAGs carry a high negative charge on the account of sulfate and carboxyl groups added to their sugar residues.
- Core protein, to which GAGs are covalently bonded at a serine residue by a tetrasaccharide bridge.
- Link protein, which noncovalently attaches proteoglycan to hyaluronic acid, the principal carbohydrate polymer of the extracellular matrix.

Proteoglycan monomers interact specifically though noncovalently with hyaluronic acid to form very high molecular weight "aggregates." The major proteoglycan of cartilage is aggrecan, of which the core protein may have covalently attached as many as 100 chondroitin sulfate and 50 keratan sulfate GAGs. Cartilage also contains small, nonaggregating proteoglycans, including decorin, which "decorates" the surface of type II collagen fibrils, and biglycan, of which the core protein bears "two" chondroitin sulfate GAGs. The molecular structure and negative charge of proteoglycans enable them to occupy a large volume for mass and to attract water according to the Gibbs-Donnan equilibrium. They form a porous hydrated gel, which resists compression and regulates the passage of molecules and cells through the extracellular matrix. By contrast, collagen fibrils form a scaffold, which maintains the structural integrity of the extracellular matrix and primarily resists tensile forces.

There are several types of mucopolysaccharidoses. Type II is X-linked. Type III is predominantly a neural disease. Type IV is most common. Types VI and IX may have normal intelligence.

Type	Features
Ih (Hurler) **Is (Scheie)**	Autosomal recessive mutation in α–L-iduronidase gene on 4p16.3. Scheie was formerly type V. Appear normal at birth, manifesting after 6 months. Developmental and growth retardation after 2 years. Gargoyle facies, with exophthalmos, corneal clouding, thick eye-brows and large tongue. Odontoid hypoplasia with atlanto-axial instability, 'cod-fish' vertebrae, lumbar gibbus, kyphoscoliosis. 'Oar-shaped' ribs, epiphysial deformation including hip dysplasia and genua valga. Cardiopulmonary anomalies, including myopathy and arrhythmia, hernias, hepatosplenomegaly. Dermal melanocytosis, hypertrichosis.
II (Hunter)	X-linked recessive mutation in iduronidate 2-sulfatase on Xq28. Urinary excretion of chondroitin sulfate B (dermatan sulfate) and heparitin (heparan) sulfate.
III (Sanfilippo)	Autosomal recessive mutation in N-sulfoglucosamine sulfohydrolase gene on 17q25.3 resulting in impaired degradation of heparan sulfate, excreted in urine. Severe nervous system disease with relative sparing of skeleton.
IV (Morquio)	Autosomal recessive mutation in β–galactosidase gene on 3p22.3. Urinary excretion of keratan sulfate.
VI (Maroteaux-Lamy)	Autosomal recessive mutation in arylsulfatase B gene on 5q14.1.
VII (Sly)	Autosomal recessive mutation in β–glucuronidase gene on 7q11.21. Hydrops fœtalis.
IX	Mutation in hyaluronidase gene on 3p21.31. Multiple peri-arthric masses representing hyaluronan-induced aggregation of histiocytes resulting form failure of catabolism of hyaluronan by hyaluronidase.

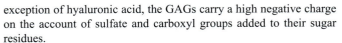

Hurler and Scheie represent a spectrum of severe to mild disease. Scheie may be so mild that diagnosis is in adulthood. The other disorders are subtyped by letter according to disease severity.

Carpal tunnel syndrome is a common feature of the mucopolysaccharidoses, due in part to excessive lysosomal storage in the flexor retinaculum. Spine [B] and hip [C] are the other foci of orthopædic care.

Anteoperative assessment must include cardiac evaluation and cervical spine imaging.

Medical treatment includes enzyme replacement and bone marrow transplantation. The latter, performed before age 2 years, prolongs survival and, while they may delay or halt extraskeletal disease progression, they may not affect skeletal manifestations.

A form of mucopolysaccharidosis, claimed to be due to glucosamine-6-sulfate sulfatase deficiency, named Di Ferrante syndrome, and given the designation VIII, was found to be erroneous and retired after the discovery of type IX.

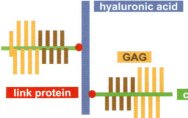

A   Extracellular matrix Proteoglycans are glycosylated proteins consisting of a core protein to which one or more types of glycosaminoglycan are covalently linked.

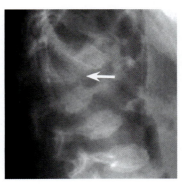

B   Lumbar gibbus in Hurler syndrome Failure of formation of upper lumbar vertebra allows the superjacent vertebra to fall forward into the deficiency space.

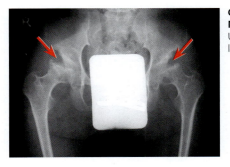

C   Hip dysplasia in Morquio syndrome Untreated hip dysplasia may lead to severe coxarthritis.

MULTIPLE ENCHONDROMATOSIS

Benign tumors of cartilage located in metaphyses of long bones, where lesions are asymmetric and deforming.

Hands and feet most involved.

Orthopedic management focuses on limb equalization and realignment osteotomy.

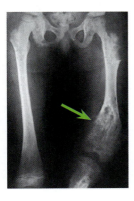

Type	Features
Ollier	Malignant transformation to chondrosarcoma 10-30%.
Mafucci	Associated with hæmangiomata. Higher rate of malignant transformation, including of extraskeletal tissue.

MULTIPLE EXOSTOSES

Also known as multiple osteochondromata and diaphyseal aclasis, describing a lesion of "bone" capped by "cartilage" showing "lack of an interruption" of the "diaphysis" from the primary bone.

There are three types, distinguished genetically.

Type	Features
I	Autosomal dominant mutation in exostosin-1 (EXT1) gene on 8q24, resulting in activation of the hedgehog signaling pathway. 70% of all cases, most morbid form.
II	Autosomal dominant mutation in exostosin-2 gene on 11p11.2.
III	Mapped to locus on 19.

Lesions arise from physis, grow away from adjacent joint, and affect long bones, flat bones (except skull), and vertebrae.

This contrasts from the solitary form of the disease:

- The exostoses are deforming, including bowing, shortening, and joint dysplasia.
- Mild short stature.
- Malignant transformation is approximately 1%. Symptoms and signs include pain and rapid growth.

Restraint is fundamental to orthopedic management.

Indications for operation include:

- Pain, such as at prominent lesions that may be struck.
- Dysfunction, such as compression of tibial nerve producing denervation of tibialis posterior muscle (red).
- Deformity, such as tethering by a shortened ulna , which may lead to radial bowing, ulnad displacement of the wrist, and head of radius dislocation.
- Unacceptable appearance.
- Concern for malignant transformation.

MULTIPLE SYNOSTOSIS SYNDROME

Three subtypes are distinguished by mutation.

Type	Features
1	Mutation in homolog of mouse Noggin gene on 17q22.
2	Mutation in growth/differentiation factor-5 on 20q11.22. GDF5 belongs to the transforming growth factor –β superfamily. Allelic with several disorders, including brachydactyly types A and C.
3	Mutation in fibroblast growth factor 9 gene on 13q12.11. FGF9 is a member of fibroblast growth factor family.

The alternate appellation facioaudiosymphalangism syndrome describes the principal clinical manifestations.

Narrow face, nasal hypoplasia, and conductive deafness due to middle ear ankylosis.

Multiple synostoses, including carpal and tarsal coalitions, brachydactyly, radial head (sub)luxation, vertebral fusion and hypoplasia producing stenosis, and pectus deformity.

Absent cutaneous creases over interphalangeal joints, aplastic/hypoplastic nails.

NAIL–PATELLA SYNDROME

Autosomal dominant mutation in LIM homeobox transcription factor 1-b on q34.1. LMX1B plays a role in dorsoventral patterning of the

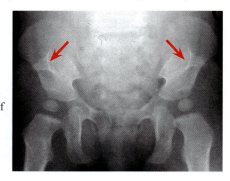

vertebrate limb and renal development. Absence or hypoplasia/dysplasia of nails and patellae, as well as of pectoralis, biceps, and quadriceps muscles, represents ventral patterning of the dorsal aspects of the limbs.

Short stature, iliac horns, limited elbow motion with radial head hypoplasia and dislocation, scapular anomaly, scoliosis, and clubfoot.

Renal disease, including glomerulonephritis with proteinuria and hematuria, ends in renal failure in 10% of patients.

Sensorineural deafness, glaucoma, cataract, and cleft lip and palate.

NEUROFIBROMATOSIS

Type	Features	
	Autosomal dominant mutation in neurofibromin gene on 17q11.2. Neurofibromin is a tumor suppressor inhibiting p21 ras oncoprotein. Also known as von Recklinghausen disease. 90% of cases with a 1:4000 incidence. Diagnosis requires 2 of the following:	
	Diagnosis - 2 features	
1 - Peripheral	*Café-au-lait* patches	≥ 6 > 5 mm before puberty > 15 mm after puberty
	Neurofibromata	> 2 subcutaneous 1 plexiform
	Freckling	axillary or inguinal
	Osseous lesion	sphenoid dysplasia scoliosis congenital pseudarthrosis
	Family history	First-degree relative with NF1
	Lisch nodule	hamartoma of iris
	Optic glioma	
2 - Central	Autosomal dominant mutation in merlin (neurofibromin 2) gene on 22q12.2. Sensorineural hearing loss, ocular anomalies but no Lisch nodules, central and peripheral neuropathy, neural tumors including vestibular schwannoma (of vestibulocochlear cranial nerve VIII), meningioma, ependymoma, astrocytoma. Central affection delays diagnosis. Stereotactic radiosurgery or microsurgical resection of vestibular schwannoma.	

Simple neurofibromata, made up of Schwann cells and fibrous tissue, rarely produce deficit. Plexiform neurofibromata, which are highly vascular, lead to disfigurement and gigantism, which may require limb equalization.

Café au lait patches have smooth or "coast of California" borders, in distinction from the rough or "coast of Maine borders" in McCune-Albright syndrome.

Scoliosis may be idiopathic or "dystrophic." The former behaves and is treated as such. The latter is characterized by short and sharp angulation, osseous erosion by intraspinal lesions and dural ectasia, and spinal instability. Bracing plays no role, and early anterior together with posterior fusion is indicated because of the risk of pseudarthrosis. Neural risk is significant, untreated or treated.

Pseudarthrosis may involve any bone, though most often the tibia, presenting as an anterolateral bow. This is treated by prophylactic bracing to avoid fracture, and operative treatment after fracture, including compressive external fixation or medullary nailing with autogenous osseous graft or vascularized fibula transference. Bone morphogenetic protein as adjuvant is controversial.

Other features include cognitive impairment, macrocephaly without hydrocephalus, seizures, and vascular anomalies. Neurofibromatosis 1 carries an increased tumor risk, including leukemia and pheochromocytoma.

While the Irish surgeon Robert W. Smith (1849) was first to report two men with "a vast number of neuromatous tumors in the subcutaneous cellular tissues," von Recklinghausen's description in tribute to his professor Rudolph Virchow gave the enduring eponym for neurofibromatosis 1.

Feature	%	
Café-au-lait patches	95	
Lisch nodules	90	
Axillary freckling	80	
Cutaneous neurofibromata	60	
Cognitive impairment	60	
Family history	50	
Scoliosis	40	
Pseudarthrosis	15	
Malignancy	10	
Spinal neurofibromata	2	

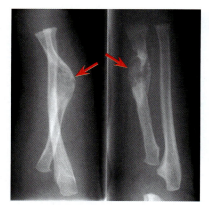

Pseudarthrosis of radius
Deformity begets dysfunction.

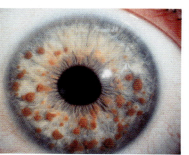

Lisch nodules These represent a yellow to brown pigmented hamartoma of the iris, consisting of dendritic melanocytes. They do not affect vision, but aid diagnosis.

OCULODENTODIGITAL DYSPLASIA

Autosomal dominant and recessive mutations in the gap junction α-1 protein gene on 6q22.31. The protein is a member of the connexin family and is a component of gap junctions, which form intercellular channels for diffusion.

Ocular: microphthalmos, glaucoma, and cataract.

Dental: hypoplastic enamel, microdontia, and premature tooth loss.

Digital: camptodactyly, syndactyly of ring and smallest fingers as well as of toes, and aphalangia.

Hip dysplasia and hyperostosis, in particular of vertebrae and skull, which can result in neural compression. Osseous involvement other than digits has given rise to the alternate appellation oculodentoosseous dysplasia.

Neural features include spasticity, dysarthria, and hearing loss.

Fine, sparse hair and orange–yellow palmoplantar keratoderma.

OSTEOGENESIS IMPERFECTA

The Dutch anatomist W. Vrolik named the condition osteogenesis imperfecta. It also is known as fragilitas ossium: "brittleness of bones."

Mutation of gene encoding type I collagen α-1 chain on 17q21.33 or α-2 chain on 7q21.3.

Collagen, derived from Greek κολλα: "glue", and the suffix -γεν: "giving rise to," is the name given to a family of proteins that comprise the principal constituents of the extracellular matrix of tissues of the musculoskeletal system. The collagen molecule is composed of three polypeptide chains, two α-1 and one α-2, and is therefore a trimer. Although the primary structure of each polypeptide chain differs among collagen types, repeating three amino acid motifs are strictly preserved, represented by the formula -(GLY-X-Y)n-. Every third residue is a glycine (Gly). X and Y can vary; however, a high proportion of amino acids at the X position tends to be proline (Pro), and a high proportion at the Y position tends to be hydroxyproline (Hyp). Those portions of a collagen chain, which follow this typical motif, are helical and are known as collagenous domains; those that do not are termed noncollagenous domains. The individual chains may be identical, encoded by the same gene, in which case they form a homotrimer, or they may be different gene products, forming a heterotrimer. Cleavage of amino terminal and carboxyl terminal propeptides during or after secretion converts procollagen to collagen. The tertiary structure of each collagen chain is a left-handed helix, and the three chains wrap around one another to form a right-handed super helical molecule.

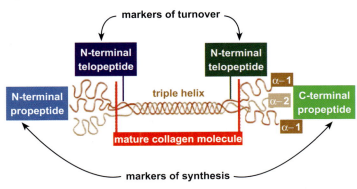

Mutations may result in exclusion or inclusion of an allelic product. In heterozygous-excluded mutations (haploinsufficiency), failure of secretion and incorporation into a protein trimer, or of synthesis (null alleles), of a polypeptide chain, produce mild disease due to a quantitative reduction of normal molecules. In the homozygote, the severity of disease is proportional to the amount of allelic product excluded. Included mutations (dominant negative), such as deletions, insertions, duplications, point mutations, rearrangements, and exon-skipping mutations, result in a more morbid phenotype because the abnormal allelic product

is expressed in the extracellular matrix where it "poisons" all molecules into which it is incorporated. Severe phenotypes result from glycine mutations, because this is the smallest and only amino acid (lacking a side chain) that can fit in the center of the triple helix. Assembly of the collagen molecule commences at the carboxyl terminus. This produces a "phenotypic gradient": mutations in the carboxyl terminal region produce more severe phenotypes based upon a greater potential for disruption of the triple helix. Exceptions to these principles exist: for example, certain mutations are lethal, which do not involve glycine and regardless of location.

Osteogenesis imperfecta is the most common lethal skeletal dysplasia. Phenotype reflects distribution of type I collagen.

Tissue distribution	Feature
Bone	• Osteopenia, with trabecular loss, cortical thinning and gracility of long bones. • Fracture (e.g., of long bones, avulsion of olecranon). • Deformity, including accordion femora, saber tibiae, scoliosis, cod-fish vertebrae, protrusio acetabuli, basilar invagination (type III). • Conductive deafness due to otosclerosis. Wormian bones
Dentin	Blue-grey discoloration, brittleness and excessive wear, malocclusion, late tooth eruption, constricted coronal radicular junctions, obliterated pulp cavities and caries.
Skin	Easy bruisability, bleeding. Decreased elasticity, distensibility, hysteresis.
Connective tissue	• Translucency with visualization of underlying choroidea produces "Wedgewood blue" sclerae. • Ligamentous laxity. • Muscle rupture (e.g., of patellar tendon).

Increased turnover, woven to lamellar bone ratio, and hypercellularity conspire to weaken bone. Fracture healing and postoperative union are unretarded, often with "luxuriant" callus, although the quality of the new bone remains poor. Fracture rate is bimodal: childhood, decreases after puberty, and rises after menopause.

Hearing loss, which affects 50% of patients, begins in second decade as conductive, from osseous fragility in the middle ear, and evolves with age to sensorineural. Otosclerosis also produces vertigo.

Ole Worm, Professor of Anatomy at Copenhagen (1558 to 1654), described intrasutural bones, which may be more numerous in disease states characterized by delayed or deficient ossification.

Mechanism of operative malignant hyperthermia remains unclear.

Four clinical types are distinguished. They are subtyped as A or B based upon absence or presence, respectively, of dentinogenesis imperfecta.

Type	I	II (Vrolik)	III	IV
Mutation	α–1 or α–2 chain of type I collagen			
Inheritance	dominant	new mutation	recessive	dominant
Frequency	50%	5%	25%	20%
Severity	mild	lethal	progressive deforming	variable
Sclerae	blue	blue	blue or white	white
Hearing loss	50%	—	yes	no
Ambulation	yes	—	wheel-chair	yes
Stature	normal	—	very short	short

Ambulatory potential proportional directly to age of onset and inversely to deformity.

Several additional types have been distinguished that are characterized by brittle bones but that are caused by mutations other than of type I collagen.

Type	Features
V	Mutation of interferon -induced transmembrane protein-5 on 11p15.5. Moderate. Normal sclerae, normal teeth. Calcification of interosseous membrane of forearm, dislocation of head of radius, radiodense metaphyseal bands. Osseous histology shows 'mesh-like' pattern.
VI	Mutation of pigment epithelium-derived factor (serine protease inhibitor F1) on 17p13.3. 'Fish scale' lamellæ and hyperosteoidosis suggest defect of mineralization.
VII	Mutation of cartilage associated protein on 3p22.3. First Nations community of northern Quebec.
VIII	Mutation of leprecan on 1p34.2. Concentration in cases of West African origins.
IX	Mutation of peptidylprolyl isomerase B (cyclophilin B) on 15q22.31. Overhydroxylation suggests overmodification of type I collagen.
X	Mutation of serine protease inhibitor H on 11q13.5.
XI	Mutation of FKBP10 member of peptidyl-prolyl cis/ trans isomerase family on 17q21.2.
XII	Mutation of C_2H_2-type zinc finger transcription factor SP7 on 12q13.13.
XIII	Mutation of bone morphogenetic protein 1 on 8p21.3. Resembles type III.
XIV	Mutation of transmembrane protein 38B on 9q31.2.
XV	Mutation of wingless-type MMTV integration site family, member 1, on 12q13.12. Intermediate between type III and type IV.

Types V, VI, and XI may phenotypically be likened to type IV. Type XV may have features of both type III and type IV. The other types resemble type III. Discovery of additional mutations and typing represents an area of flux.

Diagnosis is aided by analysis of type I collagen production by cultured dermal fibroblasts.

Osteogenesis imperfecta leads the differential diagnosis of nonaccidental trauma.

Minimize type and duration of immobilization for fracture in order to reduce sequelae of exacerbated osteopenia, stiffness, and weakness. Recurrent fractures and progressive deformity may be addressed by corrective osteotomy and fixation with either solid or telescoping medullary nails. Scoliosis is treated with early fusion because natural history is progression despite bracing and bone fragility undermines fixation. Symptomatic basilar invagination is treated by posterior with or without anterior decompression followed by posterior fusion.

Audiologic examination and electronystagmography are indicated for hearing loss.

Bisphosphonates are synthetic analogs of pyrophosphate, a natural inhibitor of osteoclastic bone resorption. Cyclic intravenous administration decreases bone turnover; increases bone mineral density, cortical width, and trabecular number; delays onset and reduces number of fractures; improves ambulation; and increases height. Physes are unaffected.

Osteogenesis imperfecta has been described in an Egyptian mummy of the twenty-first dynasty (1,000 BC). The nineteenth-century Viking king and invader of England Ivar Benløs (Ivar the Boneless), who had blue eyes and was carried into battle seated on a shield of bronze, is said to have had "gristle in the limbs where other men had bones."

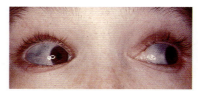

Blue sclerae Subjacent vascular plexus tinges thinned connective tissue.

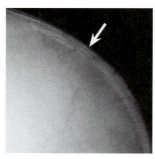

Wormian bones Multiple intrasutural bones of the skull.

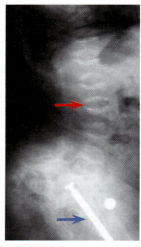

Spine and operative treatment Biconcave vertebral end plates resemble "codfish" (*red*). Telescoping Bailey-Dubow rod (*blue*) strengthens femur against fracture and corrects deformity while allowing for longitudinal growth.

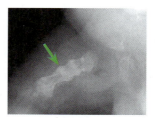
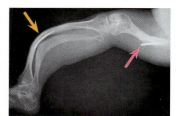

Deformity of long bones Multiple fractures of the femur with hypertrophic callus give the appearance of an accordion (*green*). Bowing of the tibia due to microfragility has been likened to a saber (*orange*). Note migration of Rush rod out of femur (*pink*).

OSTEOPETROSIS

Autosomal recessive also may be referred to as infantile malignant, to describe presentation in childhood and severity of clinical presentation, including death from myelophthisis. Autosomal dominant forms are more benign and typically present in adulthood. Several subtypes have been distinguished, principally based upon mutation. Autosomal dominant 2 was described by Albers-Schönberg and is known as "marble bone disease" after the radiographic appearance.

Osteoclast dysfunction leads to defective resorption of immature bone.

Encroachment upon bone marrow results in pancytopenia and infection, which of the jaw results in dental caries.

Cranial nerve compression results in blindness, deafness, and facial palsy.

Extramedullary hematopoiesis leads to hepatosplenomegaly.

Abnormal bone turnover results in morbid fractures and deformity, which are the foci of orthopedic management. Complication rate is high. Osteosynthesis may be hindered by sclerosis. Arthroplasty is complicated by loosening and infection. Osseous union may be delayed.

Mainstay of medical treatment is bone marrow transplantation. Recombinant human interferon gamma-1b to increase superoxide generation by leukocytes and bone-resorbing agent calcitriol are indicated while awaiting, or for patients who are not candidates for, bone marrow transplantation.

Type	Features
AD 1	Mutation of low density lipoprotein receptor-related protein 5 on 11q13.2, with full penetrance. Osteosclerosis predominates in craniofacial skeleton. Only type not associated with fractures.
AD 2	Mutation of chloride channel-7 protein on 16p13.3, with incomplete penetrance. Same mutation as AR 4. Osteosclerosis predominates in axial and appendicular skeleton. Sclerosis of upper and lower end-plates described as 'sandwich vertebrae' and 'rugger jersey spine'. Differential osteosclerosis produces 'bone within bone' or 'endobones' in the limbs. Confirm diagnosis by elevated serum levels of tartrate-resistant acid phosphatase and BB isoenzyme of creatine kinase. 50% patients require orthopædic surgery.
AR 1	Mutation of V-type proton ATPase subunit of the vacuolar proton pump on 11q13.2. Impairment in calcium homeostasis results in tetanic seizure and secondary hyperparathyroidism.
AR 2	Mutation of receptor activator of nuclear factor kappa-B ligand (RANKL) on 13q14.11. RANKL is an osteoclast cell surface receptor that binds RANK. Clinical mildness resembles dominant forms.
AR 3	Mutation of carbonic anhydrase II, which is expressed in kidney and brain, on 8q21.1. Renal tubular acidosis. The appellation 'marble brain disease' describes mental retardation associated with intracranial calcifications. Originated in Arabian peninsula.
AR 4	Mutation of chloride channel-7 protein on 16p13.3. Same mutation as AD 2.
AR 5	Mutation of osteopetrosis-associated transmembrane protein-1, which prevents acidification of osteoclast resorption lacuna, on 6q21.
AR 6	Mutation of pleckstrin homology domain-containing family M member 1 on 17q21.31. Intermediate form.
AR 7	Mutation of receptor activator of nuclear factor kappa-B (RANK) on 18q21.33. Hypogammaglobulinæmia.
AR 8	Mutation of sorting nexin 10 on 7p15.2.

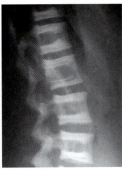

Spine Endplate sclerosis leads to sandwich vertebrae that give the appearance of a rugger jersey.

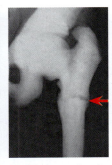

Marble bone Despite the epithet, osseous fragility manifests as morbid fracture.

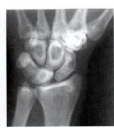

Wrist Bone within bone, or endobones.

OTOPALATODIGITAL SYNDROME

Gain-of-function mutation in filamin A gene on Xq28.

Skeletal Short stature; pectus excavatum; "coat hanger" wavy, short ribs; scoliosis; hip dysplasia; joint contractures; radial head dislocation; long bone bowing; carpal and tarsal fusion; brachydactyly; secondary ossification center at base of second metacarpal and metatarsal; wide spacing between broad toes with persistent fetal pads creates "tree frog" feet; and nail dystrophy.

Craniofacial Cleft palate, conductive deafness caused by ossicular anomalies, and dental dysplasia.

Four disorders are distinguished, representing a phenotypic spectrum of a single entity. Frontometaphyseal dysplasia adds urogenital anomalies, including hydronephrosis/hydroureter, hypospadias, and cryptorchidism.

Perinatal lethal due to cardiopulmonary insufficiency.

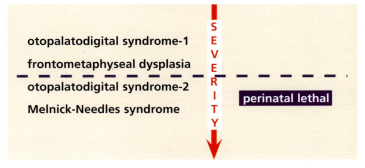

POLAND SYNDROME

Most sporadic, though autosomal dominant pedigrees have been reported.

Ipsilateral aplasia/hypoplasia of pectoralis major and/or minor muscle, which may be associated with Sprengel anomaly; hypoplastic or fused ribs; aplasia/hypoplasia of nipple; symbrachydactyly or oligodactyly, including of thumb; and aplasia/hypoplasia of other shoulder muscles. Anteoperative MRI aids assessment of reconstructive options.

Association with Klippel-Feil syndrome (*q.v.*) and Möbius syndrome (*q.v.*) has led to the hypothesis that a vascular insult during embryogenesis is causative, termed subclavian artery supply disruption sequence.

Boys thrice as common as girls. 75% of cases are right-sided. Left-sided anomalies may be associated with dextrocardia. One bilateral case has been reported, which may be better classified as a type of thoracic dysplasia.

Unilateral gluteal hypoplasia and symbrachydactyly of the foot, due to *in utero* external iliac artery supply disruption sequence, may represent the lower limb equivalent of the Poland syndrome.

PRADER-WILLI SYNDROME

Microdeletion of paternal copies of imprinted small nuclear ribonucleoprotein polypeptide N and necdin within region 15q11-q13.

Most cases are sporadic. Paternal hydrocarbon exposure has been implicated.

Prenatal delayed onset of fetal activity.

Neonatal poor suck and swallow reflexes lead to failure to thrive, which is followed by hyperphagia and obesity and ultimately alimentary diabetes. Psychomotor delay with behavioral problems such as anger, picking, and related to food.

Hypersalivation, hypotonia, hypopigmentation, hypogonadism, reduced bifrontal diameter, ocular anomalies, cardiac insufficiency, hypoventilation, intracranial morphologic abnormalities on MRI, and dysthermia.

Kyphoscoliosis, which is the focus of orthopedic surgery, and small hands and feet with clinodactyly–syndactyly, in particular thumb adduction over index.

Medical treatment includes psychotherapy, dietary control, and growth hormone to improve growth, tone, and respiration and to reduce fat.

PROTEUS SYNDROME

Mosaicism for a somatic-activating mutation in the protein kinase AKT1 gene on 14q32.3.

Sporadic occurrence and progressive course.

Variable asymmetric, disproportionate, localized tissue hypertrophy leading to gigantism of trunk and/or limbs.

Lymphatic and vascular tumors in skin and subcutaneous tissue, including characteristic "cerebriform" connective tissue nevi having grooves and gyrations.

Hyperostosis of craniofacial skeleton, in particular of external auditory meatus.

Limb equalization for hemihypertrophy.

Fusion for spine deformity and decompression for spine stenosis, which may be due to kyphoscoliosis or tumor infiltration.

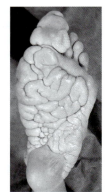

The disorder is named after the ancient Greek Sea God Proteus, "the polymorphous," who could change his shape like the ever-changing nature of the sea.

Joseph Carey Merrick (1862–1890), advertized as "Half a Man and Half an Elephant" by his showmen, may have been affected by this condition.

PYLE DISEASE

This also is known as metaphyseal dysplasia.

Autosomal recessive.

The distinguishing feature is bizarre röntgenographic changes, including "unremodeled" appearance of long bones, with minimal clinical consequences. Erlenmeyer flask deformity of proximal tibia and distal femur and genu valgum.

PRUNE BELLY SYNDROME

Autosomal recessive mutation in cholinergic receptor, muscarinic 3 gene on 1q43.

The disorder is named for absence of abdominal muscles with overlying skin, which is thin and lax with multiple creases due to redundancy.

Urogenital anomalies, including megacystis with disorganized detrusor muscle, hydronephrosis, and cryptorchidism.

Urinary obstruction in the fetus may produce distension and maldevelopment of abdominal wall.

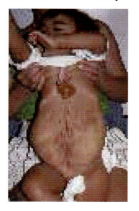

Musculoskeletal manifestations include hip dysplasia with dislocation due to laxity, segmentation defects of the spine producing congenital scoliosis and of the chest such as costal fusion, clubfoot, and vertical talus.

Other management includes self-catheterization or vesicostomy, orchiopexy, and potentially dialysis and renal transplantation.

PSEUDOACHONDROPLASIA

Autosomal dominant mutation of cartilage oligomeric matrix protein gene on 19p31.11.

Allelic with epiphysial dysplasia, multiple, of Fairbanks, which is milder.

The appellation derives from a resemblance to achondroplasia, including rhizomicromelia, trident hand, and lumbar hyperlordosis.

Distinguishing features are:
- Normal presentation at birth, with diagnosis rarely before 2 years.
- Normocephaly, including calvaria and face.
- Epiphysial involvement leading to premature osteoarthritis, with arthroplasty common by the fourth decade.
- Odontoid hypoplasia producing cervical spine instability and myelopathy, requiring stabilization.
- Absence of lumbar spine stenosis.

PTERYGIUM SYNDROME

The term derives from Greek πτερυξ: "wing," after the appearance of the skin as it stretches across a joint.

Pterygia result in primary growth disturbance and secondary physical distortion:

Musculoskeletal Kyphoscoliosis due to vertebral anomaly; articular contracture with (sub)luxation in particular of hip, knee (white), and elbow; hypoplasia of patellae and innominate bones; clubfoot; vertical talus; syndactyly and synostosis of feet more than hands; cutaneous dimples over extension side of elbows and knees; and pyramidal cutaneous overgrowth of halluceal nails.

Craniofacial Cleft lip and palate, paramedian mucous cyst of lower lip, syngnathia, ankyloblepharon filiforme adnatum, and hearing loss.

Genitourinary Bifid scrotum (blue), cryptorchidism, and hypoplasia.

Visceral Cardiopulmonary anomaly and diaphragmatic, abdominal, and inguinal hernias.

Three principal types are distinguished, with broader involvement and increasing severity.

Early pterygium release because neurovascular structures limit extent and rate of recurrence is high. Add external fixator for gradual correction after index release.

Phenotypic overlap with arthrogryposis and Freeman-Sheldon syndrome.

Type	Features
Popliteal - faciogenitopopliteal syndrome	Autosomal dominant mutation in interferon regulatory factor-6 gene on 1q32-q41. Pterygium may extend from ischium to calcaneus as it crosses the popliteal fossa.
Multiple - Escobar syndrome	Autosomal recessive mutation in the gene encoding the gamma subunit of acetylcholine receptor on 2q37.1. Dysmorphology caused by transient inactivation of neuromuscular end-plate. Pterygium colli distinctive.
Lethal - Bartsocas-Papas syndrome	Autosomal recessive mutation in receptor-interacting serine-threonine kinase-4 gene on 21q.22.3. Clustering in Mediterranean ancestry. Death from pulmonary hypoplasia and insufficiency.

PYCNODYSOSTOSIS

From Greek πυκνος: "close-packed, dense, thick," after the radiodensity of bone.

Autosomal recessive mutation of cathepsin K on 1q21.3. Cathepsin K belongs to the papain cysteine protease superfamily, among which it is unique in having an expression restricted to a specific cell type, the osteoclast.

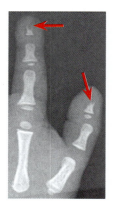

Abnormal proteolysis in the organic matrix leads to bone sclerosis and fragility, resulting in phenotypic overlap with osteopetrosis.

Delayed suture closure, hypodontia, and caries.

Aplasia or hypoplasia of clavicle, scoliosis, spondylolysis and spondylolisthesis, brachydactyly and acroosteolysis of distal phalanges, and onychodysplasia.

RICKETS

Named after involvement of the spine, from Greek ραχις: "spine."

Defective bone mineralization due to hypocalcemia and hypophosphatemia.

In the liver, vitamin D 25-hydroxylase adds -OH to vitamin D at carbon 25. In the kidney, 1-alpha-hydroxylase adds a second -OH to produce the active metabolite $1,25(OH)_2D3$, which binds and activates the nuclear vitamin D receptor.

Four types are distinguished.

Type	Features
Hypophosphatæmic - autosomal	• Dominant mutation in fibroblast growth factor 23 on 12p13. • Recessive mutations in dentin matrix acidic phosphoprotein 1 on 4q21 and in ectonucleotide pyrophosphatase phosphodiesterase 1 on 6q22-q23.
Hypophosphatæmic - X-linked	• Dominant mutation in phosphate regulating endopeptidase homolog on Xp22.11. • More severe recessive mutation in chloride channel exchange transporter 5 on Xp11.22.
Vitamin D-deficient	Mutation in: • type 1A: 25-hydroxyvitamin D3-1-alpha-hydroxylase on 12q14. • type 1B: vitamin D 25-hydroxylase on 11p15.2.
Vitamin D-resistant	Mutation in: • type 2A: vitamin D receptor on 12q13.11, resulting in end organ insensitivity. • type 2B: nuclear ribonucleoprotein C, which interferes with the function of vitamin D receptor.

Rickets also may result from malnutrition, including inadequate consumption of vitamin D2 (ergocalciferol) in plants and lack of sunlight, of which ultraviolet radiation is necessary for synthesis of vitamin D3 (cholecalciferol), the inactive precursor.

Short stature; osteomalacia; "soft" fracture, for example, greenstick (red); long bone bowing, physeal widening with metaphyseal irregularity; bone and joint pain; calcification of entheses; spinal stenosis; and craniotabes (soft skull).

"Bulging" epiphyses lead to articular enlargement, and hypertrophic costochondral junctions produce the "rachitic" rosary (white).

Indentation of soft ribs at the insertion of the diaphragm is known as "Harrison groove."

Muscle weakness, alopecia, and caries.

Hypocalcemia may result in seizure, hypercalciuria in nephrocalcinosis, and secondary hyperparathyroidism in subperiosteal erosions.

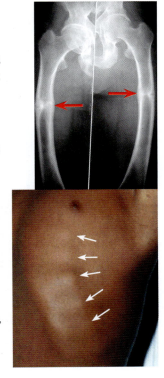

RILEY-DAY SYNDROME

See familial dysautonomia.

RUBINSTEIN-TAYBI SYNDROME

Autosomal dominant mutation of the transcriptional coactivator cAmp response element-binding (CREB) protein on 16p13.3.

Also known as broad thumb–hallux syndrome, after these features and the characteristic facies (heavy high-arched eyebrows, long eyelashes, low ears, grimacing smile) emphasized in the original report.

Congenital scoliosis, slipped capital femoral epiphysis, patellar and other joint instability, single palmar and plantar creases, and polydactyly.

Psychomotor delay; ocular (glaucoma, cataract), cardiac (valvular regurgitation, septal defect, pulmonic stenosis, aortic coarctation), and genitourinary (cryptorchidism) anomalies; and hirsutism. Five percent of patients develop a tumor, including neural, rhabdomyosarcoma, leukemia, and pheochromocytoma. The rate is similar to neurofibromatosis I.

Floating-Harbor syndrome (named for Boston Floating Hospital and Harbor General Hospital in Torrance where the first two cases were observed) is caused by mutation in SNF2-related CBP-activator protein, which is a coactivator of CREB protein. Its features resemble the craniofacial features of Rubinstein-Taybi syndrome.

SECKEL SYNDROME

Autosomal recessive mutation in ataxia–telangiectasia and Rad3-related protein gene on 3q22.1 (type 1). Six other subtypes distinguished by mutation.

The German pathologist and polymath Rudolph Carl Virchow (1821 to 1902) called this "bird-headed" dwarfism, after the characteristic microcephaly, large eyes, prominent sharp nose, and small chin and ears.

Scoliosis, hip dysplasia, hypoplasia of proximal radius and proximal fibula, and flexion contractures.

Central nervous system anomalies result in psychomotor delay and seizures.

SILVER-RUSSELL SYNDROME

DNA hypomethylation at the telomeric imprinting control region on 11p15.5, involving adult skeletal muscle and insulin-like growth factor 2 genes. Ten percent represent maternal uniparental disomy, in which child receives two copies of chromosome 7 from mother.

Characteristic triangular facies with broad forehead ("pseudohydrocephalic"), wide mouth, and small chin.

Body asymmetry, including hemihypertrophy; hand and foot anomalies, including second metacarpal pseudoepiphysis; congenital scoliosis; and hip dysplasia.

Genital malformations and gastrointestinal symptoms.

Tumor risk, including Wilms (nephroblastoma), hepatocellular, and craniopharyngioma.

Opposite epimutations, in which the same chromosomal region is hypermethylated, are associated with Beckwith-Wiedemann syndrome and Wilms tumor type 2.

Associated with assistive reproductive technologies.

SMALL PATELLA SYNDROME

Also called ischiopatellar dysplasia and coxopodopatellar syndrome, which are more inclusive descriptors.

Autosomal dominant mutation in T-box 4 on 17q23.2. T-box 4 encodes a transcription factor with a DNA-binding T-box domain that plays a role in lower limb development.

Patellar aplasia/hypoplasia and instability, ischial hypoplasia with delayed ossification of ischiopubic junction, wide and flat proximal femoral epiphyses, infra-acetabular notching, and widened first to second web spaces in the feet.

Nails are normal, ṣnd while the pelvis is significntly involved, iliac horns are absent, which distinguish this from nail–patella syndrome.

SPLIT HAND/SPLIT FOOT MALFORMATION

This also is known as ectrodactyly, from Greek εκτρωσις: "wound resulting in loss, abortion."

Designated a malformation to emphasize a primary structural lesion, in comparison with deformity, which is secondary.

Aplasia/hypoplasia of central rays produce clefts in hands and feet resembling a "lobster claw" or "ostrich foot." Preaxial loss may produce monodactyly.

Preaxial upper limb involvement is a locus discriminator, affecting approximately 50% of types 3 and 5 and <5% of others.

Variable orofacial clefting and mental retardation.

Six types are distinguished.

Type	Features
1	Mutation in distal-less homeobox 5 on 7q21.3. Sensorineural hearing loss.
2	Linkage to Xq26.
3	Contiguous gene duplication linked to 10q24 trisomy. Renal hypoplasia.
4	Mutation in tumor protein p63 on 3q28.
5	Mutation in 2q31
6	Mutation in wingless-type MMTV integration site family member 10B on 12q13.

SPONDYLOEPIMETAPHYSEAL DYSPLASIA

Dysplasia of long bones, both epiphyses and metaphyses, and spine, after Greek σπονδυλοι = Latin *vertebra*.

Skeletal Metaphyseal flaring and cupping, epiphysial irregularity, kyphoscoliosis, and anterior vertebral "tongues."

Hip, knee, and head of radius dislocation and clubfoot.

Ocular Blue sclerae, dislocation of lens, and cleft palate.

Cardiac anomalies account for demise.

Other "Doughy" skin and variable mental retardation.

Type	Features
Joint laxity type 1 (Beighton)	Autosomal recessive mutation in β–1,3 galactosyltransferase 6 on 1p36.33. Allelic to progeroid form of Ehlers-Danlos.
Joint laxity type 2 (Hall)	Autosomal dominant mutation in kinesin family member 22 on 16p11.2. Distinguished by leptodactyly.
Strudwick	Autosomal dominant mutation in type II collagen on 12q13.11. Allelic to spondyloepiphysial dysplasia, form which it may be distinguished by 'dappled' metaphyses due to alternating regions of osteosclerosis and osteopenia. Dens axis hypoplasia with C1-C2 instability.
Missouri	Mutation in matrix metalloproteinase 13 on 11q22.2. Spontaneous improvement by 2nd decade.
Shohat	Hepatosplenomegaly distend abdomen.
Aggrecan	Mutation in aggrecan on 15q.26.1.
Abnormal dentition	Oligodontia with discoloration.
Genevieve	Autosomal recessive. Hirsutism, ataxia.
Irapa	Described in Yukpa tribe of Irapa, Venezuela.

Type	Features
X-linked	Without or with central nervous system anomalies, psychomotor dysfunction.
Matrilin-3	Linkage to 2p24.1. Allelic to epiphysial dysplasia, multiple, type 5.
Hypotrichosis (Whyte)	Congenital absence of hair follicles, tarda skeletal involvement.
Sponastrime	Term derived from '**spon**dylar and **nas**al alterations with **stri**ated **me**taphyses', to emphasize distinguishing features.
Micromelia	Sub-type with most severe skeletal involvement.

SPONDYLOEPIPHYSIAL DYSPLASIA

Heterogeneous group affecting spine and epiphyses.

Congenita results from mutation of COL2A1 gene, which produces both α-1 chain of type II collagen and the α-3 chain of type XI collagen. Type II collagen is a homotrimer of polypeptide chains encoded by the COL2A1. The principal tissues of distribution are cartilage and vitreous humor, hence the phenotypic expression in bone (by morbid endochondral ossification), joint, and eye. This subtype is allelic with Kniest dysplasia and Stickler syndrome, which bound a spectrum from severe to mild, respectively.

Skeletal Microcormia. Abnormal epiphysial ossification leads to premature osteoarthritis. Dens hypoplasia risks atlantoaxial instability. Thoracic kyphoscoliosis, lumbar hyperlordosis, and platyspondyly with anterior body "tongue" (red). Coxa vara produces a waddling gait (green). Articular contractures, genua valga and vara, clubfoot, and brachydactyly.

Ocular Myopia, retinal detachment, vitreoretinal degeneration, and corneal dystrophy.

Craniofacial Cleft palate and sensorineural hearing loss.

Type	Features
Congenita	Mutation in α–1 chain of collagen type II on 12q13.11.
Tarda (onset > 5 years)	Mutation in tracking protein particle complex, subunit 2 on Xp22.2. Autosomal dominant and recessive forms identified.
Maroteaux	Mutation in transient receptor potential cation channel subfamily V member 4 on 12q24.11. Allelic to brachyolmia type 3, metatropic dysplasia and spondylometaphyseal dysplasia of Kozlowski.
Kimberley	Mutation in aggrecan-1 on 15q26.1.
Omani type	Mutation in carbohydrate sulfotransferase-3 on 10q22. Multiple joint dislocations. Congenital heart disease.

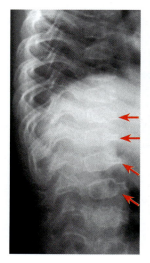

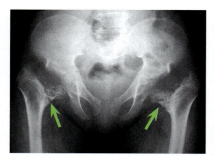

Coxa vara Capital femoral epiphyses are severely deformed. Proximal femoral physeal–shaft angles >60 degrees.

Spinal deformity Vertebral bodies give rise to projections, which have been likened to a "tongue."

SPONDYLOMETAPHYSEAL DYSPLASIA

Heterogeneous group characterized by spinal and metaphyseal changes of variable pattern and severity.

Kyphoscoliosis, dens hypoplasia with atlantoaxial instability, and vertebral bodies extend beyond pedicles like an "open staircase." Flaring of long bone metaphyses results in articular deformity such as coxa vara and may resemble rickets.

Type	Features
Kozlowski	Autosomal dominant mutation in transient receptor potential cation channel subfamily V member 4 on 12q24.11. Allelic to brachyolmia type 3, Charcot-Marie-Tooth type IIc, metatropic dysplasia, spondylo-epiphysial dysplasia (Maroteaux), spinal muscular atrophy. Carpal and tarsal ossification delay.
Sedaghatian	Autosomal recessive. Cardiorespiratory insufficiency. Central nervous system anomalies. Perinatal demise.
Richmond	X-linked. Sclerosis of skull base.
Sutcliffe	Autosomal dominant. Corner and bucket handle fractures. Mild spine involvement.
Goldblatt	Dentinogenesis imperfecta. Joint laxity.
Axial	Autosomal recessive. Retinitis pigmentosa.
Cone-rod dystrophy	Without or with central nervous system anomalies, psychomotor dysfunction.
A4	Severe changes in neck of femur.
East African	Similar to A4 without anterior vertebral tongues.
Algerian	Severe genu valgum.
Bowed forearms and facial dysmorphism	

STICKLER SYNDROME

The descriptive alternate appellation "arthroophthalmopathy" reflects tissue distribution of types II, IX, and XI collagens in cartilage and vitreous humor.

Mildest spondyloepiphysial dysplasia, including normal stature, with ocular disease most prominent.

Marfanoid habitus.

Type	Features
I	Autosomal dominant mutation in α-1 chain of type II collagen on 12q13.11.
II	Autosomal dominant mutation in α-1 chain of type XI collagen on 1p21.1. Allelic to Marshall syndrome.
III	Autosomal dominant mutation in α-2 chain of type XI collagen on 6p21.3. Allelic to otospondylomegaepiphysial dysplasia and Weissenbacher-Zweymuller syndrome.
IV	Autosomal recessive mutation in α-1 chain of type IX collagen on 6q13.
V	Autosomal recessive mutation in α-2 chain of type IX collagen on 1p34.2.

STREETER DYSPLASIA

See amniotic band syndrome.

THANATOPHORIC DYSPLASIA

The term, derived from Greek θανατος: "death" and φορεω: "I bring," describes a neonatal lethal skeletal dysplasia in the family of FGFR3 receptor mutations. See achondroplasia.

THROMBOCYTOPENIA–ABSENT RADIUS (TAR) SYNDROME

Autosomal recessive mutation of RNA-binding motif protein 8A on 1q21.1.

Thrombocytopenia is critical in first 2 years, when it can be lethal, is managed with platelet transfusion, and improves with age.

Radial aplasia and clubhand (red) with preservation of thumb (white).

Variable involvement of lower limbs, including hip dysplasia, patellar instability, absent fibula, carpal hypoplasia, and synostosis.

Cardiovascular, renal, and central nervous system anomalies.

Distinguished from Fanconi syndrome by absence of panmyelopathy, leukemia, thumb anomalies, and pigmentary changes.

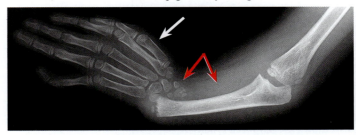

TRICHORHINOPHALANGEAL DYSPLASIA

Craniofacial Thin "hair" (Greek θριξ, τριχο-), piriform "nose" (Greek ρις, ρινο-) with bulbous tip, and dental dysgenesis.

Skeletal Conoid phalangeal epiphyses with brachydactyly, scoliosis, hip dysplasia, pes planus, and koilonychia/leukonychia.

Three types are distinguished.

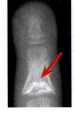

TURNER SYNDROME

One type of gonadal dysgenesis, characterized by amenorrhea, sterility, and delayed sexual development.

Partial (p deletion or mosaicism) or complete absence of X chromosome (45X, XO).

Mild psychomotor delay, lymphedema, low hairline and ears, webbed neck, and "shield chest" with broadly spaced nipples.

Short stature, cubitus valgus, patellofemoral instability, scoliosis, Madelung deformity, and fourth and fifth brachydactyly.

Cardiac and renal anomalies, hypothyroidism, otitis media, and celiac disease.

Type	Features
I	Autosomal dominant haplo-insufficiency in zinc finger transcription factor on 8q23.3.
II (Langer-Giedion)	Autosomal dominant loss of functional copies of zinc finger transcription factor gene and exostosin 1 gene on 8q24.11. Phenotype combines trichorhinophalangeal syndrome and multiple exostosis.
III (Sugio-Kajii)	Autosomal dominant haplo-insufficiency in zinc finger transcription factor on 8q23.3. Distinguished from type I by severity of phalangeal and metacarpal involvement. Distinguished from Ruvalcaba syndrome by absence of mental retardation and microcephaly.

VACTERL ASSOCIATION

Expanded acronym from VATER, representing a nonrandom association of independent disorders rather than a single etiologic entity. Diagnosis requires three anomalies.

Vertebral Hemivertebrae produce congenital scoliosis and spinal dysrrhaphism.

Anal atresia

Cardiac Septal defects, patent ductus arteriosus, tetralogy of Fallot, and transposition of the great arteries.

Tracheoesophageal fistula

Renal Renal aplasia/dysplasia, vesicoureteral reflux, and ureteropelvic obstruction.

Limb Radial aplasia/hypoplasia, radioulnar synostosis, thumb hypoplasia, polysyndactyly, and tibial field defects.

Three types are distinguished.

Type	Features
VACTERL	Mutation in the Homeobox D13 gene on 2q31.1 identified in 1 patient.
VACTERL-X	X-linked. Mutation in zinc finger protein of cerebellum 3 on Xq26.3.
VACTERL-H	Associated with hydrocephalus. Mutation in the phosphatase and tensin homolog on 10q23.31 identified in 1 patient

VACTERL may be a feature of Fanconi anæmia.

VELOCARDIOFACIAL SYNDROME

Also known as Shprintzen syndrome.

Autosomal dominant mutation in T-box 1 on 22q11.21. Allelic to DiGeorge syndrome.

Craniofacial Pierre Robin sequence including cleft palate, micrognathia, and velopharyngeal insufficiency. Most common palatal anomaly syndrome. Ocular anomalies include tortuous retinal vessels and posterior embryotoxon. "Hooded" eyelids and asymmetric crying are characteristic.

Cardiac Septal defects and conotruncal anomalies.

Skeletal Arachnodactyly, scoliosis, Sprengel anomaly, and articular laxity.

Other Psychiatric disorders and hypocalcemia.

von WILLEBRAND DISEASE

Mutation in von Willebrand factor on 12p13.31.

Type	Features
1	Quantitative *partial* (5-30% normal levels) deficiency. 75% of cases.
2	Qualitative abnormality of von Willebrand factor. 20% of cases. Further subdivided according to whether platelet function is affected or whether there is a defect in factor VIII binding.
3	Quantitative *severe* (< 1% normal levels) deficiency. < 5% of cases

vWF binds platelets, which it promotes to adhere, and factor VIII, which degrades when not bound.

Treat with the vasopressin analog desmopressin acetate (1-deamino-8-D-arginine vasopressin; dDAVP).

Orthopedic management focuses on hemarthropathy—compare hæmophilia.

WHISTLING FACE SYNDROME

See Freeman-Sheldon syndrome.

WAARDENBURG SYNDROME

Autosomal dominant mutation of paired box gene 3 on 2q36.1.

The gene product is a transcription factor essential to ear, eye, and pigmentary development.

Craniofacial Sensorineural hearing loss. Dystopia canthorum giving appearance of wide-set eyes due to lateral displacement of inner canthi (W index > 2), heterochromia iridis, and synophrys.

Pigmentary Albinism, including poliosis.

Skeletal Spina bifida, winged or elevated scapulae.

Subtypes reflect heterogeneity.

Type	Features
1	Craniofacial malformations.
2	Absence of dystopia canthorum.
3	Upper limb anomalies.
4	Visceral involvement such as Hirschsprung disease.

ARTHRITIS, JUVENILE IDIOPATHIC

Disease of a joint is termed *arthritis*, from Greek αρθρον: "joint." *Arthralgia*, from Greek αλγος: "pain," is used when pain is the predominant feature, in contrast with swelling. *Arthrosis*, from Greek suffix -ωσις: "condition of," originated in anatomy in the work of Galen, who distinguished different types of articulations as diarthrosis ("in all directions"), amphiarthrosis ("in two directions or planes"), and synarthrosis (when bones are "joined together" such as at a suture). The term has been adopted into pathology to distinguish noninflammatory disease of joints, reserving arthritis for joint inflammation, which is indicated by Greek suffix -ιτις. Inflammation at a site of "insertion" of a ligament or a tendon is referred to as *enthesitis*, from Green εν-: "in" and τιθεναι: "to place."

The term juvenile idiopathic arthritis is an inclusive term. "Rheumatoid" has been abandoned because most subtypes lack this factor.

JUVENILE IDIOPATHIC ARTHRITIS		
Current	**Former**	
	"Rheumatoid"	
Oligo-articular	Pauciarticular	
Poly-articular	Rheumatoid factor positive	Polyarticular
	Rheumatoid factor negative	
Systemic	Still disease	
Enthesitis associated	Spondyloarthropathy, including ankylosing spondylitis Reiter syndrome	
Psoriatic	Psoriasis	
Undifferentiated		

Oligo-, from Greek ολιγος: "few," is defined as <5 joints. It has replaced pauci-, from Latin *paucus*: "few," to be consistent with poly-, from Greek πολυς: "much, many," and after the convention that Greek is the language of disease.

Chronic iridocyclitis (inflammation of the anterior uvea) often is asymptomatic, necessitating referral to an ophthalmologist for slit-lamp examination. Early-onset disease and positive ANA are at greatest risk.

Psoriasis is characterized by a dry, silvery, scaly rash, from Greek ψαω: "I rub (away), crumble."

Chronic juxta-articular inflammation may produce hyperemic osseous overgrowth in early-onset disease and premature physeal closure in late-onset disease. Discrepancy does not exceed 5 cm.

Orthopedic management includes:

- Arthrocentesis. This is the best step to diagnosis.
- Physiotherapy and bracing for contracture and weakness.
- Limb equalization by physeodesis, in up to half of patients.
- Arthroplasty. Overall, disease burden limits activity and prolongs implant survival.

Medical treatment includes:

- Nonsteroidal anti-inflammatory agents
- Articular injection of corticosteroid
- Disease-modifying antirheumatic drugs, such as methotrexate
- Biologics, such as tumor necrosis factor-α blockers and anti-interleukin-6 inhibitors

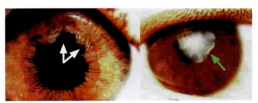

Iridocyclitis
Irregular pupil (*white*) and cataract (*green*)

	OLIGOARTICULAR	POLYARTICULAR	SYSTEMIC	ENTHESITIS associated
Frequency	60%	30%	10%	
Gender	♀	♀	♂ = ♀	♂
Age (years)	< 5	Early < 5 Late > 10	All	> 10
Joints	Large (e.g., knee) > small	Small (e.g., fingers) > large	all (including hip)	"Spondylo-arthropathy": spine + sacro-iliac + other
Presentation	Joint, iridocyclitis	Unhappy: morning stiffness, fatigue, poor appetite, weight loss, anæmia.	Systemic: "saw-tooth" fever (daily rapid return to normal temperature); "salmon-colored" migratory rash, lymphadenopathy, visceral involvement including serositis, hepatosplenomegaly, disseminated intravascular coagulation.	Syndesmophytes create a "bamboo" appearance of the spine, and reduce excursion during maximal respiration and flexion (Schober sign). Inflammatory bowel disease. Bath Ankylosing Spondylitis Disease Activity Index assesses fatigue, pain, enthesitis and morning stiffness.
ESR	→	↗	↑	↗
CRP	→	↗	↑	↗
ANA	60%	30%	15%	
RF		50% (late onset)	5%	(-)
HLA-B27				(+)

Albers–Schönberg H. Roentgenbilder einer seltenen knochenerkrankung. *Münch. Med. Wschr.* 51:365, 1904.

Albright F, Butler AM, Hampton AO, Smith P. Syndrome characterized by osteitis fibrosa disseminata, areas of pigmentation and endocrine dysfunction, with precocious puberty in females: report of five cases. *N. Eng. J. Med.* 216:727–746, 1937.

Apert ME. De l'acrocephalosyndactylie. *Bull. Mem. Soc. Med. Hôp. Paris* 23:1310–1330, 1906.

Bartsocas CS, Papas CV. Popliteal pterygium syndrome: evidence for a severe autosomal recessive form. *J. Med. Genet.* 9:222–226, 1972.

Beals RK, Hecht F. Delineation of another heritable disorder of connective tissue. *J. Bone Joint Surg.* 53A:987, 1971.

Beals RK. Auriculo–osteodysplasia, a syndrome of multiple osseous dysplasia, ear anomaly, and short stature. *J. Bone Joint Surg.* 49-A:1541, 1967.

Beckwith JB. Macroglossia, omphalocele, adrenal cytomegaly, gigantism, and hyperplastic visceromegaly. *Birth Defects Orig. Art. Ser.* V(2):188–196, 1969.

Bick EM. The classic: on hereditary cleidocranial dysostosis (transl.). *Clin. Orthop.* 58:5–7, 1968.

Biggs R, Douglas AS, Macfarlane RG, Dacie JV, Pitney WR, Merskey C, O'Brien JR. Christmas disease: a condition previously mistaken for haemophilia. *Brit. Med. J.* 2:1378–1382, 1952.

Bruck A. Über eine seltene Form von Erkrankung der Knochen und Gelenke. *Dtsch. Med. Wsch.* 23:152–155, 1897.

Byers PH. Osteogenesis imperfecta. In: Royce PM, Steinmann B. *Connective Tissue and Its Heritable Disorders: Molecular, Genetic, and Medical Aspects.* New York: Wiley-Liss; 1993.

Caffey J, Silverman W. Infantile cortical hyperostosis, preliminary report on new syndrome. *Am. J. Roentgen.* 54:1–16, 1945.

Canton E. Arrest of development of the left perpendicular ramus of the lower jaw, combined with malformation of the external ear. *Trans. Path. Soc. London.* 12:237, 1861.

Carpenter G. Two sisters showing malformation of the skull and other congenital abnormalities. *Rep. Soc. Study Dis. Child (London).* 1:110, 1901.

Conradi EJ. Vorzeitiges Auftreten von Kochen und eigenartigen Verkalkungskernen bei Chondrodystrophia fötalis hypoplastica. Histologische und Röntgenuntersuchungen. *Kinderheilk.* 80:86, 1914.

De Barsy AM, Moens E, Dierckx L. Dwarfism, oligophrenia and degeneration of the elastic tissue in skin and cornea. A new syndrome? *Helv. Paediat. Acta* 23:305–313, 1968.

De Lange C. Sur un type nouveau de dé–génération (typus Amstelodamensis). *Arch. Med. Enfant.* 36:713, 1933.

Diab M, Raff M, Gunther DF. Osseous fragility in Marshall-Smith syndrome. *Am. J. Med. Genet.* 119-A:218–222, 2003.

Down JL. *Mental Affections of Childhood and Youth.* London, UK: Churchill; 1887:172.

Down JLH. Observations on an ethnic classification of idiots. *Clin. Lect. Rep. London Hosp.* 3:259–262, 1866.

Dyggve HV, Melchior JC, Clausen J. Morquio–Ulrich's disease; An inborn error of metabolism? *Arch. Dis. Child.* 37:525, 1962.

Eagle JF Jr, Barrett GS. Congenital deficiency of abdominal musculature with associated genitourinary abnormalities: a syndrome: report of nine cases. *Pediatrics* 6:721–736, 1950.

Ehlers E. Curtis laxa, Neigung zu Haemorrhagien in der Haut lockerung meherer Artikulationen. *Dermatol. Z.* 8:173, 1901.

Ellis RBW, Van Creveld S. A syndrome characterized by ectodermal dysplasia, polydactyly, chondrodysplasia, and congenital morbis cordis: report of three cases. *Arch. Dis. Child.* 15:65, 1940.

Escobar V, Bixler D, Gleiser S, Weaver DD. Gibbs T. Multiple pterygium syndrome. *Am. J. Dis. Child.* 132:609–611, 1978.

Fairbank HAT. Dysplasia epiphysealis multiplex. *Proc. Roy. Soc. Med.* 39:315–317, 1945.

Farabee WC. *Hereditary and Sexual Influence in Meristic Variation: A Study of Digital Malformations in Man.* PhD thesis. Cambridge, MA: Harvard University; 1903.

Foulkes GD, Rienker K. Congenital constriction band syndrome: a seventy-year experience. *J. Pediatr. Orthop.* 14:242, 1994.

Freeman EA, Sheldon JH. Cranio-carpotarsal dystrophy: undescribed congenital malformation. *Arch. Dis. Child.* 13:277–283, 1938.

Friedreich N. Über degenerative Atrophie der spinalen, Hinterstränge. *Arch. Anat. Physiol.* 26:391, 1863.

Frölich F. *Der Mangel der Muskeln, insbesondere der Seitenbauchmuskeln.* Dissertation. Germany: Wurzburg; 1839.

Gaucher PCE. De l'epithelioma primitif de la rate, hypertrophie idiopathique de la rate sans leucemie. *Thesis, Faculte-de Medicine Paris*; 1882.

Giedion A. Das Tricho-rhino-phalangeal Syndrom. *Helv. Paediatr. Acta.* 21:475–482, 1966.

Goldenhar M. Associations malformatives de l'oeil et de l'oreille: en particulier, le syndrome: dermoide epibulbaire-appendices auriculaires—fistula auris congenita et ses relations avec la dysostose mandibulo-faciale. *J. Genet. Hum.* 1:243-282, 1952.

Golding FC. Chondro-osteodystrophy. *Brit. J. Radiol.* 8:457, 1935.

Gorlin RJ, Cervenka J, Moller K, Horrobin M, Witkop CJ Jr. Malformation syndromes: a selected miscellany. *Birth Defects Orig. Art. Ser.* 11:39–50, 1975.

Gross H, Groh C, Weippl G. Kongenitale hypoplastische thrombopenie mit radius-aplasie, ein syndrom multipler Abartungen. *Neue Oest Z Kinderheilk.* 1:574, 1956.

Guillain G, Barré JA, Strohl A. Le réflexe médico–plantaire: Étude de ses caracteres graphiques et de son temps perdu. *Bull. Soc. Med. Hôp. Paris.* 40:1459, 1915.

Hall JB, Reed SD, Dricoll EP. Amyoplasia: a common, sporadic condition with congenital contractures. *Am. J. Med. Genet.* 15:571, 1983.

Hernandez RM, Miranda A, Kofman-Alfaro S. Acrodysostosis in two generations: an autosomal dominant syndrome. *Clin. Genet.* 39:376, 1991.

Holt M, Oram S. Familial heart disease with skeletal malformations. *Br. Heart J.* 22:236, 1960.

Horton WA. Molecular genetic basis of the human chondrodysplasias. *Endocrinol. Metab. Clin. N. Am.* 25:683, 1996.

Hünermann CZ. Chondrodystrophia calcificans congenita als abortive form der chondrodystrophie. *Kinderheilk.* 51:1, 1931.

Hunter C. A rare disease in two brothers. *Proc. R. Soc. Med.* 10:104–106, 1917.

Hunter J. *The Works of John Hunter.* Vol 1. London, UK: Longman, Rees, 1835.

Jackson WPU, Albright F. Metaphyseal dysplasia, epiphyseal dysplasia, diaphyseal dysplasia, and related conditions. I. Familial metaphyseal dysplasia and craniometaphyseal dysplasia: their relation to leontiasis ossea and osteopetrosis: disorders of 'bone remodeling'. *Arch. Intern. Med.* 94:871, 1954.

Jansen M. Über atypische Chondrodystrophie (Achondroplasie) und ueber eine noch nicht beschriebene angeborene Wachstumsstoerung des Knochensystems: Metaphysaere Dysostosis. *Z. Orthop. Chir.* 61:253–286, 1934.

Kantaputra PN, Gorlin RJ, Langer LO Jr. Dominant mesomelic dysplasia, ankle, carpal, and tarsal synostosis type: a new autosomal dominant bone disorder. *Am. J. Med. Genet.* 44:730–737, 1992.

Kaplan FS, Xu M, Seemann P, Connor JM, Glaser DL, Carroll L, Delai P, Fastnacht-Urban E, Forman SJ, Gillessen-Kaesbach G, Hoover-Fong J, Koster B, Pauli RM, Reardon W, Zaidi S-A, Zasloff M, Morhart R, Mundlos S, Groppe J, Shore EM. Classic and atypical fibrodysplasia ossificans progressiva (FOP) phenotypes are caused by mutations in the bone morphogenetic protein (BMP) type I receptor ACVR1. *Hum. Mutat.* 30:379–390, 2009.

Kitoh H. Antley-Bixler syndrome: a disorder characterized by congenital synostosis of the elbow joint and the cranial suture. *J. Pediatr. Orthop.* 16:243, 1996.

Klippel M, Feil A. Un cas d'absence des vertebres cervicales avec cage thoracique remontant jusqua à la base du crane (cage thoracique cervicale). *Nouv. Icon. Salpetière.* 25:223, 1912.

Klippel M, Trenaunay P. Du naevus variqueux osteo-hypertrophique. *Arch. Gen. Med.* 185:641–672, 1900.

Kniest W. Zur Abgrenzung der Dysostosis enchondralis von der Chondrodystrophie. *Z. Kinderheilk.* 43:633–640, 1952.

Kozlowski K, Maroteaux P, Spranger JW. La dysostose spondylo-metaphysaire. *Presse Med.* 75:2769–2774, 1967.

Lamy M, Maroteaux P. Le nanisme diastrophique. *Presse Med.* 68:1977, 1960.

Larsen LJ, Schottstaedt ER, Bost FC. Multiple congenital dislocations associated with characteristic facial abnormality. *J. Pediatr.* 37:574, 1950.

Léri A, Weill J. Une affection congenitale et symetrique du developpement osseux: la dyschondrosteose. *Bull. Mem. Soc. Med. Hôp Paris.* 53:1491–1494, 1929.

Lesch M, Nyhan WL. A familial disorder of uric acid metabolism and central nervous system function. *Am. J. Med.* 36:561–570, 1964.

Lewis T. Hereditary malformations of the hands and feet. IIa. Hereditary split foot. *Treasury of Human Inheritance* 1:6–17, 1912.

Lohmann W. Beitrag zur Kenntnis des reinen Mikrophthalmus. *Arch. Augenheilk.* 86:136–141, 1920.

Marfan AB. Un cas de deformation congenitale des quatre membres, plus prononcee aux extremites, caracterisee par l'allongement des os avec un certain degre d'amincissement. *Bull. Mem. Soc. Med. Hôp. Paris.* 13:220–226, 1896.

Maroteaux P, Bouvet JP, Briard ML. La maladie des synostoses multiples. *Nouv. Presse Med.* 1:3041–3047, 1972.

Maroteaux P, Leveque B, Marie J, Lamy M. Une nouvelle dysostose avec elimination urinaire de chondroitine-sulfate B. *Presse Med.* 71:1849–1852, 1963.

Maroteaux P, Spranger JW, Wiedemann H-R. Der metatropische Zwergwuchs. *Arch. Kinderheilk.* 173:211–226, 1966.

Maroteaux P. La metachondromatose. *Z. Kinderheilk.* 109:246–261, 1971.

Maroteaux P. Le syndrome campomelique. *Presse Med.* 22:1157–1162, 1971.

Marshall RE, Graham CB, Scott CR, Smith DW. Syndrome of accelerated skeletal maturation and relative failure to thrive: a newly recognized clinical growth disorder. *J. Pediatr.* 78:95–101, 1971.

McCune DJ. Osteitis fibro-cystica: The case of a nine year old girl who also exhibits precocious puberty, multiple pigmentation of the skin and hyperthyroidism. *Am. J. Dis. Child.* 52:743, 1936.

McKusick VA, Eldridge R, Hosteler JA, Ruangwit U, Egeland JA. Dwarfism in the Amish. II. Cartilage-hair hypoplasia. *Bull. Johns Hopkins Hosp.* 116:285–326, 1965.

Meier Z, Rothschild M. Ein Fall von Arthrogryposis multiplex congenita kombiniert mit Dysostosis mandibulofacialis (Franceschetti-Syndrom). *Helv. Paediat. Acta* 14:213–216, 1959.

Melnick JC, Needles CF. An undiagnosed bone dysplasia: a two family study of 4 generations and 3 generations. *Am. J. Roentgen.* 97:39–48, 1966.

Möbius PJ. Über angeborene doppelseitige Abducens-Facialis-Laehmung. *Münch. Med. Wschr.* 35: 91–94 and 108–111, 1888.

Nievergelt K. Positiver Vaterschaftsnachweis auf grund erblicher Missbildungen der Extremitaeten. *Arch. Klaus Stift Vererbungsforsch.* 19:157, 1944.

Nowaczyk MJ, Huggins MJ, Fleming A, Mohide PT. Femoral-facial syndrome: prenatal diagnosis and clinical features. Report of three cases. *Am. J. Med. Genet.* 152-A:2029–2033, 2010.

Otto JC. An account of an hemorrhagic disposition existing in certain families. *M. Repository* 6:1, 1803.

Penttinen RP, Lichtenstein JR, Martin GR, McKusick VA. Abnormal collagen metabolism in cultured cells in osteogenesis imperfecta. *Proc. Nat. Acad. Sci.* 72:586–589, 1975.

Poland A. Deficiency of the pectoral muscle. *Guys Hosp. Rep.* 6:191, 1841.

Prader A, Labhart A, Willi H. Ein Syndrom von Adipositas, Kleinwuchs, Kryptorchismus und Oligophrenie nach Myatonieartigem Zustand im Neugeborenenalter. *Schweiz. Med. Wschr.* 86:1260–1261, 1956.

Prockop DJ, Kivirikko KI. Heritable diseases of collagen. *N. Eng. J. Med.* 311:376–386, 1984.

Pyle E. Case of unusual bone development. *J. Bone Joint Surg.* 13:874–876, 1931.

Quan L, Smith DW. The VATER association: vertebral defects, anal atresia, tracheoesophageal fistula with esophageal atresia, radial dysplasia. *Birth Defects Orig. Art. Ser.* 8(2):75–78, 1972.

Ribbing S. Studien ueber hereditaere, multiple Epiphysenstoerungen. *Acta Radiol. Suppl.* 34:7–107, 1937.

Riley CM, Day RL, Greeley DM, Langford WS. Central autonomic dysfunction with defective lacrimation: report of five cases. *Pediatrics* 3:468–478, 1949.

Rock MJ, Prenen J, Funari VA, Funari TL, Merriman B, Nelson SF, Lachman RS, Wilcox WR, Reyno S, Quadrelli R, Vaglio A, Owsianik G, Janssens A, Voets T, Ikegawa S, Nagai T, Rimoin DL, Nilius B, Cohn DH. Gain-of-function mutations in TRPV4 cause autosomal dominant brachyolmia. *Nat. Genet.* 40:999–1003, 2008.

Rubinstein JH, Taybi H. Broad thumbs and toes and facial abnormalities. *Am. J. Dis. Child.* 105:588–608, 1963.

Russell A. A syndrome of intra-uterine-dwarfism recognizable at birth with cranio-facial dysostosis, disproportionate short arms, and other anomalies (5 examples). *Proc. Roy. Soc. Med.* 47:1040–1044, 1954.

Scheie HG, Hambrick GW Jr, Barness LA. A newly recognized forme fruste of Hurler's disease (gargoylism). *Am. J. Ophthal.* 53:753–769, 1962.

Schmid F. Beitrag zur Dysostosis enchondralis metaphysarea. *Mschr. Kinderheilk.* 97:393–397, 1949.

Shprintzen RJ, Goldberg RB, Young D, Wolford L. The velo-cardio-facial syndrome: a clinical and genetic analysis. *Pediatrics* 67:167–172, 1981.

Sillence DO, Senn A, Danks DM. Genetic heterogeneity in osteogenesis imperfecta. *J. Med. Genet.* 16:101–116, 1979.

Silver HK, Kiyasu W, George J, Deamer WC. Syndrome of congenital hemihypertrophy, shortness of stature, and elevated urinary gonadotropins. *Pediatrics* 12:368–376, 1953.

Sly WS, Quinton B, McAlister WH, Rimoin DL. Beta-glucuronidase deficiency: report of clinical, radiologic, biochemical features of a new mucopolysaccharidosis. *J. Pediatr.* 82:249–257, 1973.

Stern AM, Gall JC Jr, Perry BL, Stimson CW, Weitkamp LR, Poznanski AK. The hand-foot-uterus syndrome: a new hereditary disorder characterized by hand and foot dysplasia, dermatoglyphic abnormalities, and partial duplication of the female genital tract. *J. Pediatr.* 77:109–116, 1970.

Streeter GL. Focal deficiencies in fetal tissues and their relation to intra-uterine amputation. *Contrib. Embryol.* 22(126):1–144, 1930.

Trélat V. Sur un vice conformation trés-rare de la lévre inférieure. *J. Med. Chir. Pract.* 40:442, 1869.

Trevor D. Tarso-epiphysial aclasis: a congenital error of epiphysial development. *J. Bone Joint Surg.* 32-B:204–213, 1950.

Turner HH. A syndrome of infantilism, congenital webbed neck, and cubitus valgus. *Endocrinology* 23:566–74, 1938.

Turner JW. An hereditary arthrodysplasia associated with hereditary dystrophy of the nails. *JAMA* 100:882–884, 1933.

von Recklinghausen F. Über die multiplen Fibrome der Haut und ihre Beziehung zu den multiplen Neuromen. Berlin, Germany: August Hirschwald; 1882.

Waardenburg P. A new syndrome combining developmental anomalies of the eyelids, eyebrows and nose root with pigmentary defects of the iris and head hair and with congenital deafness. *Am. J. Hum. Genet.* 3:195–253, 1951.

Weber FP. Angioma formation in connection with hypertrophy of limbs and hemihypertrophy. *Brit. J. Derm.* 19:231–235, 1907.

Wheaton SW. Two specimens of congenital cranial deformity in infants associated with fusion of the fingers and toes. *Trans. Path. Soc. Lon.* 45:238–241, 1894.

Wiedemann H-R, Burgio GR, Aldenhoff P, Kunze J, Kaufmann HJ, Schirg E. The Proteus syndrome: partial gigantism of the hands and/or feet, nevi, hemihypertrophy, subcutaneous tumors, macrocephaly or other skull anomalies and possible accelerated growth and visceral affections. *Europ. J. Pediatr.* 140:5–12, 1983.

Wood VE, Peppers TA, Shook J. Cleft-foot closure: a simplified technique and review of the literature. *J. Pediatr. Orthop.* 17:501, 1997.

INDEX

Note: Page numbers in italics refer to illustrations

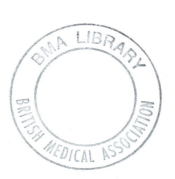